Introduction to
Pharmacology

Introduction to Pharmacology

PR Sengupta

MD, MPhil (Medical)

former

Professor of Pharmacology
RG Kar Medical College, Kolkata, WB
National Medical College, Kolkata, WB
MGM Medical College, Kishanganj, Bihar

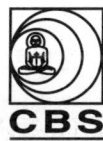

CBS

CBS Publishers & Distributors Pvt Ltd

New Delhi • Bengaluru • Chennai • Kochi • Kolkata • Mumbai

Bhopal • Bhubaneswar • Hyderabad • Jharkhand • Nagpur • Patna • Pune • Uttarakhand • Dhaka (Bangladesh)

Introduction to
Pharmacology

ISBN: 978-93-85915-55-0

Copyright © Author and Publisher

First Edition: 2016

Reprint: 2019

Published by Satish Kumar Jain and produced by Varun Jain for

CBS Publishers & Distributors Pvt Ltd

4819/XI Prahlad Street, 24 Ansari Road, Daryaganj, New Delhi 110 002, India.
Ph: 23289259, 23266861, 23266867   Fax: 011-23243014   Website: www.cbspd.com
e-mail: delhi@cbspd.com; cbspubs@airtelmail.in.

Corporate Office: 204 FIE, Industrial Area, Patparganj, Delhi 110 092
Ph: 4934 4934   Fax: 4934 4935   e-mail: publishing@cbspd.com; publicity@cbspd.com

Branches

- **Bengaluru:** Seema House 2975, 17th Cross, K.R. Road,
  Banasankari 2nd Stage, Bengaluru 560 070, Karnataka
  Ph: +91-80-26771678/79   Fax: +91-80-26771680   e-mail: bangalore@cbspd.com
- **Chennai:** 7, Subbaraya Street, Shenoy Nagar, Chennai 600 030, Tamil Nadu
  Ph: +91-44-26680620, 26681266   Fax: +91-44-42032115   e-mail: chennai@cbspd.com
- **Kochi:** 42/1325, 1326, Power House Road, Opposite KSEB Power House,
  Ernakulam 682 018, Kochi, Kerala
  Ph: +91-484-4059061-65   Fax: +91-484-4059065   e-mail: kochi@cbspd.com
- **Kolkata:** 6/B, Ground Floor, Rameswar Shaw Road, Kolkata-700 014, West Bengal
  Ph: +91-33-22891126, 22891127, 22891128   e-mail: kolkata@cbspd.com
- **Mumbai:** 83-C, Dr E Moses Road, Worli, Mumbai-400018, Maharashtra
  Ph: +91-22-24902340/41   Fax: +91-22-24902342   e-mail: mumbai@cbspd.com

Representatives

Bhopal	0-8319310552	**Bhubaneswar**	0-9911037372	**Hyderabad**	0-9885175004
Jharkhand	0-9811541605	**Nagpur**	0-9021734563	**Patna**	0-9334159340
Pune	0-9623451994	**Uttarakhand**	0-9716462459	**Dhaka (Bangladesh)**	01912-003485

Printed at: Rashtriya Printers, Dilshad Garden, Delhi, India

Preface

This edition of *Introduction to Pharmacology* has been thoroughly revised and updated as per MCI curriculum. The practical part of the book has been modified to help the students during their practical examination. In general, this book will be useful to medical students to learn the subject in a short time.

Pharmacology is an everchanging subject like medicine. I have tried to write this book in concise form with modern concepts, so that the students are able to read and learn this subject. The book contains all essential drugs, rational basis of therapeutics and recent advances in pharmacology. I have consulted several standard textbooks of pharmacology. While writing this book, I have followed the new syllabus of pharmacology of MBBS course in different Indian Universities. It will be helpful to medical students as well as the students of pharmacy, dental sciences, allied health sciences and nursing, to acquire the basic principles necessary for rational use of drugs. Any suggestion for further improvement of this book will be highly appreciated.

I express my sincere thanks to CBS Publishers & Distributors for publishing this edition of the book for the students and doctors.

PR Sengupta

Acknowledgements

I express my gratitude and thanks to Mr SK Jain, Managing Director, CBS Publishers & Distributors, for publishing this book. I am grateful to him for taking pains in bringing out this book. I thank all the staff members of CBS Publishers & Distributors. I express my acknowledgements to the authors/editors of reference books and some of my teachers Prof K Ahmed, Prof M Imam, Prof S Sikdar, Dr NM Roy, Prof BP Mukherjee and Prof RC Majumdar. Last, I express my thanks to my wife Mrs Gopa Sengupta and daughter Dr (Mrs) Susmita Roy for their constant encouragement and moral support during the writing of this book.

PR Sengupta

Contents

Part 2

Section II: ENDOCRINE PHARMACOLOGY

Section III: CHEMOTHERAPY

Section IV: IMMUNOPHARMACOLOGY

Section V: MISCELLANEOUS DRUGS

Section VI: TOXICOLOGY

Part 3

Section I: PRACTICAL PHARMACOLOGY

Section II: CLINICAL PHARMACOLOGY

National Essential Drugs List (1996)

Part 1

Section I

GENERAL PHARMACOLOGY

1. Introduction to Pharmacology
2. Routes of Drug Administration
3. Pharmacokinetics
4. Clinical Pharmacokinetics
5. Pharmacodynamics
6. Quantitative Aspects of Pharmacodynamics and Assay of Drugs
7. Drug Interactions
8. Adverse Drug Reactions
9. Development and Evaluation of New Drugs

Introduction to Pharmacology

INTRODUCTION

Pharmacology is a branch of medical science which deals with drugs. It is derived from two Greek words, viz. *pharmacon* (means drug) and *logos* (means studies). It contains the knowledge of history, source, physical and chemical properties, compounding, biochemical and physiological effects, mechanism of action, absorption, distribution, biotransformation and excretion and therapeutic and other uses of drugs. The first book of pharmacology was written by Samuel Dale in 1693. Oswald Schmiedeberg (1838–1921) is known as the Father of Modern Pharmacology.

Drug and Medicine

A drug is a chemical substance that affects processes in living organism and used for the treatment, prophylaxis (prevention) or diagnosis of the disease. It is derived from a French word *Drogue* (means dry herb). According to WHO (World Health Organization), a drug is a chemical substance or biological product that is used or intended to be used to modify or explore physiological systems or pathological states for the benefit of the recipient. A drug cannot create a new function but can modify (increase or decrease) an already existing function. When a drug is used in proper dosage form for safe administration in a recipient, then it is called a medicine. All medicines are drugs but all drugs are not medicines. There are thousands of drugs, but all drugs are not essential.

Essential Drug Concept

It was introduced by WHO in 1977 to avoid the complications of drug use faced by the physician. A list containing essential drugs is available for the physicians in clinical practice. Essential drugs are those drugs which satisfy the healthcare needs of the majority of the population and they should, therefore, be available at all times in adequate amounts, in appropriate dosage forms and at reasonable cost. Drugs which do not fulfill these criteria are not essential drugs. List of essential drugs is given in the last pages of this book.

- Orphan drugs are those drugs which are used for the treatment, prevention or diagnosis of rare diseases like kala-azar, cancers, viral diseases, etc. and in digoxin, heavy metal or other drug, e.g. digoxin specific fab antibodies, T_3, BAL, etc. poisoning. Though they may be life-saving for some patients, but they are less produced commercially due to high cost of manufacture and small number of patients requiring the drug.

Drug Nomenclature

A drug has more than one name, for example:

- **Acetylsalicylic acid (chemical name)**
  - Aspirin (official name)

– Dispirin (proprietary/brand name)
– Salicylate (generic name).

- **Chlorphenothiazine propyldiamine (chemical name)**
  – Chlorpromazine (official name)
  – Largactil (brand name/trade name)
  – Phenothiazine (generic name).

Drug Therapy

It is of three types:

1. **Rational therapy:** It is the logical treatment of diseases by drugs based on pharmacological effects of drugs correlated with pathological aspects of diseases, e.g. digoxin in congestive cardiac failure, ferrous sulphate in iron deficiency anaemia, antibiotics in bacterial infections, etc.

2. **Empirical therapy:** It is the treatment of diseases based on experience, belief or guess and without any pharmacological explanation, i.e. uses of homeopathic drugs for curing diseases.

3. **Accessory therapy (alternative medicine):** It is the treatment of diseases by other means besides drugs, e.g. use of physiotherapy in arthritis, administration of suitable foods in malnutrition, etc.

Branches of Pharmacology

These are described as follows:

1. **Pharmacokinetics (*Kinesia* meaning movement):** It deals with the absorption, distribution, metabolism and excretion of drugs. It is what the body does to the drug.

2. **Pharmacodynamics (*Dynamics* meaning power):** It deals with the biochemical and physiological effects of drugs and their mechanisms of action. It is what the drug does to the body.

3. **Pharmacotherapeutics (therapeutics):** It is the use of drugs in the prevention and treatment of diseases.

4. **Toxicology:** It deals with adverse reactions of drugs and their treatment.

5. **Clinical pharmacology:** It deals with the study of drug effects in human beings (normal and patients).

6. **Experimental pharmacology:** It deals with the study of drug effects in laboratory animals (rats, guinea pigs, rabbits, etc.).

7. **Pharmacy:** It is the collection, compounding and dispensing of drugs for use in man or animal.

8. **Posology:** It deals with the dosage of drugs.

Pharmacopoeia

It is an official book published by the authorised body in a country containing description of commonly used drugs with their sources, properties, uses, doses and tests of identity, purity and potency, e.g. Indian pharmacopoeia (I.P.), British Pharmacopoeia (B.P.), United States Pharmacopoeia (U.S.P.). Extra pharmacopoeia (Martindale), etc. It is revised every five years to contain newly developed and essential drugs. Harmful drugs that have better substitutes are omitted in the new edition. Drugs contained in pharmacopoeia are called official drugs.

Sources of Drugs

Drugs are obtained from various sources. According to sources they are as follows:

1. **Natural drugs:** These are obtained from:
   a. Plants, for example:
      - Morphine from poppy capsules
      - Atropine from belladonna leaves
      - Quinine from cinchona barks
      - Castor oil from castor seeds.
   b. Microorganisms, for example:
      - Penicillin from *Penicillium notatum* (a fungus).
      - Streptomycin from *Streptomyces griseus* (a soil dwelling organism)
      - Bacitracin from *Bacillus subtilis* (a bacteria)
      - Diastase from *Aspergillus oryzae* (a fungus)
   c. Animals, for example:
      - Insulin from pig or ox pancreas
      - Thyroxine from pig or ox thyroid gland

- Heparin from pig or ox liver
- Cod liver oil from cod fish liver.

d. Minerals, for example:
- Calcium, magnesium, aluminium, sodium, potassium and iron salts.
- Liquid paraffin from petroleum.

2. **Synthetic drugs:** These are prepared by chemical synthesis in pharmaceutical laboratories, e.g. sulphonamides, quinolones, salicylates, barbiturates, benzodiazepines, etc.

3. **Semisynthetic drugs:** These are prepared by chemical modification of natural drugs in pharmaceutical laboratories, e.g. ampicillin from penicillin-G, cephalexin from cephalosporin-C, dehydroemetine from emetine, dihydroergotamine from ergotamine.

4. **Biosynthetic drugs:** These are prepared by cloning of human DNA into the bacteria like *E. coli*. Cloning means production of identical subjects like the parent. The technique is called recombinant DNA technology or genetic engineering, for example:
- Human insulins (insulin-S, insulin-I)
- Human growth hormones (somatrem, somatropin)
- Human interferons (interferon-α, interferon-β)
- Tissue plasminogen activator (alteplase)
- Human BCG vaccine
- Human hepatitis B vaccine, etc.

Gene-based Therapy (Gene Therapy)

It is the introduction of functional genetic material (DNA) into the target cells to replace or supplement the defective genes. It can impart new functions to cells. By it many diseases which are now only palliated can be cured, e.g. cancers, Alzheimer's disease, Parkinson's disease, diabetes mellitus, hypertension, hyperlipidaemia, haemophilia, cystic fibrosis, muscular dystrophy, Gaucher's disease, sickle cell anaemia, dwarfism, multiple sclerosis, HIV infections, etc.

Chemical Natures of Drugs

Plant Products

The pharmacologically active substances (principles) of plants are as follows:

1. **Alkaloids:** These are organic nitrogenous substances containing cyclic nitrogen and also carbon, hydrogen and sometimes oxygen obtained from plants. These are basic substances (bases) which are insoluble in water but when combined with mineral acids, they form acidic salts, which are soluble in water. Their names end with "ine", e.g. atropine, morphine, nicotine, pilocarpine, emetine, caffeine, etc. Most alkaloids are solid and nonvolatile but some alkaloids are liquid and volatile, e.g. pilocarpine, nicotine, lobeline and amphetamine. Animal alkaloids are called amines, e.g. adrenaline, noradrenaline, dopamine, histamine and 5-hydroxytryptamine.

2. **Glycosides:** These are organic non-nitrogenous substances containing C, H, O and sometimes S obtained from plants. They are neutral or slightly acidic substances which are soluble in water. They do not combine with acids to form salts. When they are heated with mineral acids they hydrolyze and split up into two components, viz. sugar and non-sugar (aglycone or genin). Sugar component is responsible for water and lipid solubility, cell permeability, tissue fixation and potency, while non-sugar component is responsible for pharmacological actions, e.g. digoxin is obtained from leaves of digitalis lanata, sinigrin is obtained from mustard seeds, senna is obtained from senna leaves and picrotoxin is obtained from fish berries (*Anamirta cocculus*).

3. **Oils:** These may be fixed oils or volatile oils obtained from plants. Fixed oils are glycerides of oleic, palmitic and stearic acids. They are obtained from seeds of plants by expression. They are insoluble in water and cannot be distilled. Many of them are edible and have food (caloric) value. They are used for cooking, e.g.

mustard oil, sunflower oil, peanut oil and coconut oil. Some are used for pharmacological actions, e.g. castor oil is used as purgative and olive oil is used as emollient and cholagogue (to cause evacuation of gallbladder by contraction). Fixed oils of animal origin are cod liver oil, shark liver oil, halibut liver oil, butter, lard (animal fats), etc. Fats are fixed oils which remain solid due to presence of more stearin (solid) than palmitin (semi-solid) and olein (liquid). Oils contain more olein than others. Volatile oils are obtained from flowers, leaves, fruits and seeds of plants by distillation. They contain the hydrocarbon "terpene" or some polymers of it, which serves as a diluent or solvent of the active compound. They are soluble in water and impart to it their taste and smell. They are volatalized by heat and possess aromas (smell). They have no food (caloric) value. They are used as carminative, flavouring agent, antiseptic, anodyne or counter-irritant, e.g. cardamom oil, peppermint oil, thymol, clove oil or turpentine oil respectively. Some volatile oils remain solid at ordinary temperature. They are called stearoptenes, e.g. camphor, menthol and thymol. Mineral oils are mixture of hydrocarbons of the methane and related substances obtained from petroleum by fractional distillation, e.g. liquid paraffin, soft paraffin and hard paraffin. Liquid paraffin is used as emollient laxative, while soft and hard paraffins are used as ointment bases.

4. **Tannins:** These are organic non-nitrogenous substances obtained from plants. They have astringent action upon the mucous membrane and thus exert a protective action. They are soluble in water and have astringent taste. They are used as tincture, e.g. tincture of catechu is used as anti-diarrhoeal agent (releases tannic acid in intestine) and tincture of Kalmegh is bitter and is used as appetizer in hepatic dysfunction.

5. **Resins:** These are solid nonvolatile substances formed by oxidation or polymerization of volatile oils in plants. They are insoluble in water but soluble in alcohol, e.g. jalap and colocynth (previously used as drastic purgatives). Podophyllum resins (20% suspension in liquid paraffin) is used as cauterising agent in venereal warts. Oleoresin is a mixture of resin with volatile oil, e.g. male fern extract (previously used to remove tapeworms from the intestine).

6. **Antibiotics:** These are antibacterial substances derived from fungi, actinomycetes and bacteria, e.g. penicillin, streptomycin and bacitracin respectively.

7. **Vitamins:** Majority of vitamins are obtained from plants, e.g. vitamins B complex, C, E, K, etc.

The pharmacologically inert (inactive) substances of plants are:

- **Gums:** These are secretory products of plants. These are colloidal carbohydrates (polysaccharides). These are dispersible in water and form thick mucilaginous colloids, e.g. gum acacia and gum tragacanth are used as emulsifying or suspending agents for preparation of emulsions or suspensions in pharmacy.

- **Waxes:** These are waxy or plastic substances obtained from various plants (vegetable wax) or from animals, e.g. sheep wool (wool wax/lanolin) and honeycomb deposited by bees (beeswax). These are esters of long chain fatty acids with higher, usually monohydroxy alcohols. Beeswax is yellow. It is converted to white wax by bleaching with chlorine. Waxes are used in pharmacy for preparing ointments, creams, suppositories, etc.

Animal Products

These are hormones, enzymes, fixed oils, vitamins and waxes. These have been discussed in respective chapters.

2

Routes of Drug Administration

Drugs can be administered by different routes for local and systemic effects.

Factors Deciding the Route of Choice

- **Physicochemical properties** of the drug, i.e. whether the drug is solid (tablet, capsule, powder, pessary and suppository), liquid (mixture, syrup, lotion, enema and injection) or gas, soluble or insoluble, irritant or nonirritant, etc.
- **Type** of desired effect, i.e. systemic or local effect for which the drug is used.
- **Rapidity** of desired effect, e.g. oral, IM, etc. for routine treatment, IV for emergency treatment.
- **Quality** of desired effect, e.g. magnesium sulphate given orally is a purgative, but when given rectally lowers intracranial tension.
- **Condition** of the patient, i.e. whether the patient is conscious or unconscious, vomiting or not vomiting, etc.

Local Routes

These are used for localized lesions at accessible sites. Systemic absorption of the drug from these sites is minimum or absent. Thus a high concentration of the drug is attained at the desired site without exposing the rest of the body. This minimizes systemic adverse effects or toxicity of the drug. The drug is applied on the skin and various mucous membranes as ointment, cream, lotion, drops, jelly, powder, tablet, suppository, or pessary. Injections in deeper tissues include intra-articular (in joint cavity), e.g. hydrocortisone hemisuccinate; intrathecal (into subarachnoid space of L 2–3 or L 3–4), e.g. lidocaine, isoniazid, amphotericin B, etc. intramedullary (into bone marrow), e.g. hematinics; intra-arterial (into artery of limbs), e.g. anticancer drugs in limb cancer; retrobulbar (behind the eyeball), e.g. hydrocortisone hemisuccinate/acetate; intrapleural (inside pleural cavity), e.g. antitubercular drugs, anticancer drugs and intraperitoneal (inside peritoneal cavity), e.g. antitubercular drugs, inhalation have been discussed later on anticancer drugs.

Systemic Routes

These are used for systemic effects of drugs. The drug is absorbed into blood and distributed all over the body including the site of action through circulation (Flow Chart 2.1). These routes are:

Enteral (GIT)

These are given as follows:

a. **Oral (ingestion of drug):** It is most convenient and economical. It is more safe than other routes. It requires patient's cooperation. The absorption of the drug may be variable and erratic. Drugs that are poorly soluble, slowly absorbed, unstable or extensively metabolized by the liver

Flow Chart 2.1: Routes of drug administration

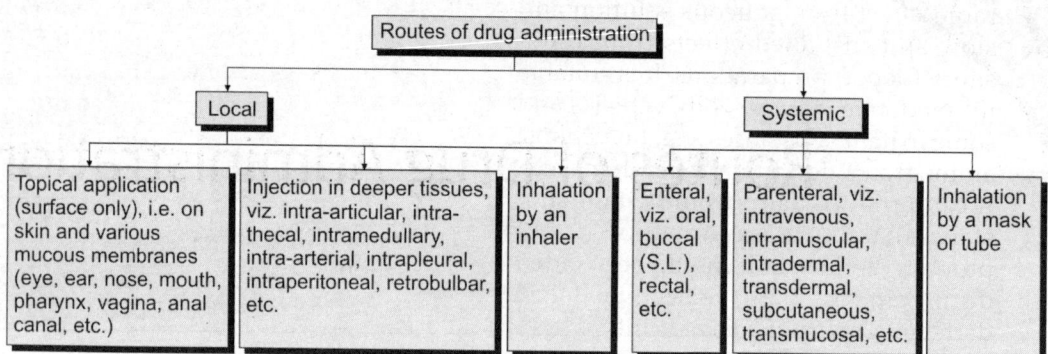

have low bioavailability. The drug is administered as tablet, dragee, capsule, powder, syrup, mixture, suspension or emulsion. Majority of drugs are administered orally as self-administration is possible and adverse effects appear slowly.

b. **Buccal (sublingual):** In it, the drug (as tablet) is placed under the tongue, where from it is absorbed and reaches the systemic circulation directly without passing via the liver (thus avoiding first pass metabolism in the liver and gut wall). Only lipid-soluble and non-irritant drugs can be administered by this route, e.g. glyceryl trinitrate, isosorbide dinitrate, nifedipine, buprenorphine, clonidine, isoprenaline, methyl testosterone, etc. The drug is rapidly absorbed producing prompt effect. Quick termination of drug effect can be done by spitting the remaining portion of the drug from the mouth and so adverse effects can be avoided but on frequent use may produce ulceration locally.

c. **Rectal:** Some irritant and unpleasant drugs can be put in rectum (as suppository or enema) for systemic effects. This route is also used when the patient is having re-current vomiting the drug is absorbed from lower rectum (by external haemorrhoidal veins), then it directly reaches systemic circulation bypassing first pass metabolism in the liver. If the drug is absorbed from upper rectum (by internal haemorrhoidal veins) then it cannot bypass liver. Drugs administered rectally are bisacodyl, glycerine, indomethacin and phenylbutazone as suppository and paraldehyde, tribromoethanol, prednisolone, soap water or barium sulphate as enema. This route is inconvenient and embarrassing and sometimes can cause rectal inflammation.

Parenteral ('Par' meaning away, 'Enteron' meaning intestine)

These include all types of injections and controlled release drug delivery systems.

Injections

i. **Intravenous (IV) injection:** It produces immediate effect, as absorption is not required. It is valuable for emergency use and in seriously ill patients. It permits titration of dose, of the drug. It is usually required for high molecular weight proteins and peptide drugs. It is suitable for large volume and for irritant drugs when diluted. It is not suitable for oily solutions or insoluble substances. It can be given as a bolus or vary slowly (as drip). With it, there is increased risk of adverse reactions. Thrombophlebitis commonly occurs. Lack of sterility in the procedure may cause viral hepatitis or AIDS. Drugs like thiopentone sodium, diazepam, frusemide, diazoxide, sodium nitroprusside, etc. are administered IV for quick effects in emergency conditions.

ii. **Intramuscular (IM) injection:** It produces rapid effect from aqueous solution and slow and sustained effects from repository (depot) preparations. It is suitable for moderate volumes, oily vehicles and some irritant substances, e.g. penicillins, aminoglycosides, iron preparations, etc. It can produce pain (from irritant substances) and abscess formation (if not properly sterilized). It should be avoided during anticoagulant medication. It may damage a nerve if injected into it producing severe pain and paresis.

iii. **Subcutaneous (SC) injection:** It produces rapid effect from aqueous solution and slow and sustained effects from repository preparations as IM injection. It is suitable for some insoluble suspensions and for implantation of solid pallets. It is not suitable for large or moderate volumes of drugs. It can produce pain or necrosis of tissue from irritant substances. Drugs like insulin, adrenaline, heparin (low M.W.), tetanus toxoid, etc. are administered subcutaneously.

Pellet implantation: The drug as solid pellet is introduced into the subcutaneous tissue with the help of a trocar and cannula. It provides a sustained release of the drug for several weeks or months, e.g. testosterone, DOCA, etc.

iv. **Intradermal injection:** In it, the drug is injected into the layers of skin by raising a bleb or multiple puncture of epidermis (by a needle), e.g. BCG or smallpox vaccination. It is also used for testing of drug sensitivity, e.g. penicillin, ATS, etc.

v. **Controlled release drug delivery systems:** These are given as follows:

a. *Transdermal (transcutaneous) drug delivery system (TDS):* It is used for percutaneous absorption of some drugs, e.g. glyceryl trinitrate, isosorbide dinitrate, scopolamine, clonidine, insulin, verapamil, timolol, digoxin, fentanyl, nicotine, prostaglandin, oestradiol, testesterone, etc. The drug is held in a reservoir of suitable materials are applied on the surface of the skin in the form of adhesive patches of various shapes and sizes (5–20 cm sq.), which deliver the incorporated drug at a constant rate into the systemic circulation *via* the skin by diffusion. A single patch can ensure continuous low grade absorption for about 7 days. Common sites of application of adhesive patches are chest, abdomen, upper arm, lower back, buttock, mastoid region and behind the ear (pinna). Its advantages are longer duration of action, decreased frequency of administration, relatively stable plasma concentration, minimum adverse effects (local irritation and oedema) and better patient compliance. The patch can be removed if adverse effects (local inflammation and oedema) appear. Other types of transdermal drug delivery system are dermojet injection, iontophoresis, inunction and implantable miniature syringe pump. Iontophoresis provides penetration of drug into deeper tissues from surface of the skin by galvanic current, e.g. salicylates in arthritis. Inunction provides absorption of drugs into blood by rubbing the drug on the surface of the skin, e.g. nitroglycerine ointment in angina pectoris. Dermojet is a type of transdermal drug delivery system in which needle is not used. A high velocity jet of drug solution is projected from a microfine orifice using a gun-like implement. The drug passes through the layers of skin and gets deposited in the subcutaneous tissue. It is painless and suitable for mass inoculation of vaccines. Implantable computerized miniature syringe pump is used for adminiztration of drugs like insulin, glyceryl trinitrate, etc.

b. *Transmucosal drug delivery system:* It is used for slow mucosal absorption of some drugs, e.g. pilocarpine, progesterone, etc. Ocular insert (ocusert) of pilocarpine is placed directly under the eyelid and delivers a small amount of the drug at a steady rate for about 7 days without causing any discomfort. It thus avoids the need of repeated eye drops application. Progestasert is an intrauterine contraceptive device which provides controlled release of small amount of progestrone within the uterus for about one year.

vi. **Inhalation:** Volatile liquid and gaseous anaesthetics and therapeutic gases (O_2, CO_2 and He) are administered by inhalation. Amylnitrate pearl is broken in handkerchief and inhaled. Other devices like dry powder inhaler spinhaler (of chromolyn sodium), metered dose aerosol inhaler (of salbutamol, beclomethasone, etc.) and compressed air-driven nebulized solution inhaler/nebulizer (of salbutamol, acetylcysteine, etc.) are also available for inhalation. In it, the irritant substances can cause inflammation of respiratory tract.

3

Pharmacokinetics

INTRODUCTION

Pharmacokinetics is the study of movements of the drug in the body. It includes absorption, distribution, metabolism and excretion (ADME) of the drug. It is what the body does to the drug **(Fig. 3.1)**.

Pharmacokinetic Processes

These are given as follows:

Absorption of Drugs

Absorption is the transfer of the drug across the biological (cell) membrane, from the site of administration into the blood. When a drug is administered orally, it passes through the mucous membrane of the gut and capillary endothelium to reach the blood. When it is given by injection, it passes only through capillary endothelium, except given intravenously, when it reaches the blood directly.

Biological (cell) membrane is a lipoprotein (lipoidal) membrane. The lipid portion of the membrane is bimolecular (bilayer) and made of phospholipid and cholesterol molecules. Protein molecules are adsorbed on the outer and inner surfaces of the lipid layer. The membrane contains many aqueous pores (water filled channels), through which filtration of small drug molecules occur.

Absorption of the drug can occur by following processes (mechanisms):

i. **Passive (simple) diffusion:** A drug which is lipid-soluble can cross the cell membrane easily by diffusion, e.g. ether, propranolol, thiopentone, diazepam, etc. cross the cell membrane by dissolving in the lipid matrix of the membrane. The rate

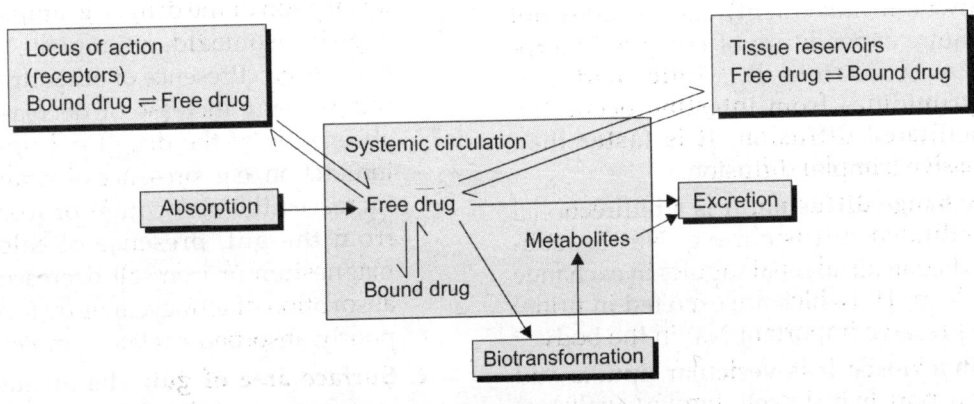

Fig. 3.1: Pharmacokinetics of the drug

of transfer of the drug is proportional to lipid/water partition coefficient of the drug. Greater the coefficient of the drug, higher the concentration of the drug in the membrane and faster the diffusion of the drug through the membrane. Ionized drugs are not lipid-soluble and cannot easily cross cell membrane by diffusion.

ii. **Filtration:** It is the passage of the drug molecule through the aqueous pores in the cell membrane or through inter-epithelial gaps (paracellular spaces). Water-soluble drugs of low molecular weights whether ionized or unionized can easily pass through the membrane pores and enter intracellular or extracellular space or excreted in urine by glomerular filtration, e.g. atenolol, heparin, alcohol, mannitol, etc.

iii. **Active transport:** It is the movement of the drug molecule across the cell membrane against the concentration gradient (uphill movement) requiring expenditure of energy (ATP). It is carrier mediated, i.e. carried by a specific carrier called a transport protein. It can be inhibited by metabolic poisons (antimetabolites). Absorption of glucose, iron and amino acids from intestine occurs by active transport process.

iv. **Facilitated diffusion:** In it, the drug molecule crosses the cell membrane by the help of a carrier protein but the movement of the drug molecule is towards the concentration gradient (i.e. downhill movement) and so does not require expenditure of energy. Absorption of vitamin B_{12}, folic acid and pyrimidines from intestine occurs by facilitated diffusion. It is faster than passive (simple) diffusion.

v. **Exchange diffusion:** It is a bidirectional facilitated diffusion, e.g. Na^+ is reabsorbed in distal renal tubules in exchange of K^+ or H^+ (which are excreted in urine) to preserve important Na^+ in the body.

vi. **Pinocytosis:** It is vesicular uptake and transport. In it, the cell engulfs (swallows) a large size drug molecule (polypeptide, lipoprotein, etc.) by an infolding process of a small portion of a cell membrane forming a vesicle and transports it. It requires expenditure of energy like active transport. It occurs mainly in liver cells.

Factors influencing the rate of absorption of drugs from GIT are as follows:

i. *Biological factors (intrinsic factors):* These are gut (GIT) related factors.

a. **Local pH of gut:** Most drugs are either weak acids or weak bases and exist in aqueous solution as a mixture of ionized and unionized forms. Ionized form is lipid-insoluble, whereas unionized form is lipid-soluble. Acidic drugs like salicylates, barbiturates and sulphonamides are rapidly absorbed from the stomach as they are poorly ionized in the acid pH (less than 5) of stomach and thus remain mostly in unionized form. Basic drugs like morphine, quinine, chloroquine, amphetamine and ephedrine are not absorbed from the stomach, but absorbed from the small intestine in the alkaline pH where they remain mostly in unionized form in the alkaline pH (more than 7) of small intestine.

b. **Presence of food and other drugs in gut:** Most drugs are better absorbed in empty stomach. Presence of food in the stomach dilutes the drug and retards absorption of the drug, e.g. ampicillin, aspirin, isoniazid, rifampicin, tetracycline, etc. Presence of other drugs in the gut may increase or decrease the absorption of the drug by drug-drug interaction, e.g. presence of vitamin C increases the absorption of iron salt from the gut, presence of calcium, magnesium or iron salt decreases the absorption of tetracyclines by forming poorly absorbed chelate complexes.

c. **Surface area of gut:** The greater the surface area of the absorbing surface on which the drug is spread, the more rapid is the rate of absorption. Drugs are better absorbed from the small intestine than the stomach due to the greater surface area. Decrease in surface area due to gastrectomy or enterectomy reduces absorption of drugs.

d. **Motility of gut:** Increase in gut motility as in diarrhoea, decreases absorption of drugs due to rapid elimination in faeces. Decrease in gut motility as in shock or CCF slows absorption of drugs. Vomiting also decreases absorption of drugs.

e. **Local circulation (blood flow) in gut:** Increase of blood flow in gut due to vasodilation increases absorption of drugs. Decrease of blood flow in gut due to vasoconstriction as in haemorrhagic shock decreases absorption of drugs.

f. **First pass effect:** Some drugs, e.g. glyceryl trinitrate, isosorbide dinitrate, isoprenaline, propanolol, chlorpromazine, etc. undergo first pass metabolism in gut wall and liver during passage through portal circulation which decreases their therapeutic effects. These drugs are better administered sublingually to reach the systemic circulation directly by passing gut wall and hepatic metabolism.

ii. *Pharmaceutical factors (extrinsic factors):* These are drug related factors:

a. **Physical state of drug:** Drugs given in liquid dosage forms are better and rapidly absorbed from gut than when given in solid dosage forms. Colloids are slowly absorbed than crystalloids.

b. **Water or lipid solubility of drug:** Drugs given in aqueous solution mix more readily with the aqueous phase of the absorbing surface than when given in oily solution and so rapidly absorbed from gut. At the cell surface, a lipid-soluble drug penetrates the cell

membrane more easily than a water-soluble drug and so better absorbed from gut.

c. **Particle size of drug:** Solid dosage forms of drugs that contain smaller particles (microfine crystals) are better absorbed from gut, e.g. aspirin, griseofulvin, chloramphenicol, warfarin, tolbutamide, corticosteroids, etc. They should be given in smaller dose to avoid systemic toxicity. Solid dosage forms that contain larger particles, e.g. bephenium, streptomycin, neomycin, etc. are very little absorbed from gut and so used for local effects. Larger tablet breaks down more quickly than the highly compressed small tablet and so more rapidly absorbed from gut.

d. **Disintegration time of drug:** It is the time taken for a solid dosage form (e.g. tablet) of a drug to disintegrate (break down) into finer particles in the gut completely. It depends on the type of drug and the excipient (binding agent) used in it. If the disintegration time is longer, the absorption of the drug is delayed.

e. **Dissolution time of drug:** It is the time taken for a solid dosage form (e.g. tablet) of a drug to go into the solution in the gut after it has been disintegrated. Solution as a rule is absorbed faster than the solid form.

f. **Enteric coating of drug:** Some tablets or dragees are made enteric coated by means of cellulose, acetate or phthalate, which resist disintegration and dissolution of the drug in the gut by acid gastric juice but permit disintegration and dissolution of the drug by the alkaline intestinal juice. This produces an uniform and sustained blood level of the drug without requiring too frequent dosing. Some sustained release (S.R.) and time release (T.R.) capsules are now available that release the active drug over an extended period of time. These contain drug particles covered with different coatings, that are dissolved at different time intervals in the gut. This produces uniform medication for a prolonged period.

Distribution of Drugs

After a drug is absorbed or injected into the bloodstream, it is distributed to various fluid compartments of the body such as interstitial, transcellular and intracellular fluids. Transcellular fluids are CSF, aqueous humour, endolymph, GIT fluids and joint fluids. In the initial phase of distribution of drugs, the heart, liver, kidney, brain and other highly vascular (well perfused) organs receive most of the drugs during first few minutes after absorption. In the later phase of distribution of drugs, the muscle, viscera, skin, connective tissue and adipose tissue receive a much lower proportion of the drug. Ultimately, the drug in all tissues achieve equilibrium with the drug present in the blood. It takes several minutes to several hours to attain the steady state concentration. Diffusion of drug into interstitial compartment occurs rapidly because of the highly permeable nature of capillary endothelial membrane (except in brain). Lipid-insoluble drugs that permeate membrane poorly are restricted in their distribution. Distribution is also limited to drugs that bind with plasma proteins, particularly albumin for acidic drugs and α_1-acid glycoprotein for basic drugs. A drug that is extensively and strongly bound with plasma proteins has limited excess to cellular sites of action and is metabolized and excreted slowly. Drugs may accumulate in tissues in higher concentrations than would be expected from diffusion equilibria as a result of pH gradients, binding to intracellular constituents or partitioning into lipid. Drug that has accumulated in a given tissue may act as a reservoir, which prolongs drug action. Drug reservoirs are body compartments in which a drug accumulate, e.g. plasma proteins and cellular reservoirs.

Many drugs are bound to plasma proteins. This binding is usually reversible. Free drug + protein $\rightleftharpoons$ drug protein complex. Irreversible (covalent) binding may occur with reactive drugs like alkylating agents.

Cellular reservoirs: Many drugs accumulate in muscle, fat, liver, bone, etc. in higher concentrations than in the extracellular fluids. Accumulation of drugs in cells may be due to active transport or due to binding with cellular constituents. Tissue binding of drugs occurs with proteins, phospholipids or nucleoproteins and is generally reversible.

CNS transfer of drugs: Some drugs can be present in the blood but they cannot reach the brain as they are prevented to reach. The brain by a barrier called the blood–brain barrier (BBB). However, some drugs can cross the BBB. Endothelial cells of the brain capillaries do not possess intracellular pores and pinocytotic vesicles. Presence of tight junctions and pericapillary glial cells restrict the passage of drugs into the brain. Highly lipid-soluble drugs like thiopentone can easily cross the BBB producing rapid action (within a minute after IV injection). As there is little binding of the drug to the brain constituents, so its action is terminated rapidly by redistribution to less vascular tissues of the body (muscle, viscera, adipose tissue, etc.).

Placental transfer of drugs: This is important because some drugs (e.g. phenytoin, prednisolone, warfarin, etc.) can cause congenital anomalies (malformation of foetus) by crossing the placental barrier by simple diffusion. Some drugs (e.g. morphine, barbiturates, etc.) when administered before delivery may cause serious adverse effects on the neonate. Lipid-soluble, unionized drugs readily enter the foetal blood from the maternal circulation. Drugs that are ionized or have low lipid solubility cannot cross placental barrier.

Biotransformation of Drugs

Biotransformation of the drug within a living organism means alteration of chemical structure of the drug. In simple words, it is the metabolism of the drug molecule in the body. The fate of a drug in the body is metabolism and then excretion mainly as metabolites. Drugs are treated by the body as foreign substances (xenobiotics), which the body tries to remove from the body by metabolism and excretion. Drugs may be lipid-soluble (lipophilic) or water-soluble (hydrophilic). Lipid-soluble drugs are nonionizable (nonpolar) and can easily cross the cell membrane. They are metabolized in the liver as they can easily enter the liver cells (hepatocytes). They are not excreted in urine, as they are reabsorbed in renal tubules. They are to be converted to water-soluble metabolites in order to eliminate them from the body. Water-soluble drugs are ionizable (polar). They are little metabolized in the liver and excreted in urine as they are not reabsorbed in renal tubules.

Sites of metabolism of drugs: These are liver, GIT, plasma, kidneys, lungs and skin. In the liver, the metabolic reactions occur mainly in the smooth endoplasmic reticulum (microsomes). The enzymes for metabolism of drugs are collectively called cytochrome P-450 (CYP). They are haeme-containing membrane proteins (haemoproteins), present in the microsomes of liver and other cells. They catalyze a wide variety of oxidative and reductive reactions. There are three types of CYP, viz. CYP_1, CYP_2 and CYP_3 each of which has four subtypes (A, B, C and D), e.g. CYP_1A, CYP_1B, CYP_2C and CYP_2D. These have different substrate specificities.

Metabolic reactions of drugs: These are of two types:

i. Phase I reactions (non-synthetic/functionalization reactions): These are oxidation, reduction and hydrolysis of drugs. Here, the metabolites formed are active or inactive.

ii. Phase II reactions (synthetic/conjugation reactions): These are conjugation (union) of drugs with endogenous water-soluble substances like glucuronic acid, acetic acid, methionine, glutathione, glycine, etc. Here, the metabolites formed are inactive (inert).

A drug may undergo following reactions to form metabolites for excretion in urine or bile **(Fig. 3.2)**.

If the metabolites formed in phase I reactions are highly ionized (polar), they will be excreted in urine or bile. If the metabolites formed in phase I reaction are poorly ionized (nonpolar) then they will undergo phase II reactions to become water-soluble products, which are then excreted in urine or bile.

Enzymes responsible for metabolic reactions are microsomal and nonmicrosomal enzymes. Microsomal (cytosolic, mitochondrial, etc.) enzymes catalyze most oxidation and reduction reactions, some hydrolysis reactions and glucuronide conjugation reaction. Nonmicrosomal enzymes catalyze some oxidation and reduction reactions, many hydrolysis reactions and all conjugation reactions except glucuronidation.

Oxidative reactions: Oxidation is the process of addition of oxygen or negatively charged radical to a drug molecule or removal of hydrogen or positively charged radical

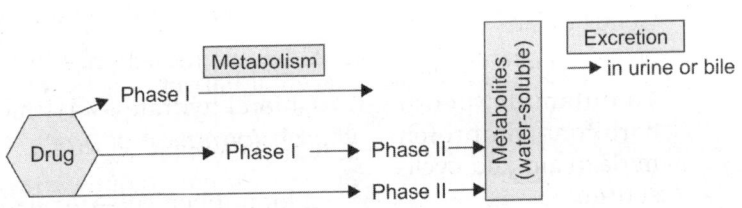

Fig. 3.2: Phases of drug metabolism

from a drug molecule. It occurs most commonly within the microsomes of liver cells. The enzyme system which oxidizes the drug is called mixed function oxidase (MFO) system or mono-oxygenase (MO) system. The system consists of cytochrome oxidase enzyme (cytochrome P-450), NADPH (a coenzyme), NADPH-cytochrome P-450 reductase and molecular oxygen. The drug (substrate) reacts with the oxidized (Fe^{3+}) form of cytochrome P-450 to form an enzyme substrate complex. The cytochrome P-450 reductase accepts an electron from NADPH, which in turn, reduces the oxidized cytochrome P-450 substrate complex. The reduced (Fe^{2+}) cytochrome P-450 substrate complex then reacts with molecular oxygen and a second electron from NADPH donated through the same flavoprotein reductase to form an activated oxygen species. In the final step, one atom of oxygen is released as H_2O and the second atom of oxygen is transferred to the substrate. Upon release of the oxidized substrate, the oxidized cytochrome P-450 enzyme is regenerated. There are several types of oxidation reactions:

1. N-Dealkylation, e.g.

Imipramine	→	Desmethylimipramine
Diazepam	→	Desmethyldiazepam.
Other drugs	:	Codeine, erythromycin, morphine, theophylline and tamoxifen.

2. O-Dealkylation, e.g.

Codeine	→	Morphine
Phenacetin	→	Paracetamol
Other drugs	:	Indomethacin and dextromethorphan.

3. Aliphatic hydroxylation, e.g.

Salicylic acid	→	Gentisic acid
Meprobamate	→	Hydroxymeprobamate
Other drugs	:	Tolbutamide, pentobarbitone, ibuprofen, midazolam and cyclosporin.

4. Aromatic hydroxylation, e.g.

Phenobarbitone	→	P-hydroxyphenobarbitone
Phenytoin	→	Hydroxyphenytoin
Other drugs	:	Propranonol, phenylbutazone and ethinylestradiol.

5. N-Oxidation, e.g.

Mephobarbitone	→	Phenobarbitone
Chlorphenteramine	→	Phenteramine
Other drugs	:	Chlorpheniramine, guanethidine, quinidine and acetaminophen.

6. S-Oxidation, e.g.

Cimetidine	→	Cimetidine sulphoxide
Other drugs	:	Chlorpromazine and thioridazine.

7. Deamination, e.g.

Amphetamine	→	Benzyl methyl ketone (phenylacetone).
Other drugs	:	Diazepam and flurazepam.

Deamination of adrenaline and noradrenaline by MAO is nonmicrosomal enzyme reaction occurring in mitochondria.

Reduction reactions: Reduction is the process opposite to that of oxidation. Here also both microsomal and nonmicrosomal enzymes are involved. There are several types of reduction reactions.

1. Azoreduction, e.g.

Prontosil → Sulphanilamide.

2. Aldehyde reduction, e.g.

Chloral hydrate → Trichloroethanol.

3. Nitroreduction, e.g.

Chloramphenicol → Arylamine.

4. Ketoreduction, e.g.

Cortisone $\rightarrow$ Hydrocortisone.

5. Chlororeduction, e.g.

Halothane $\rightarrow$ Trifluoroethanol.

6. Disulphide reduction, e.g.

Disulfiram $\rightarrow$ Diethyldithiocarbamic acid.

Hydrolysis reactions: Hydrolysis is the cleavage (division) of a drug molecule by addition of a molecule of water. It occurs with the help of the enzymes esterase, amidase and peptidase in the ester, amide and polypeptide respectively in liver and plasma. Here also both microsomal and nonmicrosomal enzymes are involved, e.g.

$$\text{Acetylcholine} + H_2O \xrightarrow[\uparrow]{} \text{Acetic acid} + \text{Choline}$$

(Cholinesterase)

$$\text{Procaine} + H_2O \xrightarrow[\uparrow]{} \text{PABA} + \text{Diethylaminoethanol}$$

(Procaine esterase)

$$\text{Procainamide} + H_2O \xrightarrow[\uparrow]{} \text{PABA} + \text{Diethylamino-ethanolamine}$$

(Procaine amidase)

$$\text{Meperidine} + H_2O \xrightarrow[\uparrow]{} \text{Meperidinic acid} + \text{Ethanol}$$

(Peptidase)

Other drugs: Aspirin, clofibrate, lidocaine and indomethacin.

Conjugation reactions: Conjugation is the addition of an endogenous water-soluble molecule (group) to the parent drug or its oxidized metabolite by the help of transferase enzyme leading to termination of biological activity of the drug and elimination of it in urine. These are given as follows:

1. Glucuronide conjugation, e.g.

$$\text{Morphine} + \text{Glucuronic acid} \xrightarrow[\uparrow]{} \text{Morphine-glucuronide}$$

(Glucuronidation)   (Glucuronyl transferase)

Other drugs: Diazepam, aspirin and acetaminophen.

2. Sulphate conjugation, e.g.

$$\text{Chloramphenicol} + H_2SO_4 \xrightarrow[\uparrow]{} \text{Chloramphenicol ethereal sulphate}$$

(Sulphation) (Sulphotransferase)

Other drugs: Acetaminophen, oestrogen and other steroids and methyldopa.

3. Acetate conjugation, e.g.

$$\text{Sulphanilamide} + \text{Acetic acid} \xrightarrow[\uparrow]{} \text{Acetyl sulphanilamide}$$

(Acetylation)   (Acetyltransferase)

Other drugs: Isoniazid, dapsone and clonazepan.

4. Methyl conjugation, e.g.

$$\text{Adrenaline} + CH_3 \xrightarrow[\uparrow]{} \text{Methyladrenaline}$$

(Methylation)   (Transmethylase)

Other drugs: Noradrenaline, dopamine and histamine.

5. Glycine conjugation, e.g.

$$\text{Salicylic acid} + \text{glycine} \xrightarrow[\uparrow]{} \text{Salicyluric acid}$$

(Glycinetransferase)

Other drugs: PAS, cholic acid and benzoic acid.

Types of metabolic product (metabolites):

These are given as follows:

1. **Formation of active metabolites** from active drugs, e.g.

Chloral hydrate $\longrightarrow$ Trichloroethanol

Phenyl butazone $\longrightarrow$ Oxyphenbutazone

Other drugs: Aspirin, phenacetin, codeine, imipramine, amitriptyline, diazepam, propranolol, chloroquine and spironolactone.

2. **Formation of active metabolites** from inactive drugs (prodrugs), e.g.

Levodopa $\longrightarrow$ Dopamine

Acyclovir $\longrightarrow$ Acycloguanosine

Other drugs: Prednisone, proguanil, enalapril, sulindac, cyclophosphamide, talampicillin, diazepam, benorylate and vitamin D.

3. **Formation of inactive** or toxic metabolites from active drugs. These are most drugs,

Morphine $\rightarrow$ Morphine glucuronide (inactive).

Isoniazid $\rightarrow$ Acetyl isoniazid (toxic).

Paracetamol → N-acetyl benzoquinone-imine (toxic).

Oestrogen → Oestrogen ethereal sulphate (inactive).

Factors influencing biotransformation of drugs are:

a. Genetic factors: Inter individual variations in the biotransformation of the drug within a population is due to genetically determined differences (genetic polymorphism) in the rate of metabolism (by oxidation and conjugation) in the liver, e.g. propranolol, metaprolol, isoniazid, hydralazine, primaquine, succinylcholine, etc. Phenotypic differences in the amount of drug excreted through a polymorphically controlled pathway lead to the classification of individuals as extensive (rapid) or poor (slow) metabolizers. Most deficiencies in drug metabolizing activity are inherited as autosomally recessive traits. Due to deficiency of corresponding metabolizing enzyme in some persons, the metabolism of the drug is decreased leading to increased therapeutic effect or toxicity of the drug. Pharmacogenetics deals with the genetically mediated variations in drug metabolism and responses (will be discussed with drug effects).

b. Environmental factors: Exposure to certain chemicals and environmental pollutants leads to increased biosynthesis of cytochrome P-450. This enzyme induction leads to an increased rate of metabolism and corresponding decrease in the availability of the parent drug. Drugs that are metabolized to reactive compounds by enzyme induction can produce increased toxicity. Some drugs can induce both the metabolism of other drugs and its own metabolism, e.g. carbamazepine and phenobarbitone. These are called **autoinducers.** Inhibition of drug metabolizing enzyme results in increased concentration of the parent drug, prolonged pharmacological effects and increased toxicity.

c. Physiological factors: Drugs produce greater and more prolonged effects at the extremes of age (elderly persons and infants) due to decreased rate of metabolism of drugs or lack of ability of conjugation of drugs (due to enzyme deficiency). Deficiency of nutritional factors (protein, fat, vitamins and minerals) in diet decreases the rate of drug metabolism. Drugs that are highly plasma protein bound are slowly metabolized in the body as they cannot reach the site of metabolism (especially liver) by diffusion.

d. Pathological factors: In liver and heart diseases, the metabolism of drugs is decreased. In hyperthyroidism, the metabolism of drugs is increased and in hypothyroidism the metabolism of drugs is decreased. In malnutrition, the metabolism of drugs is decreased.

Excretion of Drugs

Drugs are excreted from the body either unchanged or as metabolites. Excretory organs of drugs are kidneys, liver, lungs, intestine, breasts, skin, salivary and lacrimal glands. Lipid-soluble drugs are not readily excreted until they are metabolized to polar (ionized) compounds.

Renal excretion: Kidneys are most important organs for excretion of drugs and their metabolites by glomerular filtration, active tubular secretion and passive tubular reabsorption. The amount of drug entering the tubular lumen by filtration is dependent on its plasma protein binding and GFR. In the proximal renal tubules some organic anions and cations enter the glomerular filtrate by active, carrier mediated tubular secretion. Many organic acids such as penicillins and metabolites such as glucuronides are transported to tubular urine by the active transport system, that secretes uric acid. Organic bases such as tetraethyl ammonium are transported by a separate active transport system, that secretes choline, histamine and other endogenous bases. In the proximal and distal renal tubules, the unionized forms of weak acids and bases undergo passive reabsorption. The concentration gradient for back diffusion is produced by reabsorption of water with Na^+ and other inorganic ions. As the tubular cells are less permeable to the ionized forms of weak electrolytes, so passive reabsorption of these substances is pH dependent. When tubular urine is made more alkaline, weak acids are excreted more rapidly, because they are more ionized and passive reabsorption is decreased. When the tubular urine is made more acidic, the excretion of weak acids is decreased but excretion of weak bases is increased.

Biliary and faecal excretion: Many metabolites of drugs are excreted into the intestinal tract from the liver via bile. These metabolites are either excreted in the faeces or reabsorbed into the blood and ultimately excreted in urine.

Excretion in other routes: Anaesthetic gases and vapours, alcohol, paraldehyde and occasionally small quantities of other drugs or metabolites are excreted by lungs. Some drugs are excreted through breast milk and may cause adverse effects in the nursing infants, e.g. penicillins, sulphonamides, tetracyclines, chloramphenicol, isoniazid, morphine, sedative-hypnotics, anticancer drugs, etc. Some drugs are excreted in small amounts in sweat, saliva and tears, e.g. lithium, potassium iodide, potassium thiocyanate, rifampicin and heavy metals (like arsenic and mercury) but this is quantitatively unimportant.

4

Clinical Pharmacokinetics

Commonly used pharmacokinetic parameters are:

- Bioavailability
- Volume of distribution
- Clearance
- Half-life.

BIOAVAILABILITY

Bioavailability means the availability of a biologically active drug. It is the fraction of unchanged drug that reaches the blood (systemic circulation) or the site of action following administration by any route. When a drug is administered IV, all the drugs are available for biological activity and so bioavailability is 100%. When a drug is administered IM or SC, the bioavailability of the drug is usually complete (100%) or may be incomplete (<100%) due to local tissue binding of the drug. When a drug is administered orally, then the bioavailability of the drug may vary from 0 to 100% due to nonabsorption, partial absorption or complete absorption of the drug. Conventionally, bioavailability is applied for oral bioavailability.

Importance of Bioavailability

It is necessary to know bioavailability of each drug, because it will determine whether the drug can be administered orally or not, and if it can be administered orally, then what should be the oral dose in comparison to IV dose of the drug.

Determination of Bioavailability

To determine bioavailability of a drug, the drug is first administered IV and its plasma concentrations are measured at one hourly intervals. The plasma concentration–time curves following IV and oral administration of the same dose of the drug are plotted in graph paper (as shown in **Fig. 4.1**). From these curves, the area under the curve (AUC) is measured for IV and oral dose of the drug. Bioavailability is determined by the formula:

$$BA = \frac{AUC\ after\ an\ oral\ dose}{AUC\ after\ an\ IV\ dose}$$

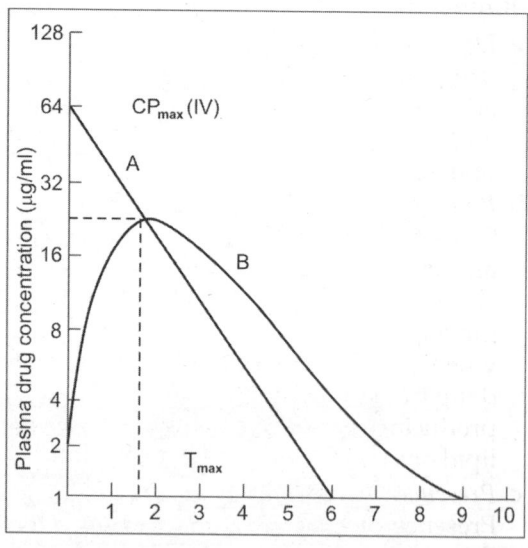

Fig. 4.1: AUC after oral and IV dose of a drug

(where BA is the bioavailability and AUC is the area under curve). It is always expressed in percentage (%). A is the plasma concentration–time curve following IV administration of a drug. B is the plasma concentration–time curve following oral administration of a drug.

CP_{max} is peak (maximum) plasma concentration following IV/oral administration of a drug. T_{max} is the time of peak plasma concentration following oral administration of a drug.

For the sake of convenience, instead of measuring plasma concentrations of the drug by repeated injections, the total urinary excretion of the drug at one hourly intervals can be measured if the drug is primarily excreted in urine.

Bioavailability determined by these methods is called absolute bioavailability. Relative bioavailability is determined by comparing the AUC of oral dose of the test preparation with the AUC of oral dose of the standard preparation of the drug without IV administration.

Factors Modifying Bioavailability

These are given as follows:

1. **Route of administration of the drug:** Bioavailability of a drug is 100% after IV administration and less than 100% after oral or other route of administration.

2. **Biological (intrinsic) factors like:**
   a. *Degradation of the drug in gut (GIT)*: Some drugs such as benzyl penicillin, insulin, adrenaline, etc. are destroyed in the gut and so they have low bioavailability after oral administration.
   b. *Route of absorption of the drug from gut*: Some drugs, e.g. streptomycin, neomycin, aluminium hydroxide, magnesium trisilicate, etc. are poorly absorbed from the gut and so they have poor bioavailability when administered orally. Water-soluble drugs are absorbed easily from GIT producing greater bioavailability than the lipid-soluble drugs.
   c. *Presence of food and other drugs in gut*: Presence of food in stomach dilutes the drug and retards the absorption of the drug. Presence of calcium, magnesium,

aluminium or iron salts decreases the absorption of tetracyclines by forming poorly absorbed chelate complexes and thus reduces bioavailability. Cholestyramine resin binds with thyroxine, warfarin or other acidic drugs in gut and decreases their bioavailability.

   d. *First pass (presystemic) metabolism of the drug*: Some drugs are metabolized in the gut wall and liver by enzymes before reaching the systemic circulation, e.g. GTN, isosorbide dinitrate, isoprenaline, nifedipine, buprenorphine, etc. and their bioavailability is low after oral administration. So, they are administered sublingually for systemic action.
   e. *Enterohepatic circulation (recycling)*: Some drugs undergo enterohepatic circulation, e.g. tetracylines, erythromycin, ampicillin, rifampicin, digitoxin, oral contraceptives, etc. and so their bioavailability is decreased.

3. **Pharmaceutical (extrinsic) factors:** Pharmaceutical factors like physicochemical properties of drugs, dosage forms, particle size of drugs, type of excipient used, disintegration time and dissolution rate of drugs influence bioavailability of drugs. Drugs administered as microcrystalline form, e.g. aspirin, griseofulvin, nitrofurantoin, etc. are rapidly absorbed producing greater bioavailability than when administered as coarse particles.

Bioequivalence

It means equal therapeutic effectiveness of two or more drug products (formulations) manufactured by different pharmaceutical laboratories due to same bioavailability of the active ingredient. Differences in bioavailability (low or high) of drug formulations can reduce therapeutic effect or increase toxicity of the drug. For this reason, a clinician must be careful while changing one brand (drug formulation) to another brand (drug formulation) of the same drug. It is of great clinical significance in drugs with narrow safety margin, e.g. digoxin, quinidine, phenytoin, warfarin, salbutamol, glibenclamide, lithium, etc.

VOLUME OF DISTRIBUTION

The volume of distribution of a drug means the fluid volume that would be required to contain all the drugs in the body at the same concentration as in blood or plasma. The total volume of the fluid compartments of the body into which a drug may be distributed is about 40 litres in an adult (70 kg). These fluid compartments are extracellular fluid (20 L) including plasma water (5 L) interstitial fluid (10 L) and transcellular fluid (5 L) and intracellular fluid (20 L). The fluid volume into which a drug is supposed to be distributed is called volume of distribution (Vd). It is calculated by the formula:

$$Vd = \frac{\text{Amount of the drug in the body (D)}}{\text{Concentration (C) of the drug in the blood or plasma}}$$

where Vd is the apparent volume of distribution of the drug after IV administration. Vd calculated by this method is not real but hypothetical (imaginary) and so it is called apparent volume of distribution.

From this estimated Vd, some useful conclusions can be drawn:

i. Drugs which remain mostly confined within the blood or plasma and cannot go beyond the vascular compartment, e.g. heparin, warfarin, phenytoin, aspirin, frusemide, etc. have small Vd (5–10 L). Such drugs can be removed easily by haemodialysis (dialysis of plasma) in case of poisoning.

ii. Drugs which go beyond the vascular compartment and are distributed in the tissue fluids, e.g. ampicillin, cephalexin, sulphamethoxazole, etc. have large Vd (10–20 L).

iii. Drugs which are present not only in blood and tissue fluid, but are heavily dissolved in adipose tissue (e.g. thiopentone, pethidine, etc.) or concentrate in tissue proteins of liver or other organs, e.g. chloroquine, mepacrine, etc. have very large Vd (500–50,000 L).

iv. Lipid-soluble (nonionized) drugs which can readily cross cell membranes and distributed throughout the body fluids have large Vd and water-soluble (ionized) and highly plasma proteins bound drugs have small Vd.

v. When the Vd exceeds the total volume of body water (40 L), then there is uptake and binding of the drug within the tissue such as adipose tissue, muscle, liver, brain, heart and bone.

One compartmental vs. multicompartmental models: For some drugs, the body may be considered to consist of a single (one) homogeneous compartment made of blood and tissues. In this, all drug administration occurs directly into the body compartment and distribution of drug is instantaneous through the body fluid volume. Clearance of drug from this compartment occurs by first order kinetic, i.e. the amount of drug eliminated per unit time depends on the amount (concentration) of drug in the body compartment. In it, a plot of the logarithm of the concentration of drug in plasma against time will be straight line **(Fig. 40.2a)**.

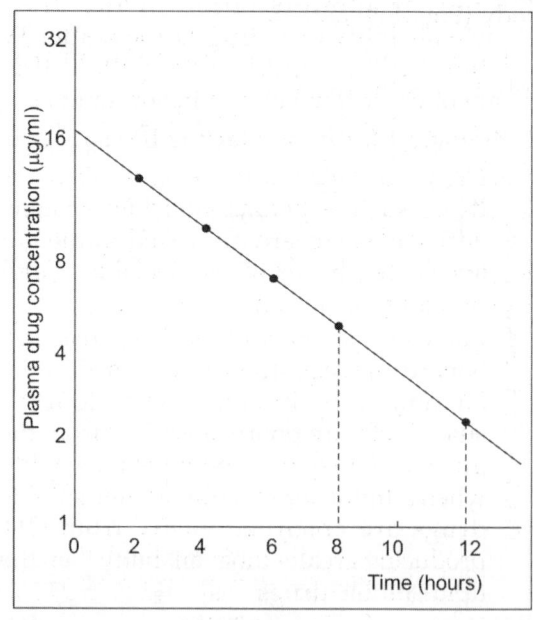

Fig. 4.2a: One compartment model after IV administration

For most of the drugs, the body is considered to be consisting of multiple (two) compartments. The first compartment is called central compartment and consists of blood and some organs like heart, brain, liver, lung and kidney, which are highly vascular and where the drug can enter very easily from the vascular compartment. The second compartment is called peripheral compartment and consists of mostly muscles and adipose tissue, where the vascularity is less (poor) in comparison to first compartment. When a drug is administered by IV bolus, it is rapidly distributed in the central compartment and after sometime it enters the peripheral compartment.

Clearance of drug from these compartments occurs by multiple exponential kinetics. In it, a plot of the logarithm of the concentration of drug in plasma against time will be a curved line. The curve shows two phases—an initial rapid decline phase of the plasma concentration of drug due to distribution to the tissue and then a slow and uniform decline phase of the plasma concentration of drug due to elimination from the body **(Figs 4.2b and c)**.

Factors influencing the volume of distribution of the drug are:

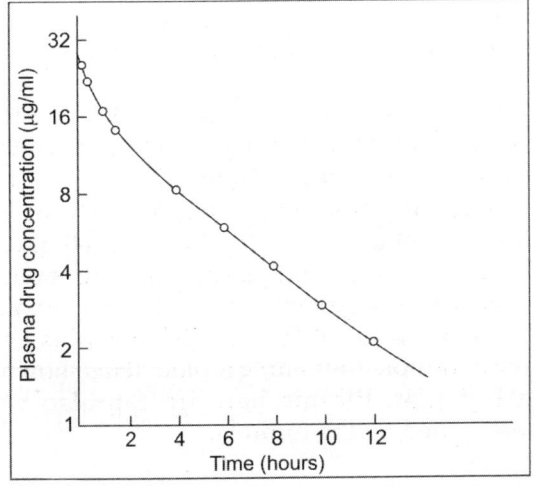

Fig. 4.2b: Multicompartment model after IV administration

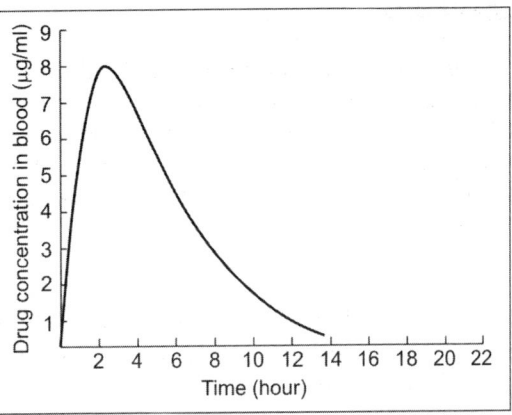

Fig. 4.2c: One compartment model after oral administration

i. **pKa of the drug:** It is the negative logarithm of dissociation (ionization) constant 'Ka', i.e. pKa = – log Ka. For an acidic drug,

$$pKa = pH + \log \frac{\text{Unionized acid}}{\text{Ionized base}}$$

and for a basic drug,

$$pKa = pH + \log \frac{\text{Ionized base}}{\text{Unionized acid}}$$

(Handerson-Hassalbalch equation)

Generally acidic drugs have a lower pKa value (2.5–6) and basic drugs have a higher pKa value (6–10). As a general rule, acidic drugs (e.g. aspirin) are more ionized, lipid-insoluble and less diffusible in a relatively alkaline medium (e.g. intestine), whereas they are more nonionized, lipid-soluble and more diffusible in relatively acidic medium (e.g. stomach). Similar is the relationship between the basic drug and the environmental pH. Thus, pKa of drug influences volume of distribution of a drug.

ii. **Degree of binding of the drug with plasma proteins or with other tissue proteins:** The greater the binding, the less the volume of distribution of the drug.

iii. **Lipid solubility of the drug:** The higher the lipid solubility of the drug, the greater is the volume of distribution of the drug.

iv. **Patient's age, gender, disease and body composition:** These can also change volume of distribution of the drug.

CLEARANCE

Clearance is the measure of body's ability to eliminate a drug. It is the rate of elimination of a drug by all routes normalized to the concentration of drug in the biological fluid (blood or plasma). It is calculated by the formula.

$$CL = \frac{\text{Rate of elimination of drug (vol/min)}}{\text{Concentration of drug in blood or plasma}}$$

where CL is the clearance of drug. It indicates the volume of biological fluid (blood or plasma) that would have to be completely freed of drug to account for the elimination. It is expressed as a volume per unit of time. It may be blood clearance (CL_p), plasma clearance (CL_p) or clearance based on the concentration of unbound (free) drug (CL_u) depending on the concentration measured (C_b, C_p or C_u). The organs of elimination can only clear drug from the blood or plasma with which they are in direct contact. Clearance by means of various organs of elimination is additive. Elimination of drug may occur as a result of processes that occur in the kidney (renal clearance), liver (hepatic clearance) or other organs. Dividing the rate of elimination of each organ by a concentration of drug (e.g. plasma concentration) will give the respective clearance by that organ. Total systemic clearance is the sum of all these separate clearances.

Steady state concentration (C_{ss}): When a drug is administered at a constant rate, then a steady state concentration will be achieved ultimately. At this point, the rate of elimination of a drug is equal to the rate of drug availability. If the drug is administered as intermittent doses (e.g. 250 mg every 8 hours), then during each interdose interval the concentration of drug rises or falls. At steady state, the entire cycle is repeated identically in each interval **(Fig. 4.3)**. For steady state concentration of a drug 4 or 5 plasma half-lives are required.

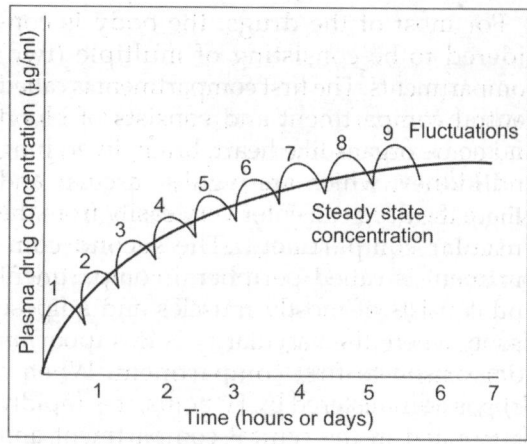

Fig. 4.3: Steady state concentration of drug

HALF-LIFE ($t^1/_2$)

Half-life of a drug is the time taken for the plasma concentration or the amount of drug in the body to be reduced to half (50%) of its original (peak) concentration or amount. It is a simple parameter, which indicates the rate of elimination of a drug from the body. After single dose of a drug, plasma concentration of the drug rises to its peak value. Then it begins to fall due to elimination of the drug by the kidneys or by any other route. The time when the concentration of the drug becomes exactly half of the peak value is the plasma half-life. It is a time and is expressed in terms of units of time (minutes/hours/days). It is not dependent upon the value of plasma concentration of the drug. For complete elimination of a drug from the body 5 plasma half-lives are required **(Table 4.1)**.

Determination of plasma half-life of a drug: A single intravenous bolus injection of the drug is given and plasma concentrations of the drug are estimated at one hour interval. From the data obtained, the log plasma concentration–time curve is plotted (as shown in **Fig. 4.4**). Plasma half-life can also be determined by the formula:

$$t\frac{1}{2} = 0.693 \times \frac{V}{CL},$$

where V is the volume of distribution and CL is the clearance of the drug.

In one compartmental model [as shown in **Fig. 4.2(a)**], the plasma t½ can be determined readily. As it follows first order kinetics, so it is always same, irrespective of the value of its peak concentration. In multi (two) compartmental model [as shown in **Fig. 4.2(b)**] drug concentrations in plasma follow a multi-exponential pattern of decline. Initially there is rapid decline phase due to distribution of the drug to tissue and later on a slow and uniform decline phase due to elimination of the drug. Thus two half-lives, viz. α-t½ (distribution half-life) and β-t½ (elimination half-life) can be calculated from the two slopes (α and β).

Table 4.1: Plasma half-life of a drug

1. Plasma t½ means 50% drug is eliminated.
2. Plasma t½ means 75% (50 + 25) drug is eliminated.
3. Plasma t½ means 87.5% (50 + 25 + 12.5) drug is eliminated.
4. Plasma t½ means 93.75% (50 + 25 + 12.5 + 6.25) drug is eliminated.
5. Plasma t½ means 96.87% (50 + 25 + 12.5 + 6.25 + 3.12) drug is eliminated.

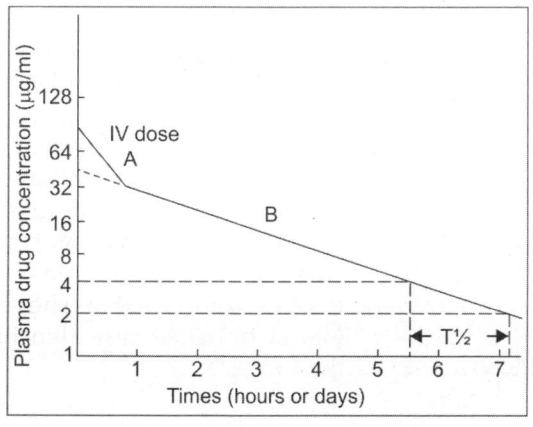

Fig. 4.4: Plasma half-life of a drug

Importance of Plasma Half-life

It is necessary:
- To know the duration of effect and frequency of administration of a drug.
- To determine the dosage schedule of a drug. A drug with short half-life requires frequent daily dosing, while a drug with long half-life requires one or more daily dosing.
- To know the steady state concentration of a drug.
- To assess the therapeutic efficacy of a drug.
- To assess the adverse effects of a drug.

Plasma Half-lives of Some Drugs

Glyceryl trinitrate (20 minutes), penicillin-G (30 minutes), insulin (40 minutes), amoxycillin (1 hour), aspirin (4 hours), tolbutamide (5 hours), doxycycline (20 hours), digoxin (40 hours), diazepam (43 hours), phenylbutazone (60 hours), sulphadoxine/digitoxin (7 days).

Factors Influencing Plasma t½

These are as follows:
- **Rate of clearance of drug:** Faster the clearance, shorter the plasma t½ of a drug.
- **Metabolic degradation of drug:** Faster the metabolism, shorter the plasma t½ of a drug.
- **Enterohepatic circulation (cycling) of drug:** It increases plasma t½ of a drug.
- **Plasma protein binding of drug:** High plasma protein binding of a drug increases the plasma t½ of a drug.
- **Distribution and storage of drug:** A drug which is widely distributed in the body and stored in tissues, has long plasma t½.

Other Terms

Biological half-life: It is the time taken for the biological activity of a drug in the body to be reduced to 50% of its original value (activity). It is measured with the help of radioactive isotope administered IV.

Biological effect of half-life: It is the time taken for the pharmacological effect of a drug in the body to be reduced to 50% of its original value (effect). It is measured in hit and run drugs, e.g. reserpine, MAO-inhibitors, organophosphorus compounds and anticancer drugs, which have short plasma half-life but long biological effect half-life.

Kinetics of drug clearance (elimination): Drugs are eliminated from the body by first order kinetics or zero order kinetics.

i. **First order kinetics (exponential kinetics):** Here, the elimination of a drug is directly proportional to its plasma concentration. In it a constant fraction (%) of a drug present in the body is eliminated per unit time (hour). This occurs with most of the drugs including penicillins, tetracyclines, sulphonamides, digitalis glycosides, calcium channel blockers, β-blockers, etc. It is nonsaturable and dose independent kinetics. Graphically, decline in plasma concentration of the drug which follows first order kinetics is shown in **Fig. 4.2(a)**. It shows a straight line.

ii. **Zero order kinetics (saturation kinetics):** Here, the elimination of a drug is not proportional to its plasma concentration. In it a fixed amount of the drug present in the body is eliminated per unit time irrespective of plasma concentration of the drug. It occurs with few drugs like phenytoin, alcohol, warfarin, aspirin, phenylbutazone, aminophylline, paraldehyde and general anaesthetics in higher doses. In these drugs, elimination occurs by first order kinetics in lower plasma concentrations but by zero order kinetics in higher plasma concentrations. This is because the reacting enzyme for the metabolism of the drug is limited and gets saturated at higher dose of the drug. These drugs have no constant plasma t½, which rises with the increase of plasma concentration of the drug. Special care is needed to increase the dose of these drugs to avoid adverse effects. Graphically, decline in plasma concentration of the drug which follows zero order kinetics is shown in **Fig. 4.2(b)**. It shows a curved line.

5

Pharmacodynamics

INTRODUCTION

Pharmacodynamics is the study of bio-chemical and physiological effects of drugs and their mechanisms of action. It deals with the targets of drug action; types, sites and natures of drug action and factors modifying/influencing drug action. It is what the drug does to the body.

Sites (Targets) of Drug Action

These are receptors, ion channels, enzymes, carrier proteins and structural proteins (as shown in **Fig. 5.1**).

i. **Drug receptors:** These are regulatory macromolecular proteins or nucleic acids present in the cell (in different cellular constituents including cell membrane). These are specific in size, shape and structure and allow interaction with specific ligands or substrates including drugs. Only specific drugs bind with specific receptors. If the forces (i.e. chemical bonds) that bind the drugs with receptors are weak (e.g. ionic bond, hydrogen bond, hydrophobic bond and Van der Waals bond), the binding will be reversible but if the forces involved are strong (e.g. covalent bond) then the binding will be almost irreversible. Drug receptor interaction involves two steps. First, the drug binds with the receptor and then generates stimulus, which in turn produces the effect. The combining capacity of the drug with the receptor is called affinity and the power to generate the stimulus or to produce action (effect) is called efficacy or intrinsic activity. A large number of receptors have been identified in the body. These are physiolo-gical and nonphysiological receptors. Physiological receptors mediate res-ponses to transmitters, hormones, auta-coids and other endogenous regulatory ligands, e.g. cholinergic, adrenergic, histaminergic, serotonergic, prosta-glandins, steroid hormones, thyroid hormones and other growth factors. Nonphysiological receptors are true drug receptors, e.g. benzodiazepine receptor, cardiac glycoside receptor, thiazide receptor, etc. Drugs can act on both physiological and nonphysiological receptors. Receptors and drug action will be discussed later on.

ii. **Ion channels:** These are minute pores present in the cell membrane. Common ion channels are of Na^+, K^+, Ca^{2+} and Cl^-. These are modulated (open or block) by drugs in different ways. Most of the ion channels are modulated by binding of drugs directly to the parts of channel protein in the cell. Some are ligand gated receptor mediated ion channels and others are modulated indirectly involving G-proteins or other intermediaries. Opening of Na^+ or Ca^{2+} channels by drugs produces depolarization of cell mem-

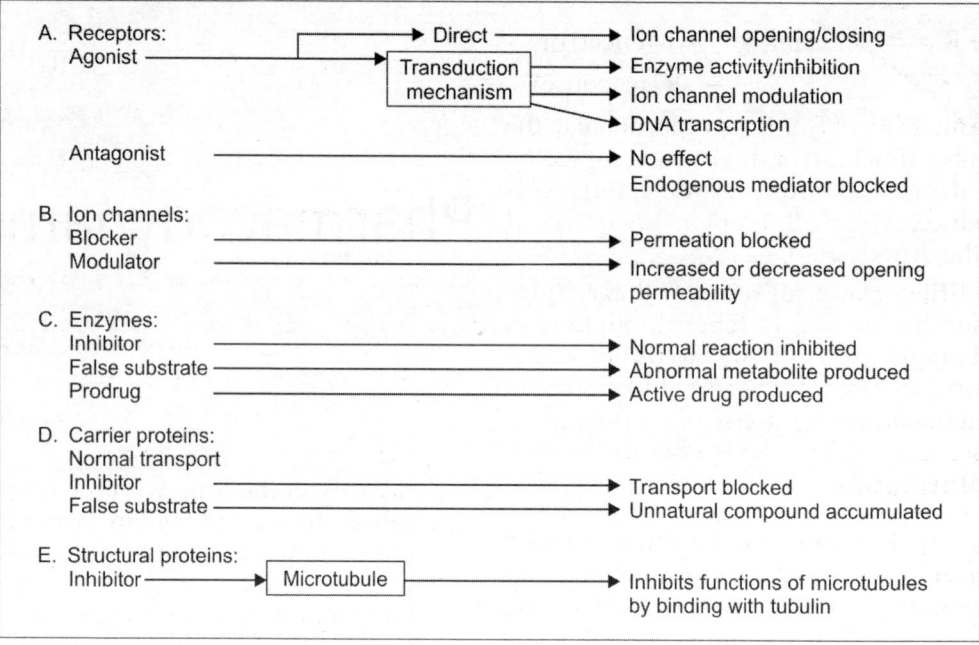

Fig. 5.1: Mechanisms of action (MoA) of drugs

brane, whereas opening of K^+ or Cl^- channels produces hyperpolarization of the cell membrane.

iii. **Enzymes:** These are biocatalysts present in the cell. These are targets for many drugs. Most commonly the drug molecule acts as a substrate analogue, which acts as a competitive inhibitor of the enzyme. Common target enzymes are cholinesterase (ChE), monoamine oxidase (MAO), cyclo-oxygenase (COX) and angiotensin converting enzyme (ACE). In some cases, the inhibition can be irreversible, e.g. organophosphorus compounds on acetylcholinesterase (AChE) and aspirin on platelet cyclo-oxygenase (COX).

iv. **Carrier molecules:** These are carrier proteins which transport ions and small organic molecules across the cell membrane. These are targets for some drugs. Common carrier molecules are of myocardial Na^+ pump (Na^+/K^+-ATPase pump), gastric proton pump (H^+/K^+- ATPase pump), neuronal noradrenaline uptake pump and apoferritin (in intestine)/transferrin (in blood) in iron transport.

v. **Structural proteins:** A few drugs act on structural proteins of cells, e.g. 5-fluorouracil incorporates into mRNA of cells; colchicine, paclitaxel and vinca alkaloids (vinblastine and vincristine) bind with the protein 'tubulin' of microtubules of cells.

Discussion in Detail

Receptors and Drug Action

Paul Ehrlich (1901) introduced the concept of receptor for drug action. He described drug-receptor interaction as a lock and key system. Many theories have been proposed from time to time to explain drug-receptor interaction. Of these receptor theories, three are popular.

a. **Receptor occupation theory (proposed by Clark in 1933):** According to this theory, drug action is due to occupation of receptors by specific drugs. The interaction between the drug (D) and receptor (R) is governed by the law of mass action as follows:

$$D + R \rightleftharpoons DR \text{ complex} \rightarrow E \text{ (effect) or}$$
$$R \text{ (response)}$$

The intensity of E or R is proportional to the number (fraction) of receptors occupied by the drug. Maximum response (effect) is produced when all receptors are occupied by the drug.

b. **Modified (classical) receptor theory (proposed by Ariens, Furchgott, Nickerson and Stephenson in 1957):** According to this theory, all receptors need not be occupied for a maximum response of a drug. Spare (reserve) receptors, which are majority of total receptors are responsible for maximum response (full agonist action) of the drug. They also introduced the concept of affinity and intrinsic activity (efficacy) in relation to drug action through receptors. Affinity is the ability of the drug to combine with the receptor and intrinsic activity (efficacy) is the ability of the drug to produce action (effect) by combining with the receptor. An agonist has both affinity and intrinsic activity (efficacy), while an antagonist has affinity but no intrinsic activity (efficacy).

c. **Rate theory of drug action (proposed by Paton in 1961):** According to this theory, the effect of a drug depends on the rate of drug-receptor interaction (combination) to produce drug-receptor complex and subsequently breakdown (dissociation) of the drug from the receptor and not to the number (fraction) of receptors occupied by the drug. It provides the basis for "Fade Phenomenon", i.e. the response of an agonist is initially high but decreases (fades) later on in spite of continued presence of the agonist.

Functions of Receptors

(1) Ligand binding (Latin: *Ligure* meaning binding) and (2) Message propagation, i.e. to propagate regulatory signals to the target (effector) cells either directing or indirectly through intermediary cellular molecules called transducers. The receptor, its cellular target and any intermediary molecule are called receptor-effector system or signal transduction pathway. Receptors and their associated effector and transducer proteins also act as integrators of extracellular information as they coordinate signals from multiple ligands with each other and with the metabolic activities of the cell. An important property of physiological receptors, which make them an excellent target for drugs is that they act catalytically and so they are biochemical signal amplifiers. The catalytic nature of physiological receptors is obvious when the receptor itself is an enzyme, e.g. (1) when a signal ligand molecule binds to a receptor that is an ion channel and opens it causing flow of many ions through the channel, (2) when a single steroid hormone molecule binds to its receptor and initiates transcription of many copies of specific mRNA, which in turn can give rise to multiple copies of a single protein.

Types of drug receptors: These are of three types:

a. **Pharmacoreceptors:** These are receptors with which the drug molecules first interact (combine) to produce effects.

b. **Spare (reserve) receptors:** These are receptors with which the drug molecules next interact to produce effects. These are majority of receptors (about 80%).

c. **Silent (storage) receptors:** These do not produce pharmacological effects. These are involved in binding of drugs to plasma proteins, cellular proteins or enzymes for distribution and metabolism of drugs.

Again, drug receptors may be cell surface receptors or intracellular receptors. Cell surface receptors are ligand gated receptor mediated ion channels, G-protein coupled receptors and tyrosine (protein) kinase linked receptors.

a. **Ligand gated receptor mediated ion channels:** The natural ligands which act by regulating transmembrane flow of ions are acetylcholine, GABA, glutamic acid and aspartic acid, which are synaptic transmitters. When these ligands bind to the specific receptor channel, the gate opens and the respective ion flows along the concentration gradient and thereby alter the electric potential across the membrane, e.g. acetylcholine opens Na^+ channel, GABA opens Cl^- channel and glutamate and aspartate open K^+ channels.

b. **G-protein coupled receptors:** Many receptors in the cell membrane regulate distinct effective protein through the mediation of a group of GTP-binding proteins called G-proteins. These are present at the inner surface of the cell membrane. Receptors for biogenic amines, eicosanoids and many peptide hormones are G-protein coupled receptors. They act by facilitating the binding of GTP to specific G-protein (Gs or Gi). GTP binding activates the G-protein, which regulates the activity of specific effectors through second messengers. The effector includes enzymes such as adenylcyclase and phospholipases (A_2, C and D) and ion channels that are specific for Na^+, K^+, Ca^{2+} or Cl^- (as shown in **Fig. 5.2**). An individual cell may express multiple G-proteins. Each of these may respond to several different receptors and regulate several different effectors with a characteristic pattern of selectiveness.

c. **Thyrosine (protein) kinase-linked receptors:** These membrane bound receptors mediate the action of insulin, epidermal growth factor, platelet derived growth factor and certain lymphokines. Insulin by acting through these receptors triggers uptake of glucose and amino acids and regulates metabolism of glycogen and triglycerides in the cell.

Intracellular (cytosol and nuclear) receptors: These are receptors which regulate gene expression (DNA transcription). They have no second messenger. Receptors for steroid hormones, thyroid hormones, vitamin D and retinoids are soluble DNA binding proteins, which regulate the transcription of specific genes leading to synthesis of particular proteins and production of cellular effects.

Second messengers: These are produced by the 1st messenger, i.e. original ligand (natural hormone or drug mimicking the naturally occurring ligand), e.g. cAMP, cGMP, IP_3, DAG and Ca^{2+}, etc. These are ultimately degraded.

Response (Effect) of Drug Receptor Interaction

If a drug has affinity for the receptor and if it is in close proximity of the receptor site, then receptor occupancy takes place. This drug-receptor interaction (coupling) leads to a variety of responses (effects) depending on the nature of drug molecules, which are:

Agonists

These are drugs that resemble the natural transmitter or hormone and activate the concerned receptors leading to responses (effects). They have affinity for the receptors

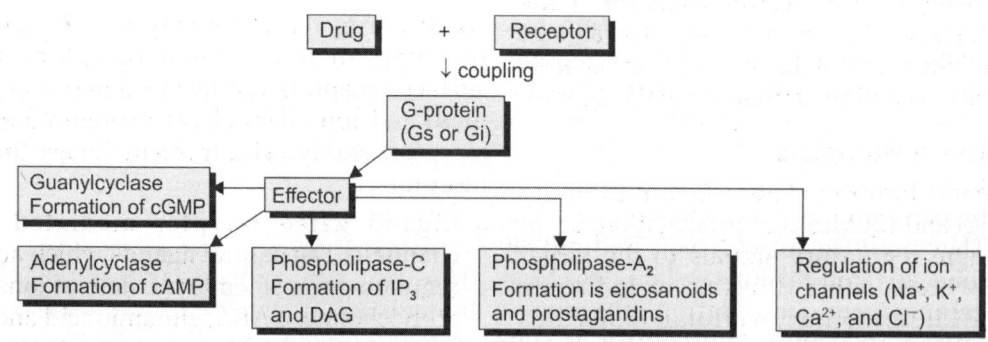

Fig. 5.2: Drug action through G-protein

and maximal efficacy/intrinsic activity (discussed before), e.g. acetylcholine, noradrenaline, histamine, 5-HT, angiotensin, prostaglandins and their chemical analogues.

Antagonists

These are drugs that antagonize or block responses (effects) of the concerned agonists. They have affinity for the receptors but no efficacy/intrinsic activity. These are three types:

i. **Reversible (competitive) antagonists:** For example, atropine for acetylcholine, phentolamine/propranolol for adrenaline/noradrenaline, mepyramine for histamine, naloxane for morphine, flumaxenil for diazepam, etc.

ii. **Irreversible (noncompetitive) antagonists:** For example, organophosphorus compounds for acetylcholine, phenoxybenzamine for adrenaline/noradrenaline, papaverine/decamethonium/α-bungarotoxin for acetylcholine, etc.

iii. **Partial agonists:** These are drugs that have both agonist and antagonist actions. They have affinity for the receptors but submaximal efficacy (intrinsic activity). They competitively antagonize the effect of a full agonists but in the absence of the agonist they can produce some responses (effects) like that of the agonist, e.g. succinylcholine for acetylcholine, nalorphine for morphine, saralasin for angiotensin II, etc.

iv. **Inverse agonists (negative antagonists):** These are drugs that have affinity for the receptors but negative efficacy (intrinsic activity). They produce effects opposite to those of agonists (e.g. β-carbolines like dimethoxyethyl-carbomethoxy (β-carboline/DMCM)) produce effects opposite to that of benzodiazepines (e.g. diazepam) by occupying benzodiazepine receptors. They produce anxiety, increased muscle tone and convulsions, while benzodiazepines produce sedation, anxiolysis, muscle relaxation and control of convulsions. Both these types of drugs act on

benzodiazepine (BDZ) receptors by modulating the effects of the neurotransmitter GABA. Actions of both groups of drugs can be blocked by specific BDZ antagonist "Flumazenil".

Ion Channels and Drug Action

Some drugs act by influencing ion channels and modulating passage of ions across the cell membrane. Ion channels can be voltage dependent ligand gated (indirect) or direct. In the former type, combination of the drug with the receptor results in opening or blocking of ion channels. G-protein (Gs or Gi) are commonly involved in such interactions, e.g. opening of Na^+ channels by DDT, aconitine, veratradine, etc.; blocking of Na^+ channels by minoxidil, diazoxide, cromakaline, etc.; blocking of K^+ channels by sulphonylureas, amiodarone, sotalol, etc.; blocking of Ca^{2+} channels by calcium channel blockers (verapamil, nifedipine, diltiazem, etc.); opening of GABA-receptor chloride channel by benzodiazepines (diazepam, alprazolam, lorazepam, etc.). Some drugs can also combine with specific channel protein directly.

Enzymes and Drug Action

Enzymes are protein in nature and catalyze biological reactions. Substrates are substances that are acted upon by the enzymes. The drug (substrate) combines with an enzyme forming a complex and mediating the resultant drug effect.

The enzyme substrate complex producing effect can be reversible (competitive) or irreversible (noncompetitive) (as shown in **Table 5.1**).

Some drugs stimulate the activity of some endogenous cellular enzymes, e.g. adrenaline and noradrenaline stimulate adenylcyclase, pyridoxine stimulates decarboxylase (DC), etc. Some drugs stimulate the synthesis of microsomal enzymes and thus increase metabolism of other drugs, e.g. phenobarbitone, phenytoin, carbamazepine, rifampicin, phenyl butazone, diphenhydramine, prednisolone and other glucocorticoids, DDT, etc. These are microsomal enzyme inducers. Auto-inducers

Table 5.1: Drug and enzyme inhibition

Drug	Enzyme	Effect
Physostigmine	Cholinesterase	Inhibition (reversible)
Organophosphorus compounds (D, F, P, etc.)	Cholinesterase	Inhibition (irreversible)
Hemicholinium	Choline-acetyl transferase	Inhibition of acetylcholine synthesis by acting as false substrate (reversible)
Methyldopa	Dopa-decarboxylase	Inhibition of noradrenaline synthesis by acting as false substrate (reversible)
Allopurinol	Xanthine oxidase	Inhibition (reversible)
Sulphonamides	Folate synthetase	Inhibition of growth of bacteria (reversible)
Aspirin	Cyclo-oxygenase	Inhibition (irreversible)
Acetazolamide	Carbonic anhydrase	Inhibition (irreversible)
Digoxin	Na^+/K^+-ATPase	Inhibition (irreversible)
Theophylline	Phosphodiesterase	Inhibition (irreversible)
MAO inhibitors	Monoamino oxidase (MAO)	Inhibition (irreversible)

are drugs which stimulate their own metabolism by inducing microsomal enzymes, e.g. phenobarbitone and carbamazepine. Again some drugs inhibit the synthesis of microsomal enzymes and thus decrease the metabolism of other drugs, e.g. cimetidine, isoniazid, allopurinol, amiodarone, ciprofloxacin in metronidazole, erythromycin, choloramphenicol, alcohol, etc. These are microsomal enzyme inhibitors.

Carrier Molecules and Drug Action

Some drugs are carried to the site of action by binding with carrier protein molecules, e.g. passage of glucose across the cell membrane by glucokinase, iron transport by apoferritin and transferrin, uptake of neurotransmitters (noradrenaline, acetylcholine, etc.) or other precursor carrier proteins can act by inhibition of transport process, e.g. blockade of organic acid transport in renal tubules by probenecid causing delay in penicillin excretion and enhancement of urate excretion.

Carrier proteins have specific recognition sites, which bind to and carry the permitting molecules, e.g. digoxin blocks sodium pump (Na^+/K^+-ATPase pump), omeprazole blocks proton pump (H^+/K^+-ATPase pump), imipramine blocks noradrenaline uptake, etc.

Structural Proteins and Drug Action

Discussed before.

Types of Drug Action

Drugs may produce their effects on cell by stimulation, depression, irritation or cytotoxic action on cells or may act as replacement agent or by modification of immune status (as shown in **Table 5.2**).

Natures of Drug Action

Drugs may act by one or more of the following ways:

1. **Primary action:** It is the action of drug in unchanged (intact) form, e.g. aluminium hydroxide as a gastric antacid and magnesium sulphate as a purgative.
2. **Secondary action:** It is the action of a drug in changed form, i.e. after metabolic degradation, e.g. hexamine as an urinary antiseptic

Table 5.2: Types of drug action

Process	Drugs	Site of action
Stimulation	Adrenaline, isoprenaline, dopamine Pilocarpine and physostigmine	Cardiac muscle Exocrine glands
Depression	Barbiturates, alcohol, morphine and other opioids Quinidine and procainamide	CNS Cardiac muscle
Irritation	Purgatives (irritant)	GIT
Cytotoxic action	Antimicrobials Anticancer drugs	Parasitic cells Neoplastic (cancer) cells
Replacement Immunomodulation	Hormones Sera and vaccines (immunostimulants) Glucocorticosteroids, cyclosporine, azathioprine, cyclophosphamide (immunosuppressants)	Endocrine system Immunity system Immunity system

after being converted to formaldehyde, proguanil as an antimalarial after being converted to cycloguanil.

3. **Topical (local) action/antimicrobial action:** It is the action of a drug at the site of contact with the tissue to kill the microorganisms, e.g. silver sulphadiazine cream in skin burn, miconazole cream in fungal infection of skin and sulphacetamide drops in ocular infection.

4. **Systemic (remote) action:** It is action of a drug after absorption and distribution to the site of action, e.g. digoxin on heart, diazepam on CNS and ergometrine on uterus.

5. **Reflex action:** It is the action of a drug modified through reflex pathway, e.g. potassium iodide as reflex expectorant, ipecacuanha as reflex emetic and kalmegh (bitter) as reflex stomachic.

6. **Salt action:** It is the action of a drug produced by the physical property of the salt form of the drug, e.g. magnesium sulphate as osmotic purgative and mannitol as osmotic diuretic.

7. **Ionic action:** It is the action of a drug produced by the liberated ions (especially cations) from the drug, e.g. Ca^{2+} from calcium gluconate in tetany and Fe^{2+} from ferrous sulphate in iron deficiency anaemia.

8. **Chelating action:** It is the action of the drug produced by formation of chelate complex (ring-like structure) with metallic ions, e.g. dimercaprol in arsenic poisoning and penicillamine in copper poisoning.

Structure-Activity Relationship (SAR) and Drug Design

Both the affinity of a drug and its intrinsic activity (efficacy) are determined by its chemical structure. This relationship is called structure-activity relationship. It was first proposed by Crum Brown and TS Frazer in 1968: Change of chemical structure of the drug produces following changes in drug responses (effects):

1. Relatively minor modification in the drug molecule may result in major changes in pharmacological properties of the drug, e.g. procaine (aLA) to procainamide (a potent cardiac antiarrhythmic drug with prolonged duration of action), atropine (an anticholinergic drug) to homatropine (a mydriatic and cycloplegic with short duration of action on eye) and chlorthiazide (a diuretic) to polythiazide (a more potent diuretic).

2. Chemical modification of the structure of a drug has lead to development of congeners with less side effects and toxicity, e.g. nicotinic acid (vitamin B_3) to nicotinamide

(vitamin B_4), which does not produce flushing or itching, chlorpromazine (a tranquilizer) to trioflupromazine (a more potent tranquilizer with negligible antihistaminic and hypotensive actions) and testosterone (an androgen) to nandrolone (an anabolic steriod with negligible androgenic action).

3. Chemical modification of structure of a drug also has lead to development of competitive antagonists, e.g. morphine to nalorphine, naloxone or naltrexone, para-aminobenzoic acid (PABA) to para-aminobenzene sulphanilamide (sulphonamide) or para-aminobenzene salicylic acid (PAS).

4. The study of SAR of series of agonists and antagonists has enabled the identification of receptors and their subtypes for various neurotransmitters (ligands) and synthesis of specific drugs for each receptor subtypes, e.g. acetylcholine acts on muscarinic (M_1 to M_5) and nicotinic (N_N and N_M) receptors. Atropine, pirenzepine, etc. are muscarinic antagonists, while hexamethonium, d-tubocurarine, etc. are nicotinic antagonists. Adrenaline acts on α (α_1 and α_2) and β (β_1, β_2 and β_3) receptors.

Phenoxybenzamine, prazosin, etc. are α-receptor antagonists, while propranolol, atonolol, etc. are β-receptor antagonists.

Stereoselectivity of Drugs

Drug molecules are not flat structures as depicted on paper, but they have three dimensional configuration. This special orientation is important for drug receptor interaction. Only a limited portion of a drug molecule interacts with the receptor depending on electrostatic binding sites. For this reason, sometimes diverse chemical substances can react with the same receptor, e.g. diethyl stilbestrol and oestradiol on the oestrogen receptor.

Many drugs have one or more asymmetric centres in their structures. These drugs exit in two nonidentical mirror image forms, viz. d-form (dextroform) and l-form (levoform), which can exhibit different biological activities, e.g. d-amphetamine is more active than l-amphetamine and l-hyoscyamine is more active than d-hyoscyamine. Similarly, S (sensitive) isomer form of warfarin is more active than R (resistant) isomer form of warfarin. In all these cases chemical structure may be the same, but due to a change in 3-dimensional configuration, the biological activities are changed.

Regulation of Receptors

In a cell the total number of functionally active receptors may be high or low. When high, the state is called upregulation and when low, the state is called downregulation of receptors. Change in the receptor population is a homeostatic mechanism of the tissue to maintain a physiological state in tissue function. Drug responsiveness changes with increase or decrease in receptor population, due to increased synthesis or degradation of receptors respectively.

1. **Upregulation of receptors:** Prolonged administration of an antagonist, e.g. propranolol (a β-blocker) leads to formation of new receptors causing increased tissue sensitivity. This phenomenon leads to hyperactivity (supersensitivity) of receptors to an agonist following sudden withdrawal of the antagonist after prolonged treatment, e.g. rebound hypertension, appearance of angina pectoris or cardiac arrhythmias following sudden withdrawal of propranolol or other β-blockers. Other drugs like clonidine (a central α_2-agonist), glucocorticoids and opioids can produce upregulation of receptors after prolonged administration and their sudden withdrawal leads to dangerous withdrawal reactions. This will be discussed with the respective drugs.

2. **Downregulation of receptors:** Prolonged administration of an agonist (ligand) leads to decrease in number of receptors, causing decreased tissue sensitivity. This phenomenon leads to hypoactivity (hyposensitivity) of receptors to an agonist after prolonged treatment. Ligand binding of receptors

induces accelerated endocytosis (internalization) of receptors, followed by degradation of those receptors. When this process occurs at a rate faster than denovosynthesis of receptors, then the total number of cell surface receptors is decreased, causing diminished responsiveness of the tissue. This produces tachyphylaxis or tolerance due to diminished drug effects after continued use of drugs like coronary dilators (e.g. nitrites and nitrates), bronchodilators (e.g. ephedrine, theophylline and salbutamol) or centrally active drugs (e.g. cocaine, morphine, phenobarbitone, etc.).

Potency and Efficacy of Drugs

Potency (strength) of a drug is the concentration (amount) of the drug in relation to its therapeutic effect. It is generally used to compare two or more drugs having similar biological activity (effect). Drugs with low potency are used in higher doses and vice versa, e.g. anti-inflammatory potency of some NSAIDs like piroxicam (daily dose 20 mg), diclofenac (daily dose 100 mg) and ibuprofen (daily dose 200 mg). So they have high, moderate and low potencies respectively.

Efficacy (therapeutic effectiveness) of a drug depends not only on its potency but also the type of response (maximum, moderate or poor/low) produced by the drug, e.g. full agonists produce maximum response and partial agonists produce moderate or low response.

Factors Modifying Drug Action and Therapeutic Outcome

These can be divided into two groups, *viz.* subject related factors and drug related factors.

Subject (Patient) Related Factors

These are given as follows:
1. **Age:** At extremes of age (infants and old people), there is increased sensitivity to the drug than in the adults. Infants are more sensitive to some drugs, e.g. chloramphenicol, gentamicin, morphine or other narcotics and thyroxine or other hormones. It is due to immaturity of drug metabolizing enzyme system, lower plasma protein binding of the drug, incomplete development of excretory system and smaller tissue mass, e.g. gray baby syndrome occurring in neonates after administration of chloramphenicol in large dosage. Thus infants require smaller amount of drugs than children. Similarly, old people require less amount of drugs than adult due to inability to metabolize the drug properly and degenerative changes in brain, liver, kidney and other organs of the body.

2. **Body weight/surface area:** The concentration of a drug at the site of action depends on the ratio between the body weight or surface area and the amount of the drug administered. Thus, the dose of a drug should be suitably adjusted for abnormally lean or obese persons and for those who are markedly dehydrated or oedematous (i.e. underweight or overweight persons).

3. **Sex:** The metabolism of a drug is slow in female due to more adipose tissues. Drugs that cause pelvic congestion, e.g. irritant purgatives like castor oil, senna, etc. should be avoided during menstruation and pregnancy. Drugs like antithyroids (e.g. carbimazole, propyl thiouracil, etc.), antimetabolites (e.g. methotrexate, mercaptopurine, etc.) and CNS depressants (e.g. phenobarbitone, morphine, etc.), should be avoided during pregnancy as they can effect the foetus.

4. **Race/species:** Indians tolerate thiacetazone (an antitubercular drug) more than Europeans. Japanese people suffer from subacute myelo-optic neuropathy (SMON) by taking diiodohydroxyquin and iodochlorohydroxyquin, but not Indian people. Negroes require higher concentrations of atropine and ephedrine to dilate pupil than Mongolians (Caucasians). These variations are due to different race. Similarly, animals like rabbits are more sensitive to d-tubocurarine than cats due to different species. Rats and mice are resistant to digoxin, but not dogs and cats.

5. **Genetic variations (genetic polymorphism):** There is interindividual variation in the rate of drug metabolism and the effect and toxicity of some drugs, e.g. propranolol, isoniazid, primaquine, phenobarbitone, halothane, succinylcholine, etc. This is mainly due to different rates of drug metabolism, as the amount of hepatic microsomal enzymes is genetically controlled. There is also differences in the target tissue/organ sensitivity. This will be discussed with the respective drugs. Pharmacogenetics deals with genetically mediated variation in drug action.

6. **Psychological/emotional state:** It can affect drug effects specially in CNS acting drugs, e.g. more general anaesthetics are required in nervous and anxious persons, higher doses of chlorpromazine (500 to 1000 mg/day) is required to produce tranquillization in schizophrenic persons than in normal individuals. Placebos (inert dosage form to please some persons) sometime produce therapeutic benefits in patients of psychosomatic disorders like angina pectoris and bronchial asthma, who are placebos reactors (easily respond to placebos).

7. **Physiological state:** Effects of some drugs vary with the physiological state, e.g. salicylates reduce body temperature only in presence of fever, uterus is more sensitive to the effect of oxytocin during pregnancy, irritant purgatives like castor oil and senna should be avoided during pregnancy as they can cause abortion. Drugs which are secreted in milk, e.g. tetracyclines should be used with caution in lactating mothers as they may affect infants. Children require smaller dosage than the adult due to many differences in the physiological functions (especially in pharmacokinetics) between the child and the adult.

8. **Pathological state:** Presence of diseases alter the effects of drugs, e.g. thiazides induce more marked diuresis in oedematous patients than in normal persons, adrenaline and digoxin induce more car-diac arrhythmias in patients of myocardial infarction, hypothyroid patients are more sensitive to the effects of digoxin, morphine and CNS depressant drugs, myasthenic patients are more sensitive to d-tubo-curarine and other curaremimetic drugs. Hypnotics given in patients with severe pain may cause mental confusion and delirium. Presence of hepatic and renal diseases impair metabolism and excretion of many drugs leading to toxicity.

Drug Related Factors

These are given as follows:

1. **Dose of a drug (drug dosage):** It is the appropriate amount of a drug needed to produce a certain degree of response in a patient. It is expressed in terms of weight (g, mg, μg), volume (ml) or unit (IU). It is given in range because of individual variation. It can be prophylactic dose, therapeutic dose or toxic dose depending on the concentration of the drug. If the dose is too small, there will be no effect and if too large, toxic effects will be produced. There are some formulas for calculation of child dose (1–12 years).

a. *According to age—*
Young's formula:

$$\text{Child dose} = \frac{\text{Age}}{\text{Age} + 12} \times \text{Adult dose}$$

Dilling's formula:

$$\text{Child dose} = \frac{\text{Age}}{20} \times \text{Adult dose}$$

b. According to body weight (BW)—Clark's formula:

$$\text{Child dose} = \frac{\text{Body weight (kg)}}{70} \times \text{Adult dose}$$

c. According to body surface area (BSA) — Duboi's formula:

$$\text{Child dose} = \frac{\text{BSA (m}^2)}{1.7} \times \text{Adult dose}$$

Body surface area (m²) = Body weight (kg) × Height (cm) × 0.008

Last two formulas are more accurate for calculating paediatric dose, because total body weight, extracellular fluid volume and metabolic activity are considered here.

Types of dosage of drugs

a. *Standard dose:* It is the dose which is given in most paetients due to wide margin of safety of the drug, e.g. penicillin, albendazole, etc.

b. *Loading dose:* It is the dose given at the onset of therapy with the aim of achieving the target concentration of the drug rapidly. It is required during the use of some drugs, e.g. digoxin, digitoxin, chloroquine, thiouracils, etc.

c. *Maintenance dose:* It is the dose given to maintain steady state concentration of drug in plasma within a given therapeutic range. It is required during the use of above drugs after giving in loading dose.

d. *Target level dose:* It is the dose required to produce target steady state concentration of the drug. It is adjusted by monitoring of plasma concentration of the drug. It is required during the use of antiepileptic drugs, antidepressants, lithium, digoxin, etc.

e. *Titrated dose:* It is the optimal dose required to produce maximum therapeutic effect with tolerable adverse effects. It is calculated by giving high initial dose and downward titration. (in critical situations) or low initial dose and upward titration (in most non-critical situations). Optimal dose is arrived at by titrating it with an acceptable level of adverse effects. It is required during the use of anticancer drugs, corticosteroids, levodopa, etc.

f. *Regulated dose:* It is the dose which is accurately adjusted by repeated measurement of the affected physiological parameter. It is required during use of antihypertensives, anticoagulants, hypoglycaemics, diuretics, etc.

2. **Form of a drug**: When a drug is administered in the form of injection, it is rapidly absorbed and produces rapid effect. Among the oral preparations, mixtures and powders are more rapidly absorbed than tablets and capsules and so produce rapid effects.

3. **Route of administration of a drug:** It can alter the effects of a drug, e.g. magnesium sulphate when given orally acts as a purgative, when given rectally lowers intracranial tension and when given parenterally (IV) produces CNS and cardiac depressant effects. N-acetylcysteine when given by inhalation is a mucolytic agent and when given parenterally (IV) is useful in paracetamol poisoning. Drugs like insulin and adrenaline are not effective by oral route and so administered parenterally (SC or IM) to produce effects.

4. **Time of administration of a drug:** It can alter the effect of a drug, e.g. hypnotics administered at night produce better effects than when taken during daytime, corticosteroids administered as a single morning dose cause less pituitary adrenal suppression than when taken in divided doses in the whole day.

5. **Fixed dose drug combination:** Combined use of two or more drugs in fixed dose produces **synergism** (Greek: *syn* meaning together and *ergon* meaning work). It means synergistic effect (similar effect) of two or more drugs. It can be—

Additive effect: Here, the total effect of two or more drugs is equal to the sum of the effect of the individual drug, e.g. combination of antacids, analgesics, antihypertensives, diuretics, bronchodilators or chemotherapeutic agents.

Supra-additive effect (Potentiation): Here, the total effect of two or more drugs is more than the sum of the effect of the individual drug, e.g. combination of levodopa and carbidopa, sulphamethoxazole and trimethoprim, acetylcholine and physostigmine or penicillin and probenecid. This effect occurs when one drug increases the action of another drug either by acting in different mechanism or delaying metabolism or excretion of the other drug.

Antagonism (Infra-additive effect): Here one drug decreases or inhibits the effect of another drug by opposite action, i.e. the two drugs have action in opposite direction. It can be:

a. **Physical antagonism:** It is due to physical properties of drugs, e.g. activated charcoal in alkaloidal poisoning (charcoal adsorbs alkaloid and prevent their absorption from the GIT).

b. **Chemical antagonism:** It is due to chemical interaction in solution between two drugs, e.g. acid (HCl) and alkalies ($NaHCO_3$), chelating agents (BAL) and heavy metal (arsenic), etc.

c. **Physiological antagonism:** It is due to opposite effects of two drugs on the same physical function, e.g. histamine and adrenaline on B.P. or bronchial muscle, insulin and glucagon on blood sugar level, hydrochlorothiazide and triamterene on urinary K^+ excretion, etc.

d. **Pharmacological antagonism:** It is due to opposite effects of two drugs binding to the same receptor. It can be competitive antagonism or noncompetitive antagonism.

Competitive antagonism is usually reversible and can be overcome (surmountable/equilibrium type) by increasing the dose of agonist, e.g. acetylcholine (agonist) and atropine d-tubocurarine (antagonist), adrenaline (agonist) and tolazoine/propranolol (antagonist), histamine (agonist) and mepyramine/cimetidine (antagonist), morphine (agonist) and nalorphine/naloxone (antagonist), diazepam (agonist) and flumazenil (antagonist), etc. It can be irreversible, if the binding occurs by covalent bond, e.g. adrenaline (agonist) and phenoxy benzamine (antagonist), acetylcholine (agonist) and decamethonium (antagonist). Noncompetitive antagonism is irreversible and cannot be overcome (unsurmountable/nonequilibrium type) by increasing the dose of the agonist, e.g. acetylcholine (agonist) and decamethonium/papverine/α-bungarotoxin (antagonist), diazepam (agonist) and bicuculine (antagonist), etc. Differences between competitive antagonism and noncompetitive antagonism is shown in **Table 5.3**.

6. **Drug cumulation (cumulative action):** Repeated administration of some drugs lead to accumulation of the drug in the body tissues, if the rate of administration of the drug is more than the rate of elimination. This produces cumulative toxicity, e.g. digoxin, digitoxin, emetine, chloro-

Table 5.3: Comparison between competitive and noncompetitive antagonisms

Parameter	Competitive antagonism	Noncompetitive antagonism
1. Receptor binding	Reversible (by hydrogen bond or van der Waals bond)	Irreversible (by covalent bond)
2. Agonist-antagonist interaction	Competitive	Noncompetitive
3. Dose response curves of agonist in presence of antagonist	Parallel shifting to the right side without change in slope	Not so
4. Antagonism	Surmountable (maximum response is produced by increasing the dose)	Unsurmountable (maximum response is diminished inspite of increasing the dose)
5. Duration of action	Short (depends on drug clearance)	Long (depends on new receptors synthesis)

quine, arsenic and other heavy metals, etc. To avoid cumulation, these drugs should be administrated at a maintenance dose and checking of hepatic and renal functions must be done before and during drug administration as hepatic and renal diseases delay metabolism and excretion of these drugs.

7. **Drug tolerance:** It is the gradual decrease in responsiveness of tissue (*in vivo*) to a drug on repeated administration. It may be acute tolerance (tachyphylaxis), which develops within a few minutes or hours and chronic tolerance, which develops within a few days or weeks. Tachyphylaxis can be demonstrated in experimental animals, e.g. ephedrine on B.P. of cat or dog (due to depletion of catecholamine stores in adrenergic neurons).

Types of Tolerance

These are of following types:

1. **Pharmacokinetic (drug dispositional tolerance):** This is due to changes in drug absorption, distribution, metabolism and excretion leading to decreased availability of the drug at the target tissue, e.g. barbiturates after repeated administration increase their own metabolism by stimulating the microsomal enzyme systems in the liver (enzyme induction). Decreased rate of absorption of drugs occurs in diarrhoea (apparent or pseudotolerance) leading to decreased effects of drugs.

2. **Pharmacodynamic (functional) tolerance:** This is due to changes in the functions of the larger tissue, which make them less sensitive to the drug. It is often associated with some cellular or tissue changes. With some drugs this may occur due to decrease in drug-receptors (downregulation of receptors), e.g. CNS depressants like morphine, barbiturates, alcohol, etc.

3. **Pharmacogenetic tolerance:** This is due to genetic (inherited) factors like enzyme variation in the body leading to decreased metabolism of the drug, e.g. isoniazid, halothane, succinylcholine, etc.

4. **Racial/species tolerance:** Some human races and animal species are tolerant to some drugs due to racial/species variation, e.g. Negroes are tolerant to ephedrine, atropine and other mydriatics. Rabbits can tolerate large doses of atropine due to presence of the enzyme atropine esterase in their liver and plasma.

5. **Cross-tolerance:** If a person initially develops tolerance to a drug belonging to a particular group, he also develops tolerance to other drugs belonging to the same group due to similar chemical structure. This is called cross-tolerance, e.g. between alcohol and general anaesthetics, between glyceryl trinitrate and isosorbide dinitrate, between morphine and pethedine, etc.

6. **Drug resistance** is the tolerance of microorganisms (bacteria) to some antibiotics, e.g. staphylococci may develop resistance to penicillins and tetracyclines.

7. **Drug dependence:** It is the compulsive use of some drugs. It arises due to periodic, repeated or continuous administration of some drugs like opioids, barbiturates, cocaine, alchohol, amphetamines, caffeine, nicotine, canabis indica, LSD, etc. that produce harm to the individual and to the society. It is characterized by tolerance, psychic dependence and physical dependence. Tolerance is the reduced effect of the drug due to repeated use and is due to cellular or tissue adaptation of central neurons. Psychic (psychological) dependence is a condition in which a drug produces a feeling of satisfaction and pleasure (psychic drive) by periodic or continuous administration of the drug, e.g. caffeine, amphetamines, nicotine, canabis indica, LSD, etc. produce habituation (psychic dependence). Physical (physiological) dependence is a condition in which the body (especially CNS) achieves an adaptive state that manifests itself by intense physical disturbances when the drug is suddenly withdrawn (withdrawal or abstinence syndrome). Previously the term

addiction was used to denote both psychic and physical dependence on drugs. It is now called drug abuse (detrimental use of drugs). It is characterized by an overpowering desire (intense craving) to continue use of the drug, a tendency to increase the dose of the drug and occurrence of severe withdrawal symptoms, which are not only debilitating but may sometimes prove fatal, e.g. opioids, barbiturates, alcohol, cocaine, etc. produce addiction (drug abuse).

Outline of a treatment of drug dependence (addiction):

1. Hospitalization of the patient.
2. Gradual withdrawal of the drug.
3. Substitution therapy, e.g. methadone for morphine.
4. Specific drug therapy, e.g. antabuse for alcohol.
5. Correction of nutritional deficiencies.
6. Psychotherapy and occupational therapy.
7. Rehabilitation of the patient.

Quantitative Aspects of Pharmacodynamics and Assay of Drugs

PHARMACODYNAMIC PARAMETERS

These are given as follows:

1. Dose response relationship of agonists.
2. Antagonism of agonist response by antagonists.
3. Therapeutic index and protective index.
4. Therapeutic efficacy and therapeutic window.

As there are wide quantitative variations in drug responses in different species and in the same species under different conditions, so different methods have been devised to study the phenomenon of biological variation in drug response and to minimize the errors of prediction in clinical use of drugs. These are useful in study of drug effects in animals and men.

Dose Response Relationship of Agonists

Two types of dose response relationship are commonly seen:

a. **Graded dose response relationship:** In it, as the dose of a drug is increased, the response (effect) of the tissue or organ is also increased. The individual units of the responding system are capable of producing progressively increasing responses with increase of the dose of a particular drug. The increase in response can be measured. With increase of dose, at first there is considerable increase in the response and there are smaller increments

as the response approaches the maximum limit. After the maximum response has been reached, no further increase in the response can be obtained with further increase of dose (as shown in **Fig. 6.1a**). This phenomenon is called **ceiling response** (effect).

If the graded responses are plotted in a graph paper against the doses in arithmetic units, then a hyperbolic dose response curve is obtained (as shown in **Fig. 6.1b**). When the graded responses are plotted in a graph paper against the doses in logarithmic units, then a sigmoid (s-shaped) dose response curve is obtained with a straight line (linear shaped) in the middle (as shown in **Fig. 6.1c**).

The log dose response curve is particularly useful for the comparison of potencies of different compounds as in bioassays. The linear relationship in the middle has the advantage that a given increase in the log dose always corresponds to the same increase in the response.

b. **Quantal or all-or-none dose response relationship:** Here responses follow all-or-none phenomenon, i.e. the individual of the responding system either respond to their maximum limit or not at all to a dose of a drug and there is no gradation of response. This type of relationship is observed when the presence or absence of some drug induced phenomena such as

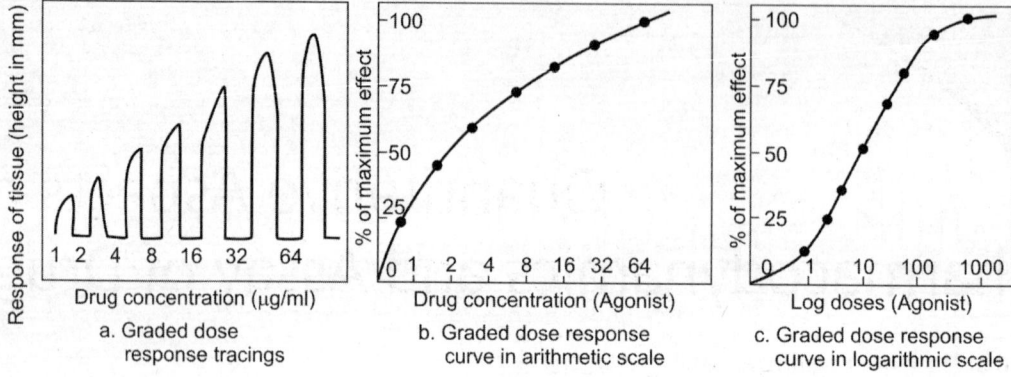

a. Graded dose
response tracings

b. Graded dose response
curve in arithmetic scale

c. Graded dose response
curve in logarithmic scale

Fig. 6.1

convulsion, death, etc. is determined in a population of animals as in toxicity studies. Different doses of the drugs are used in different groups of animals and the percentage of positive responses (data) are recorded. Here also the log dose response curve is sigmoidal (s-shaped) with a straight line (linear shaped) in the middle. The Gaussian or the normal nature of the quantal log dose response curve is usually bell-shaped or symmetrical (as shown in **Fig. 6.2**). This suggests that the observed differences are due to polygenic random variations in the responsiveness of the animals as well as non-random but inter-coupled events like other actions of the drug.

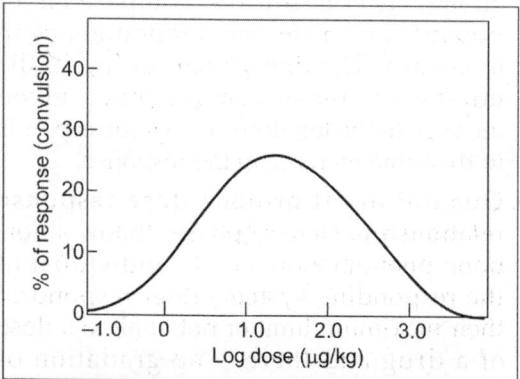

Fig. 6.2: Bimodal quantal dose response curve

Antagonism of Agonist Response by Antagonists

An agonist is a drug that has both affinity for the receptor and efficacy. The result of the agonist-receptor interaction is a drug response (effect). Antagonists are drugs that have affinity for the receptor but has no efficacy (i.e. incapable of producing biological response). Antagonists can interact directly at the same receptor site as the agonist or affect other reactions necessary for the drug response. There are two main types of pharmacological antagonism.

a. **Competitive antagonism:** If the inhibitory action of an antagonist can be overcome by increasing the concentration of the agonist, thereby achieving the same maximum response, the inhibition is called **competitive antagonism.** It can reversibly bind to the same receptor site as the agonist (as shown in **Fig. 6.3**), e.g. acetylcholine and atropine, histamine and chlorpheniramine, etc. or irreversibly bind to a remote receptor site that influences the affinity of the agonist for its receptor, e.g. acetylcholine and decamethonium, adrenaline and phenoxybenzamine, etc.

A competitive antagonist shifts the dose-response curve to the right but does not reduce the slope of the curve and the maximum response of the agonist (as shown in **Fig. 6.4a**).

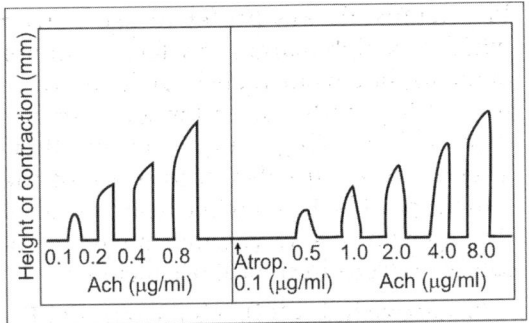

Fig. 6.3: Tracings showing competitive antagonism of acetylcholine by atropine

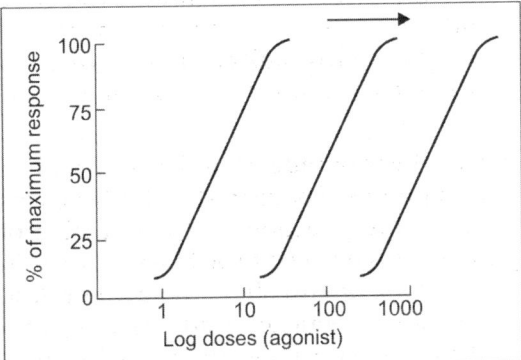

Fig. 6.4a: Curves showing competitive antagonism

b. **Noncompetitive antagonism:** If the inhibitory action of an antagonist cannot be overcome by increasing the concentration of the agonist, thereby not achieving the maximum response, the inhibition is called noncompetitive antagonism. A noncompetitive antagonist decreases the capacity of the agonist to combine with its receptor. This can occur by binding of the noncompetitive antagonist to either the agonist receptor site or another site that influences the capacity of the agonist that combines to its receptor, e.g. acetylcholine (agonist) and papaverine (antagonist); acetylcholine (agonist) and α-bungarotoxin (antagonist) and diazepam (agonist) and bicuculine (antagonist).

A noncompetitive antagonist does not shift the dose response curve to the right but reduces the slope of the curve and diminishes the maximum response of agonist (as shown in **Fig. 6.4b**).

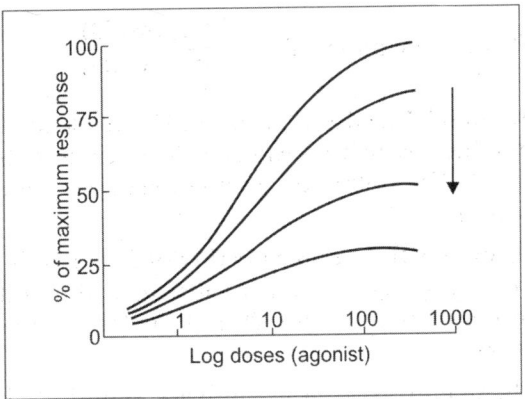

Fig. 6.4b: Curves showing noncompetitive antagonism

c. **Partial agonists:** Partial agonists are compounds with affinity for the receptors but with low or moderate efficacy. A partial agonist with high affinity can competitively inhibit the action of full agonist. Partial agonists thus have both agonist and antagonist properties, e.g. nalorphine, pentazocine, propiram, profadol, etc. of morphine.

A partial agonist produces characteristic dose response curve by increasing of dose (as shown in **Fig. 6.5a**).

Therapeutic Index (TI)

It is the ratio of the median lethal dose (MLD or LD_{50}) to the effective dose (MED or ED_{50})

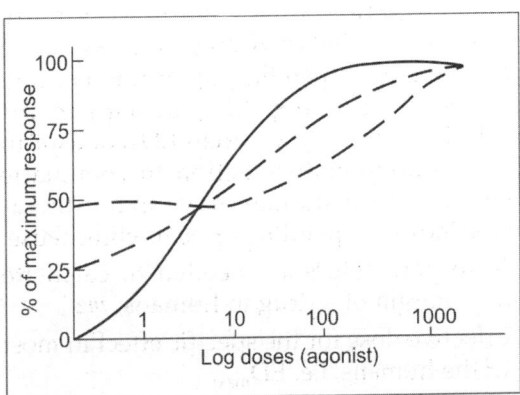

Fig. 6.5a: Curves showing effects of partial antagonism

$$\text{Therapeutic index (TI)} = \frac{\text{LD}_{50} \text{ (MLD)}}{\text{ED}_{50} \text{ (MED)}}$$

Median lethal dose (MLD or LD_{50}) is the dose (mg/kg), which is expected to kill one half (50%) of an unlimited population of the same species.

Median effective dose (MED or ED_{50}) is the dose (mg/kg), which produces a desired response in one half (50%) of the test population.

Therapeutic index is a number and indicative of margin of safety in animals studied. As the drug metabolism varies from species to species, so the therapeutic index would also vary in a similar fashion. It supplies reliable information when both LD_{50} and ED_{50} are determined for the same strain belonging to the same species. It is not a useful guide for the safety of a drug in humans (in clinical use), because LD_{50} is not a good guide to toxicity in the therapeutic setting and ED_{50} is often not definable, since it depends on what measure of effectiveness is used. Therapeutic index in humans can be calculated by the formula:

$$\text{TI} = \frac{\text{Maximum nontoxic dose}}{\text{Median effective dose}}$$

The greater the therapeutic index, the safer is the drug. For safe therapeutic use of a drug, its therapeutic index must be more than one, e.g. penicillin has a high therapeutic index, while digoxin has a low therapeutic index. In clinical practice, toxic symptom is more relevent than lethality. A drug may have more than one ED_{50} depending upon the measure of effectiveness, e.g. ED_{50} of aspirin for headache is much lower than ED_{50} of aspirin for anti-inflammatory action in rheumatic fever. Thus a drug may have many therapeutic indices depending upon its clinical use.

Two parameters are needed to calculate safety margin of a drug in humans, *viz.*

1. Effective dose for the specific effect in most of the humans, i.e. ED_{max}.
2. Maximum tolerated dose, which does not produce any adverse reactions, i.e. TD_0.

Physicians always prefer to use a drug which has high margin of safety for minor ailments, but in emergencies, where a drug is used for short-term or for some limited disease (e.g. CCF), drugs with low therapeutic index are also used. Care of the patient must be taken while using drugs of low margin of safety. Other measures of safety of drugs in clinical use include:

a. **Protective index (PI):** It is the ratio of ED_{50} of neurological impairment to ED_{50} of seizure (convulsion) protection of a drug in humans. A drug with a protective index of 5 (e.g. diazepam) is more promising anticonvulsant than a drug of protective index of 3 (e.g. phenobarbitone).

b. **Risk-benefit index:** It is the estimation of proportions of patients showing beneficial or harmful reactions, i.e. the number of patients who need to be treated (NNT) in order for one to show the given effect, whether beneficial or adverse, e.g. in a study of pain relief by antidepressant drugs compared with placebo, the findings were for benefit (relief of pain) NNT = 3, for minor unwanted effect NNT = 3 and for major adverse effects NNT = 22. Thus, if 100 patients treated, an average of 33 patients showed benefit from the drug, 33 patients showed minor unwanted effects and 4 or 5 patients showed major adverse effects.

Therapeutic Efficacy (Effectiveness)

It is the maximum effect that can be produced by a drug in humans, e.g. sodium depleting activity of potassium sparing diuretics (up to 5%), thiazide diuretics (up to 10%) and high ceiling diuretics (up to 20%) indicates that the therapeutic efficacy of these drugs are low, moderate and high respectively.

Therapeutic Window

It is the range of effective and safe concentrations of a drug in plasma. It is an unusual feature seen in certain drugs, e.g. tricyclic antidepressants (imipramine, amitriptyline, etc.) produce optimum therapeutic effects, when their plasma concentrations are maintained between 50–200 ng/ml. Clonidine produces lowering of BP when its plasma concentrations are maintained between 0.2–2 ng/ml (above which BP will rise). Therapeutic window may be narrow or wide. Drugs like digoxin, lignocaine, phenytoin ethosuximide, theophylline, imipramine, lithium and aminoglycosides (e.g. gentamycin) have narrow therapeutic window. So slight overdose of these drugs can produce toxicity. To avoid toxicity, frequent measurement of plasma or serum concentrations of these drugs is essential.

ASSAY OF DRUGS

It is the estimation of concentration or potency of drugs by chemical or biological methods. Chemical assay methods are commonly used because of convenience and reproducibility. But in some cases they are not suitable and unreliable due to presence of closely related inert chemicals. Biological assay (bioassay) methods (by measuring of biological responses produced by drugs) are highly sensitive and selective. They are used for following purposes:

1. To measure the pharmacological activity of new or chemically undefined substances.
2. To investigate the function of endogenous mediators, e.g. neurotransmitters.
3. To measure unwanted effects and toxicity of drugs.

Bioassay is essential in the development of new drugs. The activity of a new compound must be compared in various test systems with that of standard (known) compounds. The choice of suitable test systems for the preliminary bioassay is important. The test must be simple and quick. They must also be as specific as possible for the type of biological activity that is being sought.

General Principles of Bioassays

These are given as follows:

1. **Use of standards:** Bioassays are designed to measure the relative potency of the standard and the unknown (test) preparations. The standard is usually a pure substance. International standards have been developed for all drugs which are biologically standardized and their potency are described. When it is not possible to estimate accurately the exact amount of the active principle, then unit system is adopted to signify potency. One unit is a measure of fixed amount of particular biological activity, e.g. one IU of insulin is the biological activity in 0.5 mg of standard insulin preparation, one IU of heparin is the biological activity in 0.0077 mg of standard heparin sodium.

2. **Design of bioassays:** In any biological assay procedure, proper planning is absolutely necessary. The important points that should be considered are as follows:
   a. Selection of a correct reference standard preparation.
   b. Selection of a highly sensitive biological preparation (tissue or animal).
   c. A knowledge of variable factors. The response of the same organ or tissue to the same drug may vary widely due to biological variation depending upon the species, sex, age, weight, breeding, diet and environmental factors. Therefore, in the selection of animals, all the above factors must be born in mind. An ideal bioassay will be in the same animal or on the same tissue which has been treated with the standard drug as well as with the unknown drug, e.g. assay of acetylcholine on isolated frog's rectus muscle, assay of histamine on isolated guinea pig's ileum, assay of adrenaline on anaesthetized cat's BP, assay of 5-HT on isolated rat's uterus, etc.

3. **Graded or quantal responses:** An assay may be based on graded response (e.g. change of blood glucose concentration, contraction of a strip of smooth muscle, change in the time taken for a rat to run to a maze, etc.) or quantal (all-or-none) responses (e.g. death, loss of righting reflex, success in maze running within a stipulated time, etc.).

Types of Bioassays

These are of two types:

1. **Direct bioassay (matching/bracketing assay):** In it, by repeated trial and error, one dose each of standard (S) and unknown (U) samples of a drug are so identified that they produce the same response. It is difficult to determine and may give inaccurate result. It cannot be subjected to statistical analysis for estimation of margin of error, e.g. histamine bioassay on isolated guinea pig's ileum, posterior pituitary extract assay in isolated rat's uterus.

2. **Indirect bioassays:** In these bioassays, comparisons are made between standard (S) and unknown (U) samples of drug by two dose response curves (parallel line assay). The procedure is based on the following basic principles of dose response relationship.
   a. Log dose response curve in each case is linear in the middle portion (25–75% of maximum response).
   b. Log dose response curves of the standard and unknown drug having the same active principle are parallel. These are mainly of two types:
      • **4-point assay** (as shown in **Fig. 6.5b**): It is an accurate bioassay system, but it is time consuming. In it, 2 doses (low and high of standard (S) and 2 doses (low and high) of unknown (U) samples of a drug are so selected that

the ratio of doses are same, i.e. $S_1 : S_2 = U_1 : U_2$ and the responses produced by these 4 doses produce fall within the middle portion of the log dose response curves.

The sequence of 4 doses (S_1, S_2, U_1 and U_2) is usually given as Latin square design ($S_1S_2U_1U_2$, $S_2U_1U_2S_1$, $U_1U_2S_1S_2$ and $U_2S_1S_2U_1$). 16 responses (4 of each) are recorded and the data is analyzed statistically. If the log dose response curve of standard and unknown drugs are not parallel, then the responses are not produced by the same drug.

From ED_{50} ratio of unknown and standard, the potency of unknown sample of drug is determined, i.e.

$$\text{Potency of U} = \frac{ED_{50}U}{ED_{50}S}$$

The potency of unknown sample of drug is determined from the log dose response curve of the standard. It can also be calculated by the formula:

$$M = \frac{(S_1 - U_1) + (S_2 - U_2)}{(S_1 + U_1) - (S_2 + U_2)} \times d$$

where "d" is the log of ratio of high to low dose, i.e. $\log 2 = 0.301$.

Antilog of "M" is the potency of standard sample to unknown sample of the drug.

   • **3-point assay** (as shown in **Fig. 6.5c**): It is a quicker system than 4-point assay. It is often used when the unknown sample is very small and repeated doses cannot be given. In it, 2 doses (low and high) of standard (S) sample of a drug are so selected that the responses fall within the middle portion of the dose response curve. Then the dose of unknown (U) sample of the drug is determined whose response fall within the range of responses produced by two doses of standard sample of the drug. The concentration of unknown sample of drug is deter-

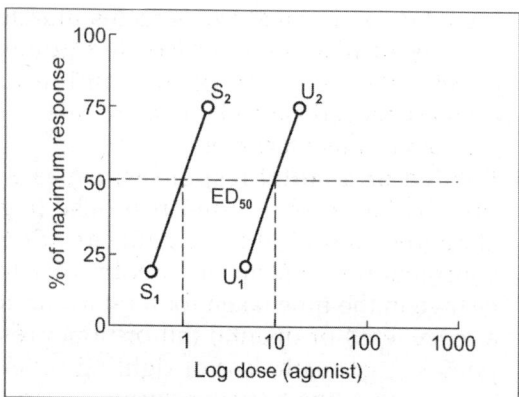

Fig. 6.5b: 4-point assay

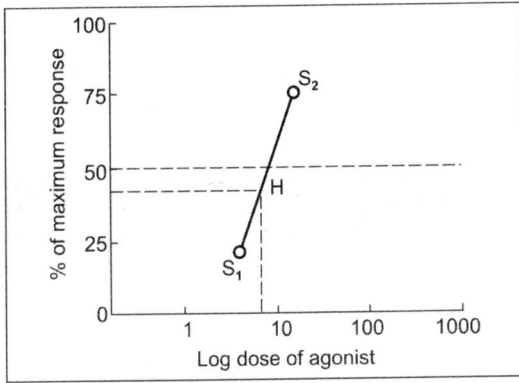

Fig. 6.5c: 3-point assay

mined from the log dose response curve of the standard.

Bioassays in man: These are done when animal tests fail to predict human responses, especially when the responses are subjective in nature and not measurable in animals. These can be done both in normal subjects and in diseased persons. These are most rational and realistic and include clinical trial and sequential trial. Clinical trial is a special type of bioassay in man to compare objectively the results of two or more therapeutic procedures. To minimize bias in clinical trial, randomization and double bind technique are adopted. For new drugs, clinical trial is carried out during phase-II of clinical development. Sequential trial is done in cases of analgesics, cough suppressants, hypotensives, etc. where the subject (patient) and the drug to be used in the same subject are alloted sequentially. This is only possible if the results of treatment can be determined after short time and the test drug or placebo can be given as a crossover design. In it, total number of subjects needed is relatively small.

7

Drug Interactions

INTRODUCTION

Drug interaction is the alteration of the drug effect when two or more drugs are administered simultaneously in the body. It is also called drug-drug interaction. Drug-food interaction can occur during the use of some drugs with some foods, e.g. MAO inhibitors like phenelzine and iproniazid with cheese, meat, yeast, wine, beer and citrous fruits containing tyramine can produce hypertensive crisis (cheese reaction).

DRUG-DRUG INTERACTION

Interaction between two drugs may produce a desired (beneficial) effect or an undesired (harmful) effect. Examples of useful drug interactions are combination of antibiotics or antihypertensives. Examples of harmful drug interactions are many and are discussed below. Drug-drug interaction that occurs *in vitro* (outside the body) is called physicochemical interaction. Drugs may be inactivated or precipitated from solution if mixed in the same syringe or added to blood or infusion fluid prior to administration, e.g. succinylcholine with thiopentone sodium mixed in the same syringe produces complex formation. Protamine zinc insulin containing excess of protamine interacts with soluble insulin if mixed in the same syringe. Ampicillin, benzyl penicillin, heparin and aminophylline are unstable with the acidic pH

of dextrose solution and should not be administered with it. Noradrenaline solution cannot be infused with normal saline and can be infused with dextrose solution as it is stable at acidic pH. When noradrenaline solution is to be infused with normal saline, vitamin C should be added to the reservoir to prevent oxidation of noradrenaline. Hydrocortisone hemisuccinate or gentamicin should not be administered with ampicillin, methicillin, carbenicillin or tetracycline in the same infusion bottle, as they loss potency. No drug can be administered with blood, plasma, sodium bicarbonate, lactate or mannitol solution in the same transfusion or infusion bottle.

Drug-drug interactions that occur *in vivo* (inside the body) are of two types: pharmacokinetic interaction and pharmacodynamic interaction.

Pharmacokinetic Interaction

It occurs by altering the concentration of one drug by the other in the tissue or tissue fluid. It may occur during absorption, distribution, biotransformation or excretion of drugs. It occurs by following mechanisms:

1. Interference with the gastrointestinal absorption of one drug by another, e.g. gastric antacids containing magnesium and calcium salts decrease the absorption of tetracyclines and iron salts. Prokinetic drugs (metoclopramide, domperidone,

etc.) decrease the absorption of anticholinergics, antihistaminics, opiates and phenothiazines by increasing gastric emptying time and GIT motility. Sucralfate decreases absorption of phenytoin and liquid paraffin decreases absorption of fat-soluble vitamins (A, D, E and K).

2. Displacement of plasma protein binding of one drug by another, e.g. aspirin phenylbutazone, oxyphenbutazone, indomethacin or clofibrate can displace warfarin sodium from the binding sites leading to severe bleeding episode. Salicylates, sulphonamides and oral anticoagulants (warfarin, dicumarol, etc.) can displace oral antidiabetics (tolbutamide, chlorpropamide, etc.) from the binding sites leading to hypoglycemic coma. Salicylates and sulphonamides (long-acting) can displace bile pigments from the binding protein, especially in neonates producing kernicterus (jaundice). Similarly, digoxin is diplaced by quinidine, verapamil, nifedipine or amiodarone; phenytoin is displaced by NSAIDs; methotrexate is displaced by salicylates or sulphonamides producing severe toxicity.

3. Inhibition of adrenergic neuronal uptake of one drug by another, e.g. imipramine and chlorpromazine inhibit the neuronal uptake of guanethidine and bethanidine and, therefore, interfere with the antihypertensive activity of the latter drugs.

4. Depletion of catecholamines from adrenergic neurons, e.g. reserpine depletes catecholamines from adrenergic neurons and decreases sympathetic activity of ephedrine or metaraminol.

5. Alteration of metabolism of one drug by another by microsomal enzyme induction or inhibition. Enzyme inducers, e.g. phenobarbitone, phenytoin, carbamazepine, rifampicin, griseofulvin, etc. increase metabolism of warfarin, dicoumarol, etc. and therefore, decrease anticoagulant effect of latter drugs. Rifampicin increases metabolism of oral contraceptive drugs leading to decreased contraceptive activity and failure of contraception. Similarly, carbamazepine decreases the effect of phony ton; pyridoxine decreases the effect of levodopa; phenobarbitone, phenytoin or rifampicin decreases the effect of warfarin, digoxin or prednisolone. Enzyme inhibitors, e.g. phenylbutazone, cimetidine, metronidazole, isoniazid, chloramphenicol, etc. decrease metabolism of warfarin, tolbutamide or phenytoin leading to increased toxicity. Similarly, cimetidine increases the toxicity of diazepam, morphine, theophylline or lignocaine. Allopurinol (xanthine oxidase inhibitor) increases the toxicity of mercaptopurine or azathioprine.

6. Alteration of renal excretion of one drug by another, e.g. probenecid decreases renal excretion of penicillins leading to prolonged duration of action. Similarly, aspirin decreases uricosuric effect of sulphinpyrazone, NSAIDs decrease excretion of lithium and, therefore, increase the toxicity.

Pharmacodynamic Interaction

It occurs by modification of the pharmacological effect of one drug by another without altering the concentration of the drug in the tissue or tissue fluid. It may occur at receptor or nonreceptor site.

Receptor Site

Drugs acting on the same receptor or at different active receptors may enhance or decrease the response by additive, synergistic or antagonistic effect, e.g. d-tubocurarine with aminoglycoside antibiotics (e.g. streptomycin) may increase the block at neuromuscular junction and can produce respiratory muscle paralysis. Combined administration of morphine and barbiturates (e.g. phenobarbitone sodium) can produce marked CNS depression by additive/synergistic action, d-tubocurarine and succinylcholine at neuromuscular junction and morphine and pentazocine (partial agonist) as analgesics (by blocking μ receptors) produce antagonistic (opposite) actions. Examples of pharmacodynamic interactions are many and are described in respective chapters.

Nonreceptor Site

Drugs may interact by changing fluid and electrolyte balance or due to opposite chemotherapeutic action, e.g. diuretics causing potassium depletion can increase toxicity of digoxin by producing hypokalemia. Again hypokalemia can antagonize the antiarrhythmic activity of phenytoin, lignocaine, quinidine or procainamide. Hyperkalemia produced by potassium sparing diuretics, captopril, enalapril and NSAIDs may decrease the clinical efficacy of digoxin. Combined administration of bactericidal antibiotics (e.g. penicillins) and bacteriostatic antibiotics (e.g. tetracyclines) decrease therapeutic effect of each other.

Importance of Knowledge of Drug Interaction

Drug interaction is a vital problem in clinical practice nowadays. A physician who uses multiple drugs in a prescription must be alert about the possibility of drug interaction. He must be aware of both risky drugs and susceptible patients to avoid drug interaction. Risky drugs are those drugs that affect the vital processes in the body (e.g. warfarin, morphine and chlorpromazine), that have saturable (zero order) kinetics (e.g. phenytoin, theophylline and aspirin), that have a steep dose response curve (e.g. verapamil, levodopa and chlorpropamide), that show dose dependent toxicity (e.g. digoxin, lithium, methotrexate and aminoglycoside antibiotics), where the patient depends on the prophylactic action (e.g. oral contraceptives and cyclosporin) and where the loss of effect leads to a breakthrough of disease (e.g. quinidine, antiepileptics and glucocorticosteriods). Susceptible patients are elderly patients, patients with unstable disease (e.g. epileptics, brittle-diabetics, dementia patients and patients with cardiac arrhythmias) and patients dependent upon drug treatment for survival (e.g. transplant recipients and patients with Addison's disease).

8

Adverse Drug Reactions

INTRODUCTION

All drugs whether used systemically or topically can produce adverse drug reactions ranging from mild inconvenience to serious toxicity or even death. The incidence of adverse drug reactions (ADRs) in hospital indoor patients is about 10%.

Types of Adverse Drug Reactions

These are of two types:
1. **Predictable (Type I)** reactions, e.g. side effects, secondary effects, drug withdrawal reactions and toxic effects. These are based on pharmacological properties of the drug. These are more common and dose dependent reactions.
2. **Unpredictable (Type II)** reactions, e.g. intolerance, idiosyncrasy and allergic (hypersensitivity) reactions. These are based on the peculiarity of the patient and not on drug's own action. These are less common and dose independent reactions. These are generally more serious and often require withdrawal of the drug. Some adverse reactions are avoidable, e.g. gastric irritation produced by some drugs (e.g. iron salts, theophylline, NSAIDs, etc.) can be avoided by giving the drug after meals. Other adverse reactions are unavoidable, which are due to:
   a. Pharmacological effects in therapeutic doses, e.g. dryness of mouth and skin with anticholinergics, palpitation and tachycardia with catecholamines, etc.

   b. Sequelae of pharmacological effects in therapeutic doses, e.g. postural hypotension with prazosin, hydralazine, trimethaphan, etc. throbbing headache and syncope produced by nitrites and nitrates.
   c. Low safety margin of some drugs, e.g. digoxin, lithium carbonate, anticancer drugs, etc.

Discussion of Individual Adverse Effects or Reactions of Drugs

1. **Side effects**: These are extension of pharmacological effects of drugs in therapeutic doses, i.e. due to excess of normal pharmacodynamic effects. These are predictable and dose related effects and usually trivial in nature. These constitute about 80% of all adverse reactions, e.g. dryness of mouth and skin by anticholinergic drugs (e.g. atropine), postural hypotension by some antihypertensive drugs (e.g. prazosin), hypokalemia by loop diuretics (e.g. frusemide) and thiazide diuretics (e.g. hydrochlorothiazide), constipation by morphine and verapamil, throbbing headache by nitrites and nitrates (e.g. GTN), sedation by antihistaminics (e.g. promethazine) and systemic acidosis by carbonic anhydrase inhibitors (e.g. acetazolamide).

2. **Secondary effects**: These are indirect consequences of primary drug action, e.g. superinfection and vitamin deficiency due to suppression of normal bacterial flora in

the gut by broad spectrum/extended spectrum antibiotics, e.g. tetracyclines, chloramphenicol, ampicillin, etc.; activation of latent tuberculosis by administration of corticosteroids due to weakening of host defence mechanism.

3. **Drug withdrawal reactions:** Sudden withdrawal of certain drugs may produce worsening of the clinical condition for which the drug was being used, e.g. acute adrenal insufficiency may be precipitated by sudden withdrawal of corticosteroid. Severe hypertension and sympathetic overactivity may occur after sudden withdrawal of clonidine. Worsening of angina pectoris or myocardial infarction may occur after sudden withdrawal of β-blockers (e.g. propranolol). Frequency of seizures may increase on sudden withdrawal of anti-epileptic drugs (e.g. phenytoin). These manifestations are also due to adaptive changes and can be minimized by gradual withdrawal of the drugs.

4. **Toxic effects (toxicity):** These are due to overdose of drugs producing excessive pharmacological effects (acute toxicity) or prolonged repeated use of drugs producing organ/tissue toxicity (chronic toxicity), e.g. coma produced by barbiturates and alcohol, complete heart (AV) block by digoxin, bleeding by heparin, respiratory depression by morphine and myocardial damage by emetine are due to overdose of the respective drug.
   Ototoxicity and nephrotoxicity produced by aminoglycoside antibiotics (e.g. streptomycin) and high ceiling diuretics (e.g. ethacrynic acid), oculotoxicity by chloroquine, ethambutol, methanol, etc. and neurotoxicity by isoniazid, hydralazine, vincristine, etc. are due to prolonged use of the respective drug. These are predictable and dose related effects and usually serious in nature, demanding prompt treatment.

5. **Intolerance:** It is the appearance of characteristic adverse reaction of a drug in an individual at therapeutic dose. It is due to low threshold to pharmacological action of a drug, e.g. a single dose of chloroquine may produce vomiting and abdominal pain in some patients. A single dose of triflupromazine may produce muscular dystonias in some patients. A few doses of phenobarbitone may cause excitement and mental confusion in some patients.

6. **Idiosyncrasy:** It is a genetically determined abnormal reaction to a chemical (drug). It is due to total absence or reduced activity of some enzymes in an individual, e.g. haemolytic anaemia produced by oxidizing agents like primaquine and sulphonamides in individuals due to deficiency of the enzyme glucose-6 phosphate dehydrogenase in RBCs (glutathione present in RBCs is a highly reducing agent. Lack of glutathione leads to brittleness of RBCs). Prolonged apnoea and respiratory paralysis produced by succinylcholine in individuals whose sera contain atypical cholinesterase. Acute porphyria is produced by phenobarbitone, alcohol or chloramphenicol in individuals due to induction of the enzyme delta-amino laevulinic acid (ALA) synthetase, which forms porphyrin precursor ALA for heme synthesis. Intolerance like salicylism, iodism and cinchonism are idiosyncratic reactions. Aspirin can produce bronchial asthma in some patients. Idiosyncratic reactions are harmful and sometimes may be fatal. They may appear in low doses.

7. **Allergic (hypersensitivity) reactions (allergenicity, immunotoxicity):** Drug allergy is an immunologically mediated reaction producing serotype symptoms which are unrelated to the pharmacological effects and doses of the drug. These reactions occur only in a minority of patients (5–10%) exposed to the drug and cannot be produced in other patients at any dose. Prior sensitization of the cells is needed and a latent period of at least one to two weeks is required after the first exposure. The drug or its metabolite acts as antigen or hepten (incomplete antigen), which becomes complete antigen after binding with the endogenous protein and induces production of antibodies by sensitized

lymphocytes. Re-exposure of the body tissue to the drug produces antigen antibody reaction which may be mild to serious and reversible in most occasions. The chief target organs of drug allergy are skin, respiratory tract, gastrointestinal tract, blood and blood vessels. All drugs are not allergenic and all patients do not manifest allergy. Chemically related drugs often show cross-sensitivity. One drug can produce different types of allergic reactions in different patients, whereas widely different drugs can produce same type of reaction. The course of drug allergy is also variable. A patient previously sensitive to one drug may subsequently tolerate it without any reaction.

Drug Poisoning and Treatment

Poison is a substance which endanger life by severely effecting one or more vital functions in the body. Drug in large dosage (either accidentally or for suicidal or homicidal purpose) can produce poisoning effects.

Treatment of a Poisoned Person

These include:

1. **Identification of the poison:** This is done by taking history from the relatives or from the patient (if conscious). Estimation of blood level of poison (e.g. barbiturate, morphine, etc.) is also important for identification of the poison.

2. **Termination of exposure of the poison:** This is done by removing the patient to fresh air (in case of inhaled poison) and washing of skin and eyes of the patient (in case of poison entering from the surface).

3. **Prevention of further absorption of the poison:** This is done by using an emetic, e.g. ipecac syrup or apomorphine injection (if the patient is conscious), gastric lavage by stomach tube (in conscious or unconscious patient) and universal antidote (suspension of activated charcoal in water or mixture of burnt toast, strong tea and milk of magnesia in the ratio 2:1:1) for removing the ingested poison from GIT.

Emetics should not be used in patients of corrosive poisoning (for fear of perforation of stomach).

4. **Use of specific antidotes where possible:** These are use of receptor antagonists (e.g. naloxone in morphine poisoning, atropine and pralidoxime in organophosphorus compound poisoning), chelating agents (e.g. dimercaprol in arsenic poisoning, desferrioxamine mesylate in iron poisoning) and specific antibodies (e.g. digoxin-FAB-antibody in digoxin poisoning).

5. **General supportive measures and symptomatic treatment:**

   a. Maintenance of airway and adequate ventilation by oxygen inhalation or artificial respiration are done if required.

   b. Maintenance of BP and heartbeat by fluid infusion (normal saline or 5% dextrose saline), vasopressor agents (noradrenaline, mephentermine, etc.) and cardiac stimulants (dopamine, dobutamine, etc.) are done if required.

6. **Hastening of the elimination of the poison:** Altering the urinary pH to alkaline side (alkalinization) by using sodium bicarbonate, potassium citrate, etc. orally helps in excretion of acidic drugs like barbiturates, salicylates, etc. in urine and to acidic side (acidification) by using ammonium chloride, vitamin C, etc. orally helps in excretion of basic drugs like chloroquine, amphetamine, etc. in urine. Forced alkaline diuresis (by using frusemide or mannitol and sodium bicarbonate solution IV) is very useful in removing phenobarbitone, aspirin, etc. from the body.

7. **In serious poisoning,** peritoneal dialysis or haemodialysis can be done in a hospital for removal of the poison from the body.

Organ/Tissue Toxicity

These are chronic toxicities due to prolonged use of drugs (as shown in **Table 8.1**). Withdrawal of the respective drug helps in cure of the condition. In some cases administration of substances that prevent toxicity of drugs

Table 8.1: Organ/tissue toxicity of drugs

Type of toxicity	Produced by drugs
Nephrotoxicity	Aminoglycoside antibiotics, loop diuretics, sulphonamides, tetracyclines, corticosteroids, cephaloridine, amphotericin-B, heavy metals, phenacetin, phenylbutazone, phenytoin, pentamidine, hydralazine, procainamide, lithium, isoniazid, methysergide, penicillamine, NSAIDs, anticancer drugs.
Hepatotoxicity	Isoniazid, rifampicin, tetracyclines, pyrazinamide, paracetamol, pheylbutazone, chlorpromazine, chlorpropamide, erythromycin estolate, halothane, thiacetazone, PAS, sulphonamides, valproic acid, phenytoin, indomethanin, chloroform, alcohol, methyldopa, salicylates.
Haematological/ myelotoxicity (bone marrow depression)	Chloramphenicol, sulphonamides, sulphones, heavy metals, thiouracils, phenothiazines, NSAIDs, quinidine, procainamide, phenytoin, imipramine, doxapine, clozapine, radioactive isotopes, anticancer drugs.
Ototoxicity	Aminoglycoside antibiotics, loop diuretics, salicylates, quinine, chloroquine, minocycline, quinidine, anticancer drugs.
Oculotoxicity	Ethambutol, chloroquine, quinine, diodoquin, methanol, thioridazine, digoxin, mechlorethamine.
Behavioural toxicity	Reserpine, clonidine, propranolol, amphetamine, cocaine, glucocorticoids, marijuana, LSD, mescaline.
Neurotoxicity	Isoniazid, hydralazine, nalidixic acid, nitrofurantoin, vincristine.
Skin toxicity	Heavy metals, drugs producing allergic reactions (see later on).
Cardiotoxicity	Emetine, digoxin, quinidine, lithium, adrenaline, halothane, chloroform.
Pulmonary toxicity	Acetylcysteine, sodium chromoglycate, captopril, morphine.
Endocrine toxicity	Chlorpromazine, oral contraceptives, glucocorticoids.
Carcinogenicity	Anticancer drugs, radioactive isotopes, nicotine, oestrogens.
Mutagenicity	Anticancer drugs, metronidazole.

can be used, e.g. pyridoxine in isoniazid neurotoxicity.

Teratogenicity (Greek Word "Teros" Means Monster)

A teratogen is an agent which can cause physical malformation in foetus, when administered to the pregnant women during the period of organogenesis (18th–60th days of foetal life). After that period, during the remainder days of pregnancy, exposure of foetus to foetotoxic drugs may cause functional disability or in alteration in growth of organs or foetus but no physical defects. The sedative hypnotics, thalidomide prescribed in pregnant women for relief of morning sickness was found to produce various types of developmental anomalies in the newborns (1958–61). This thalidomide disaster has lead to imposement of strict teratogenicity tests on new drugs before their clinical uses **(Table 8.2)**.

Types and Mechanisms of Allergic Reactions to Drugs

These are humoral reactions and cell mediated reactions.

Humoral Reactions

These are of three types:

Type I (immediate hypersensitivity/anaphylatic) reactions: Here on re-exposure to the drug, reactions develop within a few

Table 8.2: Drugs producing teratogenicity

Drug	Abnormality in foetus of man
Thalidomide	Amelia (total absence of limbs), phochomelia (seal limbs or short limbs), multiple defects.
Anticancer drugs (methotrexate, etc.)	Multiple defects, foetal death.
Androgens (testosterone, etc.)	Virilization; limb, oesophageal and cardiac defects.
Progestins (progesterone, etc.)	Virilization of female foetus.
Oestrogens (stilbestrol, etc.)	Vaginal carcinoma in teenaged female offspring.
Warfarin	Nose, eye and hand defects; retardation of growth.
Corticosteroids (prednisolone, etc.)	Cleft palate and lip, cardiac defects.
Tetracyclines	Deformed and discoloured teeth, retarded bone growth.
Antithyroid drugs (carbimazole, etc.)	Foetal goitre, hypothyroidism.
Phenytoin	Hypoplastic phalanges, cleft lip or palate, microcephaly.
Carbamazepine	Neutral tube defects, other abnormalities.
Valproic acid	Spina bifida, neural tube defects.
Lithium	Foetal goitre, cardiac abnormality.
Phenobarbitone	Various malformations.
Aspirin/Indomethacin	Premature closure of ductus arteriosus.

minutes and the manifestations include urticaria, pruritus, rhinitis, bronchospasm (asthma) and anaphylactic shock. IgE antibodies are formed, which get fixed to the mast cell surface and release mediators of allergy like histamine, leukotrienes (LTs), prostaglandins (PGs) and platelet-activating factor (PAF). The most serious and life-threatening reaction is anaphylactic shock, which is manifested as urticaria, pruritus, angioedema, bronchospasm and hypotension. It is treated by prompt administration of adrenaline solution (1:1000) in the dose of 0.5 to 1 mg SC or IM and repeated after five minutes if required. It is a rapidly acting drug producing dramatic response. An antihistaminic drug and a glucocorticoid can be used IM or IV but they are slowly acting drugs. An intradermal (skin) test may forewarn type I allergic reactions.

Type II (autoallergic/cytolytic) reactions: Here the drug combines with a body protein, so that the body no longer recognizes the protein as self and treats it as a foreign protein and then form antibodies (IgG and IgM). The antigen-antibody reaction leads to activation of complement, which damages cells, including blood cells and their precursors by cytolysis leading to granulocytopenia, thrombocytopenia, aplastic anaemia and haemolytic anaemia. Collagen diseases like systemic lupus erythematosus (SLE) may be due to type II reactions.

Type III (retarded/arthus) reactions: Here antigen and antibody (IgG) form large complexes and activate complement, which precipitates on vascular endothelium giving rise to destructive inflammatory response of small blood vessels. The manifestations are serum sickness (1–3 weeks later producing fever, athralgia and lymphadenopathy), nephritis, vasculitis and pulmonary disease. These reactions usually subside after 1–2 weeks.

Cell Mediated Reactions

These are discussed as follows:

Type IV (delayed cell mediated) reactions: Here antigen specific receptors develop on T lymphocytes. On contact with antigen these T cells produce lymphokines, which attract granulocytes and then produce an inflammatory response. The manifestations are contact dermatitis, some skin rashes, pneumonitis and photosensitization of skin to UV radiation (sunray). These reactions develop after 48 hours of antigen exposure and subside gradually.

Examples of drugs that frequently producing allergic reactions: Penicillins, cefalosporins, erythromycin, tetracyclines, chloramphenicol, sulphonamides, rifampicin, isoniazid, cocaine, procaine, lidocaine, insulin, heparin, NSAIDs, sulphonylureas, phenothiazines, chloroquine, quinine, quinidine, thiouracils, methyldopa, levodopa, phenytoin, carbamazepine, hydralazine, captopril, allopurinol, halothane, streptokinase, ATS, ADS, ACS, etc.

Care should be taken in prescribing drugs for patients suffering from allergic disorders, because in them the incidence of drug allergy is more.

Treatment of Drug Allergy

The offending drug must be immediately stopped. Most mild reactions like skin rashes subside by themselves and do not require specific treatment. In some type I reactions like urticaria, pruritus, rhinitis, swelling of lips and eyelids, antihistaminics are beneficial. In case of anaphylactic shock adrenaline is the drug of choice (discussed before).

Special Adverse Drug Reactions

1. **Drugs causing unmasking or exacerbations of some diseases:** Drugs can unmask a latent condition or exacerbate an already existing disease, e.g. glucocorticoids may unmask latent diabetes or exacerbate an existing peptic ulcer or tuberculosis. Isoniazid may unmask latent epilepsy.
2. **Drugs producing new diseases (iatrogenic diseases):** Sometimes, drug themselves may produce certain diseases after prolonged use. These are called iatrogenic diseases (physician made diseases, Greek word "iatros" meaning physician), e.g. parkinsonism is produced by chlorpromazine and reserpine; peptic ulcer is produced by NSAIDs (aspirin, etc.) and corticosteroids; hypertension is produced by glucocorticoids; candidiasis is produced by broad spectrum antibiotics; glaucoma is produced by anticholinergic drugs and ocular glucocorticoids; hepatitis is produced by isoniazid, rifampicin and pyrazinamide; systemic lupus erythematosus (SLE) is produced by hydralazine and procainamide, etc.
3. **Toxicity due to drug interactions:** This can occur when two or more drugs are administered simultaneously to a patient (discussed in Drug Interactions).

Factors Influencing Adverse Drug Reactions (ADRs)

These are given as follows:

1. **Drug related factors:** Chemical and physical properties of drugs; presence of vehicles, adjuvants, binding agents or coating agents with drugs; margin of safety (low or wide) of drugs and drug-drug interactions can modify adverse drug reactions.

2. **Routes of drug administration:** The toxicity of an orally administered drug is generally greatest when it is given in an empty stomach and least when it is given after food. Drugs given by slow IV infusion produce less toxicity than when given by rapid single injection. Some drugs produce toxicity even in contact with skin by percutaneous absorption, e.g. organophosphorus compounds.

3. **Subject susceptibility (age, sex and pregnancy):** Neonates and old persons are more prone to adverse drug reactions. Women are more susceptible to adverse drug reactions than men. Teratogenic drugs should be avoided during pregnancy.

4. Disease states: Presence of diseases of liver or kidney, presence of congestive cardiac failure, cardiovascular shock, hypertension, bronchial asthma, diabetes mellitus, thromboembolic disorders, gastritis or peptic ulcer can precipitate adverse drug reactions by altering pharmacokinetics of drugs.

5. Racial differences: Persons of some races (e.g. Egyptians, Swedenese, etc.) are poor acetylators and so drugs like isoniazid, hydralazine, etc. can produce neurotoxicity in them, whereas persons of some races (e.g. Eskimos, Japanese, etc.) are rapid acetylators and so isoniazid, hydrallazine, etc. can produce hepatotoxicity in them. Again persons of some races (e.g. American Negroes) often suffer from haemolytic anaemia by using primaquine, quinine and other oxidant drugs due to deficiency of the enzyme, glucose-6-phosphate dehydrogenase in RBCs (discussed in Pharmacogenetics).

Toxicity Studies in Animals

To assess the safety of a drug, various toxicity studies are carried out in animals (mice, rats, guinea pigs, dogs and monkeys) under varying conditions of drug administration. The tests done are:

Acute Toxicity Tests

In these tests, the drug is tested for the effects of single dose by injecting graded doses in different groups of animals. Detailed observations are made on the effects of the drugs on locomotion, behaviour, respiration and production of convulsion and vomiting. This is followed by autopsy and histological examination. The studies are conducted in at least two species of animals (usually mice and rats) and two routes of administration of the drug (one by intended route of use) are used. Animals of both sexes and various age groups are subjected to such tests. These studies determine LD_{50}, ED_{50} and therapeutic index for the drug under investigation.

Subacute Toxicity Tests

In these tests, a drug is tested for the effects of daily doses for a shorter period of time (usually 14 to 21 days) to save time. Usually two species (rats and dogs) are used and the route of administration is according to the intended route of use. Evaluation of the state of health of the animals is done weekly. All animals are subjected to autopsy and histological examination of all organ systems like chronic toxicity tests.

Chronic Toxicity Tests

In these tests, a drug is tested for the effect of daily doses for a longer period of time (usually 3 months to 1 year). Usually 2 species (rats and dogs) are used and the route of administration is according to the intended route of use. Evaluation of the state of health of the animals is done weekly. All animals are subjected to autopsy and histological examination of all organ systems. In chronic toxicity studies following observations are made:

- Observation of gross changes like increase or decrease of body weight, loss of fur, behavioural effects (abnormalities), skin and eye effects and changes in mating behaviour of the animals.
- Examination of effects of the drug on the individual organs like liver, kidney, heart, adrenal and bone marrow after autopsy (by histopathology). Estimation of enzyme activities and liver function tests are carried out in animals.
- Examination of effects of the drug on the reproductive system, including teratogenicity (in animals like rats, mice or rabbits).
- Carcinogenicity and mutagenicity of the drug (in animals like rats, mice or rabbits).
- Dependence liability of the drug (in animals like cats, dogs or monkeys).

9

Development and Evaluation of New Drugs

INTRODUCTION

New drugs are continuously introduced in the market. They are developed mainly by three ways:

1. Drug designing (on the basis of chemical structures and their biological actions).
2. Modification of the chemical structure of a known drug.
3. Systemic pharmacological screening of different natural products and synthetic compounds.

Most new drugs are discovered by testing (screening) a large number of natural products or synthetic compounds for varieties of biological actions. Once a compound is found to have an effect, numerous chemical modifications are made and tested until one is found to be suitable for further evaluation. Current drug development highly focusses on prospective designing for a specific chemical effect.

Before introducing a new drug in clinical practice, the risk benefit ratio of the drug must be satisfactory. This risk benefit ratio varies from drug to drug, e.g. high risk sedative hypnotic is unacceptable, but a high risk anticancer drug is acceptable. To develop or introduce a new drug following tests are carried out:

Preclinical Tests

Preclinical tests are done in animals (like rats, mice, guinea pigs, rabbits, dogs, cats and monkeys) for following purposes:

a. *Pharmacological studies:* These are carried out in animals using *in vivo* or *in vitro* techniques. These studies bring out specific biological activities (effects), mechanisms of action, pharmacokinetics and effective dosage range of test compounds.

b. *Toxicity studies:* These should be done with compounds which have showed positive pharmacology. These include acute, subacute and chronic toxicity tests, therapeutic index, effects on reproductive system including teratogenicity; carcinogenicity and mutagenicity of drugs and mechanism of toxicity (discussed previously).

Clinical Evaluation (in Humans)

When the studies in animals predict that a new chemical compound may be a useful medicine, then it is put to clinical pharmacology (in healthy human volunteers) and clinical trial (in patients). These human studies are carried out in four phases (one after another).

Phase I (preliminary pharmacologic evaluation): In it; pharmacokinetics, safety and effects of a new drug are studied in healthy human volunteers.

Phase II (controlled clinical evaluation): In it; pharmacokinetics, safety and therapeutic efficacy of the new drug are studied in small numbers of selected patients using single blind (patient) design (procedure).

Phase III (controlled clinical trials): In it; safety and therapeutic efficacy of the new drug are studied in large numbers (hundreds) of selected patients using double blind (patient and doctor) design (procedure) with a cross-over design. After satisfactory completion of this phase, application is made to the drug controller for permission to market the new drug.

Phase IV (postmarketing surveillance for some drugs): It begins after obtaining the approval of the drug controller to market the drug. It constitutes a vigilant postmarketing surveillance to monitor ADRs and safety of the new drug including detection of rare toxicity reported by the physicians from various clinics and hospitals. The new drug is also compared with an already used drug for efficacy and safety.

All pharmacological, clinical and toxicological data should be subjected to statistical analysis to detect the utility of the new drug.

In connection with the clinical evaluation and trials following terms should be noted:

1. **Placebo:** Placebo (Latin word, means "I please") is a dummy medication (an inert substance, i.e. without pharmacological action, but harmless) used to please a patient. It looks like the drug and when administered to patient or a healthy volunteer, the subject remains under the impression that he has received a drug. Some persons may develop temporary improvement from some diseases (angina pectoris, hypertension, diabetes, etc.) even after receiving the placebo. Placebo therapy is used during single blind and double blind studies.

To minimize bias in clinical trials, randomization (random selection of subjects) and double blind design are adopted.

2. **Single blind design:** In it, some of the patients get drug to be tested and others get the placebo and the patient is blind about the drug or the placebo. After getting the drug or the placebo, the patients report to the doctor (investigator) about their improvement or symptoms.

3. **Double blind design:** In it, neither the patient nor the doctor (investigator) knows who has received what (drug or placebo). The drug and the placebo are supplied by a third man under a code. This avoids bias of the investigator.

4. **Cross-over design:** In it, some patients get the drug to be tested and others get the placebo by a third man and both the patients and the doctor are blind about the drug or placebo. After getting reports of the patients about their improvement or symptoms, the third man supply the drug and the placebo to the patients in alternate phases and the reports are monitored by the doctor (investigator).

Ethics in the Development of New Drugs

Majority of toxicity tests in animals, which are subjected to ethical criticism are based on studies in whole animals, because only in them it is possible to approach the complexity of organization of body systems of humans, to explore any consequence of variable drug absorption, metabolism and excretion and to reveal direct and indirect toxic effects of drugs. Use of animals for toxicity tests would be unjustified if results useful to man could not be obtained. Animals are similar to man in many respects and so they are used initially for toxicity tests. To exclude the need for tests in whole animals, *in vitro* tests are being introduced, which are scientifically highly satisfactory. The idea to exclude whole animal tests is not only ethical but also economical, because whole animals are very costly to breed in house and to keep them healthy. It is better to choose non-whole animal methods, if they are scientifically satisfactory and practically available.

In clinical trials using humans, the comfort, health and food of the subject must be satisfactory and there should not be any bias in choosing the subject.

Section II

ANS PHARMACOLOGY

10

General Considerations

Nervous system is very complex and highly integrated system. It is divided into central nervous system (CNS) and peripheral nervous system (PNS). Peripheral nervous system is again divided into somatic nervous system (SNS/voluntary nervous system) and autonomic nervous system (ANS/involuntary nervous system). Central nervous system includes brain and spinal cord, while peripheral nervous system includes 12 pairs of cranial nerves and 31 pairs of spinal nerves, which are distributed throughout the body. Autonomic nervous system is a part of peripheral ntervous system. It was named by Langley in 1898 (*Autos* means self and *normos* means governing). Unlike somatic nervous system it is not under the control of will, i.e. it is independent of volitional control. It has some degree of autonomy. It controls the activities (functions) of the heart, blood vessels, smooth muscles of viscera and exocrine glands. Somatic nervous system controls the activities (functions) of the skeletal muscles.

Autonomic nervous system is divided into parasympathetic nervous system and sympathetic nervous system. There are differences between these two systems **(Table 10.1).**

The two systems remain in a state of dynamic equilibrium in the body to maintain homeostasis (internal environment) as most of the organs of the body receive both parasympathetic and sympathetic (dual) supplies. Dominance of parasympathetic

Table 10.1: Differences between parasympathetic NS and sympathetic NS

	Parasympathetic NS	*Sympathetic NS*
1. Origin	Craniosacral outflow ($C_{3,7,9 \text{ and } 10}$, S_{2-4})	Thoracolumbar outflow (T_{1-12}, L_{1-3})
2. Distribution	Limited (1 or 2 postganglionic fibres)	Wide (5 to 50 post-ganglionic fibres)
3. Ganglia	On or close to the organ	Away from the organ
4. Preganglionic nerve fibre	Long, myelinated	Short, myelinated
5. Postganglionic nerve fibre	Short, nonmyelinated (ratio of length 20:1)	Long, nonmyelinated (ratio of length 1:2).
6. Neurotransmitter	Acetylcholine	Noradrenaline (major) Acetylcholine (minor)

Contd.

Table 10.1: Differences between parasympathetic NS and sympathetic NS (Contd.)

	Parasympathetic NS	Sympathetic NS
7. Important functions	Conservation of body energy, regulation of tissue building processes (digestion and assimilation of food).	Utilization of body energy, tackling of stress and emergency and preparing the individual for fight or flight.
8. Importance of the system	Vital for life. Man or animal cannot survive without it as functions of all organs stop.	Not so vital for life. Man or animal can survive without it.

system occurs in placid state whereas dominance of sympathetic system occurs in stressful and emergency situation.

Control of ANS

It is under higher control of hypothalamus and reticular activating system (RAS). Limbic system coordinates emotions with autonomic reactions. Final coordination between somatic and autonomic functions occur in cerebral cortex.

Neurotransmission

It occurs by axonal conduction (passage of a nerve impulse along an axon or muscle fibre) and junctional transmission (by chemical substance). Nerve impulses elicit response in smooth, cardiac and skeletal muscles, exocrine glands and postsynaptic neurons (effector tissues) through liberation of specific chemical transmitters like acetylcholine and nor-adrenaline. Junctional regions in ANS are:

1. **Synaptic junction:** It is the junctional region between two neurons, where information from one neuron is relayed to the other neuron, but there is no protoplasmic continuity between two neurons. Synapses are present in the autonomic ganglia and enteric nervous system ganglia.

2. **Neuroeffector junction:** It is the junctional region between a postganglionic autonomic nerve fibre with the effector tissue (smooth muscle, cardiac muscle or exocrine gland).

3. **Myoneuronal junction:** It is the junctional region between a somatic nerve fibre and the skeletal muscle fibre. In all these junctional sites neurotransmission occurs by chemical transmission with the help of neurotransmitter.

Neurotransmitter (Neurohumor)

It is a chemical substance which is synthesized and stored in the nerve endings and released from there by nerve stimulus (impulse/NAP). It stimulates or inhibits the postsynaptic neuron. It has short latency (onset of action) and short duration of action. Acetylcholine is the neurotransmitter in parasympathetic nervous system and nor-adrenaline is the major neurotransmitter and acetylcholine is the minor neurotransmitter in sympathetic nervous system. Common features (properties) of a neurotransmitter are:

- It should be present in the presynaptic nerve fibre and its distribution should be discrete rather than uniform.
- It should be synthesized in the presynaptic nerve fibre by specific enzyme and stored in synaptic vesicles or storage granules.
- It should be released from the nerve endings by nerve impulse (NAP).
- It should interact with specific receptors on the effector cells/tissues.
- Its effects should be terminated by enzymatic destruction (metabolism), diffusion from the site of receptors or reuptake by the nerve endings (in intact or broken form).
- It should have agonists and antagonists to produce desired effects.
- It should produce identical responses when used externally (extrinsically) to the tissue

or organ (isolated or intact) as produced by stimulation of the nerve, wherefrom it is released.

Steps in Neurohumoral Transmission

These are discussed as follows:

- Synthesis of the neurotransmitter in the nerve fibre by specific enzyme.
- Storage of the neurotransmitter in the synaptic vesicles or storage granules of nerve endings.
- Release of the neurotransmitter into the synaptic cleft or other medium by nerve impulse (NAP).
- Interaction of the neurotransmitter with the receptor on the effector cell membrane producing response (effect).
- Rapid removal of the neurotransmitter from the site of receptor by enzymatic destruction, diffusion from the site or reuptake mechanism.
- Recovery of the effector cell to the state that preceded transmitter action.

Neuromodulator (Cotransmitter)

It is a chemical substance which is not synthesized and stored in the nerve endings but present in non-neuronal sites. It modulates, i.e. modifies (increases or decreases) the response (effect) of the neurotransmitter on the target sites. It has longer latency and longer duration of action than neurotransmitter, e.g. prostaglandins (PCs), nitric oxide (NO), circulating steroids and CO_2 ammonia (NH_3) are neuromodulators.

Neuromediator

It is a chemical substance which is present in synapses or in effector cells and acts as a second messenger in mediating intracellular events following postsynaptic activity (stimulation or inhibition) by a neurotransmitter, e.g. cyclic nucleotides (cAMP and cGMP), inositol triphosphate (IP_3), diacylglycerol (DAG) and calcium ions of autonomic Receptors. These are:

1. **Postsynaptic receptors:** These are present on the postsynaptic membrane of effector cell or tissue and produce pharmacological effects by binding with the transmitters or agonists, e.g. cholinergic receptors (M_1/M_2/M_3, N_M and N_N) and adrenergic receptors (α_1, α_2, β_1, β_2 and β_3).

2. **Presynaptic autoreceptors:** These are present on the presynaptic membrane of the effector neuron and respond to the transmitter released from nerve endings and regulate the release of transmitters from the nerve endings by autoinhibitory feedback mechanism, e.g. M_2 receptor at adrenergic enteric nervous system and α_2 receptor at adrenergic nerve fibres produce inhibitory effects (i.e. decrease in release of neurotransmitters). N_M receptor at cholinergic somatic motor nerve fibres and β_2 receptor at adrenergic nerve fibres and cholinergic somatic motor nerve fibres produce excitatory effects (i.e. increase in release of neurotransmitters). They have no pharmacological effects.

Denervation Supersensitivity

If a nerve supply to a target organ/tissue (skeletal muscle/smooth muscle/cardiac muscle) is cut, after some weeks it will be found that application of the neurotransmitter to the target organ produces unusually strong effect. This phenomenon of increased sensitivity of a tissue or organ after denervation is called denervation supersensitivity, e.g. a skeletal muscle, after cutting the motor nerve becomes highly sensitive to acetylcholine and the nictitating membrane, after cutting its postganglionic sympathetic supply becomes highly sensitive to noradrenaline. There are three probable mechanisms for it:

1. Increase in number of receptors of the denervated tissue or organ.
2. Abolition of reuptake mechanism of the neurotransmitter.
3. Increase in post-receptor binding effect of the neurotransmitter.
   Sites of cholinergic and adrenergic transmission (as shown in **Fig. 10.1**).

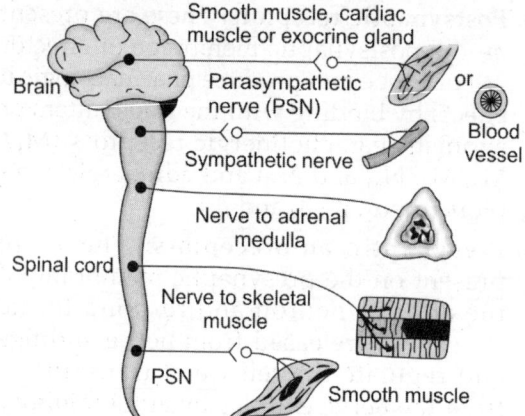

Fig. 10.1: Sites of cholinergic and adrenergic transmission

Cholinergic Transmission

Here acetylcholine is the neurotransmitter.

Sites

- All preganglionic parasympathetic and sympathetic nerve fibres.
- All postganglionic parasympathetic nerve fibres.
- Postganglionic sympathetic nerve fibres supplying sweat glands, hair follicles and few blood vessels (arterioles) of skin of face and neck (vasodilator fibres), where acetylcholine is the neurotransmitter.
- Nerve fibres supplying adrenal medulla.
- Somatic motor nerve fibres supplying skeletal muscles.
- Certain synapses in CNS (brain and spinal cord).

Adrenergic Transmission

Here noradrenaline and adrenaline are neurotransmitters.

Sites

- All postganglionic sympathetic nerve fibres except those supplying sweat glands, hair follicles and few blood vessels of skin, where acetylcholine is the neurotransmitter.
- Certain synapses in CNS (brain and spinal cord).

Cholinergic System (Parasympathetic Nervous System)

Acetylcholine is the neurotransmitter in this system.

Synthesis, Storage, Release and Degradation (Destruction) of Acetylcholine

The substrates for the synthesis of acetylcholine are glucose and choline. Glucose enters the neuron by facilitated diffusion and is converted to pyruvate. Choline is almost completely ionized at body pH and enters the neuron by active transport. Pyruvate from cytosol (cytoplasm) enters into mitochondria of neuronal cell and is converted into acetate. Acetate then combines with coenzyme A (CoA) by the help of the acetyl kinase enzyme forming acetyl CoA in the mitochondria. Acetyl CoA is transported to cytosol and combines with choline by the help of the enzyme, choline acetyl transferase (choline acetylase) forming acetylcholine and CoA (as shown in **Fig. 10.2**).

Acetylcholine is then transported to synaptic vesicles for storage. It is released from the synaptic vesicles by exocytosis (bursting of vesicles) due to arrival of nerve impulse (producing nerve action potential (NAP)). It then crosses the synaptic cleft by diffusion and interacts with specific receptors (muscarinic and nicotinic) on the effector cells to produce responses (effects) (as shown in **Fig. 10.2**). The released acetylcholine is rapidly hydrolyzed to choline and acetate by the enzyme, choline esterase (ChE). About 50% of choline is taken up by the neuron by active transport (reuptake mechanism) and utilized in the synthesis of acetylcholine. The rest is carried away in circulation as follows:

There are two types of cholinesterases, which cause destruction of acetylcholine and other choline esters. These are as follows:

1. Acetylcholinesterase (true/specific cholinesterase).
2. Butyryl cholinesterase (pseudo/ nonspecific cholinesterase).

There are differences between these cholinesterases (as shown in **Table 10.2**).

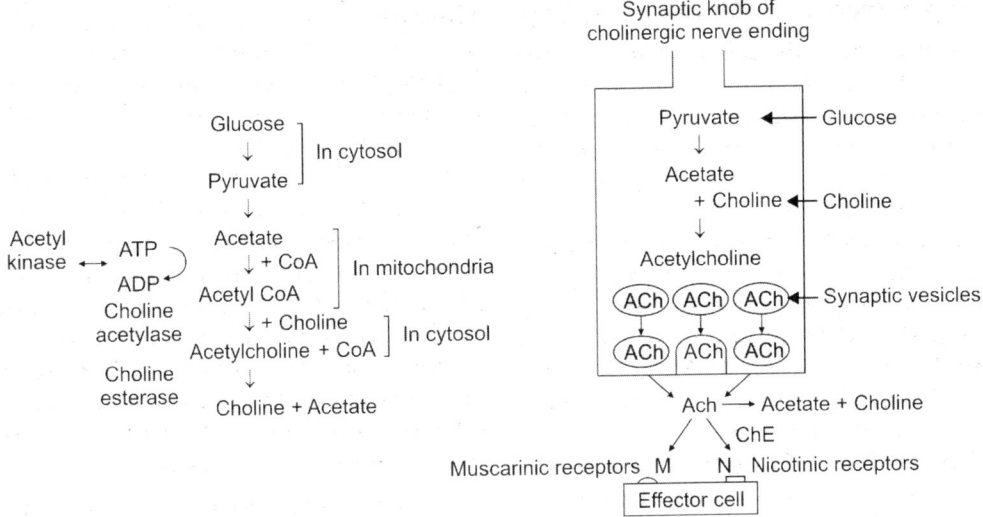

Fig. 10.2: Synthesis and degradation of acetylcholine

Table 10.2: Differences between cholinesterases

	Acetylcholinesterase	*Butyrylcholinesterase*
1. Location (sites)	Neurons, ganglia, myoneuronal junctions and RBCs.	Plasma, liver, intestine and other organs including brain (white matter).
2. Functions	Rapidly hydrolyzes acetylcholine and slowly hydrolyzes methacholine but not butyrylcholine, benzoylcholine and succinylcholine.	Rapidly hydrolyzes butyrylcholine, benzoylcholine and succinylcholine; and slowly hydrolyzes acetylcholine and methacholine.
3. Inhibitors	Anticholinesterases. More sensitive to reversible anticholinesterases than irreversible anticholinesterases.	Anticholinesterases. More sensitive to irreversible anticholinesterases than reversible anticholinesterases.

Drugs influencing (modifying) cholinergic transmission. These are as follows:

- Drugs inhibiting synthesis of acetylcholine in cholinergic nerve endings (by blocking active uptake of choline), e.g. hemicholinium, vesamicol and triethylcholine.
- Drugs inhibiting release of acetylcholine from cholinergic nerve endings (by blocking exocytosis), e.g. procaine, streptomycin, verapamil, magnesium sulphate and botulinus toxin (Type I).
- Drugs potentiating (increasing) the action of acetylcholine (by causing accumulation of acetylcholine at cholinergic receptor sites), e.g. anticholinesterases (physostigmine, neostigmine and diisopropyl fluorophosphate).
- Drugs antagonizing (decreasing) the action of acetylcholine (by blocking cholinergic receptors), e.g. anticholinergic drugs (atropine, scopolamine, etc. at muscarinic receptor sites).
- Neuromuscular blockers (d-tubocurarine, gallamine, etc. at nicotinic N_M receptor site).
- Ganglionic blockers (hexamethonium, trimethaphan, etc. at nicotinic N_N receptor site).

Cholinergic Receptors (Cholinoreceptors)

These are present on the cell membrane of the effector cells, with which acetylcholine (endogenous or exogenous) interacts to produce responses (effects). These are two types, *viz.* muscarinic (M) receptors and nicotinic (N) receptors.

a. **Muscarinic (M) receptors:** These are so-called as they are stimulated (activated) by muscarine. They are five subtypes, *viz.* M_1, M_2, M_3, M_4 and M_5 receptors (as shown in **Table 10.3a**); of these; M_1, M_2 and M_3 are physiological/functional. They are blocked by atropine receptors.

b. **Nicotinic (N) receptors:** These are so-called as they are stimulated (activated) by nico- tine. They are two subtypes, *viz.* N_M and N_N receptors (as shown in **Table 10.3b**). They are blocked by neurotoxins.

Molecular mechanism of action at cholinergic receptor level (molecular basis of cholinergic receptor functions)

Muscarinic receptors are G-protein coupled receptors. Stimulation (activation) of M_1 and M_3 receptors causes stimulation (activation) of the membrane bound enzyme, phospholipase-C (PLC) leading to increased formation of inositol triphosphate (IP_3) and diacylglycerol (DAG), which act as second messengers. They cause increased release of calcium ions (Ca^{2+}) from sarcoplasmic reticulum into the cytoplasm of effector cells and produce stimulation of these cells. Stimulation (activation) of M_2 receptor opens the potassium ion (K^+) channels and cause increased concentration of K^+ in the effector cells (myocardium) leading to depression (inhibition) of heart.

Nicotinic receptors (N_M and N_N) enclose a cation (Na^+/Ca^{2+}) channel, which is ligand gated. Stimulation (activation) of nicotinic receptors causes opening of cation channels leading to increased concentration of cations in the effector cells. This produces stimulation of effector cells.

Table 10.3a: Muscarinic receptors

Receptor	Location (Sites)	Functions	Selective agonists	Selective antagonists
M_1 receptor	Neurons (CNS and PNS), ganglia, gastric glands	Stimulation of neuronal and ganglion cells	Oxotremorine	Unknown
		Stimulation of gastric secretion	Unknown	Pirenzepine Telenzepine
M_2 receptor	Heart (myocardium)	Depression of heart	Methacholine	Methoetramine Tripitramine
M_3 receptor	Vascular smooth muscle Exocrine glands	Relaxation, contraction Increase secretion	Bethanechol	Derifenacin

Table 10.3b: Nicotinic receptors

Receptor	Location (Sites)	Functions	Selective agonists	Selective antagonists
N_M receptor	Skeletal muscles (neuromuscular junction/motor end plate)	Contraction of skeletal muscles (by stimulation of skeletal muscle cells)	Phenyltrimethyl ammonium (PTMA)	d-tubocurarine Gallamine
N_N receptor	Neurons, ganglia, adrenal medulla	Stimulation of neuronal and ganglion cells, release of catecholamines	Dimethylphenyl piperazinium (DMPP)	Hexamethonium Trimethaphan

Adrenergic System (Sympathetic Nervous System)

Noradrenaline is the major neurotransmitter in this system and acetylcholine is the minor neurotransmitter.

Synthesis, storage, release and degradation of noradrenaline

The substrate for the synthesis of nor-adrenaline is tyrosine (an amino acid). It is present in diet and also synthesized in the liver from phenylalanine (an amino acid). Tyrosine is taken up (by an active transport process) from circulation (blood) by the adrenergic neuronal cells and chromaffin cells of adrenal medulla. In the cytoplasm of these cells tyrosine is converted to dihydroxyphenyl-alanine (DOPA) by the enzyme tyrosine hydroxylases and DOPA is converted to dopamine by the enzyme DOPA decar-boxylase. Dopamine is taken up (by an active transport process) from the cytoplasm by the storage vesicles (adrenergic granules) and is converted to noradrenaline by the enzyme, dopamine β-hydroxylase. In the cytoplasm of chromaffin cells of adrenal medulla, nor-adrenaline is converted to adrenaline by the methylating enzyme phenylethanolamine N-methyl transferase (as shown in **Fig. 10.3**).

For the induction of phenyl ethanolamine N-methyl transferase, glucocorticoids are required. Chromaffin cells of adrenal medulla situated very close to the cortical cells of adrenal cortex (secreting corticosteroids) synthesize adrenaline vigorously from nor-adrenaline, as the blood vessels draining the adrenal cortex supply the chromaffin cells of adrenal medulla.

Most of the noradrenalines stored in the storage vesicles of adrenergic neurons are complex with ATP (in the ratio of 1:4), calcium and a protein (chromogranin-A). On arrival of a nerve impulse (NAP is generated), noradrenaline is released from adrenergic nerve endings by fusion of some storage granules to the inner surface of neuronal membrane (by Ca^{2+}) leading to bursting of storage granules and exocytosis of granular content into the synaptic cleft (neuroeffector junction). The released noradrenaline then acts

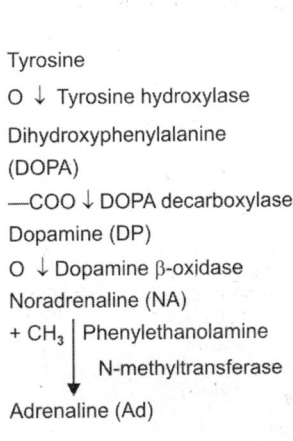

Tyrosine

O ↓ Tyrosine hydroxylase

Dihydroxyphenylalanine (DOPA)

—COO ↓ DOPA decarboxylase

Dopamine (DP)

O ↓ Dopamine β-oxidase

Noradrenaline (NA)

+ CH₃ | Phenylethanolamine
         N-methyltransferase

Adrenaline (Ad)

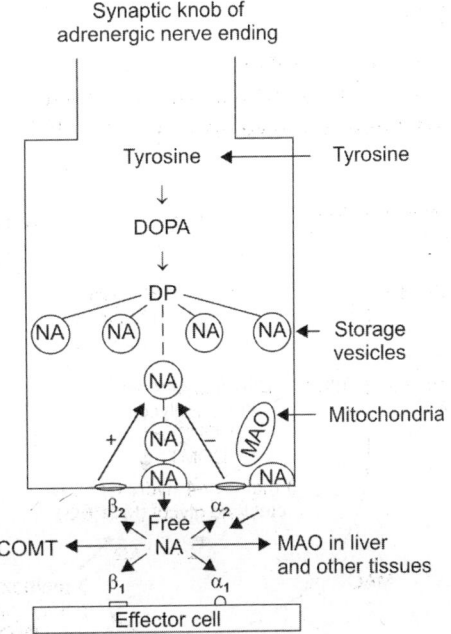

Fig. 10.3: Steps in the synthesis of catecholamines

on postsynaptic adrenergic receptors (α and β) on the effector cells to produce responses (effects). A part of noradrenaline acts on presynaptic autoreceptors (α_2 and β_2), which exert inhibitory or stimulatory effect on the release of noradrenaline from storage vesicles. About 80% of noradrenaline released into the synaptic cleft is rapidly taken up (by active transport process) by the adrenergic nerve endings (reuptake mechanism) and stored in storage granules and vesicles. Some amount of noradrenaline (also adrenaline) is metabolized by enzymes like catecholorthomethyl transferase (COMT) and monoamine oxidase (MAO). COMT is a cytoplasmic enzyme and MAO is a mitochondrial enzyme. Steps in the metabolism of noradrenaline and adrenaline are shown in the **Fig. 10.4**.

Active metabolites like VMA and MOPEG are conjugated with glucuronic acid and sulphate in the liver and excreted in urine as glucuronide and ethereal sulphate respectively.

In pheochromocytoma (adrenal medullary tumour), the urinary excretion of VMA is highly increased (used as diagnostic test).

Drugs Influencing (Modifying) Adrenergic Transmission

These are given as follows:
- Drugs inhibiting synthesis of noradrenaline in adrenergic nerve endings (by utilizing/competing for the same synthetic pathway), e.g. α-methylparatyrosine, α-methyldopa.
- Drugs inhibiting storage of noradrenaline (by blocking vesicular uptake of noradrenaline and causing depletion of NA from the storage site), e.g. reserpine.
- Drugs inhibiting release of noradrenaline (by blocking neuronal uptake of noradrenaline), e.g. cocaine, imipramine, guanethidine, bretylium.
- Drugs promoting release of noradrenaline from the storage site (storage vesicles), e.g. tyramine, amphetamine.

- Drugs inhibiting metabolism of noradrenaline. These are:
  - COMT inhibitors, e.g. pyrogallol, and tropolone.
  - MAO inhibitors, e.g. clogyline (MAO-A inhibitor).
  - Selegiline (MAO-B inhibitor).
  - Pargyline (both MAO-A and MAO-B inhibitors).

Adrenergic Receptors (Adrenoreceptors)

These are present on the cell membrane of effector cells, with which noradrenaline and other adrenergic drugs interact to produce responses (effects). These are two types, viz. α receptors and β receptors:

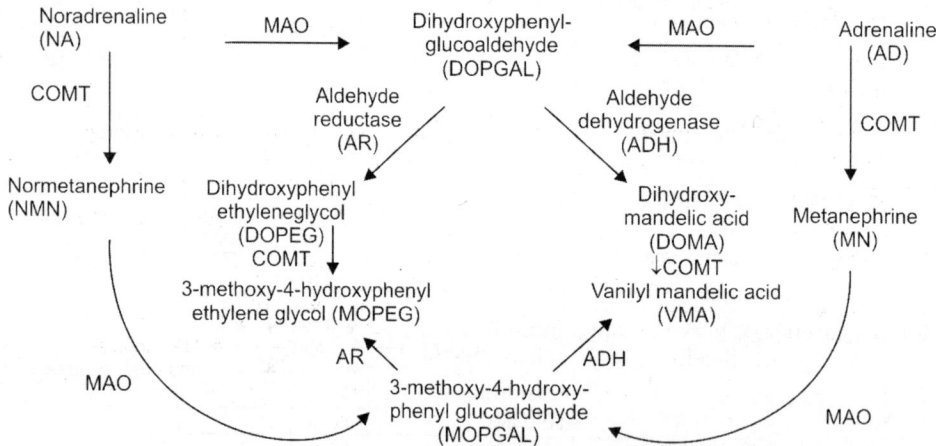

Fig. 10.4: Steps in the metabolism of noradrenaline and adrenaline

a. Alpha (α) receptors: They are two subtypes, *viz.* α_1 and α_2 receptors (as shown in **Table 10.4a**).

b. Beta (β) receptors: They are three subtypes, *viz.* β_1, β_2 and β_3 receptors (as shown in **Table 10.4b**).

Molecular mechanism of action at adrenergic receptor level (molecular basis of adrenergic receptor functions):

Adrenergic receptors are G-protein coupled receptors. Activation (stimulation) of adrenergic receptors produce G-protein mediated effects leading to generation of second messengers and activation of cation channels (Ca^{2+}, Na^+, K^+). There are three types of G-proteins, *viz.* G_q, G_s and G_i in the cell membrane, which lead to generation of second messengers (cAMP, cGMP, IP_3 and DAG), IP_3 stimulates the release of calcium ions (Ca^{2+}) from intracellular stores (at sarcoplasmic reticulum) by a specific receptor mediated pathway. DAG is a potent activator of cellular protein kinase, which is also activated by cAMP and Ca^{2+}.

Following responses (effects) are produced by interaction of the agonist with the concerned receptor:

• Occupation of α_1 receptor by the agonist produces G protein mediated effects leading to activation (stimulation) of phospholipase-C (PLC) and increasing formation of IP_3 (from IP_2) and DAG (from phosphatidic acid). This leads to increased release of Ca^{2+} from intracellular stores and produces responses (effects) of the effector cells.

• Occupation of α_2 receptor by the agonist produces G protein mediated effects leading to inhibition of adenylcyclase and decreasing formation of cAMP (from ATP). This leads to decreased formation and activity of cellular protein kinase causing decreased formation of cellular proteins and produces inhibitory responses (effects) of the effector cells.

Occupation of β-receptors (β_1, β_2 and β_3) by the agonist produces G_s protein mediated effects leading to activation (stimulation) of adenylcyclase and increasing formation of cAMP (from ATP). This leads to increased formation and activity of cellular protein kinase causing increased formation of cellular proteins and also activation of voltage sensitive Ca^{2+} channels in the cell membrane

Table 10.4a: Alpha receptors

Receptor	Location (sites)	Functions	Selective agonists	Selective antagonists
α_1 receptor	Vascular smooth muscle	Contraction	Phenylephrine, methoxamine	Prazosin, terazosin
	Nonvascular smooth muscles (in sphincters, radial muscle of iris, piloerector muscle, etc.)	Contraction		
	Heart (myocardium) Liver	Increase rate and force of contraction Glycogenolysis Gluconeogenesis		
α_2 receptor	Adrenergic nerve ending, Pancreatic β-cells	Inhibition of NA release Inhibition of insulin release	Clonidine, α-methyldopa	Yohimbine, rauwolsine
	Platelets	Aggregation of platelets		

Table 10.4b: Beta receptors

Receptor	Location (sites)	Functions	Selective agonists	Selective antagonists
β_1 receptor	Heart (myocardium)	Stimulation (increase rate and force of contraction)	Dobutamine, prenalterol	Atenolol, metoprolol
	Juxtaglomerular cells of kidney	Increase release of renin		
β_2 receptor	Vascular and non-vascular smooth muscles (in bronchi, GIT, urinary bladder, etc.)	Relaxation	Salbutamol, terbutaline	Butoxamine, α-methyl propranolol
	Adrenergic nerve ending	Stimulation of NA release		
	Liver	Glycogenolysis Gluconeogenesis		
	Skeletal muscle	Glycogenolysis, uptake of K^+		
β_3 receptor	Adipose tissue	Lipolysis in adipocytes	BRL-37344	ICI-118551

of cardiac and skeletal muscles producing influx of Ca^{2+} and responses (effects) of the effector cells.

Autonomic Drugs

These are drugs that act on autonomic receptors.

These are of 6 groups:

1. Cholinergic drugs/parasympathomimetic drugs, e.g. acetylcholine, physostigmine, neostigmine, DFP, etc.

2. Anticholinergic drugs/parasympatholytic drugs, e.g. atropine, scopolamine, dicyclomine flavoxate, etc.

3. Neuromuscular blocking agents, e.g. d-tubocurarine, gallamine, pancuronium, succinylcholine, etc.

4. Ganglion stimulating/blocking agents, e.g. nicotine/hexamethonium, etc.

5. Adrenergic drugs/sympathomimetic drugs, e.g. adrenaline, noradrenaline, isoprenaline, ephedrine, etc.

6. Antiadrenergic drugs/sympatholytic drugs:
   – α receptors blocking drugs, e.g. phenoxybenzamine, phentolamine, prazosin, yohimbin, etc.
   – β receptors blocking drugs, e.g. propranolol, atenolol, metoprolol, butoxamine, etc.

11

Cholinergic Drugs/ Parasympathomimetic Drugs

INTRODUCTION

Cholinergic drugs produce effects similar to those of acetylcholine either acting directly on cholinergic receptors or indirectly by inhibiting the enzyme cholinesterase and causing accumulation of acetylcholine at cholinergic receptor sites. As their effects mimic (like) the effects of stimulation of parasympathetic nervous system, so they are called parasympathomimetic drugs.

Classification

These are of two groups:

i. **Directly acting cholinergic drugs (cholinergic agonists):** They act directly on cholinergic receptors.
- *Choline esters*
  e.g. Acetylcholine] Natural drug

  Methacholine⎤
  Carbachol ⎬ Synthetic drugs
  Bethanechol ⎦

- *Cholinomimetic alkaloids*
  e.g. Pilocarpine⎤
  Muscarine ⎬ Natural drugs
  Arecholine ⎦

- *Miscellaneous drugs*
  e.g. Oxotremorine ⎤ Synthetic drugs
  Metoclopramide⎦

ii. **Indirectly acting cholinergic drugs (anticholinesterases):** They act indirectly on cholinergic receptors.
- *Reversible anticholinesterases:* They produce reversible inhibition of cholinesterase.
  e.g. Physostigmine] Natural drug

  Carbamates:
  Neostigmine
  Pyridostigmine
  Rivastigmine
  Edrophonium ⎬ Synthetic drugs
  Ambenonium
  Demecarium
  Acridine:
  Tetrahydroaminoacridine⎦

- *Irreversible anticholinesterases*: They produce irreversible inhibition of cholinesterase. They are synthetic drugs. They are two groups:
  - Organophosphorus compounds, e.g. diisopropyl fluorophosphate (DFP), octamethyl pyrophosphotetramide (OMPA) and echothiophate (used as miotics in glaucoma), parathion, malathion and diazinon (used as insecticides and pesticides), tabun, sarin and soman (used as nerve gases in war field).
  - Carbamate esters, e.g. carbaryl and propoxur (used as insecticides and pesticides).

Choline Esters

Acetylcholine is an ester of choline with acetic acid. Methacholine is an ester of β-methyl-choline with acetic acid. Carbachol is an ester of choline with carbamic acid. Bethanechol is an ester of betamethylcholine with carbamic acid. The base choline also possesses properties like acetylcholine but the amount required to produce equivalent effect is large. Esterification of choline increases the activity markedly. Chemically these are quaternary ammonium compounds and their specific action is due to the presence of trimethyl-ammonium $[R{-}N^+ (CH_3)_3]$ grouping. Chemical structures of choline esters are shown in **Fig. 11.1**.

Pharmacokinetics

They are polar compounds and have low lipid solubility. They are poorly absorbed from GIT and cannot cross blood–brain barrier easily. Their hydrolysis by cholinesterase is variable. Acetylcholine is quickly hydrolyzed (and hence degraded) but methacholine is slowly hydrolyzed and carbachol and bethanechol are fairly resistant to cholinesterase.

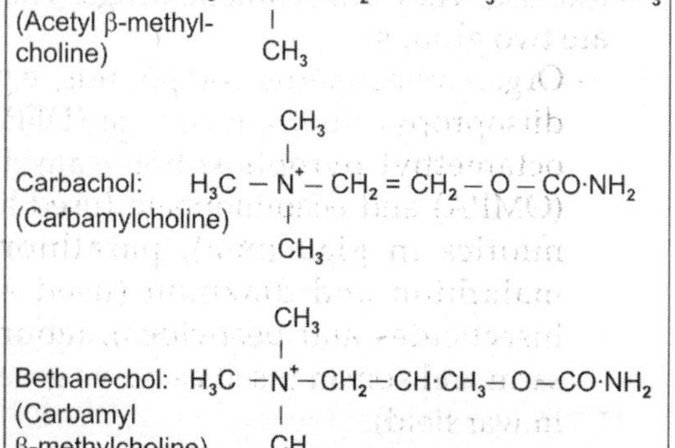

Acetylcholine: $H_3C-N^+-C_\alpha H_2-C_\beta H_2-O-CO-CH_3$ with CH_3 groups

Methacholine: $H_3C-N^+-CH_2-CH{\cdot}CH_3-O-CO{\cdot}CH_3$ with CH_3 groups
(Acetyl β-methyl-choline)

Carbachol: $H_3C-N^+-CH_2=CH_2-O-CO{\cdot}NH_2$ with CH_3 groups
(Carbamylcholine)

Bethanechol: $H_3C-N^+-CH_2-CH{\cdot}CH_3-O-CO{\cdot}NH_2$ with CH_3 groups
(Carbamyl β-methylcholine)

Fig. 11.1: Chemical structures of choline esters

DISCUSSION OF DRUGS

Acetylcholine

It is a cholinergic neurotransmitter. It is discussed as a prototype drug of cholinergic agonists. It is a natural choline ester. It has very short duration of action, because it is rapidly hydrolyzed by acetylcholinesterase to choline and acetate.

Pharmacological Actions

It has two types of actions, *viz.* muscarinic actions (like muscarine) and nicotinic actions (like nicotine). Muscarinic actions are exerted on heart muscle, smooth muscles, exocrine glands and CNS by interacting with muscarinic receptors. Nicotinic actions are exerted on autonomic ganglia, adrenal medulla, skeletal muscles and CNS by interacting with nicotinic receptors. It produces following effects:

1. *Cardiovascular effects*

   a. **On heart (M-receptors):** It depresses heart by acting on M_2 receptors in myocardium, which are inhibitory in nature. It slows heart rate (negative chronotropic action) and decreases force of cardiac contraction (negative inotropic action) leading to decrease in cardiac output. It produces hyperpolarization of the cells of SA node and decreases the rate of spontaneous diastolic depolarization. As a result, it decreases the rate of impulse generation in heart leading to brady-cardia, heart block and even cardiac arrest. It slows AV conduction velocity and increases refractory period. It shortens the duration of action potential (AP) of heart muscle. It decreases the force of atrial contraction more than that of ventricular contraction (as ventricles have little cholinergic/vagal fibres).

   b. **On blood vessels (M_3 receptors):** It relaxes vascular smooth muscles and dilates all blood vessels in the body, though only a few blood vessels (in skin of face and neck) have cholinergic innervation. When it is administered by rapid IV injection in anaesthetised animals like cat it produces sharp fall of BP and then rapid recovery (due to rapid metabolism). In contrast other choline esters produce slow recovery of BP due to slow metabolism (as shown in **Fig. 11.2**).

It produces vasodilation by interacting with M_3 receptors in blood vessels leading to release of a substance called endothelial derived relaxating factor (EDRF), which is probably nitric oxide (NO), a potent vasodilator. It also inhibits the release of noradrenaline from adrenergic nerve endings by stimulating presynaptic M_2 receptors in nerve endings.

2. *Effects on nonvascular smooth muscles (M_3 receptors)*

   a. **Eye:** It produces miosis (constriction of pupil) and spasm of accommodation (cyclospasm) of eye by interacting with M_3 receptors present in circular muscle of iris and ciliary muscle of eye respectively. As a result of contraction of circular muscle of iris, the iris becomes thin. As a result of contraction of ciliary muscle, the suspensory ligaments attached to the capsule of lens become relaxed and so anterior surface of lens is bulged out decreasing the focal length of lens. So the eye is accommodated for near vision and distant vision becomes blurred. Due to thinning of iris, the iridocorneal angle becomes widened leading to increased drainage of aqueous humour through the canal of Schlemm and other venous channels and thus decreases intraocular pressure especially in glaucoma.

   b. **Bronchus:** It causes contraction of bronchial smooth muscle, leading to bronchospasm and dyspnoea. Asthmatics are highly sensitive to it and precipitation of acute attack of bronchial asthma occurs.

   c. **GIT:** It contracts smooth muscles of GIT and increases tone and peristalsis (motor activity) but it relaxes gut sphincters. It can cause intestinal cramps and even defecation.

   d. **Urinary tract:** It contracts smooth muscles of ureters and increases tone and peristalsis. It contracts detrusor muscles of urinary bladder but relaxes trigonal sphincter. This causes urgency of urination and voiding of urine.

3. *Effects at exocrine glands (M_3 receptors):* It increases secretion of all exocrine glands, which have cholinergic innervation. It thus produces sweating, salivation, lacrimation and tracheobronchial secretion. It increases gastric secretion by acting mainly on M receptors and can aggravate peptic ulcer. It has little effect on intestinal and pancreatic secretions. It does not affect bile and milk secretion.

4. *Effects at autonomic ganglia and adrenal medulla (N_N receptors):* It stimulates both sympathetic and parasympathetic ganglia in high doses leading to release of noradrenaline and acetylcholine respectively from nerve endings. When muscarinic receptors are blocked by atropine, it produces only rise of BP by the action of noradrenaline (as

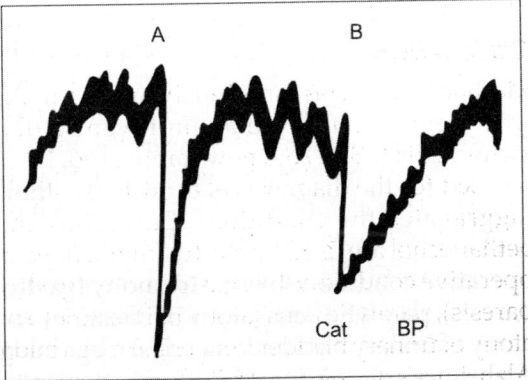

Fig. 11.2: Effects of acetylcholine (A) and carbachol (B) on anaesthetized cat BP

shown in **Fig. 11.3).** Acetylcholine released from parasympathetic ganglia then cannot cause fall of BP.

It stimulates adrenal medulla (which is embryologically a sympathetic ganglia) in high doses leading to increased secretion of adrenaline and noradrenaline.

5. *Effects at skeletal muscles (N_M receptors):* It stimulates motor end plate of skeletal muscle in high doses leading to contraction of skeletal muscle. It can produce twitchings and fasiculations of skeletal muscle when administered parenterally.

6. *CNS effects (M_1 and N_N receptors):* It cannot cross blood–brain barrier and does not produce any CNS effects when administered parenterally. When it is injected directly into the brain by intraventricular cannulation, it produces a complex pattern of stimulation and depression by acting on M_1 and N_N receptors in the brain and spinal cord.

Clinical Uses

It has no clinical use, because it has very short-lasting effect, which is widespread and nonspecific. It is used as experimental stool to demonstrate its effects on animals (cats/dogs/guinea pigs/rats, etc.). It is available as acetylcholine chloride powder for making solution.

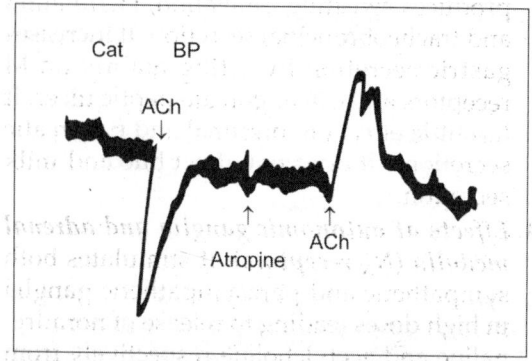

Fig. 11.3: Muscarinic and nicotinic effects of acetylcholine on anaesthetized cat BP

Adverse Reactions

These are due to extension of pharmacological actions and include flushing, headache, sweating, salivation, lacrimation, increased tracheobronchial secretion, belching, visual disturbances, urge for micturition and defecation, bradycardia, hypotension, fainting, cardiac arrhythmias, cardiac arrest and vascular collapse.

Antagonists of Acetylcholine

Adrenaline is the physiological antagonist of acetylcholine. Atropine is the competitive antagonist at muscarinic receptor sites. Hexamethonium and d-tubocurarine are competitive antagonists at nicotinic receptor sites (N_N receptors in autonomic ganglia and N_M receptors in skeletal muscles).

Other Choline Esters

These are methacholine, carbachol and bethanechol.

These are synthetic compounds. Chemically they are quaternary ammonium compounds like acetylcholine (as shown in **Fig. 11.1).** They are cholinergic agonists (acting directly on cholinergic receptors). They can be administered orally as they are absorbed from GIT to some extent. They have longer duration of action than acetylcholine, as they are resistant to cholinesterase. They have some clinical uses. Comparative pharmacological effects of choline esters are shown in **Table 11.1.**

Clinical Uses

Methacholine was previously used for the treatment of paroxysmal supraventricular tachycardia (PSVT) but now rarely used. It can be used for the diagnosis of bronchial asthma (aggravates the condition). Carbachol and bethanechol are used for the treatment of postoperative conditions like gastricatony (gastroparesis), paralytic ileus (atony of intestine) and atony of urinary bladder, congenital megacolon, Alzheimer's disease (presenile/ senile dementia) and glaucoma (as miotic drops).

Table 11.1: Comparative pharmacological effects of choline esters

Drug	Susceptibility to acetylcholines- terase	Muscarinic effects				Nicotinic effects
		CVS	GIT and UT	Eye	Sweating	
Acetylcholine	Marked (+++)	Moderate (++)	Moderate	Slight	Marked	Moderate
Methacholine	Slight (+)	Marked	Moderate	Slight	Slight	Slight
Carbachol	Nil (–)	Slight	Marked	Moderate	Slight	Marked
Bethanechol	Nil (–)	Slight	Marked	Moderate	Slight	Nil

Preparations and Dosage

- Carbachol tablet (1 mg)—1 to 4 mg daily.
- Carbachol injection (0.25 mg/ml)—0.25 to 0.5 mg SC
- Carbachol eye drops (3% soln)
- Bethanechol tablet (5 or 10 mg)—10 to 30 mg, 3–4 times daily.

Adverse Reactions

Similar to acetylcholine. Atropine sulphate is used as antidote (antagonist) in acute poisoning.

Contraindications of Choline Esters

- Bronchial asthma—as they precipitate or aggravate the condition.
- Hyperthyroidism—as they precipitate cardiac arrhythmias.
- Peptic ulcer—as they increase gastric secretion and aggravate the condition.
- Angina pectoris—as they decrease coronary blood flow and aggravate the condition.
- Myocardial infarction—as they produce hypotension and AV conduction block.

CHOLINOMIMETIC ALKALOIDS

These are pilocarpine, muscarine and arecoline. These are natural drugs acting as cholinergic agonists.

Pilocarpine

It is an alkaloid obtained from the leaves of South American shrubs—*Pilocarpus microphyllus* and *Pilocarpus jaborandi*. It is a tertiary amine and so well absorbed orally. It has prominent muscarinic actions and slight nicotinic actions. It stimulates autonomic ganglia by acting on ganglionic muscarinic (M_1) receptors. By muscarinic actions, it produces profuse salivation, lacrimation, sweating and other exocrine glands secretions. It increases tone and peristalsis of GIT and urinary tract (UT). It dilates blood vessels and causes hypotension. It can produce tachycardia and hypertension in high dosage by stimulating sympathetic ganglia. It has prominent action on eye. It produces miosis and spasm of accommodation. It lowers intraocular pressure (IOP), especially in glaucoma when applied as eye drops. By crossing blood-brain barrier it produces initial CNS stimulation followed by CNS depression.

Clinical Uses

It is too toxic for systemic use. It is mainly used as eye drops in the treatment of both narrow angle (acute congestive) glaucoma and wide angle (chronic simple) glaucoma to reduce intraocular pressure. It is also used to antagonise (reverse) the mydriatic effect of atropine and to break the adhesion between iris with cornea or lens in anterior or posterior synechia alternating with a mydriatic drops. Systemically (SC) it was previously used for the treatment of xerostomia (dryness of mouth) and high fever (by increasing sweating/diaphoresis) but now not used.

Preparation and Dosage

Pilocarpine nitrate (Pilocar) eye drops (1 to 4% soln). Pilocarpine ocusert is a drug delivery system for slow absorption of pilocarpine (over a period of seven days) but it is more costly.

Adverse Reactions

These are similar to acetylcholine but it can produce CNS toxicity after systemic use. Atropine sulphate is used as antidote (antagonist) in acute pilocarpine poisoning. (1 to 2 mg IM or IV 8 hourly).

Muscarine

It is an alkaloid obtained from the mushroom, *Amanita muscaria* or other species. It is a quaternary ammonium compound like acetylcholine. It has only muscarinic actions. It has no clinical use. It has toxicological importance, because mushroom poisoning is quite common.

Mushroom Poisoning

It occurs due to consumption (ingestion) of poisonous mushroom. It is of two types depending on the species of mushroom consumed:

- **Early onset mushroom poisoning (muscarinic type):** It occurs within ½ to 1 hour. If it is due to consumption of poisonous mushroom like *Amanita muscaria* (which contains low concentration of muscarine), then mild cholinergic symptoms like nausea, vomiting, salivation, lacrimation, headache, visual disturbances, bronchospasm, abdominal cramps and diarrhoea occur. It is treated by administration of atropine sulphate in therapeutic doses (0.5 to 1 mg IM twice daily). When it is due to consumption of poisonous mushroom like Inocyba or Clitocyba (which contain high concentration of muscarine) then severe cholinergic symptoms like bradycardia, dyspnoea, hypotension, weakness, confusion, cardiac arrhythmias, cardiovascular collapse, convulsions and coma occur. It is treated by administration of high dosage of atropine sulphate (2 to 3 mg IM every hour till improvement) and supportive measures for maintenance of respiration and BP.

- **Late (delayed) onset mushroom poisoning (neurogenic type):** It occurs within 6 to 15 hours. It is due to ingestion of poisonous mushroom like *Amanita phalloides* or related species (which contain GABA antagonists like muscimol and ibotenic acid). It is manifested by initial CNS stimulation producing irritability, restlessness, nausea, vomiting, ataxia, hallucination and delirium and later on CNS depression producing sedation, drowsiness and sleep. It has no specific treatment. Only supportive measures are done to maintain respiration and BP. To control CNS excitation diazepam (5 mg IM) may be used. Administration of atropine sulphate (IM) is contraindicated here, because it may produce convulsions and even death. Gastric lavage and administration of activated charcoal may be done to remove the poison from the gut.

Arecholine

It is an alkaloid obtained from the betel-nut, *Areca catechu*. It is a tertiary amine with ester linkage. It has both muscarinic and nicotinic actions. It has no clinical use. It has toxicological importance. Arecholine poisoning is treated by administration of atropine sulphate in therapeutic dosage (0.5 to 1 mg IM twice daily).

Miscellaneous Drugs

Oxotremorine and metoclopramide are synthetic drugs. They are muscarinic (M_1) agonists. They have no nicotinic actions. Oxotremorine is a tremor producing agent and acts by stimulation of CNS muscarinic (M_1) receptors. It is used as experimental tool to produce tremors in experimental animals like monkeys to evaluate antiparkinsonism drugs. Metoclopramide is a potent antiemetic drug which stimulates GIT muscarinic (M_1) receptors to increase the tone and peristalsis of GIT causing closure of oesophageal sphincter.

Anticholinesterases (Cholinesterase inhibitors)

These are drugs that inhibit cholinesterase, which destroys acetylcholine. They are indirectly acting cholinergic drugs, as they act through acetylcholine on cholinergic receptors at different sites. They have longer duration of action than acetylcholine. They cause accumulation of acetylcholine at cholinergic receptor sites and prevent its destruction by cholinesterase. Their classification is given with cholinergic drugs.

Chemistry: Reversible anticholinesterases bear a structural resemblance to acetylcholine. Physostigmine is a tertiary amine and lipid-soluble. Tetrahydroamine acridine is an acridine derivative and lipid-soluble. Neostigmine and other carbamates are quaternary ammonium compounds and lipid-insoluble. Of the irreversible anticholinesterases, organophosphorous compounds are highly lipid-soluble, except echothiophate which is water-soluble. Carbamates are lipid-soluble. Drugs which are lipid-soluble (lipophilic) are easily absorbed from various sites and can easily cross blood–brain barrier (BBB) to produce CNS effects.

Mechanism of Action

They act by inhibiting cholinesterase (ChE), which has two sites (anionic site and esteratic site) to bind with the substrate (acetylcholine or anticholinesterase). The binding of acetylcholine and anticholinesterases with cholinesterase and their inactivation is shown in **Fig. 11.4**. Acetylcholine binds with cholinesterase at two sites (anionic site and esteratic site) forming acetylated cholinesterase (an unstable complex). The esteratic site is freed very rapidly by hydrolysis leading to splitting of choline and acetate. Carbamates, e.g. physostigmine, neostigmine, etc. except edrophonium bind with cholinesterase at two sites (anionic site and esteratic site) forming carbamylated cholinesterase, which is relatively stable than acetylated cholinesterase and undergoes slow hydrolysis to carbamate, choline and cholinesterase. Edrophonium attaches only to anionic site of cholinesterase . and has shortest duration of action. Organophosphorous compounds, except DFP

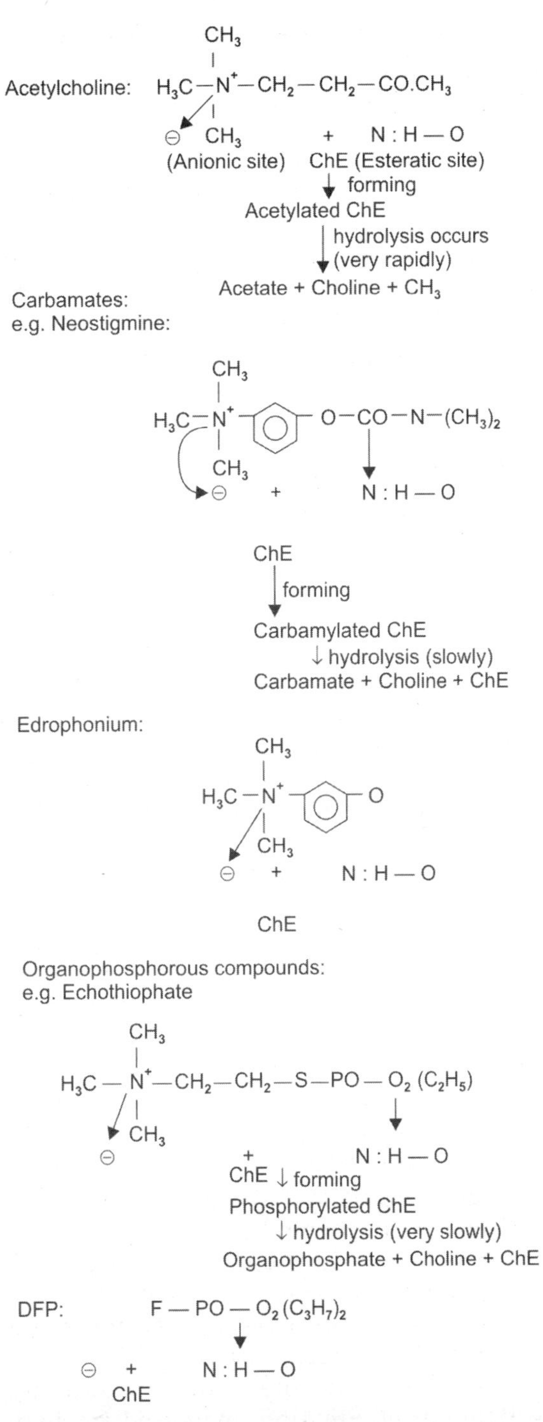

Acetylcholine: $H_3C-\overset{CH_3}{\underset{CH_3}{\overset{|}{\underset{|}{N^+}}}}-CH_2-CH_2-CO.CH_3$

(Anionic site)   ChE (Esteratic site)

$\downarrow$ forming

Acetylated ChE

$\downarrow$ hydrolysis occurs (very rapidly)

Acetate + Choline + CH$_3$

Carbamates: e.g. Neostigmine:

$H_3C-\overset{CH_3}{\underset{CH_3}{\overset{|}{\underset{|}{N^+}}}}$⟷$O-CO-N-(CH_3)_2$

ChE

$\downarrow$ forming

Carbamylated ChE

$\downarrow$ hydrolysis (slowly)

Carbamate + Choline + ChE

Edrophonium:

$H_3C-\overset{CH_3}{\underset{CH_3}{\overset{|}{\underset{|}{N^+}}}}$⟷$O$

ChE

Organophosphorous compounds: e.g. Echothiophate

$H_3C-\overset{CH_3}{\underset{CH_3}{\overset{|}{\underset{|}{N^+}}}}-CH_2-CH_2-S-PO-O_2(C_2H_5)$

ChE $\downarrow$ forming

Phosphorylated ChE

$\downarrow$ hydrolysis (very slowly)

Organophosphate + Choline + ChE

DFP: $F-PO-O_2(C_3H_7)_2$

ChE

Fig. 11.4: Binding of acetylcholine and anticholinesterases with cholinesterase and their inactivation

binds with cholinesterase at two sites (anionic site and esteratic site) forming phosphorylated cholinesterase, which is more stable than acetylated cholinesterase and undergoes very slow hydrolysis to organophosphate, choline and cholinesterase. DFP attaches to esteratic site of cholinesterase and has longest duration of action. Anionic site has negative charge and so attracts positive charge of quaternary ammonium nitrogen. Esteratic site is neucleophilic (N:H—O) and so attracts the electrophilic carbon atom of carbamyl group (–COON) of carbamate and phospharyl group of organophosphate.

DISCUSSION OF DRUGS

Reversible Anticholinesterases

Physostigmine (Eserine)

It is an alkaloid obtained from the dried ripe seed (calabar bean) of an African plant—*Physostigma venenosum*. It is a tertiary amine and lipid-soluble. It is well absorbed from GIT and can easily cross BBB. It is hydrolyzed by esterases in liver and plasma and excreted in urine. It has long-lasting action (4 to 8 hours). It is natural reversible anticholinesterase drug. It inhibits both acetylcholinesterase and butyryl cholinesterase. It acts indirectly by preventing destruction of acetylcholine released from cholinergic nerve endings by nerve stimulation and causing its accumulation at cholinergic receptor sites.

It produces muscarinic, nicotinic and CNS effects like acetylcholine. It has prominent muscarinic actions especially on eye. It produces miosis and spasm of accommodation by easily penetrating the cornea, when applied locally in the eye. It antagonizes mydriasis and cycloplegia (paralysis of accommodation) produced by atropine and other anticholinergic drugs. It increases secretion of exocrine glands producing salivation, lacrimation, increased tracheobronchial secretion and sweating. It increases tone and peristalsis of GIT and UT. It decreases heart rate and causes fall of BP (hypotension). It has less stimulant action on skeletal muscle than neostigmine and other synthetic anticholinesterase. It produces stimulation of autonomic ganglia and CNS, which is followed by depression in large dosage.

Clinical Uses

It has local and systemic uses. Locally it is used as miotic drops in the treatment of glaucoma (like pilocarpine) to reduce intraocular pressure. It is also used to antagonize (reverse) the mydriatic effect of atropine and to break the adhesion between iris and cornea or lens in anterior or posterior synechia alternation with a mydriatic drops. Systematically it is used in the treatment of belladonna (atropine) poisoning and in poisoning with phenothiazines and tricyclic antidepressants (which have anticholinergic action). It is particularly useful in patients with drug induced delirium. It is also used in Alzheimer's disease (presenile or senile dementia due to degeneration of cholinergic fibres in brain).

Preparations and Dosage

Physostigmine salicylate (Eserine) injection (2 mg/2 ml ampoule) 1 to 2 mg SC or IM and repeated after 15 minutes. If effective 2 to 4 mg may be given every 2 to 4 hours. Physostigmine salicylate eye drop (0.5 to 2% solution) or eye ointment (oculentum) is also available.

Adverse Reactions

These are similar to acetylcholine but it produces initial CNS stimulation (manifested as anxiety, restlessness, headache, giddiness, delirium and convulsions), which is followed by CNS depression (manifested as sedation, sleep and coma). Atropine sulphate is used as antidote (antagonist) in acute physostigmine poisoning (1 to 2 mg IM or IV 8 hourly).

Neostigmine

It is a synthetic anticholinesterase drug. It is a quaternary ammonium compound and lipid-insoluble. It is poorly absorbed from GIT and cannot cross BBB easily. It is hydrolyzed by esterases in liver and plasma and excreted in urine. It has short duration of action (3 to 5 hours).

It is a reversible anticholinesterase drug like physostigmine. It has also a direct action on nicotinic (N_M) receptors present in neuromuscular junction (motor end plate) of skeletal muscles. It has prominent nicotinic actions on skeletal muscles and autonomic ganglia. It is a potent anticurare drug. It antagonizes (reverses) the skeletal muscle relaxation (paralysis) produced by d-tubocurarine or other competitive neuromuscular blockers. It does not antagonize the skeletal muscle paralysis produced by succinylcholine or decamethonium (depolarizing neuromuscular blocker), where it increases the muscular paralysis by synergistic action. It stimulates autonomic ganglia in small dosage but in large dosage it blocks ganglionic transmission by persistent depolarization of ganglionic cells. It has no CNS effect.

Clinical Uses

It has only systemic uses. It is used in the treatment of myasthenia gravis to increase muscle strength. It is also used for postoperative decurarization (to reverse the skeletal muscle paralysis produced by d-tubocurarine or other competitive neuromuscular blocker) in postoperative complications (like gastric atony, paralytic ileus and urinary bladder atony) and in cobra snake bite (cobra venom has a curare-like neurotoxin). Antivenom serum is the primary treatment. Neostigmine and atropine are used to prevent respiratory muscles paralysis.

Preparations and Dosages

- Neostigmine bromide (prostigmine) tablet (15 mg)—15 to 30 mg thrice daily.
- Neostigmine methyl sulphate injection (0.5 mg/ml)—0.5 to 2 mg SC or IM.

Adverse Reactions

Adverse reactions of neostigmine are similar to acetylcholine. It has less muscarinic effects than physostigmine. It has prominent nicotinic effects on skeletal muscles and autonomic ganglia. It produces twitchings and fasciculations of muscles leading to weakness and spastic paralysis of muscles. Atropine sulphate is used as antidote (antagonist) in acute neostigmine poisoning.

Distigmine is a longer-acting neostigmine analogue. It can be used as a single daily dose (5 to 20 mg orally or IM) before breakfast.

Pyridostigmine

It is a synthetic anticholinesterase drug, which resembles neostigmine in chemical structure. It has pharmacological actions like neostigmine. It is less potent than neostigmine and has a longer duration of action.

Clinical Uses

It is used for long-term treatment of myasthenia gravis. It is claimed to be better tolerated by myasthetic patients.

Preparations and Dosages

- Pyridostigmine bromide (Destinon myastin) tablet (60 mg)— 60 to 240 mg once daily.
- Pyridostigmine methylsulphate injection (1 mg/ml)—1 to 5 mg SC or IM.

Adverse Reactions

Adverse reactions of pyridostigmine are less than neostigmine. Rivastigmine (Exless) is available as capsule (1.5, 3, 6 mg) and used once daily.

Edrophonium

It is a synthetic anticholinesterase drug. It is a quaternary ammonium compound like neostigmine. It is not absorbed from GIT. It is rapidly hydrolyzed by esterases in liver and plasma after IV injection and excreted in urine. It is the shortest-acting anticholinesterase (action persisting for only ten minutes). It has weak anticholinesterase activity as compared to neostigmine but it can increase neuromuscular transmission in small dose, which is too low to affect the smooth muscles, heart muscle and exocrine glands.

Clinical Uses

It is used for rapid postoperative decurarization (3 to 6 mg IV every 15 minutes). Edrophonium test is used for diagnostic purpose, i.e. to differentiate between myasthenic crisis and cholinergic crisis (3 mg IV produces rapid improvement/remission of myasthenia crisis but worsening/deterioration of cholinergic crisis). Cholinergic crisis is treated by atropine sulphate, pralidoxine and artifical respiration.

Preparation and Dosage

Edrophonium chloride (Tensilon) injection (10 mg/ml)—3 to 6 mg IV.

Adverse Reactions

It produces less muscarinic side effects than neostigmine which can be antagonized (reversed) by atropine sulphate.

Ambenonium

It is a synthetic anticholinesterase drug. It is a bisymmetrical quaternary ammonium compound which is more potent cholinesterase inhibitor than neostigmine. It has a more marked direct stimulant effect on skeletal muscle than neostigmine and has longer duration of action. It is used orally for long-term treatment of myasthenia gravis.

Preparation and Dosage

Ambenonium chloride (Mytelase) tablet (10 mg)— 10 to 20 mg twice daily.

Adverse Reactions

These are less than neostigmine.

Demecarium

It is a synthetic anticholinesterase drug. Structurally it is made up of two molecules of neostigmine joined through ten methylene groups. It is more potent and longer-acting than neostigmine. It is not used for the treatment of myasthenia gravis. It is used for the treatment of glaucoma, especially in resistant cases of chronic simple glaucoma for its powerful miotic action on topical instillation.

Preparation and Dosage

Demecarium bromide (Humorsol) eye drops (0.1 to 0.25% solution)—2 to 4 drops once or twice weekly.

Adverse Reactions

It can produce muscarinic side effects by passing into the nose through the nasolacrimal duct. It may rarely cause retinal detachment.

Tetrahydroaminoacridine

It is a synthetic anticholinesterase drug. It is an acridine derivative. It is lipid-soluble and can easily cross BBB. It is relatively cerebroselective anticholinesterase. It is used in Alzheimer's disease to improve memory.

Preparation and Dosage

Tetrahydroaminoacridine (Tacrine) tablet (40 mg)—40 to 80 mg twice daily.

Adverse Reactions

It can cause nausea vomiting and hepatotoxicity. Rivastigmine and donepezil are cerebroselective cholinesterase inhibitors recently introduced for the treatment of Alzheimer's disease. They are longer-acting drugs and administered once daily. They have minimum toxicity.

Irreversible Anticholinesterases

Organophosphorous compounds, e.g. DFP, echothiophate, malathion, tabun, etc. These are organic esters of phosphoric acid. They are powerful and irreversible inhibitors of cholinesterase. They inhibit butyryl cholinesterase more readily than acetylcholinesterase. They produce prolonged inhibition of both types of cholinesterase leading to accumulation of acetylcholine at cholinergic receptor sites by nerve stimulation. Their pharmacological actions are due to acetylcholine. They are lipid-soluble except echothiophate, which is water-soluble. They differ from quaternary ammonium compounds in following respects:
- They have high lipid solubility (except echothiophate).

- They can be absorbed by all routes, including intact skin, mucous membrane and lungs.
- They can easily cross BBB and produce CNS effects.
- They are inactivated (metabolized) mainly in the liver by oxidation and hydrolysis and the breakdown products are excreted in urine.

Clinical Uses

They have limited clinical uses due to their prolonged action and high toxicity. DFP and echothiophate are used as miotic drops (long-acting) in the treatment of glaucoma, especially resistant cases of chronic simple glaucoma. Other compounds are used as insecticides and pesticides in agriculture or as nerve gases in war field.

Preparations and Dosage

- DFP eye drops (0.025 to 0.05% solution in arachis oil)—1 or 2 drops applied once daily.
- Echothiophate iodide eye drops (0.05 to 0.25% soln in water)—1 or 2 drops applied once daily.

Adverse Reactions

Adverse reactions on topical use in eye—DFP can produce local irritation of eye and headache. Echothiophate causes less local irritation of eye and headache than DFP.

Organophosphorous Compound Poisoning

It is quite common due to ignorance of farmers about the correct method of handling (spraying) these compounds in agriculture as pesticides and insecticides. Acute poisoning may be occupational, accidental or suicidal due to ingestion or inhalation of the compound. It is manifested as muscarinic and nicotinic signs and symptoms of acetylcholine and also CNS effects.

1. **Muscarinic effects:** Localized exposure of eyes to the compound causes irritation of eye producing miosis, spasm of accommodation and headache. Inhalation of the compound produces bronchospasm, increased tracheobronchial secretion, cough, pulmonary oedema and a sense of tightness in the chest. Ingestion of the compound produces anorexia, nausea, vomiting, intestinal cramps, diarrhoea, excessive salivation, lacrimation, tracheobronchial secretion and sweating, constricted pupils, involuntary defecation and micturition, hypotension, bradycardia or reflex tachycardia, cardiac arrhythmias, cardiovascular collapse and respiratory failure.

2. **Nicotinic effects:** These are twitchings and fasciculations of muscles, generalized muscular weakness and a spastic type of paralysis of muscles including respiratory muscles.

3. **CNS effects:** These are excitement, restlessness, anxiety, confusion, giddiness, insomnia, ataxia, loss of reflexes, respiratory depression, convulsions and coma.

Treatment

It consists of following measures:

- **Decontamination measures:** For termination of further exposue to poison, the patient is removed from the site of exposure of the poison and placed in fresh air. Soiled clothes are removed and soiled skin, eyes and mouth are washed with water. Gastric lavage with water is done to remove poison from the stomach.

- **Supportive measures:** To maintain respiration, oxygen inhalation and in severe case; artificial respiration is given. To maintain BP and to prevent circulatory failure (shock), intravenous fluids like normal saline and vasoconstrictors like noradrenaline or dopamine are administered by IV infusion. To prevent infection, prophylactic antibiotics like ampicillin are administered. To prevent convulsions, diazepam is administered IM or IV.

- **Specific measures:** To counteract/reverse adverse effects, specific antidotes (antagonists) are administered which are:

– Anticholinergic drugs like atropine sulphate is used to counteract muscarinic and CNS effects of these compounds. Atropine sulphate is used in high dosage (2 mg IV or IM every 15 to 30 minutes).

– Cholinesterase reactivators (Oximes) like pralidoxime is used to counteract nicotinic effects, especially at neuromuscular junction (motor end plate), where atropine is ineffective. Pralidoxime chloride is used in high dosage (1 to 2 g IM or slow IV every 1 to 2 hours).

Oximes

These are synthetic drugs, e.g. pralidoxime (pyridine-2-aldoxime), obidoxime, diacetyl monoxime (DAM) and pyruvalidoxime (mono/isonitrosoacetone, MINA). These are cholinesterase reactivators used to reverse the nicotinic effects on skeletal muscles of organophosphorous compounds. They have insignificant effects on autonomic ganglia and CNS except DAM and MINA which can cross BBB.

Mechanism of Action

Organophosphorous compounds produce irreversible inhibition of cholinesterase by phosphorylation of the esteretic site of the enzyme. Oximes combine with the phosphoryl group of the phosphorylated cholinesterase by a site directed nucleophilic attack and dephosphorylate the enzyme forming a soluble complex.

This results in setting free of the phosphoryl group from the esteretic site and a reactivation of the enzyme. With the reactivation of cholinesterase, the intensified effects of acetylcholine begins to disappear. The treatment with oximes must be done within a short time (6 hours) after poisoning, because the phosphorylated cholinesterase undergoes aging process, i.e. changes to a stable complex form (by covalent bond) which cannot be reversed. So late administration of oximes is useless. Oximes are administered IV. They are metabolized mainly in liver and the breakdown products are excreted in urine.

Clinical Uses

They are used in organophosphorous compound poisoning.

Preparations and Dosage

- Pralidoxime chloride injection—1 g IV slowly and can be repeated after 1 to 2 hours.
- Obidoxime chloride injection—3 to 6 mg/kg IV slowly and can be repeated every 20 minutes (more potent than pralidoxime).
- Diacetylmonoxime chloride injection—1 to 2 g IV slowly and can be repeated after 1 to 2 hours.

Adverse Reactions

They can produce local irritation, drowsiness, giddiness, blurring of vision, diplopia, tachycardia and hypotension. In high dosage they can themselves cause neuromuscular blockade and skeletal muscle paralysis.

Chronic toxicity with organophosphorous compounds can occur due to repeated exposure to these compounds. It is manifested as peripheral neuritis (polyneuritis), demyelination of the nerve tracts of CNS and PNS, myopathy, muscular paralysis and infertility (azospermia, anovulation, etc.). There is no specific treatment for it. Recovery occurs slowly taking several years.

Diazinan (Tic–20), Carbaryl (Sevin) and Propoxur (Baygon)

They are used as insecticides and pesticides. They produce irreversible inhibition of cholinesterase. They have toxicological importance. Acute poisoning by ingestion of the poison has similar manifestations of organophosphorous compound poisoning and treated by administration of high dosage of atropine sulphate and by other supportive measures.

GLAUCOMA

Glaucoma is a condition of raised intraocular pressure (IOP) (more than 20 mmHg, which is normally 10 to 20 mmHg). It may be primary (where there is no cause/lesion) or secondary (where there is cause/lesion, e.g. iritis). Iritis produces exudation formation leading to sticking up of iris and anterior surface of lens, accumulation of aqueous humour in the posterior chamber of eye and rise of IOP. Primary glaucoma is of two types, *viz.* acute congestive (narrow angle) glaucoma and chronic simple (wide angle) glaucoma. In both types, there is obstruction of drainage of aqueous humour. Normally aqueous humour is drained by passage of it from the iridocorneal angle (situated at the lateral part of the anterior chamber of eye) to the canal of Schlemm and other venous channels. Between these channels and iridocorneal angle, the tissue consists of parallel plates like structures called trabecule, which contain holes. Aqueous humour from the anterior chamber passes through these holes and enters the canal of Schlemm and other venous channels and is thus drained. In narrow angle glaucoma, due to some reason, a portion of iris occupies the iridocorneal angle leading to impaired drainage of aqueous humour and very high rise of IOP. This may produce retinal damage and even blindness. In wide or open angle glaucoma, the blockage is due to misalignment of the trabecule obstructing the drainage of aqueous humour. It is a degenerative condition in which the patency of the trabecular meshwork is disrupted reducing the drainage of aqueous humour.

Treatment

Physostigmine, DFP, echothiophate or demecarium (eye drops), β-adrenergic blockers (timolol, betaxolol or levopunolol eye drops), carbonic anhydrase inhibitors (acetazolamide as tablet, dorzolamide eye drops) and osmotic diuretics (mannitol 20% soln or glycerol 10% soln—100 ml by IV infusion).

Acute congestive (narrow angle) glaucoma is a medical emergency. It is treated by application of miotic drops in eye, initially every ten minutes and then at longer intervals. A combination of pilocarpine nitrate (2%) with physostigmine salicylate (1% solution) is preferred. Acetazolamide (a carbonic anhy-

drase inhibitor) is used orally (0.25 to 1 g daily) as adjuvant to lower IOP. Osmotic diuretics like mannitol (20% soln) or glycerol. (10% soln) is used by IV infusion in severe cases. Once the attack is controlled a definitive surgery (partial iridectomy or sclerocorneal trepining by a special needle) is advised. Chronic simple (wide angle) glaucoma is treated by application of miotic drops (pilocarpine nitrate (2% solution), physostigmine salicylate (0.5% solution), demecarium bromide (0.25% solution), DFP (0.05% solution), echothiophate (0.25% solution) or beta adrenergic blocker drops (timolol maleate (0.5% solution)/ betaxolol hydrochloride (0.3% solution) and acetazolamide orally as an adjuvant.

MYASTHENIA GRAVIS

Myasthenia gravis (*Myo* means "muscle", *asthenia* means "weakness" and *gravis* means "great") is an autoimmune disease of skeletal muscle at neuromuscular junction (motor end plate) causing defective synaptic transmission. There is development of antibodies for nicotinic (N_M) receptors at motor end plate causing decrease in the number of N_M receptors by structural damage of the motor end plate. It is manifested as progressive skeletal muscular weakness and easy fatigability of muscles with intermittent periods of exacerbation.

Treatment

Drugs used in myasthenia gravis are anticholinesterases (neostigmine, pyridostigmine or ambenonium), adjuvant drugs (ephedrine or potassium chloride) and immune suppressants (prednisolone, azathioprine cyclophosphamide or cyclosporine). For acute therapy (short-term treatment). Neostigmine is the drug of choice in myasthenia gravis. It is administered orally as neostigmine bromide tablet in the dosage of 15 to 30 mg thrice daily and gradually increasing the dose. Its disadvantages are short duration of action (3 to 5 hours), development of tolerance and waxing and waning of muscle strength. For long-term treatments, drugs like pyridostigmine bromide (60 to 240 mg orally once daily) and amebenonium chloride (10 to 20 mg orally twice daily) are used. Ephedrine sulphate (15 to 30 mg orally thrice daily) and potassium chloride (1 to 2 g orally thrice daily) are often used as adjuvants to anticholinesterase in myasthenia gravis. Immunosuppressants like glucocorticoids (e.g. prednisolone 30 to 60 mg orally once daily), azathioprine cyclophosphamide or cyclosporine have been found effective in some patients who cannot be controlled adequately by anticholinesterases and adjuvant drugs. Plasmaparesis (to remove the causative antibodies from the plasma) may be tried in resistant cases.

Thymectomy may produce improvement in majority of cases of myasthenia gravis. Thymus contains modified muscle cells with N_M receptors on their surfaces, which may be the source of antigen for production of anti-N_M receptor antibodies in myasthenic patients.

12

Anticholinergic Drugs/ Parasympatholytic Drugs

INTRODUCTION

Anticholinergic drugs antagonise (block) the actions of acetylcholine on muscarinic receptors at different sites. They are also called antimuscarinic drugs, muscarinic blockers (antagonists) and cholinergic blocking drugs (antagonists). They are competitive and equilibrium or reversible antagonists of acetylcholine at muscarinic receptor sites.

Classification

These are of three groups:

- Natural drugs, e.g. belladonna alkaloids like atropine and scopolamine (hyoscine).
- Semisynthetic atropine/scopolamine derivatives, e.g. atropine methonitrate, homatropine hydrobromide (produce mydriasis and cycloplegia), homatropine methylbromide, scopolamine butylbromide, scopolamine methylbromide and eucatropine hydrochloride (produce mydriasis, but no cycloplegia).
- Synthetic atropine substitutes:
  - Used as mydriatics and cycloplegics in eye, e.g. cyclopentolate, tropicamide and dibutoline (produce mydriasis and cycloplegia).
  - Used as antispasmodics (spasmolytics) and antisecretory drugs.

i. Tertiary amines (lipid-soluble), e.g. Dicyclomine, oxyphencyclimine, flavoxate, oxybutynine, pirenzepine and telenzepine (selective M_1 blockers).

ii. Quaternary ammonium compounds (lipid-insoluble), e.g. propantheline, methantheline, oxyphenonium, penthienate, isopropamide, pipenzolate and glycopyrrolate.

  - Used in chronic obstructive pulmonary disease (COPD), e.g. ipratropium and tiotropium.
  - Used in parkinsonism, e.g. trihexyphenidyl (benzhexol), cycrimine, procyclidine, biperiden and benztropine.

Besides these drugs, some other drugs also possess atropine like anticholinergic activity, e.g.

i. Phenothiazines like chlorpromazine and thioridazine.

ii. Tricyclic antidepressants like imipramine and amitriptyline.

iii. Antihistaminics like promethazine and diphenylhydramine.

iv. Antiarrhythmics like quinidine and disopyramide.

v. Narcotic analgesics like pethidine and fentanyl.

Belladonna Alkaloids

These are atropine (dl-hyoscyamine) and scopolamine (l-hyoscine). Atropine is obtained from the plants *Atropa belladonna* and *Datura stramonium* and scopolamine is obtained from the plants *Hyoscyamus niger* and *Scopolia carniolica*, which are solanaceae plants. The word belladonna means "beautiful lady." It is derived from the practice of Italian ladies to dilate their pupils by applying extract of belladonna leaves to their eyes to make them look beautiful. The word atropa is derived from *atropos*, who performed the unglorious act of cutting the thread of life.

Chemistry

Atropine is an organic ester of tropic acid with the base tropine and scopolamine is an organic ester of tropic acid with the base scopine. Scopolamine differs from atropine by the presence of an oxygen bridge between carbons of the organic base (as shown in **Fig. 12.1**).

The plant synthesizes only the levorotatory isomers, which are much more active than the dextroforms. To ensure a consistent, stable product, l-hyoscyamine is recemized to dl-mixture before it is marketed as atropine.

Pharmacokinetics

Atropine and scopolamine are readily absorbed from GIT following oral administration and also absorbed from mucous membranes like conjunctiva. They are widely distributed in the body after absorption. They can cross BBB and placental barrier. They are secreted in milk and saliva. Although they are esters, but they are not hydrolyzed by cholinesterase. They are about 50% plasma protein bound. They are metabolized in the liver to the extent of 50% and are excreted in urine mainly as glucuronides. About 50% is excreted unchanged in urine. They have a plasma half-life of 4 to 12 hours but their effects in eye persist for 3 to 7 days.

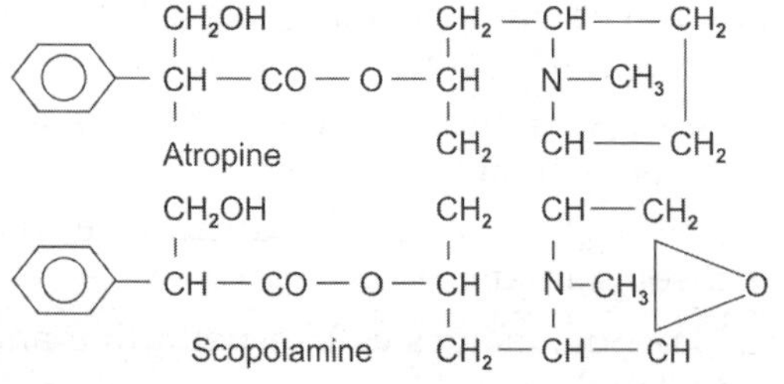

Pharmacological Actions

Mechanism of Action

They are nonselective, competitive and reversible antagonists of acetylcholine at muscarinic receptor sites. They do not interfere with the release of acetylcholine at the cholinergic nerve endings. They are more effective in blocking the effects of externally administered acetylcholine than the effects of cholinergic nerve stimulation. The dose of the drug required to produce muscarinic blockade varies from organ to organ. Thus, salivary secretion is extremely sensitive to atropine blockade, while the smooth muscle of GIT, the eye and the heart are less sensitive to atropine blockade and a relatively large doses are required to produce same effect. Although atropine can completely antagonize the effects of choline esters on the GIT, but it cannot completely antagonize the effects of vagal stimulation. In very large dosage, it can block the nicotinic action of acetylcholine at the autonomic ganglia, though it is a specific inhibitor of muscarinic effects.

Pharmacological Effects

These are qualitatively similar in atropine and scopolamine except a few differences, which are:

- Atropine is a CNS stimulant, while scopolamine is a CNS depressant producing sedation.

- Atropine has more prominent effects on the heart, GIT and bronchial smooth muscle, while scopolamine has more prominent effects on the iris, ciliary body and salivary, bronchial and sweat secretions.

- Atropine has longer duration of action than scopolamine. They produce following effects:

Fig. 12.1: Chemical structures of atropine and scopolamine

1. **Effects on exocrine secretions:** They reduce secretions of all exocrine glands except milk secretion by mammary glands. They decrease salivary secretion causing dryness of mouth (xerostomia), lacrimal secretion causing dryness of conjunctiva, tracheobronchial secretion causing dryness of respiratory tract and sweat secretion causing dry and hot skin. They inhibit gastric secretion (gastric HCl, pepsin and mucus secretion and volume of gastric juice), which is more marked when induced by cholinergic drugs. They do not inhibit gastric secretion induced by histamine, caffeine, nicotine or alcohol. They have insignificant effects on intestinal, pancreatic and biliary secretions, which are controlled by noncholinergic neurons and local hormones (secretin, pancreozymin and cholecytokinin).

2. **Effects at nonvascular smooth muscles**
   a. **Eye:** On local instillation, they produce mydriasis (dilatation of pupil) and cycloplegia (paralysis of visual accommodation). Mydriasis is due to blocking of muscarinic receptors (M_3) in the circular muscle of iris (sphincter pupillae) causing its relaxation and thus leading to unopposed sympathetic activity of the radial muscle of iris (dilator pupillae) causing its contraction. This leads to thickening of peripheral part of iris, narrowing or iridocorneal angle, prevention of drainage of aqueous humour and rise of intraocular pressure. Cycloplegia is due to blocking of muscarinic receptors (M_3) in the ciliary muscle leading to relaxation (paralysis) of ciliary muscle and thus causing tightening (increased tension) of suspensory ligaments attached to the lens capsule producing flattening of anterior curvature of lens. As a result the focal length of lens is increased making the distant vision clear and near vision blurred. So the eye is accommodated for distant vision. A person can see distant objects but cannot see near objects (cannot read newspaper). Light reflex is abolished and photophobia may occur. In elderly persons with narrow iridocorneal angle of anterior chamber of eye, an attack of acute congestive glaucoma may be precipitated due to impaired drainage of aqueous humour.

   b. **Gastrointestinal tract:** They decrease both the tone and motility of all parts of GIT resulting in prolongation of gastric emptying time, closure of sphincters and reduced intestinal movements (both propulsive and nonpropulsive). They can produce constipation by slowing the passage of chyme through the gut. They antagonize the spasmogenic action of morphine on small and large intestines and also completely abolish the excessive motility produced by cholinergic drugs.

   c. **Biliary tract:** They have a mild antispasmodic action on the biliary tract and the gallbladder. Their action on biliary sphincter is unpredictable.

   d. **Respiratory tract:** They cause bronchodilatation by relaxing smooth muscles of bronchi and bronchioles. They are particularly effective in relieving bronchoconstriction produced by cholinergic drugs. They are much less potent than adrenaline in relieving histamine induced bronchoconstriction. They reduce airway resistance in asthmatics but they are not useful in bronchial asthma, where other spasmogens like histamine, 5-HT, bradykinin, leukotrienes (LTs) and prostaglandins are involved besides acetylcholine. Moreover, they cause drying of bronchial secretion leading to accumulation of viscid and tenacious sputum in the bronchial tree, which is difficult to expectorate.

   e. **Urinary tract:** They have antispasmodic action on urinary tract. They decrease normal as well as drug induced ureteral peristalsis. They dilate renal pelvis and ureters, which is useful in relieving renal or ureteric colic. They relax detrusor muscles of urinary bladder but contract trigonal sphincter and may cause urinary retention especially in elderly males with prostatic enlargement (hyperplasia/hypertrophy).

f. **Genital tract:** They have insignificant effects on the tone and motility of the uterus, as myometrium contains small number of muscarinic receptors, although it has cholinergic innervation.

3. **Cardiovascular effects:** In therapeutic doses, they may cause a transient bradycardia (decrease in heart rate) due to their partial agonist action of acetylcholine or stimulation of the medullary vagal centres. This effect is followed by tachycardia (increase in heart rate) due to blocking of inhibitory effects of vagus nerve on the heart (by blocking M_2 receptors). This is particularly seen in young individuals who have a high vagal tone. In old people and infants this is not seen even in high doses due to low vagal tone. They rarely produce cardiac arrhythmias. They antagonize (abolish) the effects of cholinergic drugs on the heart. They have insignificant direct effects on peripheral blood vessels and BP. Even at high doses, BP and cardiac output are not altered because of compensatory haemodynamic mechanism. They can completely antagonize (reverse) peripheral vasodilatation and fall of BP produced by cholinergic drugs.

4. **CNS effects:** They interfere with muscarinic cholinergic transmission in the brain resulting in mild sedation, dysphoria or severe toxic psychoses depending on the dose. In therapeutic doses atropine causes mild CNS stimulation while scopolamine produces CNS depression leading to sedation. Atropine in moderate doses controls the tremors and rigidity in parkinsonism and in high doses produces restlessness, excitement, disorientation, irritability, hallucinations and delirium. In contrast to atropine, scopolamine in therapeutic doses produces depression of reticular activating system (RAS) causing sedation, euphoria, drowsiness, amnesia and dreamless sleep with a reduction in REM sleep. The sleep lasts for 1 to 2 hours. It also relieves motion sickness by blocking muscarinic (M_1) receptors in the motor cortex and vestibular apparatus of internal ear.

5. **Other effects:** They have some effects on autonomic ganglia but no effect on skeletal muscles. In therapeutic doses, they can produce partial block of ganglionic transmission by blocking M_1 receptors in the ganglia. In high doses, they produce complete block of ganglionic transmission by blocking N_N receptors in the ganglia. They have no effect on N_M receptors in the neuromuscular junction (motor end plate) of skeletal muscles. They can produce hyperthermia, particularly in children in high doses by inhibiting sweat secretion completely.

Clinical Uses (Indications)

They have following uses:

1. **Ocular uses:** They are used as given below:

a. Locally as eye drops or ointment to produce mydriasis and cycloplegia for fundoscopic examination of eye and to measure refractive error of eye (lens) for fitting of glasses.

b. In the treatment of acute iritis, iridocyclitis and keratitis to relieve pain in these conditions by relaxing the inflammed muscles of iris and ciliary body.

c. For prevention of anterior or posterior synechia alternating with miotic drops/ointment to break the adhesion between the iris and the lens or the cornea (due to inflammation and exudation of iris in iritis).

When maximum cycloplegia is desired, e.g. in correction of accommodative esophoria, i.e. convergent/internal strabismus (squint) producing double vision (diplopia) by deviation of axis of vision of one eye towards the other, atropine is preferred. Otherwise, short-acting atropine substitutes like homatropine may be used. Atropine is also preferred in children (due to stronger and long-lasting effect).

2. **Gastrointestinal uses:** They are used as spasmolytics to control hypermotility and colicky pain associated with diarrhoea and dysenteries. In biliary colic they are not very effective. They may relieve constipation due to spastic state of the bowel induced by morphine and lead. They were previously used in the treatment of peptic ulcer for antisecretory and antispasmodic effects but nowadays H_2-blockers (ranitidine/famotidine) and proton pump inhibitors (omeprazole/lansoprazole) are preferred due to less side effects and better acceptance by the patients.

3. **Cardiac uses:** They are useful in abolishing heart (A-V) block due to excessive vagal activity, e.g. bradyarrhythmias following myocardial infarction, cerebral strokes or head injuries or induced by cholinergic agonists like succinylcholine and general anaesthetics like ether. They are used in digitalis toxicity to control bradyarrhythmias. They are also used to counteract syncope and bradycardia in partial heart block (Stokes-Adams syndrome) due to hypersensitive carotid sinus. They may be occasionally useful in the diagnosis of accelerated AV conduction (as in Wolff-Parkinson-White syndrome) by normalizing the QRS complex duration. Atropine is more active in accelerating heart rate (thereby preventing bradycardia), whereas scopolamine (which may slow heart rate) is preferred when tachycardia must be avoided as in patients with mitral stenosis.

4. **Anaesthetic uses:** They are used as preanaesthetic medication. They reduce the stimulation of salivary and tracheobronchial secretions caused by inhalation of anaesthetics like ether and by neuromuscular blocker, succinylcholine. In addition, they prevent bradycardia, hypotension and even cardiac arrest that may result from anaesthesia or surgical procedures. For women in labour, scopolamine is preferred than atropine because it can produce tranquilization and amnesia and when combined with an opioid (e.g. pethidine) can produce a soporific state known as twilight sleep. Scopolamine has a significant sedative effect and may reduce postoperative nausea and vomiting but it produces more CNS symptoms like dizziness, hallucinations and delayed awakening from general anaesthesia, especially in elderly patients. Both atropine and scopolamine readily cross BBB and may produce the syndrome of emergence delirium in postoperative patients. For this reason, the quaternary ammonium compound glycopyrrolate, which cannot easily cross BBB and has minimum central cholinergic blocking effects is more preferred than atropine and scopolamine as preanaesthetic medication in elderly patients.

5. **Other uses:** Atropine is useful in mushroom poisoning due to muscarine. It is also used in poisoning due to cholinergic agonists, organophosphorus compounds and other anticholinesterases. Atropine and its substitutes especially flavoxate and oxybutynine are used in ureteric colic (to relieve pain) and urinary incontinence. Centrally acting atropine substitutes like trihexyphenidyl, procyclidine, benztropine are used in parkinsonism to reduce tremors and rigidity by antimuscarinic action. Scopolamine is one of the best preventives of motion sickness. It prevents nausea and vomiting in this condition by central sedative action and blocking of muscarinic (M_1) receptors in the cholinergic from the vestibular apparatus of internal ear to the vomiting centre.

Preparations and Dosage

- Atropine sulphate injection (0.6 mg/ml)— 0.6 to 2 mg SC or IM.

- Atropine sulphate tablet (0.6 mg)—0.6 to 2 mg 2 to 3 times daily.
- Atropine sulphate ointment or eye drop (0.5 to 1%).
- Scopolamine hydrobromide injection (0.3 mg/ml)—0.3 to 0.6 mg SC.
- Scopolamine hydrobromide tablet (0.3 mg)—0.3 to 0.6 mg 3 to 4 times daily.

Contraindications

These are given as follows:
- Narrow angle glaucoma in elderly patients, as they precipitate an acute attack of congestive glaucoma.
- Enlarged prostate in elderly patients, as they cause acute retention of urine due to closure of trigonal sphincter.
- Bronchial asthma and COPD, as they aggravate these conditions by reducing and drying of respiratory secretions.
- CCF with tachycardia, as they increase tachycardia and may cause anginal attack or even myocardial infarction by increasing workload and oxygen demand of the myocardium.
- Pyloric obstruction (stenosis), as they aggravate the condition by causing closure of pyloric sphincter.

Adverse Reactions

They are generally safe drugs. Their adverse effects are due to extension of pharmacological effects and are usually not serious (life-threatening). Common side effects are dryness of mouth, thirst, difficulty in swallowing, blurring of vision, photophobia, tachycardia, urinary hesitency, dizziness, fatigue and fever (hot and flushed skin). More serious adverse effects are visual disturbances, aggravation of glaucoma and marked urinary retention if the urine flow is partly obstructed due to hypertrophy of prostrate.

Acute Poisoning

It may occur accidentally by ingestion of leaves/roots of *Atropa belladonna* or seeds/ leaves of *Datura stramonium* or due to overdose of atropine/scopolamine or drugs possessing atropine-like activity. The symptoms and signs (manifestations) are mainly due to peripheral muscarinic blockade actions and CNS actions.

Peripheral effects include hot and dry skin (due to inhibition of sweating), dryness of mouth, difficulty in swallowing, intense thirst, blurring of vision, photophobia, tachycardia, palpitation, flushing, hyperthermia, urinary urgency, difficulty in micturition and even retention of urine. A rash may appear over the face, neck and upper part of the trunk leading to desquamation of skin.

Central effects include initial CNS stimulation producing excitement, restlessness, motor incoordination (ataxia), slurring of speech, disturbance of memory, confusion, hallucinations and delirium, and with very high doses convulsions. In severe poisoning CNS depression follows initial excitement leading to vasomotor centre depression, respiratory depression, coma, cardiovascular collapse and respiratory failure (due to paralysis of the respiratory centre).

The signs of acute toxicity may persist for few hours to several days.

Treatment

This includes gastric lavage (to limit further absorption of the poison from GIT if ingested), administration of antidote physostigmine salicylate (1 to 2 mg SC or IM every 2 hours till improvement) to counteract the peripheral and central effects of the poison and supportive measures to maintain respiration and BP. Ice bag or cold sponging is used to control hyperpyrexia. Diazepam (10 mg IV or IM) is used to control excitement, delirium and convulsions.

Chronic Poisoning

It is manifested by dryness of mouth, skin eruptions, tremors and speech disturbances. It subsides gradually on discontinuation of the drug.

Semisynthetic and Synthetic Atropine Substitutes

As atropine is a nonselective muscarinic blocker and produces many adverse effects in therapeutic dosage, so atropine substitutes were introduced which have selectivity in action when used locally and systemically producing less adverse effects. They are used mainly for their prominent actions. These are:

1. Mainly used in eye as mydriations and cycloplegic

They have shorter duration of action and selectively more mydriatic and cycloplegic action than atropine.

Homatropine

It is a semisynthetic derivative of atropine. It is an ester of mandelic acid with the base tropine. It has similar onset of action as atropine but has shorter duration of action than atropine and the effects persist for 1 or 2 days (in case of atropine 3 to 7 days). It does not produce complete cycloplegia and is not preferred in children. It produces less rise of intraocular pressure in comparison to atropine. It is used in ophthalmoscopic examination of retina when mydriasis with less cycloplegia is required.

Preparation: Homatropine hydrobromide (Homarin) eye drops (1 to 2% solution).

Cyclopentolate

It is a synthetic substitute of atropine. It is a superior mydriatic and cycloplegic than homatropine. It has rapid onset of action and shorter duration of action than atropine and the effects persist for 12 to 24 hours. It can increase the intraocular pressure and can produce restlessness, disorientation, ataxia, amnesia and hallucinations in children.

Preparation: Cyclopentolate (Mydrilate) eye drops (0.5 to 1% solution).

Tropicamide

It is a synthetic substitute of atropine. It is a superior mydriatic and cycloplegic than homatropine. It has rapid onset of action and

shorter duration of action than atropine and the effects persist for 1 or 2 days.

Preparation: Tropicamide (Tropisyn) eye drops (0.5 to 1% solution).

Other mydriatic and cycloplegic preparations:

- Eucatropine hydrochloride eye drops (2 to 5% soln).
- Atropine methonitrate eye drops (0.5 to 1% soln).
- Dibutoline eye drops (5 to 10% soln).

2. Mainly used as antisecretory drugs in peptic ulcer.

Pirenzepine

It is a synthetic substitute of atropine. It is a tertiary amine. It is a selective M_1 receptor blocker. It blocks gastric secretion in doses at which other antimuscarinic effects like mydriasis, inhibition of gastric emptying and tachycardia do not occur. It is used in peptic ulcer either alone or in combination with a H_2-blocker.

Preparation and Dosage

- Pirenzepine (Gastrozepin) tablet (50 mg)— 50 mg twice or thrice daily.

  It can produce dryness of mouth, blurring of vision and constipation as side effects.
- Telenzepine is more potent than pirenzepine and is used in dosage of 3 mg once daily. It has pharmacological properties like pirenzepine.

3. Mainly used as antispasmodics (spasmolytic) in peptic ulcer and intestinal colic.

Dicyclomine

It is a synthetic atropine substitute. It is a tertiary amine. It has direct spasmolytic action. It is used in peptic ulcer, infantile pyloric stenosis, intestinal colic and motion sickness. It has relatively less side effects.

Preparations and Dosage

- Dicyclomine (Colimex; Decolic) tablet (10 mg) — 10 to 20 mg twice or thrice daily.
- Dicyclomine syrup (10 mg/5 ml) — 5 to 10 mg twice or thrice daily in children.

Propantheline

It is a synthetic atropine substitute. It is a quaternary ammonium compound. It has antisecretory, antispasmodic and ganglion blocking actions. It is used in peptic ulcer, diverticulitis (to relieve pain) and diarrhoea. It is now less used because its chronic use can produce adverse effects like dryness of mouth, impotence, postural, hypotension and urinary retention. It has no central effect.

Preparation and Dosage

Propantheline bromide (Probanthine) tablet (15 mg)—15 to 30 mg thrice daily.

Oxyphenonium

It is a synthetic atropine substitute. It is a quaternary ammonium compound. It has a higher ratio of ganglion blocking activity to antimuscarinic activity than majority of other synthetic atropine substitutes. It is mainly used as antispasmodic in peptic ulcer and intestinal colic. It is now less used because its chronic use can produce adverse effects like propantheline. It has no central effect.

Preparation and Dosage

Oxyphenonium bromide (Antrenyl) tablet (10 mg) — 10 to 20 mg twice or thrice daily.

Isopropamide

It is a synthetic atropine substitute. It is a quaternary ammonium compound. It has antimuscarinic and ganglion blocking actions. It is used in peptic ulcer and diarrhoea. It has adverse effects like propantheline.

Preparation and Dosage

Isopropamide (Stelabid) tablet (5 mg) — 5 to 10 mg twice daily.

Other drugs: Methantheline (Banthine), hyoscine-N-butylbromide (Buscopan), pipenzolate (Piptal), melevoine hydrochloride, colaspa, etc.

4. **Mainly used as antispasmodics (spasmolytic) in urinary disorders.**

Flavoxate

It is a synthetic atropine substitute. It is a tertiary amine. It has anticholinergic, analgesic and local anaesthetic actions. It has a direct relaxant action on smooth muscle. It is used to treat dysuria, suprapubic pain and urinary urgency and increased frequency of urination in cystitis, prostatitis and arthritis.

Preparation and Dosage

Flavoxate (Urispan) tablet (100 mg)— 100 to 200 mg 2 to 3 times daily.

Oxybutynin

It has pharmacological properties and uses like flavoxate. It is more potent than flavoxate.

Preparation and Dosage

Oxybutynin (Ditropan) tablet (5 mg) — 5 to 10 mg 2 to 3 times daily.

5. **Mainly used in bronchial asthma, and pulmonary disease (COPDs), e.g. ipratropium bromide and tiotropium bromide as inhalation (aerosol). Discussed in respiratory system.**

6. **Mainly uses as antiparkinsonism drugs, e.g. trihexyphenydyl, cycrimine, procyclidine, biperiden and benztropine.**

These act by blocking cholinergic activity in the basal ganglia of brain which is increased in parkinsonism. Discussed in CNS.

13

Neuromuscular Blocking Agents

INTRODUCTION

Neuromuscular blockers block neuro-muscular transmission of acetylcholine by occupying nicotinic muscular (N_M) receptors at motor end plate of neuromuscular junction and produce relaxation (paralysis) of skeletal (voluntary) muscles. They are peripherally acting muscle relaxants affecting muscle tone and contraction. They are used as adjuvants to general anaesthesia to produce adequate muscle relaxation during light anaesthesia. Skeletal muscle relaxants are broadly divided into three groups:

- Peripherally acting muscle relaxants, (neuromuscular blockers), e.g. d-tubo-curarine, gallamine and succinyl choline.
- Centrally acting muscle relaxants, and others, e.g. diazepam, mephenesin and others baclofen (GABA derivative).
- Directly acting muscle relaxants, e.g. dantrolene and quinine.

Physiology of Skeletal Muscle Contraction

The process of skeletal muscle contraction consists of:

- Release of acetylcholine in relatively large amounts from the synaptic vesicles of the motor nerve endings into the synaptic cleft as a result of nerve impulse.
- Acetylcholine released into the synaptic cleft then combines with the nicotinic muscular (N_M) receptors on the motor end

plate. This combination results in the production of a localized depolarization (due to influx of Na^+ and efflux of K^+ ions from the motor end plate) and the development of an end plate potential (EPP).

- When the end plate potential reaches a sufficient magnitude, the surrounding area of the muscle fibre membrane is excited, resulting in the development of muscle action potential (MAP), which initiates contraction of the muscle (with the release of Ca^{2+} ion from the sarcoplasmic reti-culum).
- Acetylcholine is rapidly hydrolyzed by the enzyme cholinesterase and so repolari-zation of the motor end plate and the muscle fibre membrane (by reversal of ionic fluxes) occurs. The repolarized muscle is now capable of responding to a fresh nerve impulse.

Classification of Neuromuscular Blockers

These are two groups:

1. **Competitive (stabilizing) blockers:** These are of following types:
   - Long-acting drugs (1 to 2 hours), e.g. d-tubocurarine, dimethyltubocurarine, gallamine, pancuronium, alcuronium, doxacuronium and pipecuronium.
   - Intermediate-acting drugs (30 to 50 minutes), e.g. vecuronium, atracurium, rocuronium and rapacuronium.

- Short-acting drugs (10 to 20 minutes), e.g. mivacurium.
2. **Depolarizing (noncompetitive) blockers:** Succinylcholine (Suxamethonium) and decamethorium (C_{10}). These are ultrashort-acting drugs (5 to 15 minutes).

Mechanism of Neuromuscular Blocking by these Drugs

Competitive neuromuscular blockers are competitive antagonists of acetylcholine at nicotinic muscular (N_M) receptors of the motor end plate. They prevent depolarization of the motor end plate by acetylcholine by occupying N_M receptors and produce flaccid paralysis of skeletal muscles. About 90% of these receptors are to be blocked to produce failure of neuromuscular transmission. Anticholinesterase drugs like neostigmine reverse the effect of these drugs by increasing the concentration of acetylcholine (agonist) at the motor end plate. Gallamine also inhibits neuronal release of acetylcholine by acting on presynaptic muscarinic M_2 receptors. Depolarizing blockers produce persistent (prolonged) depolarization of the motor end plate, so that acetylcholine cannot act on it to produce response. There is no further generation of action potential (AP) after the initial twitchings and fasciculations and there is loss of electrical excitability at the motor end plate. They cause transient spastic paralysis of skeletal muscles followed by flaccid paralysis in man, but only spastic paralysis in chicken (due to species variation). Anticholinesterases like neostigmine cannot reverse their effect on the skeletal muscles, rather increase the block.

Clinical Uses of Neuromuscular Blockers

- They are widely used to produce skeletal muscle relaxation during surgery. They act as adjuvants to general anaesthetics to obtain relaxation of skeletal muscles particularly of the abdominal wall, so that operative manipulations are facilitated. They reduce the dose of general anaesthetic required and so a lighter level of anae-

sthesia is sufficient for doing operation. This minimizes the risk of respiratory and cardiovascular depression and postanaesthetic complications (by shortening postoperative recovery period). Long- or intermediate-acting neuromuscular blockers are used for this purpose.

- They are used to produce muscle relaxation during endotracheal intubation and in various orthopedic manipulations like correction of dislocation and setting of fractures and also in short diagnostic procedures like laryngoscopy, bronchoscopy, oesophagoscopy and endoscopy. Short-acting neuromuscular blockers are preferred here.

- They are also used during electroconvulsive therapy (ECT) and electroshock therapy (EST) in psychiatric disorders to prevent convulsions and trauma to the patients. A short-acting neuromuscular blocker with diazepam is preferred here.

- They can be used in severe cases of tetanus and status epilepticus, which are not controlled by diazepam or other drugs. A long- or intermediate-acting neuromuscular blocker is preferred here.

Administration of neuromuscular blockers: They are administered parenterally, usually intravenously. They are potentially hazardous drugs and so they should be administered to patients only by anaesthesiologists in the operation theatre, where facilities for respiratory and cardiovascular resuscitations such as respiratory pump, artificial pacemaker and defebrillator are available.

DISCUSSION OF INDIVIDUAL NEUROMUSCULAR BLOCKERS

Competitive (Stabilizing) Neuromuscular Blockers

d-tubocurarine

It is a dextrorotatory quaternary ammonium compound. It is a natural alkaloid (cyclic benzyl-isoquinoline) obtained from the plants *Chondrodendron tomentosum* and *Strychnos lethalis* that grow in Amazon region of South

America. Crude extract of curare (generic name) is a dark brown gummy mass of resinoid character and soluble in water. It is called tubo, because the native people of Amazon region used to carry it in bamboo tubes. They used it as arrow poison for hunting of wild animals. The flesh of these hunted animals can be eaten without any risk, as tubocurarine is not absorbed from GIT.

Pharmacokinetics

It is not absorbed orally and so it is administered parenterally, usually IV. It is not metabolized in the liver. About 50% of it is excreted unchanged in urine and the rest is excreted through bile. It cannot cross BBB and placental barrier. It can be safely used in obstetric surgery.

Pharmacological Actions

Mechanism of action discussed previously. It produces following effects:

- **Effects at skeletal muscles:** It initially produces weakness of muscles, which is followed by flaccid paralysis of muscles. The smaller muscles, which subserve rapid fine movements are more sensitive to it than the larger and stronger muscles, which subserve slow coarse movement. Sequence of muscle paralysis:
  - Small muscles of fingers, toes, eyes, ears, face, pharynx and larynx are affected first making it impossible to perform delicate motor tasks and producing diplopia, slurred speech and difficulty in swallowing.
  - Large muscles of limbs, neck and trunk are then affected.
  - Respiratory muscles (intercoastal muscles and diaphragm) are affected last.

  Consciousness and sensorium (sensation) are unaffected throughout the course of paralysis. Paralysed muscles still respond to direct electrical stimulation. Recovery occurs in reverse order, i.e. the respiratory muscles are recovered first and the small muscles are recovered last. This

block can be reversed by anticholinesterases (as shown in **Table 13.1**).

- **Effect on autonomic ganglia:** In therapeutic doses it has insignificant effect on autonomic ganglia. In large dosage it can block autonomic ganglia (i.e. ganglionic transmission) after a brief period of stimulation.
- **Cardiovascular effects:** In therapeutic dosage it has insignificant effect on CVS. In large dosage it produces depression of heart and fall of BP (partly by histamine release and partly by ganglionic blocking action).
- **Respiratory effects:** It can produce increased respiratory secretions and bronchospasm by releasing histamine from mast cells. In large dosage it produces respiratory paralysis.
- **GIT effects:** It can increase gastric secretion by releasing histamine. It can produce paralytic ileus by ganglionic blocking action in large dosage.

Clinical Uses

It can be used as a skeletal muscle relaxant during surgery. Its action starts within 5 minutes and lasts for 1 to 2 hours.

Preparation and Dosage

Tubocurarine chloride (Tubarine) injection (3 mg/ml in 10 ml vial)—6 to 10 mg IV and repeated if necessary.

Adverse Reactions

It can produce hypotension, excessive salivary, respiratory and gastric secretions with regurgitation of gastric juice into the oesophagus (due to paralysis of oesophageal sphincter), hypoxia and respiratory failure. Death may occur due to respiratory paralysis.

Treatment

- Administration of specific antidote (antagonist)—neostigmine methyl sulphate injection (0.5 mg/ml)—1 to 2 mg IV and repeated if necessary.
- It is administered along with atropine sulphate injection (0.6 mg/ml)—0.6 to 1.2

mg IV (to block muscarinic effects of neostigmine).

- Supportive measures to maintain respiration and BP are taken according to need.

Drug Interactions

Curaremimetic drugs potentiate the neuromuscular block and paralysis produced by d-tubocurarine. These are:

- Inhalation of general anaesthetics like ether and halothane.
- Local anaesthetics like procaine and lignocaine.
- Antibiotics like aminoglycosides (streptomycin, etc.), tetracyclines, clindamycin and lincomycin.
- Antiarrhythmic drugs like quinidine, propranolol and verapamil.
- Miscellaneous drugs like chloroquine, trimethaphan, digitalis glycosides, opioids and corticosteroids.

Dimethyl Tubocurarine

It is a semisynthetic derivative of d-tubocurarine. It is two times more potent than d-tubocurarine. It has shorter duration of action and less CVS effects than d-tubocurarine.

Preparation and Dosage

Dimethyl tubocurarine iodide (Metocurine) injection (2 mg/ml in 5 ml vial)—1 to 2 mg IV initially and repeated after 15 minutes if necessary.

Gallamine

It is a synthetic drug. It is a quaternary ammonium compound with a curare-like action. It has similar pharmacokinetics and pharmacological actions like d-tubocurarine but it differs from d-tubocurarine in following aspects:

- It is less potent.
- It has shorter duration of action as it is mainly excreted by the kidney.
- It can block parasympathetic ganglia in therapeutic dosage.

- It has vagolytic action (atropine-like action) on the heart producing tachycardia, increased cardiac output and hypertension.
- It can cross placental barrier. It should not be used during caesarean section (CS), or other obstetric surgery as it can affect foetus by crossing placental barrier.

Clinical Uses

It can be used as a skeletal muscle relaxant during surgery except CS or other obstetric surgery.

Preparation and Dosage

Gallamine triethiodide (Flexidil) injection (20 mg/ml in 2 ml ampoule)—1 mg/kg IV and repeated if necessary.

Adverse Reactions

These are like d-tubocurarine except it does not release histamine and produces allergic reactions. Synthetic quaternary ammonium steroids, e.g. alcuronium, pancuronium, atracurium and vecuronium differ from d-tubocurarine in following aspects:

- They cause less release of histamine from mast cells.
- They do not block ganglionic transmission significantly. They are now preferred as skeletal muscle relaxants during surgery.

Alcuronium

It is a synthetic drug produced by structural modification of the alkaloid toxiferine, obtained from strychnos toxifera. It has similar onset and duration of action of d-tubocurarine but it is effective in smaller dosage (i.e. more potent). It causes less release of histamine than d-tubocurarine.

Preparation and Dosage

Alcuronium chloride (Allaferin) injection (10 mg/ml in 2 ml ampoule)—0.2 to 0.3 mg/kg IV and repeated if necessary.

Pancuronium

It is a synthetic drug. It has a steroid structure with two quaternary ammonium groups. It is about five times more potent than d-tubocurarine. It has quicker onset and shorter duration of action than d-tubocurarine. It does not release histamine and does not produce bronchospasm and hypotension. It may produce tachycardia, increased cardiac output and hypertension by vagolytic action. It is preferred in patients of shock. It prolongs the action of succinylcholine by inhibiting plasma cholinesterase. It can be safely used during caesarean section or other obstetric surgery as it does not cross placental barrier.

Preparation and Dosage

Pancuronium bromide (Pavulon) injection (2 mg/ml in 2 ml ampoule)—0.04 to 0.08 mg/ kg IV and repeated if necessary.

Atracurium

It is a synthetic drug. It is symmetrical bis quaternary ester. It is as potent as d-tubocurarine but it has shorter duration of action. It can be administered safely in patients with hepatic and renal impairments, as its metabolism is not altered in these conditions. It does not release histamine like pancuronium.

Preparation and Dosage

Atracurium besylate (Tracrium) injection (10 mg/ml in 2.5 ml ampoule)—0.3 to 0.6 mg/kg IV and repeated if necessary.

Vecuronium

It is a synthetic drug. It is a monoquaternary analog of pancuronium. It is about 1.5 times more potent than pancuronium. It has similar onset but shorter duration of action than pancuronium due to rapid distribution and metabolism. It does not release histamine. It does not cause ganglionic blockade or vagal blockade. So it has little or no CVS effects.

Preparation and Dosage

Vecuronium bromide (Norcuron) injection (4 mg/ml/ampoule)—0.04 to 0.1 mg/kg IV and repeated if necessary.

Mivacurium

It is a synthetic drug. It is a benzyl isoquinoline diester compound. It is the shortest-acting competitive skeletal muscle relaxant with rapid onset of action. It is metabolized by plasma cholinesterase. It can release of histamine causing slight fall of BP.

Preparation and Dosage

Mivacurium chloride (Mivacron) injection (1 mg/ml in 2 ml ampoule)—0.01 to 0.02 mg/ kg IV and repeated if necessary.

Depolarizing (Noncompetitive) Neuromuscular Blockers

Succinylcholine

It is a synthetic drug. It is a dicholine ester. Its structure resembles two molecules of acetylcholine joined together. It has rapid onset (within 1 minute) and short duration of action (6 to 10 minutes).

Pharmacokinetics

It is not absorbed orally and so it is administered IV. It is rapidly hydrolyzed by plasma cholinesterase to succinic acid and choline. Its duration of action is prolonged in some patients with deficiency of plasma cholinesterase or due to presence of atypical (abnormal) cholinesterase (a hereditary disorder). Producing prolonged apnoea.

Pharmacological Actions

It is a depolarizing neuromuscular blocker. It produces persistent depolarization of the motor end plate, as a result acetylcholine cannot act on it. It produces following effects:

- **Effects at skeletal muscles:** It initially produces transient (for 10 to 15 seconds) spastic paralysis of muscles (phase I block) which is manifested as twitchings and fasciculations of some groups of muscles, usually in the thoracic and abdominal region. This is followed by flaccid paralysis of muscles (phase II block/desensitization block). Thus, it produces dual block. In the initial depolarization state, the block cannot be antagonized (reversed) by anticholinesterases rather they increase the block. Subsequently, with high plasma concentration of succinylcholine, the depolarization state decreases and the motor end plate is repolarized and cannot be depolarized again as long as succinylcholine is present in the receptor (N_M) site. This block can be antagonized (reversed) by anticholinesterases (as shown in **Table 13.1**).

- **CVS effects:** It initially produces hypotension and bradycardia by acting as a partial agonist of acetylcholine. On prolonged use or in high dose it may produce tachycardia and cardiac arrhythmias.

- **Other effects:** It has muscarinic and ganglionic stimulating actions in therapeutic dose and ganglion blocking effect in large dose. It does not release histamine from mast cells.

Sequence of Muscle Paralysis

- Large muscles of limbs, neck and trunk are first affected.
- Small muscles of face, eyes, ears, pharynx, larynx, fingers and toes are then affected.
- Respiratory muscles are affected last.

Consciousness and sensorium are unaffected throughout the course of paralysis. Recovery from paralysis occurs in reverse order, i.e. respiratory muscles are recovered first and large muscles are recovered last.

Clinical Uses

It is used as skeletal muscle relaxant during short surgery or diagnostic surgical procedures. It can be used during caesarean section or other obstetric surgery. It is also preferred in ECT.

Preparation and Dosage

Succinylcholine chloride (Scoline) injection (50 mg / ml in 3 ml ampoule)—1 mg/kg IV slowly.

Table 13.1: Comparative neuromuscular blocking effects of a typical competitive blocker and a depolarizing blocker

	Competitive blocker (d-tubocurarine)	Depolarizing blocker (succinylcholine)	
		Phase I block (in low conc.)	Phase II block (in high conc.)
1. Type of paralysis of muscles	Flaccid	Spastic	Flaccid
2. Effect on motor end plate	Blockade of acetylcholine induced depolarization	Persistent depolarization	Repolarization and desensitization to acetylcholine
3. Initial muscle contraction	None	Transient twitchings and fasiculations of muscles	None
4. Response to tetanic stimuli	Unsustained	Well sustained	Poorly sustained
5. Effect of ether anaesthesia	Synergistic	No effect	Additive
6. Effect of KCl on block	Transient reversal of block due to K-induced repolarization of muscle membrane	No antagonism	Reversal of block
7. Effect of anticholinesterase	Antagonism (reversal)	Additive/Synergistic	Antagonism

For its muscarinic actions, atropine is usually injected before its use.

Adverse Reactions

It can produce postoperative muscle pain (due to depolarizing effect); bradycardia, hypotension, salivation, cardiac arrhythmias and increased gut motility (due to muscarinic and ganglionic stimulating actions); hyperkalemia (due to muscle damage by persistent depolarization); succinylcholine apnoea (last for more than 15 minutes due to deficiency of plasma cholinesterase or presence of atypical cholinesterase) and malignant hyperthermia (in patients receiving halothane or ether).

Treatment

Succinylcholine apnoea is treated by administration of fresh blood containing plasma cholinesterase and by positive pressure ventilation (artificial respiration).

Malignant hyperthermia is treated by administration of dantrolene (25 to 50 mg IV), cooling of body by ice bag application and by hyperventilation (100% oxygen is administered). Other supportive measures are taken as required.

Decamethonium (Syncurine)

It is a synthetic quaternary ammonium compound. It has ten carbon atoms and so the name. It has longer duration of action than succinylcholine. Complete recovery occurs inabout 20 minutes. It is not metabolized in the body and excreted unchanged in urine. Its administration is more hazardous than succinylcholine and so it is no longer used (obsolete).

Other types of skeletal muscle relaxants:

- *Centrally acting muscle relaxants*: These are of 3 groups:

  1. Benzodiazepines, e.g. diazepam and other drugs.
  2. Mephenesin group, e.g. Mephenesin, carisoprodol, Chlorozoxazone, chlormezanone and methocarbamol.
  3. GABA derivative, baclofen.

4. Central adrenergic α_2 agonist, tizanidine.

These drugs cause muscular relaxation without loss of consciousness. They selectively depress spinal and supraspinal reflexes involved in the regulation of muscle tone without significantly affecting monosynaptically mediated stress reflex. They have some sedative properties. They have no effect on neuromuscular transmission and on the motor end plate of muscle fibres. They can reduce decerebrate rigidity, upper motor neuron spasticity and hyper-reflexia.

Benzodiazepines are discussed in CNS.

Mephenesin is an internuncial neuron blocking agent as it acts primarily in the spinal internuncial neuron, which modulates reflexes maintaining muscle tone. It was previously used in skeletal muscle spasm but now replaced by diazepam, because when given orally it causes gastric irritation and when given IV it causes thrombophlebitis, haemolysis, muscular weakness, nystagmus, drowsiness, ataxia and hypotension. It is now included in counterirritant ointments (Medicreme/Relaxyl), where its irritant property produces pain relief in the deeper tissue through axon reflex.

Carisoprodol (Carisoma) is a muscle relaxant, sedative, weak analgesic, antipyretic and anticholinergic. It is administered orally as tablet (350 mg) in the dose of 350 mg thrice daily. It can produce side effects like drowsiness, constipation, skin rash, nausea and headache.

Chlorzoxazone, chlormezanone and methocarbamol are longer-acting and better tolerated drugs than carisoprodol and administered orally as tablets.

Baclofen (Liofen) is an analogue of the inhibiting transmitter GABA. It is a selective $GABA_B$ agoinst. It acts on presynaptic $GABA_B$ receptors, which are inhibitory to Ca^{2+} influx and thereby reduce release of excitatory transmitters in the CNS, especially in the spinal cord. It also promotes the activity of glycine (an inhibitory transmitter). It is well-absorbed from GIT and has plasma half-life of 3 to 4 hours. It is used in spasticity of spinal orgin and in cerebral strokes producing hemiplegia and paraplegia. It is administered orally as tablet (15 mg) in the dose of 15 mg twice daily. It can produce side effects like drowsiness and increased seizure activity in epileptic patients.

Tizanidine (Tizan) is a clonidine congener. It inhibits the release of excitatory amino acids in the spinal interneurons. It may facilitate the inhibitory transmitter glycine. It inhibits postsynaptic reflexes, reduces muscle tone and frequency of muscle spasms without reducing muscle strength. It has efficacy similar to baclofen or diazepam. It is used in muscle spasticity due to neurological disorders and in peripheral muscle spasms of spinal origin. It is absorbed orally, undergoes first pass metabolism and is excreted by the kidney. Its plasma t½ is 2 to 3 hours. It is available as tablet (2, 4 mg) and the dose is 2 mg thrice daily. It can be combined with, ibuprofen or diclofenac. It can produce dry mouth, drowsiness, insomnia and hallucination.

- **Directly acting muscle relaxants**, e.g. dantrolene and quinine. These drugs produce muscle relaxation by acting directly on the motor end plate of the muscle fibres.
  - Dantrolene (Dantrium) is a hydantoin derivative with no effect on CNS. It acts directly on the motor end plate of the muscle fibres by interferring with the release of Ca^{++} from the sarcoplasmic reticulum. It also interferes with the excitation–contraction coupling. It is used in patients with upper motor neuron diseases like multiple sclerosis, cerebral palsy, spinal injury, hemiplegia and paraplegia. It is administered orally as capsule (25/50 mg) in the dose of 25 to 50 mg twice daily. It is also used in neuroleptic malignant syndrome and malignant hyperthermia following use of succinyl choline with halothane anaesthesia in the dose of 25 to 50 mg IV and repeated as necessary for 2 to 3 days. It can produce side effects like muscle weakness, sweating, malaise, light headedness and occasionally hepatitis.
- Quinine is an alkaloid obtained from cinchona plant bark. It acts by increasing refractory period and decreasing excitability of the motor end plate of the muscle fibres and thus decreasing responses to repetitive nerve stimulation. It decreases muscle tone in myotonia congenita. It can abolish nocturnal muscle cramps in some patients when taken at night in the dose of 200 to 300 mg orally.

14

Ganglion Stimulating and Blocking Agents

GANGLION STIMULATING AGENTS

Ganglion stimulating agents facilitate ganglionic transmission by acting on (stimulating) receptors (N_N, M_1, α_1 and D_1) in the autonomic ganglia. They have no therapeutic use.

Classification

These are of two groups:

1. Selective nicotinic (N_N) agonists, e.g. nicotine and lobeline in small doses; tetramethyl-ammonium (TMA) and dimethyl-phenyl piperazinium (DMPP). These are synthetic compounds used as experimental stools. They cause rapid stimulation of ganglia with early onset and are blocked by competitive ganglion blockers.
2. Non-selective muscarinic (M_1) agonists, e.g. muscarine, pilocarpine and methacholine.

   They cause slow stimulation of ganglia with delayed onset. They are blocked by atropine. Nicotine is discussed here in detail, as it has toxicological importance.

Nicotine

It is an alkaloid obtained from the leaves of tobacco plant, *Nicotiana tabacum* [lobeline is an alkaloid obtained from the leaves of Indian tobacco plant (*Lobelia inflata*)]. It is a colourless volatile liquid (tertiary amine) and easily penetrates mucous membranes and skin. It is soluble in water and alkaline in reaction. Tobacco smoke contains nicotine (1 to 2%), pyridine, NH_3, HCN, CO, CO_2, furfural and nitrosamine, which are irritant substances. One cigarette contains about 10 mg of nicotine, from which 1 mg reaches the systemic circulation.

Pharmacokinetics

It is absorbed from the mouth, nose, pharynx, larynx, trachea, lungs and skin. It is metabolized in the liver, lungs and kidneys to the extent of about 80% and is excreted in urine as both metabolites and unchanged form. Cotinine is the major metabolite of nicotine. It is also secreted in milk of lactating woman, who is a smoker. It has a half-life of about 2 hours.

Pharmacological Actions

Mechanism of Action

It produces inital stimulation followed by blocking of ganglionic transmission. It first stimulates and then desensitizes the nicotinic neuronal (N_N) receptors in the autonomic ganglia. It produces following effects:

- **CNS effects:** It is a CNS stimulant in small dose. It increases alertness, attention, learning and memory. It produces euphoria and decreases reaction time, tension, depression, stress, anger, aggression and appetite. These are all behavioural effects of nicotine. It also produces other CNS effects. It increases BMR and produces tremors of the hand. It stimulates hypothalamic supraoptic nucleus releasing ADH and medullary centres (vagal, vomiting, respiratory and vasomotor) by acting reflexly (through stimulation of chemoreceptors in carotid and aortic bodies) as well as directly (in large dose). It causes convulsions in large dose, which is followed by coma and respiratory depression.

- **ANS effects:** It causes initial stimulation followed by persistent blockade of autonomic ganglia (in large dose). It causes release of catecholamines from adrenal medulla in small dose and blockade of release of catecholamines in large dose.

- **CVS effects:** It causes vasoconstriction, rise of BP, tachycardia and even cardiac arrhythmias by releasing catecholamines due to stimulation of sympathetic ganglia and adrenal medulla. It causes constriction of coronary and other blood vessels by releasing ADH. It causes fall of BP in large dose.

- **GIT and respiratory effects:** It stimulates salivary, gastric and respiratory secretions. It increases tone and motility of GIT leading to defecation. In large dose, it produces opposite effects.

- **Other effects:** It increases platelet aggregation and FFAs, LDL and VLDL concentrations of blood. It is a microsomal enzyme inducer and increases metabolism of many drugs including propranolol, nifedipine, theophylline, heparin, opioids and BDZs.

Adverse Reactions

It produces tolerance and dependence. Its withdrawal symptoms appear within 24 hours of stopping smoking in a chronic smoker and manifested as craving (for smoking), difficulty in concentration, anxiety, restlessness, headache and insomnia. Clonidine is used to reduce craving and insomnia. Acute nicotine poisoning occurs in workers engaged in spraying nicotine as an insecticide. It may occur in children from accidental ingestion of cigarettes. It is manifested by salivation, nausea, vomiting, abdominal pain, diarrhoea, cold sweat, headache, dizziness, disturbed hearing and vision; weakness, mental

confusion, hypotension dyspnoea, prostation, weak and irregular pulse and collapse followed by terminal convulsions. Death may occur due to circulatory failure or respiratory depression. Treatment is symptomatic and supportive as there is no specific antidote of nicotine.

Chronic nicotine poisoning can occur in chronic smoker. Chronic smoking is detrimental to health as it increases morbidity and mortality (decreases life span). It can produce following hazards:

- Smokers respiratory syndrome due to chronic irritation of larynx and bronchi and manifested as cough, dyspnoea, wheezing, pain in chest and respiratory tract infection.

- CNS disorders like anxiety, irritability, insomnia and depression.

- Ocular disorders like toxic amblyopia (reduced visual field).

- CVS disorders—increased incidence of hypertension, ischaemic heart disease and peripheral vascular disease like thrombo-angitis obliterns.

- Reproductive disorders in females (who are smokers) like infertility abortion, pre-eclampsia and low birth weight babies.

- Increased incidence of cancers at various sites (especially oral, laryngeal, oesophageal, duodenal, pancreatic and bronchial).

GANGLION BLOCKING AGENTS

Ganglion blockers block ganglionic transmission of acetylcholine by occupying nicotinic neuronal (N_N) receptors in the autonomic ganglia. They are nonselective in action, i.e. block both sympathetic and parasympathetic ganglia.

Classification

These are of two groups:

- Competitive (stabilizing) ganglion blockers. These are given as follows:

  - Quaternary ammonium (methonium) compounds, e.g. hexamethonium, pento-

linium, tetraethylammonium (TEA), etc.
– Sulphonium compound: Trimethaphan.
– Secondary amine: Mecamylamine.
– Tertiary amine: Pempidine.
• Depolarizing (noncompetitive) ganglion blockers, e.g. nicotine and lobeline in large doses.

Pharmacokinetics

Methonium and sulphonium compounds are lipid-insoluble (water-soluble) and so irregularly and poorly absorbed from the GIT. Their distribution is limited in extracellular space. They cannot cross BBB and so do not produce CNS effects. They are little metabolized in the body and are excreted in urine mainly as unchanged form. They are administered parenterally, mainly IV. Secondary and tertiary amines are lipid-soluble and so readily and completely absorbed from the GIT. They are distributed throughout the body including the CNS and may accumulate in kidney and liver. They are little metabolized in the body and slowly excreted in urine mainly as unchanged forms. They are administered orally as well as parenterally. They have longer duration of action than other ganglion blockers.

Pharmacological Actions

Mechanism of Action

Competitive ganglion blockers compete with acetylcholine for occupying nicotinic neuronal (N_N) receptors in the ganglion cells and block transmission of nerve impulses through the ganglia from preganglionic neuron to postganglionic neuron. Depolarizing ganglion blockers produce persistent (prolonged) depolarization of the ganglionic cell membrane, so that acetylcholine cannot act on it to produce action by depolarization.

They produce blockade of both sympathetic and parasympathetic ganglia at different sites and the effects depend on the predominant tone of the structures innervated (as shown in **Table 14.1**).

They produce fall of BP by blocking sympathetic ganglia.

They can produce postural (orthostatic) hypotension with syncope due to inhibition of sympathetically mediated vasomotor reflexes and decreased cold pressure response by blocking (abolishing) compensatory circulatory adjustments (reflex pathways) with change of posture (from recumbent/lying posture to sitting/standing posture).

They can produce sexual dysfunction (impotence) in male by impairment of penile erection (due to parasympathetic ganglion blockade) and failure of ejaculation (due to sympathetic ganglion blockade).

Clinical Uses

Ganglion blockers have limited use in hypertension as they produce various adverse effects. They are used in severe or malignant hypertension and hypertensive crisis (emergency). Trimethaphan is considered as a drug of choice in hypertension associated with acute dissecting aortic aneurysm. It is also used in autonomic hyperreflexia (due to upper spinal cord injury) and to produce controlled hypotension during neurosurgery and some cardiovascular operations.

Preparations and Dosage

• Trimethaphan camsylate (Arfonad) injection (50 mg/ml in 10 ml ampoule)—Initially 50 mg of bolus injection is given IV which is followed by slow IV infusion of 1 in 1000 solution at the rate of 1 to 3 mg/minute.
• Mecamylamine hydrochloride (Inversine) tablet (2.5 and 10 mg)—2.5 to 5 mg twice daily and gradually increasing the dose.

Adverse Reactions

Common side effect is severe hypotension, which may lead to impaired cerebral circulation and impaired glomerular filtration. Other side effects include cholinergic blocking effects like dryness of mouth, visual dis-

Table 14.1: Effects of sympathetic and parasympathetic ganglion blockades by ganglion blockers

Site	Predominant tone	Effects
Arterioles	Sympathetic (adrenergic)	Vasodilation, hypotension
Veins	Sympathetic (adrenergic)	Venodilatation, peripheral pooling of blood. Decreased venous return to heart. Decreased cardiac output
Heart	Parasympathetic (cholinergic)	Tachycardia
Eye	Parasympathetic (cholinergic)	Mydriasis (incomplete), cycloplegia (partial). Eye is focused for distant vision.
GIT	Parasympathetic (cholinergic)	Decreased tone and motility of gut constipation.
Urinary bladder	Parasympathetic (cholinergic)	Retention of urine. Difficulty in micturition
Salivary and bronchial glands	Parasympathetic (cholinergic)	Dryness of mouth. Decreased bronchial secretion.
Sweat glands	Sympathetic (cholinergic)	Dryness of skin (anhydrosis).

turbances (mydriasis and cycloplegia), urinary retention, constipation, paralytic ileus and failure of erection of penis and ejaculation. Secondary and tertiary amines can produce CNS stimulation leading to tremors, mental confusion, seizures, hallucinations, mania and mental depression. With continued administration tolerance develops to the side effects.

Contraindications

- Severe coronary artery disease
- Cerebrovascular insufficiency
- Diabetes mellitus on oral hypoglycaemic drugs
- Glaucoma
- Enlarged prostate

15

Adrenergic Drugs/ Sympathomimetic Drugs

INTRODUCTION

Adrenergic drugs produce effects similar to those of adrenaline or stimulation of postganglionic sympathetic nerves. As most of them contain an amino group ($-NH_2$) in their chemical structure, so they are called sympathomimetic amines.

Classification

These can be classified in three ways:

1. **Chemical classification** (according to chemical structure). These are of two groups:

   a. *Catecholamines* (contain a catechol ring, i.e. orthodihydroxybenzene). These are given as follows:
   - Natural drugs, e.g. adrenaline, noradrenaline and dopamine.
   - Synthetic drugs, e.g. isoprenaline, dobutamine, dopexamine and prenalterol.

   b. *Noncatecholamines* (contain a benzene/ phenol ring), e.g. ephedrine, amphetamines, phenylephrine, methoxamine, mephentermine, salbutamol and terbutaline. These are synthetic drugs.

2. **Mechanistic classification** (according to mechanism of action). These are of three groups:

   a. *Directly acting drugs* (act as agonists on adrenergic receptors), *viz.*

   - Non-selective α-adrenergic agonists (act on both α_1 and α_2 receptors), e.g. adrenaline and noradrenaline.
   - Non-selective β-adrenergic agonists (act on all types of β receptors), e.g. isoprenaline and orciprenaline.
   - Selective α_1-adrenergic agonists (act on α_1 receptors), e.g. phenylephrine, methoxamine, metaraminol and mephentermine.
   - Selective α_2-adrenergic agonists (act on α_2-receptors), e.g. clonidine, α-methyldopa, guanfacine and guanabenz.
   - Selective β_1-adrenergic agonists (act on β_1 receptors), e.g. dobutamine, dopexamine and prenalterol.
   - Selective β_2-adrenergic agonists (act on β_2 receptors), e.g. terbutaline albuterol, bitolterol, salbutamol, salmeterol, ritodrine and isoetharine.

   b. *Indirectly acting drugs* (act by releasing noradrenaline from postganglionic adrenergic nerve endings, which then act on adrenergic receptors), e.g. amphetamine, methamphetamine and tyramine.

   c. *Mixed acting drugs* (act by both direct and indirect mechanisms), e.g. ephedrine and pholedrine.

3. **Clinical classification** (according to clinical uses). These are of several groups:

- Vasopressor drugs, e.g. noradrenaline, phenylephrine, methoxamine, mephentermine and metaraminol.
- Cardiac stimulants, e.g. adrenaline, dopamine, isoprenaline, dobutamine, dopexamine and prenalterol.
- CNS stimulants, e.g. ephedrine, amphetamines and methylphenidate.
- Bronchodilators, e.g. adrenaline, ephedrine, isoprenaline, orciprenaline, salbutamol and terbutaline.
- Uterine relaxants, e.g. ritodrine, isoxsuprine and salbutamol.
- Appetite suppressants (anorectic drugs), e.g. fenfluramine, phenteramine, phendimetrazine and mazindol.
- Nasal decongestants, e.g. ephedrine, phenylephrine, oxymetazoline, xylometazoline, naphazoline and 2-aminoheptane.
- Peripheral vasodilators, e.g. nylidrin and isoxsuprine.

Chemical structures of some adrenergic drugs shown in **Fig. 15.1**.

DISCUSSION OF ADRENERGIC DRUGS

Natural Catecholamines

Adrenaline (Epinephrine)

It is discussed as a prototype drug of adrenergic agonists.

Source: It is the major hormone (80%) of adrenal medulla, where it is produced by chromaffin cells. It is also released from postganglionic adrenergic nerve endings (to the extent of 20%). It is a central and peripheral neurotransmitter like noradrenaline.

Chemistry: It is a catecholamine. Its chemical structure is shown in **Fig. 15.1**.

Pharmacokinetics

It is not administered orally because it is rapidly inactivated in the gut and the liver. On inhalation, it may be absorbed into the systemic circulation in small quantity. It is administered parenterally (SC or IM and never IV which may be dangerous). It is metabolized by two enzymes—catechol-*O*-methyltransferase (COMT), located extracellularly and monoamine oxidase (MAO), situated in the mitochondria of adrenergic

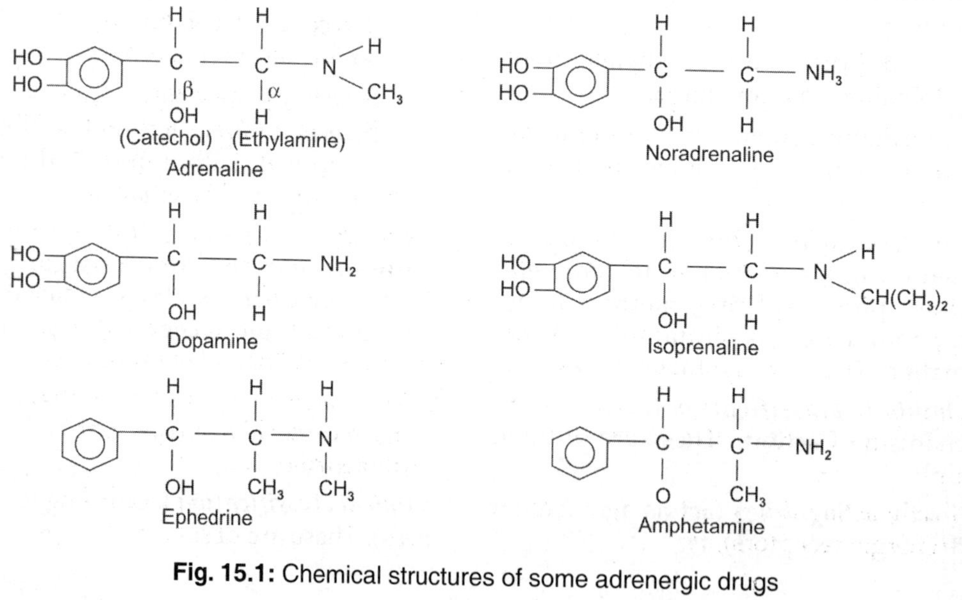

Fig. 15.1: Chemical structures of some adrenergic drugs

neurons. It is excreted in urine as ethereal sulphate and glucuronide of VMA and MOPEG. It cannot cross BBB in therapeutic dose but in high dose it can cross BBB. It has short duration of action (5 to 10 minutes after IM injection and 15 to 30 minutes after SC injection).

Pharmacological Actions

It acts as an agonist at the level of all (α_1, α_2, β_1, β_2 and β_3) adrenergic receptors. It produces following effects:

1. Cardiovascular effects

a. On heart: It is a powerful cardiac stimulant. It acts directly on the predominant β_1 receptors of the myocardium, SA node, AV node and conducting tissues. It increases the force of cardiac contractions (+ve inotropic action), heart rate (+ve chronotropic action), stroke volume and cardiac output. It makes cardiac systole shorter and more powerful. It increases work of the heart by increasing oxygen consumption of the myocardium. It thus decreases cardiac efficiency (work done relative to oxygen consumption). In high dose, it increases excitability and automaticity of the heart.

b. On blood vessels and blood pressure (BP): It is a potent vasopressor drug. It causes vasoconstriction in many vascular beds (due to the presence of α_1 receptors) especially in arterioles (precapillary resistance vessels) of skin, mucous membrane, lungs and kidneys and also of veins but it dilates blood vessels of skeletal muscles, liver, heart and mesentery (due to the presence of β_2 receptors). It increases systolic BP greater than the diastolic BP and so pulse pressure and mean pressure may or may not increase. When it is administered by rapid IV injection in anaesthetized cat or dog, it produces sharp rise of mean BP to a peak, which is proportional to the dose and then rapid recovery. Before returning to the normal level, the mean BP may fall below the normal level due to persistence of β_2 receptor action of adrenaline on blood vessels. Thus adrenaline produces biphasic response of BP (as shown in **Fig. 15.2**). Mechanisms involved in rising of BP by adrenaline are:

- Direct myocardial stimulant action (by acting on β_1 receptors) and thus increasing the force of cardiac contractions, heart rate, stroke volume and cardiac output.

- Vasoconstriction of many blood vessels (by acting on α_1 receptors). The pulse rate is first increased and then slowed, due to high rise of BP by vagal effect (compensatory vagal discharge due to stimulation of vagal centre).

Given by slow IV infusion or SC injection, it does not rise BP rather can produce fall of BP due to β_2 receptor action. It increases cerebral blood flow, when the BP is markedly increased. It decreases cutaneous blood flow especially in hands and feet by vasoconstriction.

2. Effects at nonvascular smooth muscles:
These depend on the type of adrenergic receptors present in the smooth muscles. It relaxes smooth muscles of GIT (contains β_2

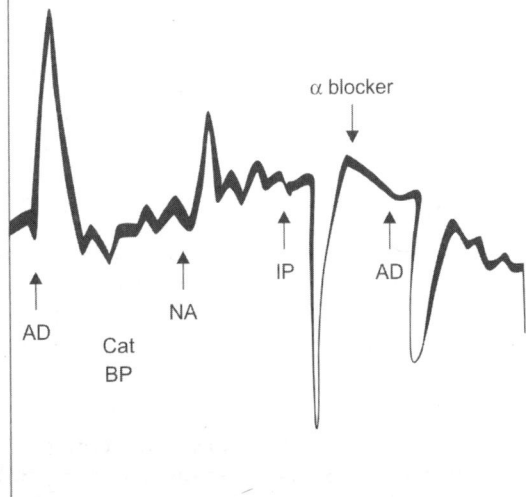

Fig. 15.2: Effects of adrenaline, noradrenaline and isoprenaline on anaesthetized cat BP and vasomotor reversal of Dale after an α blocker

receptor) and decreases tone and motility but it contracts pyloric and ileocaecal sphincters (contain α_1 receptors) if the tone of intestinal muscles is low. It causes mydriasis by contraction of radial muscles of iris (contain α_1 receptors). It does not produce cycloplegia as the ciliary muscle is devoid of adrenergic nerve fibres. It relaxes bronchial smooth muscles (contain β_2 receptors) and produces bronchodilatation. It antagonizes satisfactorily the bronchospasm produced by vagal stimulation, choline esters, histamine or an antigen antibody reaction, bradykinin, slow reacting substance (SRS) or prostaglandin $F_{2\alpha}$ or due to disease like bronchial asthma.

It relaxes detrusor muscles of the urinary bladder (contains β_2 receptors) but contracts trigonal sphincter (contains α_1 receptors) and can produce urinary retention and hesitency in urination. Its effects on uterus depend on species of animals, phase of sexual cycle and state of gestation. It contracts isolated rabbit uterus but relaxes isolated rat uterus. It contracts strips of pregnant or nonpregnant human uterus *in vitro* but relaxes human uterus *in situ/vivo*. It inhibits uterine tone and contractions during last month of pregnancy and at parturition.

It contacts (by α_1 action) vas deferens leading to ejaculation, splenic capsule leading to pouring of RBCs in circulation, piloerector muscles leading to piloerection and nictitating membrane (3rd eyelid) in cat and dog.

3. **Respiratory effects:** It is a potent bronchodilator. It is a weak stimulant of respiration. Given IV in anaesthetized animals like cat, it can produce apnoea partly by stimulating the baroreceptors and partly by a direct stimulation of respiratory centre. Given as aerosol for inhalation, it constricts pulmonary vessels and relieves bronchial congestion leading to increase of vital capacity.

4. **Metabolic effects:** It increases concentration of glucose, lactate and free fatty acids in blood by producing glycogenolysis in liver and skeletal muscles and lipolysis in adipose tissue (fat cells adepocytes). It stimulates β receptors leading to activation of the enzyme adenyl cyclase and increasing the formation of cAMP from ATP. This causes glycogenolysis (by β_2 action) due to activation of inactive phosphorylase-β to active phosphorylase-α, which causes conversion of hepatic glycogen to glucose and muscle glycogen to lactic acid. It thus produces hyperglycaemia and lactacidema but it rarely produces glycosuria. It inhibits insulin secretion by activation of presynaptic α_2 receptors (prominent action) of the β cells of pancreatic islets but it can stimulate insulin secretion by activation of β_2 receptors (less prominent action). It stimulates glucagon secretion by activation of β_2 receptors of the α cells of pancreatic islets. It decreases the uptake of glucose by peripheral tissues, partly by inhibiting insulin secretion. It produces lipolysis by stimulating β_3 receptors in adipose tissue and causing activation of triglyceride lipase leading to breakdown of triglyceride to free fatty acid (FFA) and glycerol in adipocytes (fat cells). It thus increases FFA concentration in blood. It has a calorigenic action (increases metabolism and BMR) by increasing oxygen consumption (20 to 30% more) in skeletal and other types of muscles in conventional dose.

5. **CNS effects:** In therapeutic dose it cannot cross BBB and does not produce CNS effects. In large dose or after IV administration it can cross BBB and produces CNS stimulation followed by CNS depression. When it is administered by intraventricular cannulation in anaesthetized cat or dog it produces CNS stimulation followed by CNS depression.

6. **Miscellaneous effects:** These are given as follows:
   • It modulates the secretion of insulin, glucagon, renin, parathormone, calcitonin, thyroxine and gastrin.
   • It produces platelet aggregation, eosinopenia and increased coagulability of

blood (by activating factor V/proac-celerin).

- It stabilizes mast cell membrane and decreases release of histamine and other autacoids (spasmogens) from mast cells.
- It facilitates neuromuscular transmission in skeletal muscles by stimulating pre-synaptic β_2 receptors leading to increased release of acetylcholine from cholinergic nerve endings.
- It produces skeletal muscle vasodila-tation causing antifatigue effect of stress.
- It produces muscle tremors by stimu-lating presynaptic β_2 (stimulatory) and α_2 (inhibitory) receptors in the skeletal muscle fibres (red and white respectively).
- It produces after congestion of nasal mucosa following vasoconstriction (decongestion) when applied locally. This is probably due to changes in vascular reactivity as a result of hypoxia produced by it, rather than to β receptor activity on mucosal vessels.
- It increases K^+ uptake in RBCs and muscle cells due to stimulation of β_2 receptors. This causes fall in plasma K^+ concen-tration and decreases renal excretion of K^+.

Clinical Uses (Indications)

These are given as follows:

- To produce relief of respiratoy distress due to bronchospasm as in acute bronchial asthma and drug induced bronchospasm. It produces bronchodilatation by β_2 agoinst action. It is used as aerosol or by SC in-jection.
- To produce rapid relief of hypersensitivity reactions due to drugs or other allergens. It is the drug of choice in type I hyper-sensitivity reaction (analphylactic shock), which is characterized by severe hypo-tension, bronchospasm and angioedema of larynx. It is a life-saving drug in this con-dition. It produces dramatic reversal of this condition by raising BP (due to β_1 and α_1 actions), producing bronchodilatation (due to β_2 action) inhibiting histamine release and relieving angioedema of larynx (due to β_2 action).

- To restore cardiac rhythm in patients with cardiac arrest as in partial or complete heart block, Stokes-Adams syndrome (partial heart block with syncope) and in drowning, electrocusion or carbon mon-oxide poisoning by stimulating the heart (due to β_1 action).
- For prolongation of local (infiltration) anaesthesia. It is used in combination with local anaesthetics like procaine and lignocaine to prolong their duration of action due to slow absorption as a result of vasoconstriction and decreasing blood flow.
- As a topical haemostatic agent, it controls bleeding, when applied on bleeding sur-faces such as in the nose, mouth and gum by cotton wool swab (pack) in conditions like epistaxis, tooth extraction and gum bleeding.
- As nasal decongestant, it may be used.

Preparations and Dosage

- Adrenaline hydrochloride or acid tartrate injection (1 in 1000 solution, i.e. 1 mg/ml in 1 ml ampoule)—0.5 to 1 mg SC or IM (never IV).
- Adrenaline hydrochloride solution (1%) as aerosol for inhalation.

Adverse Reactions

It can produce side effects like anxiety, fear, tenseness, restlessness, throbbing headache, tremor, weakness, dizziness, pallor, resp-iratory difficulty and palpitation. These effects subside with rest. Hyperthyroid and hyper-tensive patients are more susceptible to these effects. Its more serious adverse reactions are cerebral haemorrhage and cardiac (ven-tricular) arrhythmias due to large dose or accidental IV injection causing high rise of BP Subarachnoid haemorrhage and hemiplegia may occur even after IM injection. Ventricular fibrillation may occur if it is used during anaesthesia with halogenated hydrocarbon anaesthetic (halothane/cyclopropane) or in individual with organic heart disease. It can produce anginal pain, if it is used in patients with ischaemic heart (coronary artery) disease.

Contraindications

These are given as follows:

- Hypertension
- Hyperthyroidism
- Diabetes mellitus
- Angina pectoris
- Cardiac arrhythmias
- Arteriosclerosis
- During anaesthesia with halogenated hydrocarbon anaesthetic (which precipitates cardiac arrhythmias by sensitizing the conducting tissue of the heart to adrenaline).
- Patients receiving nonselective β-blockers like propranolol (since its unopposed action on adrenergic α_1 receptors may lead to severe hypertension and cerebral haemorrhage).

Noradrenaline/Norepinephrine

Source: It is the minor hormone (20%) of adrenal medulla, where it is produced by chromaffin cells. It is mainly released from postganglionic adrenergic nerve endings (to the extent of 80%). It is a central and peripheral neurotransmitter.

Chemistry: It is a catecholamine. Its chemical structure is shown in **Fig. 15.1**. It differs from adrenaline by lacking a methyl group ($-CH_3$) in the N of aminoradical.

Pharmacokinetics

It is ineffective orally and poorly absorbed SC. It is administered IV. It is rapidly metabolized by COMT and MAO like adrenaline and excreted in urine mainly as metabolites (ethereal sulphate and glucuronide of VMA and MOPEG) and to a small extent in unchanged form. It has a short duration of action like adrenaline.

Pharmacological Actions

It acts as an agonist at the level of α_1, α_2 and β_1 but not β adrenergic receptors. It has equipotent activity as adrenaline in stimulating β_1 receptor but it is less potent than adrenaline on α_1 receptors of most organs. It produces following effects:

- **CVS effects:** It increases systolic BP, diastolic BP, mean pressure and pulse pressure. It increases stroke volume but decreases or produces no change in cardiac output due to increase in total peripheral resistance (TPR) by vasoconstriction. It produces monophasic response of BP in anaesthetized cat or dog (as shown in **Fig. 15.3**). It increases the force of cardiac contraction but decreases heart rate by compensatory reflex, vagal activity, overcoming the direct cardioaccelerator action. It differs from adrenaline having no affinity for β_2-receptor and producing reflex bradycardia instead of tachycardia. It decreases blood flow to most organs including kidney, liver and skeletal muscles by vasoconstriction. It increases coronary blood flow by coronary dilatation, mainly due to rise of BP. It does not produce vasomotor reversal of Dale.

- **Other effects:** It has little effects on non-vascular smooth muscles. It can produce hyperglycaemia and other metabolic effects only in high dose. It produces platelets aggregation and eosinopenia like adrenaline.

Clinical Uses

It can be used as a vasopressor agent in the treatment of hypovolemic shock (due to haemorrhage and blood loss) and other hypotensive states (after spinal anaesthesia or

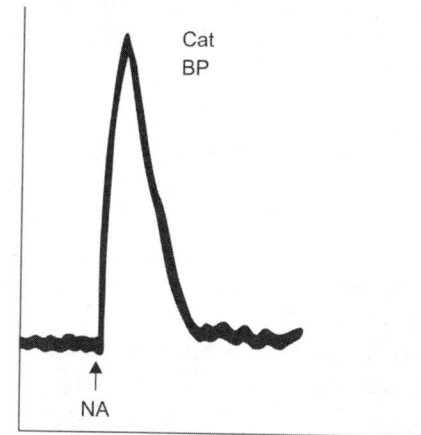

Fig. 15.3: Effect of noradrenaline on anaesthetized cat BP

surgical removal of pheochromocytoma) to raise BP but other α_1 agonists like phenylephrine, methoxamine metaraminol and meplentermine are now preferred.

Preparation and Dosage

Noradenaline bitartrate (Levoped) injection (4 mg/2 ml/ampoule)—4 mg is dissolved in 500 ml of 5% dextrose solution (acidic) and injected slowly by IV infusion at the rate of 2 mg/minute. The dose is adjusted according to the need of the patient. When BP becomes normal, the infusion is gradually tapered off.

Adverse Reactions

Its systemic toxicity is minimum in comparison to adrenaline. It can produce side effects like anxiety, respiratory difficulty, palpitation, rise of BP and headache. In hypertensive and hyperthyroid patients it can produce severe hypertension with severe headache, photophobia, anginal pain, pallor and intense sweating. During its administration, care should be taken, so that extravasation does not occur in SC tissue as it can cause necrosis, sloughing of tissue or even gangrene of the part due to severe ischaemia by vasoconstriction. It should not be used in pregnant woman because it can contract gravid uterus.

Dopamine

Source: It is the immediate metabolic precusor of noradrenaline. It is present in high concentration in basal ganglia, limbic system and hypothalamus. It is a central neurotransmitter. It is involved in the regulation of body movements.

Chemistry: It is a catecholamine. It is 3,4-dihydroxyphenylethylamine. Its chemical structure is shown in **Fig. 15.1.**

Pharmacokinetics

It is ineffective orally, as it is rapidly destroyed by COMT and MAO in the gut wall and liver. It is administered IV. It is excreted in urine mainly as metabolites and partly as unchanged form. It has extremely short plasma half-life (3 minutes).

Pharmacological Actions

It acts as an agonist on dopaminergic (D_1 and D_2) and adrenergic (α_1, β_2 and β_2) receptors. D_1 receptors are postsynaptic receptors present in few blood vessels and CNS and D_2 receptors are presynaptic receptors present in CNS, ganglia and rehal cortex (tubules). It produces following effects:

1. **CVS effects:** These are dose dependent. In small dose (1 to 5 mg/kg/min), it stimulates D_1 receptors in renal, mesenteric and coronary vessels leading to vasodilatation (by activating adenylcyclase and increasing intracellular cAMP concentration). It also causes an increase in renal blood flow, GFR and sodium excretion in urine (natriuresis). In moderate dose (5 to 10 µg/kg/min), it stimulates β_1 receptors in heart producing +ve inotropic and chronotropic actions. It also causes release of noradrenaline from nerve endings by presynaptic β_2-receptor stimulation, which contributes to its effects on the heart but it does not produce much tachycardia. It also does not produce much change of total peripheral resistance (TPR). In high dose (10 to 20 µg/kg/min), it stimulates vascular adrenergic (α_1) receptors producing a rise of BP by vasoconstriction.

2. **Other effects:** It has insignificant effects on nonvascular smooth muscles and metabolism. It cannot cross BBB and so does not produce CNS effects, but when it is administered as levodopa (precursor of dopamine), which can cross BBB and converted to dopamine, it produces antiparkinsonian effect (by stimulating D_1 receptors) in basal ganglia, emetic effect (by stimulating D_2 receptors in CTZ) and antiprolactin effect (by inhibiting prolactin secretion due to stimulation of D_2 receptors causing release of prolactin inhibitory hormone from the hypothalamus).

Clinical Uses

It is used as a vasopressor agent in the treatment of cardiogenic shock (after myocardial infarction and cardiac surgery), septic shock (due to bacteremia) and severe hypotension following removal of pheochromocytoma. It is particularly beneficial for those patients with oliguria, low cardiac output and low peripheral vascular resistance in hypovolemic shock.

Preparation and Dosage

Dopamine hydrochloride (Intropin) injection (40 mg/ml/amp)—40 mg is dissolved in 500 ml of 5% dextrose solution (acidic) and injected slowly by IV infusion at the rate of 2 to 5 μg/kg/min and gradually increased to 10 to 20 μg/kg/min according to clinical situation.

Adverse Reactions

It can produce palpitation, tachycardia, angina pectoris, hypertension, cardiac arrhythmias, renal ischaemia, nausea and vomiting. Its extravasation into subcutaneous tissue during IV administration can produce necrosis, sloughing of tissue or even gangrene of the part due to severe ischaemia by vasoconstriction. It should be avoided in patients taking MAO inhibitors as severe hypertension can occur.

Synthetic Catecholamines
Isoprenaline/Isoproterenol

Chemistry: It is a synthetic catecholamine. It is isopropyl noradrenaline. Its chemical structure is shown in **Fig. 15.1.**

Pharmacokinetics

It is ineffective orally, as it undergoes extensive first pass metabolism in gut wall and liver. It is readily absorbed when given sublingually parenterally or as an aerosol. It is metabolized in the liver and other tissues by COMT and MAO. It is a relatively poor substrate for MAO. It is excreted in urine mainly as metabolites and partly as unchanged form. It has longer duration of action than adrenaline.

Pharmacological Actions

It is a potent nonselective β-adrenergic (both β_1 and β_2 receptors) agonist. It has negligible action on α-adrenergic receptors due to low affinity for these receptors. It produces following effects:

1. **CVS effects:** It has two opposing effects on CVS, i.e. on heart and BP. It increases heart rate (by +ve chronotropic action), force of cardiac contractions (by +ve inotropic action), stroke volume and cardiac output by acting on β_1 receptors in the heart. It decreases systolic BP, diastolic BP, pulse pressure and mean pressure by acting on β_2 receptors in blood vessels. It may cause initial slight rise in mean BP due to action on β_1 receptors in the heart. It decreases total peripheral resistance (TPR) by causing dilatation of blood vessels in skeletal muscles, liver, heart and mesentery which contain β_2 receptors. It has no effect on cutaneous, mucosal, renal and splanchnic vessels and on veins, which contain α_1 receptors.

2. **Other effects:** It relaxes almost all varieties of nonvascular smooth muscles (by acting on β_2 receptors), when the tone is high. This action is most prominent in bronchial and gastrointestinal smooth muscles. It prevents or relieves bronchospasm due to various causes. It has no effect on radial muscle of iris, vas deferens and splenic capsule, which contain α_1 receptors. It causes much less hyperglycaemia than adrenaline. This is partly due to stimulation of secretion of insulin by the β-adrenergic activation of pancreatic islets (β cells). It is equally effective as adrenaline in stimulating the release of free fatty acid (FFA) from triglyceride and in energy (ATP) production.

Clinical Uses

It can be used as a cardiac stimulant in the emergency treatment of severe bradycardia, heart (AV) block or cardiac arrest, particularly during insertion of an artificial cardiac pacemaker or in patients with ventricular arrhythmias *torsades de pointes*. It is now less used in the treatment of moderate to severe bronchial asthma and in cardiogenic shock.

Preparations and Dosage

- Isoprenaline sulphate (Prenamin) tablet (10 mg)—5 to 20 mg sublingually.

- Isoprenaline hydrochloride for inhalation (Aerosol) (1:100 and 1:200 solution in normal saline)—0.5 to 1 ml by inhalation.

Adverse Reactions

It can produce buccal ulceration when used sublingually. In high dose it can produce palpitation, tachycardia, cardiac arrhythmias, angina pectoris, headache, flushing of skin and tremors. It produces less adverse effects after inhalation than sublingual administration.

It should not be used with adrenaline, as it can produce fatal ventricular arrhythmias.

Dobutamine

It is a synthetic derivative of dopamine but without dopamine receptor agonistaction. It is a selective β_1 agonist, though it has some β_2-adrenergic effects. It has a potent inotropic action but negligible chronotropic and peripheral vascular actions. If patients with low cardiac output failure, it increases the cardiac output without increasing the heart rate, BP and total peripheral resistance. Unlike dopamine, it does not cause renal vasodilatation. It is ineffective orally and so administered by IV infusion.

Clinical Uses

It is used as a cardiac stimulant in the treatment of refractory, chronic, congestive cardiac failure, unresponsive to digitalis. It can also used in the treatment of cardiogenic shock and bacteremic shock. It has a short duration of action.

Preparation and Dosage

Dobutamine hydrochloride (Dobutrex) injection (50 mg/ml in 5 ml vial)—250 mg is dissolved in 500 ml of 5% dextrose solution (acidic) and administered by slow IV infusion at the rate of 2.5 to 10 µg/kg/min.

Adverse Reactions

These are similar to dopamine. It can cause cardiac arrhythmias, which are less than dopamine.

Dopexamine (Dopacard)

It is a congener of dopamine. It is a nonselective dopaminergic (both D_1 and D_2 receptors) and β-adrenergic (both β_1 and β_2 receptors) agonist. It is used in severe heart failure cardiac surgery. It is administered by IV infusion in the dose of 0.5 to 5 µg/kg/min. It is also effective when used orally.

Adverse Reactions

These are similar to dopamine but less.

Prenalterol/Xamoterol (Corwin)

It is a phenol derivative resembling isoprenaline in chemical structure. It is a relatively selective β_1-adrenergic agonist. It increases myocardial contractility and cardiac output. Its effects on heart rate, peripheral resistance and BP are variable. It can be administered orally and parenterally. It is used in patients with postischaemic heart failure and with severe refractory chronic congestive cardiac failure. Its prolonged use may cause desensitization of β_1 receptor, thus limiting its therapeutic usefulness.

Preparations and Dosage

Prenalterol tablet (50 mg)—50 to 100 mg twice daily. Prenalterol injection (1 mg/ml) is also available.

Adverse Reactions

It can cause nausea, tachycardia and ventricular ectopic beats.

Noncatecholamines

These are synthetic drugs. These are non-polor drugs and can cross BBB. These are orally effective and long-acting. These are of following groups:

1. Nonselective Adrenergic Agonists (Stimulants)

These are discussed as follows:

Ephedrine

It is an alkaloid, which was formerly obtained from a Chinese plant, Ma huang (*Ephedra vulgaris*) and used in ancient Chinese medicines for centuries. It is now prepared synthetically. Its chemical structure resembles amphetamine (as shown in **Fig. 15.1**).

Pharmacokinetics

It is effective when administered by almost all routes. It is completely absorbed and distributed throughout the body. It has a longer duration of action (6 to 8 hours), because it is resistant to MAO. It is slowly metabolized in the liver by deamination, demethylation and conjugation. It is excreted in urine mainly as metabolites (80%) and partly as unchanged form (20%). It can cross BBB. It has a plasma half-life of 2 to 3 hours.

Pharmacological Actions

It is a mixed acting adrenergic drug that act by stimulating both α- and β-adrenergic receptors directly as well as indirectly by releasing noradrenaline from adrenergic nerve endings. It produces following effects:

- **CNS effects:** It is a potent CNS stimulant like caffeine or amphetamine. It produces restlessness, excitement, insomnia and tremors.

- **CVS effects:** It stimulates $β_1$ receptors in the heart and increases heart rate, force of cardiac contraction and cardiac output. The heart rate may be reflexly slowed. It increases both systolic and diastolic BPs like noradrenaline by vasoconstriction, increased myocardial contractility and cardiac output. In contrast to adrenaline, its pressor response occurs much slower and lasts much longer. It exhibits tachyphylaxis on repeated use.

- **Other effects:** Its effects on nonvascular smooth muscles are similar to adrenaline. It relaxes bronchial muscles but is slower in onset and less potent than adrenaline.

It relaxes detrusor muscle of urinary bladder but contracts trigonal and sphincter and increases the resistance to outflow of urine. It relaxes intestinal and uterine smooth muscles when applied locally in the conjunctiva, it produces mydriasis. It has little metabolic effects in comparison to adrenaline. It increases muscle strength by increasing metabolic rate and oxygen consumption of muscles. It is included in dope test in athletes.

Clinical Uses

It can be used in the treatment of chronic bronchial asthma, narcolepsy (amphetamine is better), Stokes-Adams syndrome (partial heart block with syncope) and myasthenia gravis (as an adjuvant to anticholinesterase drug). It is used as a nasal decongestant and as a mydriatic agent in ophthalmology.

Preparations and Dosage

- Ephedrine hydrochloride tablet (30 mg)— 15 to 30 mg thrice daily.
- Ephedrine hydrochloride injection (30 mg/ ml)—15 to 30 mg SC, IM or IV.
- Ephedrine nasal drops (1% solution).
- Ephedrine eye drops (3 to 5% solution).

Adverse Reactions

It can produce GIT upset (nausea and vomiting), difficulty in micturition, urinary retention, restlessness, excitement, insomnia, tremors, headache, psychosis, palpitation, tachycardia, cardiac arrhythmias and hypertension in large dose or after parenteral use.

Pholedrine is a mixed acting adrenergic agonist and used in hypotensive states of raised BP. It is available as veritol drops.

Amphetamine

It is a synthetic drug resembling ephedrine in chemical structure (as shown in **Fig. 15.1**). It is a racemic (d-l) β-phenylisopropylamine. Its dextroisomer form (dexamphetamine) is 3 to 4 times more potent as CNS stimulant.

Pharmacokinetics

It is well-absorbed after oral administration. It is slowly metabolized like ephedrine in the liver and excreted in urine as metabolites (60%) and unchanged form (40%). It has longer duration of action (8 to 12 hours).

Pharmacological Actions

It is an indirectly acting adrenergic drug and acts by releasing noradrenaline from adrenergic nerve endings. It has nonselective action on both α- and β-adrenergic receptors. It produces following effects:

- **CNS effects:** It is a potent CNS stimulant. It stimulates cerebrospinal axis including cerebral cortex, RAS and medullary centres. It decreases CNS depression produced by drugs. It is a potent psychomotor stimulant like caffeine. It produces wakefulness, alertness, mood elevation, talkativeness and euphoria with increased initiative, self-confidence and ability to concentrate and decreased sense of fatigue. It increases motor and speech activities and improves performance of simple mental tasks. It also improves physical performance in athletes and is often abused for this purpose. It is included in dope test in athletes. It decreases appetite by inhibiting lateral hypothalamic feeding centre and thus decreasing food intake. It does not stimulate ventromedial hypothalamic satiety centre, which produces feeling of satiety (satisfaction).

- **CVS effects:** It is less potent than ephedrine in stimulating the heart and raising BP. Heart rate is often reflexly slowed. Cardiac output is not much increased in therapeutic dose. It increases both systolic and diastolic BP. It does not change much cerebral blood flow.

- **Other effects:** It has little effects on non-vascular smooth muscles in comparison to ephedrine. It relaxes bronchial smooth muscles and contracts trigone and sphincter of urinary bladder only in large dose. It has little metabolic effects like ephedrine.

Clinical Uses

It is used in the treatment of narcolepsy, (irresistible desire to sleep) attention deficit hyperactivity disorder (ADHD) in children, (methyl phenidate is better than it), obesity (as appetite suppressant), and administered in the (dose in 5 to 10 mg daily) urinary incontinence in elderly, nocturnal enuresis in children and myasthenia gravis (to increase muscle strength).

Preparations and Dosage

- Dexamphetamine sulphate (Dexedrine) tablet (5 mg)—5 to 10 mg daily.
- Methamphetamine hydrochloride (Methedrine) tablet (5 mg)—5 to 10 mg daily.

Adverse Reactions

These are similar to ephedrine. It produces tolerance and psychological dependence on prolonged use. Withdrawal of the drug from abusers may produce symptoms of chronic fatigue and depression. Acute poisoning due to overdose is treated by acidification of urine by ammonium chloride to increase its urinary excretion. Other symptomatic treatment is done according to need.

Methamphetamine is a derivative of amphetamine. It is nearly equipotent to dexamphetamine as a CNS stimulant and is more potent than ephedrine as a pressor agent.

Methamphetamine is a piperidine derivative structurally related to amphetamine. It has mild CNS stimulant with prominent effects on mental activity than on motor activities. It is used in narcolepsy and ADHD. It has abuse liability.

Tyramine is a natural amine present in foods. It is an indirectly acting adrenergic agonist. It is responsible for cheese reaction (hypertensive crisis) when used with nonselective MAO inhibitors.

2. Selective α₁-adrenergic Agonists (Stimulants)
Phenylephrine (Neo-Synephrine)

It is a synthetic directly acting α_1-adrenergic agonist. Its oral absorption is unreliable and so it is administered parenterally and topically (in eye and nose). It cannot cross BBB and so it has no CNS effect. It has long duration of action as it is resistant to MAO and COMT. It is metabolized in the liver and excreted in urine as metabolites and unchanged form. It produces actions similar to noradrenaline, but it is less potent. It produces peripheral vasoconstriction leading to rise of BP. It can produce reflex bradycardia by vagal activation. It produces mydriasis and nasal decongestion.

Clinical Uses

It is used as a vasopressor agent in hypovolemic shock, nasal decongestant in rhinitis and sinusitis and mydriatic in ophthalmology especially in patients with glaucoma. It can also be used to treat paroxysmal atrial tachycardia.

Preparations and Dosage

- Phenylephrine hydrochloride injection (5 mg/ml/amp)—5 to 20 mg SC, IM or by IV infusion with 5% dextrose saline.
- Phenylephrine nasal or eye drops (1 to 2% solution).

Adverse Reactions

It has less adverse effects in comparison to noradrenaline.

Methoxamine

It is a synthetic directly acting α_1-adrenergic agonist. It has pharmacokinetics like phenylephrine. It causes peripheral vasoconstriction leading to rise of BP. It does not cause cardiac stimulation, but produces reflex bradycardia. It cannot cross BBB and does not cause significant CNS stimulation.

Clinical Uses

It is used as a vasopressor agent in hypovolemic shock and other hypotensive states, paroxysmal arterial tachycardia and as nasal decongestant.

Preparations and Dosage

- Methoxamine hydrochloride (Vasoxine) injection (10 mg/ml/amp)—10 to 20 mg SC, IM or by IV infusion.
- Methoxamine nasal drops (0.25 to 0.5% solution).

Adverse Reactions

These are similar to phenylephrine.

Metaraminol

It is a synthetic mixed acting α_1-adrenergic agonist. It acts directly on the adrenergic receptor. It has pharmacokinetics like phenylephrine. It causes peripheral vasoconstriction leading to rise of BP, which can cause reflex bradycardia. It also increases the force of cardiac contraction and cardiac output. It increases coronary blood flow, probably due to rise of BP.

Clinical Uses

It is used as a vasopressor agent in hypovolemic shock and other hypotensive states and in paroxysmal atrial tachycardia and as nasal decongestant.

Preparations and Dosage

- Metaraminol bitartrate (Aramine) injection (5 mg ml/amp)—5 to 10 mg IM or by IV infusion.
- Metaraminol nasal drops (0.25 to 0.5% solution).

Adverse Reactions

These are similar to phenylephrine.

Mephentermine

It is a synthetic mixed acting α_1-adrenergic agonist. It has pharmacokinetics like metaraminol. Its actions are similar to those of methamphetamine except it has weak CNS effects. It causes peripheral vasoconstriction leading to rise of BP, which can cause reflex bradycardia. It also increases the force of cardiac contraction and cardiac output. It is used as a vasopressor agent in hypovolemic shock and other hypotensive states.

Preparation and Dosage

Mephentermine hydrochloride (Mephentine) injection (5 mg/ml/amp)—5 to 20 mg IM or by IV infusion.

Adverse Reactions

These are similar to phenylephrine. In high dose it can produce cardiac depression and CNS stimulation (producing convulsions).

3. Selective α₂-adrenergic Agonists (Stimulants)

These are clonidine, α-methyldopa, guanfacine and guanabenz. These will be discussed with antihypertensive drugs in cardiovascular pharmacology.

4. Selective β₂-adrenergic Agonists (Stimulants)

These are orciprenaline, salbutamol, terbutaline, ritodrine and isoetharine. These will be discussed with bronchodilators in respiratory pharmacology.

5. Nasal Decongestants

These are adrenergic α agonists, which on topical application in nose as dilute solution produce local vasoconstriction (by $α_1$ action) in the nasal mucous membrane leading to nasal decongestion. Their chronic use causes loss of efficacy, rebound congestion (by receptor desensitization) and nasal mucosal damage.

Some Preparations

- Ephedrine hydrochloride (1% solution).
- Phenylephrine hydrochloride (0.25% solution).
- Xylometazoline hydrochloride (0.1% solution) (Otrivin).
- Oxymetazoline hydrochloride (0.05% solution) (Nasivion).
- Naphazoline hydrochloride (0.05% solution) (Privine).
- Tetrahydrazoline hydrochloride (0.05% solution).

These are used in rhinitis, sinusitis and common cold. An ideal nasal decongestant should produce a prompt, prolonged and reliable effect and should be free from tachyphylaxis, local irritation and damaging effect on nasal mucosa. It should not produce after congestion, atrophic rhinitis and anosmia (unlike ephedrine and phenylephrine).

Pseudoephedrine (Sudafed) is a stereoisomer of ephedrine. It has poor bronchodilator and CNS stimulant effects. It is given orally as tablet (60 mg) or syrup (30 mg/5 ml) as a nasal decongestant and to relieve eustachian tube congestion. It is less likely to cause tachycardia, hypertension and CNS stimulation than ephedrine.

6. Anorectic Drugs (Appetite Suppressants)

These are adrenergic drugs used in the treatment of obesity to reduce appetite by inhibiting lateral hypothalamic feeding centre and thus decreasing food intake. As amphetamines produce CNS stimulation and have abuse liability, so some drugs have been developed, which are free from these adverse effects, e.g. fenfluramine, dexfenfluramine, phenteramine, benzphenteramine, phenmetrazine, phendimetrazine, diethyl propion and mazindol.

Preparations and Dosage

- Fenfluramine (Simerex) tablet (20 mg)—20 mg thrice daily before meals.
- Dexfenfluramine (Isomeride) capsule (15 mg)—15 mg twice daily with meals.

Adverse Reactions

Fenfluramine can cause lethargy, drowsiness, palpitation, light-headedness, dry mouth, diarrhoea, loss of libido, insomnia and depression. Dexfenfluramine is better tolerated than fenfluramine and so more preferred.

7. Peripheral Vasodilators

These are nylidrin (Arlidin) and isoxsuprine (Duvadilah). These are used in peripheral vasospastic disorders as tablet or injection. Isoxsuprine is also used in cerebrovascular insufficiency, spastic occlusion of retinal vessels and as uterine relaxant. It can cause hypotension, dizziness, palpitation, nausea, vomiting, abdominal distress and skin rashes.

16

Antiadrenergic Drugs/ Sympatholytic Drugs

INTRODUCTION

Antiadrenergic drugs antagonize/prevent the responses of effector organs to endogenous as well as exogenous adrenergic drugs by blocking adrenergic receptors. These are also called adrenergic receptor blockers or adrenergic antagonists.

Classification

These are of two groups:

1. α-adrenergic receptor blockers, e.g. phenoxybenzamine, tolazoline and prazosin.
2. β-adrenergic receptor blockers, e.g. propranolol, atenolol and labetalol.

α-adrenergic Receptor Blocking Drugs (α-blockers)

These drugs block α_1 receptor mediated effects like contraction of vascular (arterial and venous) smooth muscles and some nonvascular smooth muscles (loss in pyloric ileocaecal and trigonal sphincters) and α_2 receptor mediated effects like inhibition of central sympathetic outflow, inhibition of release of noradrenaline from nerve endings, inhibition of release of insulin from pancreatic islets and facilitation of platelet aggregation. These drugs are more effective in antagonizing the alpha receptor effects of exogenously administered adrenaline and noradrenaline than those following adrenergic nerve stimulation.

Classification

These are of three groups:

1. **Non-selective α-blockers**—These are of following types:
   - *Non-equilibrium type*:
     β-haloalkylamines (alkylating agents), e.g. phenoxybenzamine and dibenzamine.
   - *Equilibrium type*:
     - Imidazolines, e.g. phentolamine and tolazoline.
     - Natural and dihydrogenated ergot alkaloids, e.g. ergotamine, ergotoxine, dihydroergotamine (DHE) and dihydroergotoxine (hydergine).
     - Miscellaneous drugs, e.g. chlorpromazine and ketanserin.
2. **Selective α_1-blockers**—These are given as follows:
   Quinazolines, e.g. prazosin, terazosin, doxazosin tamsulosin and alfazogin
3. **Selective α_2-blockers**—These are given as follows:
   Indoles, e.g. yohimbine and rauwolscine.

General Pharmacological Properties (Actions) of α-blockers

These are given as follows:

- **CVS effects:** α_1-blockers by blocking α_1 receptors in blood vessels inhibit vasoconstriction produced by catecholamines. This leads to vasodilatation in arterioles and veins causing a fall of blood pressure due to decreased peripheral vascular resistance. For most α_1-blockers, the fall of blood pressure is opposed by baroreceptor reflexes that cause increase in heart rate (tachycardia) and cardiac output and fluid retention. These reflexes are exaggerated if the blocker also blocks presynaptic α_2 receptors on peripheral sympathetic nerve endings causing increased release of noradrenaline and increased stimulation of postsynaptic β_1 receptors in the heart and juxtaglomerular cells of the kidney. They also block vasoconstriction and rise of blood pressure produced by administration of exogenous adrenergic drugs, but the pattern of effects depends on the type of adrenergic agonist that is administered, e.g. pressor response of phenylephrine is completely blocked, pressor response of noradrenaline is incompletely blocked due to residual stimulation of cardiac β_1-receptors and pressor response of adrenaline may be transformed to vasodepressor effect (vasomotor reversal of Dale) due to residual stimulation of β_2 receptors on blood vessels causing vasodilatation. α_1-blockers by blocking α_2 receptors increase central sympathetic outflow (in pontomedullary region) and also increase the release of noradrenaline from adrenergic nerve endings causing stimulation of β_1 and α_1 receptors, increase central sympathetic outflow (in pontomedullary region) and also increase the release of noradrenaline from adrenergic nerve endings causing stimulation of α_1 and β_1 receptors in the heart and peripheral blood vessels respectively with a consequent rise of blood pressure. But the net effect of both α_1 and α_2 receptors blockade is a fall of BP due to inhibition of vasoconstriction.

- **Other effects:** By blocking α_1 receptors, they antagonize the contraction of nonvascular smooth muscles in pyloric, ileocaecal and trigonal sphincters produced by adrenergic drugs. They inhibit contraction of trigonal sphincter muscles in the base of the urinary bladder leading to decreased resistance to urinary outflow. Their effect on bronchial smooth muscles is minimum, though α_1 receptors may produce contraction of bronchial muscle. They can inhibit catecholamine induced hyperglycaemia by decreasing glucose output from the liver, where both β and α receptors are involved. They may increase insulin release from pancreatic islets by blocking stimulation of α_2 receptors. They also block α_2 receptor mediated platelet aggregation.

DISCUSSION OF SOME α-BLOCKERS

Phenoxybenzamine

It is a β-haloalkylamine. It is chemically related to nitrogen mustard and produces high reactive carbonium ion in blood. It is a nonselective α-blocker. It binds with both α_1 and α_2 receptors by covalent bonds leading to irreversible blockade of the receptors. It has high affinity for α_1 receptor than α_2 receptor. It produces CVS and other effects as mentioned before. It has also antihistaminic property. It is orally effective and also administered IV. It is metabolized in the liver and excreted in urine as metabolites and unchanged form. It has long duration of action (2 to 3 days).

Clinical Uses

It is used in the long-term treatment of hypertension in patients of pheochromocytomas, which are adrenal medullary tumours secreting large quantities of catecholamines producing hypertension. Most of the pheochromocytomas are treated by surgical removal. Phenoxybenzamine is also used for preoperative preparation of patient with pheochromocytoma. It controls episodes of severe hypertension and minimizes other adverse effects of catecholamines such as contraction of plasma volume and injury to myocardium.

It can be used in the treatment of benign prostatic hypertrophy (BPH) with obstruction.

Preparations and Dosage

- Phenoxybenzamine hydrochloride (Dibenzyline) capsule (10 mg)—10 mg twice daily for 1 to 3 weeks before the operation. The dose may be increased every alternate day until the desired effect (fall of BP) is achieved.
- Phenoxybenzamine hydrochloride injection (10 mg/ml)—10 mg IV twice daily in emergency.

Adverse Reactions

It can cause postural hypotension, reflex tachycardia and cardiac arrhythmias. It also produces blurring of vision (miosis), dryness of mouth, nasal stuffiness and inhibition (failure) of ejaculation (in male). It is lipid-soluble and so crosses BBB producing sedation, giddiness, lethargy, fatigue, nausea and vomiting. It produces cumulative toxicity.

Dibenzamine is a congener of phenoxybenzamine and has similar actions but much less potent (6 to 10 times) and so rarely used.

Phentolamine

It is an imidazoline derivative. It is a nonselective α-blocker. It has similar affinity for both α_1 and α_2 receptors. It produces competitive reversible blockade of the α receptors. It has quick onset and short duration of action (2 to 3 hours).

It is poorly absorbed from GIT and so administered parenterally usually IV. It is metabolized in the liver and excreted in urine. It produces CVS and other effects as mentioned before. It has some additional effects. It blocks 5-HT receptors. It produces histaminergic actions (by releasing histamine from mast cells) and parasympathomimetic (muscarinic) actions. It blocks K^+ channels in the muscles. It stimulates gastrointestinal smooth muscle and increases GIT motility. It increases gastric secretion by an agonist action on muscarinic (M_1) receptor, which can be blocked by atropine. It also stimulates lacrimal, salivary and sweat secretions.

Clinical Uses

- It is used for short-term treatment of hypertension in patients of pheochromocytomas.
- It can be used for diagnosis of pheochromocytomas.
  Phentolamine test: Injection of phentolamine (5 mg IV) in patient of pheochromocytoma produces abrupt fall of BP (> 35 mm Hg of systolic BP and > 25 mm Hg of diastolic BP).
- It can be used locally to prevent dermal necrosis after extravasation of an α-adrenergic agonist.
- It may be used for the treatment of hypertensive crisis after sudden withdrawal of clonidine or cheese reaction due to ingestion of tyramine containing foods during the use of nonselective MAO inhibitors (e.g. phenelzine, isocarboxazid and tranylcypromine).

Preparation and Dosage

Phentolamine mesylate (Regitine) injection (5 mg/ml) 5 to 10 mg IV and repeated if necessary.

Adverse Reactions

It produces postural hypotension, reflex tachycardia, cardiac arrhythmias and ischaemic heart attack (by cardiac stimulation). It can produce nausea, vomiting, epigastric distress, diarrhoea and exacerbation of peptic ulcer (by GIT stimulation). It can produce profuse sweating and severe hypotension in large dose.

Tolazoline (Priscoline), a congener of phentolamine has similar actions but less potent and so less used.

Ergot Alkaloids

Natural amino acid ergot alkaloids, e.g. ergotamine, and ergotoxine (combination of ergocornine, ergocristine and ergocryptine) and their dihydrogenated derivatives, e.g. dihydroergotamine (DHE) and dihydroergotoxine (Hydergine) are nonselective α-receptor blockers. They produce competitive and reversible blockade of α receptors of short duration (2 to 4 hours). They are effective both orally and parenterally. They have CVS and other effects as mentioned before. They have also 5-HT antagonistic activity.

Clinical Uses

They are used in migraine and as α-adrenergic blockers.

Preparations and Dosage

- Ergotamine tartrate tablet (1 mg)—1 to 4 mg orally or sublingually.
- Ergotamine tartrate injection (0.5 mg/ml)—0.25 to 0.5 mg SC or IM.
- Dihydroergotamine injection (1 mg/ml)—1 to 1.5 mg SC or IM.

Adverse Reactions

They can produce nausea, vomiting, miosis, postural hypotension, anginal pain, vascular insufficiency and gangrene of the extremities (ergotism) due to peripheral vasospasm.

Prazosin

It is a quinazoline derivative. It is a selective α-receptor antagonist. It causes fall of BP by blocking α receptor in arterioles and veins and thus decreasing peripheral vascular resistance and venous return to the heart. It decreases cardiac preload and so it does not increase heart rate (by reflex tachycardia) and cardiac output. It depresses central sympathetic outflow. It also depresses baroreceptor reflex function in hypertensive patients. It decreases the tone of trigone and sphincter of urinary bladder leading to decreased resistance to urinary outflow in patients with benign prostatic hypertrophy (BPH). It is well-absorbed after oral administration. It is highly plasma protein bound. It is metabolized in the liver and excreted in urine mainly as metabolites. It has a moderate duration of action (4 to 6 hours). It has a plasma t½ of 2–3 hours.

Clinical Uses

- It is used in the treatment of primary (essential) hypertension and BPH (benign prostatic hyperplasia).

- It can be used in vasospastic angina pectoris and in Raynaud's disease (a vasospastic ischaemic peripheral vascular disorder).

Preparation and Dosage

Prazosin (Minipres, Prazopress) tablet (1, 2 mg)—0.5 to 1 mg twice daily and gradually increased to 2 to 4 mg twice daily according to BP response.

Adverse Reactions

It can produce first dose effect (phenomenon) characterized by severe postural hypotension and syncope due to vascular collapse. For this reason, its initial dose is given at bed time, so that the patient remains recumbent in bed for at least several hours to reduce the risk of syncopal reaction after the first dose. Later on the patient develops tolerance to this effect. Its other adverse effects include headache, dizziness, drowsiness, lethargy, nausea and constipation. Terazosin (Hytrin) and doxazosin (Doxapress) are structural analogs of prazosin. They have longer duration of action (administered once daily) but they are less potent than prazosin (require higher dosage). They have same uses and adverse effects as prazosin. Tamsulosin is more selective for receptor subtype, which accounts for about 70% of α_1 receptors in the prostate and bladder base. It is used in BPH to relieve symptoms of urinary obstruction in doses of 400 to 800 kg once daily. It does not produce postural hypotension. It can produce dizziness and retrograde ejaculation.

Yohimbine (Yacon)

It is an alkaloid obtained from the West African tree Yohimbene. It is a selective α_2-blocker. It is claimed to be an aphrodisiac (sexual stimulant) and helps about 50% of patients with impotence, but prolonged use is needed. It is administered orally as tablet (2 mg). It has short duration of action (1 to 3 hours). Rauwolfia is an alkaloid obtained from rauwolfia root. It has no aphrodisiac action.

β-adrenergic Receptor Blocking Drugs (β-blockers)

These drugs antagonize the actions of catecholamines mediated through beta receptor stimulation. They block β_1-receptor effects like cardiac stimulation and increased release of renin from juxtaglomerular cells of kidneys, β_2-receptor mediated effects like relaxation of vascular and nonvascular smooth muscles and metabolic effects (glycogenolysis and gluconeogenesis) in the liver and skeletal muscles and β_3-receptor mediated effect (lipolysis) in adipose tissue. At the cellular level, through their action on preceptors, they inhibit the activation of the membrane enzyme adenylcyclase and thus decrease the production of cAMP.

Classification

These are four groups (all are competitive blockers):

- Nonselective β-blockers (block β_1, β_2 and β_3 receptors). These are given as follows:
  - β-blockers without intrinsic sympathomimetic activity (ISA), e.g. propranolol, timolol and sotalol.
  - β-blockers with intrinsic sympathomimetic activity (ISA), e.g. pindolol, carteotolol and penbutolol.
  - β-blockers with additional alpha blocking activity, e.g. labetalol, dilevalol medroxy and bucindolol, carvedilol.
- Selective β_1-blockers (cardioselective β-blockers):
  - Without intrinsic sympathomimetic activity, e.g. atenolol, metoprolol, esmolol and nepivolol, betaxolol and bisoprlol.
  - With intrinsic sympathomimetic activity, e.g. acebutolol and celiprolol.
- Selective β_2-blockers, butoxamine.
- Selective β_3-blocker—ICI-118551 (a synthetic compound).

All groups of drugs produce competitive and equilibrium or reversible type of blockade.

Chemistry

All β-blockers have some structural similarity with the β-agonist, isoprenaline (isoproterenol). They are either lipid-soluble or water-soluble. Highly lipid-soluble β-blockers are propranolol, timolol, metoprolol, pindolol and labetalol. They can easily cross BBB. Highly water-soluble or low lipid-soluble β-blockers are atenolol, acebutolol, nadolol, sotalol and esmolol. They cannot easily cross BBB.

Affinity of β-blockers for β receptors

Nonselective β-blockers have equal affinity for β_1, β_2 and β_3 receptors.

Selective β_1-blockers have greater affinity for β_1 receptors and little or no affinity for β_2 and β_3 receptors. β-blockers with intrinsic sympathomimetic activity are not pure β-antagonists as they activate preceptors partially in the absence of catecholamines. So they are partial agonists. Labetalol, dilevatol and carved block both α_1 and β_2 receptors, whereas celiprolol blocks β_1 receptor but activates β_2 receptor (β_2-agonist action).

General Pharmacological Properties (Actions) of β-blockers

These are given as follows:

- **CVS effects**
- **Effects on heart:** β-blockers have little or no effect on the normal heart of an individual at rest but has profound effects on heart when the sympathetic control of the heart is dominant as during exercise or stress. By blocking β_1 receptors in heart, they decrease heart rate and force of cardiac contraction, i.e. they antagonize the positive chronotropic and inotropic actions of catecholamines on the heart. On short-term administration, they decrease cardiac output but increase peripheral vascular resistance by blocking vascular β_2 receptors and inhibiting compensatory sympathetic reflexes that activate vascular α_1 receptors. On long-term administration, they decrease total peripheral resistance (TPR) due

to persistent reduction in cardiac output. β-blockers that have intrinsic sympathomimetic activity can decrease peripheral vascular resistance on short-term treatment due to β_2 action. β-blockers also have significant effects on cardiac rhythm and automaticity. They decrease sinus (SA node) rate and spontaneous rate of depolarization of ectopic pacemakers, slow conduction in the atria and AV node and increase refractory period of AV node. They increase exercise tolerance in patients of angina pectoris.

- **Effects on BP:** β-blockers do not decrease BP in normal individuals (with normal BP), but they decrease BP in patients with hypertension. They lower BP by following mechanisms:
  - By blocking cardiac β_1 receptors, thus decreasing heart rate, force of cardiac contraction and cardiac output.
  - By decreasing peripheral vascular resistance on long-term use due to persistent reduction in cardiac output.
  - By blocking α_1 receptors in blood vessels (e.g. labetalol and carvedilol).
  - By central α_2 receptor stimulant (agonist) action in pontomedullary region (VMC) leading to decreased central sympathetic outflow.
  - By blocking the release of renin from the juxtaglomerular cells of kidneys (lowering of plasma renin activity), which is stimulated by sympathetic nervous system.
  - By increasing synthesis of prostacyclin (PGI_2), which is a vasodilator.

- **Respiratory effects:** Nonselective β-blockers block β_2 receptors in bronchial smooth muscle. This usually has little effect on pulmonary functions in normal individuals but in patients with bronchial asthma or chronic obstructive pulmonary disease (COPD), this can lead to life-threatening bronchoconstriction (spasm). Selective β_1-blockers and β-blockers with intrinsic sympathomimetic activity are less likely to increase airway resistance in these patients and so can be used safely.

- **Metabolic effects:** β-blockers modify the metabolism of carbohydrates and lipids. They decrease glucose tolerance capacity of the body and produce carbohydrate intolerance in prediabetic patients. They inhibit (block) catecholamine induced hyperglycaemia and hyperlipidaemia by inhibiting glycogenolysis and lipolysis. Nonselective β-blockers by blocking β_2 receptors may produce hypoglycaemia unresponsiveness or delay of recovery from hypoglycaemia in insulin dependent diabetics. So they should be used with great caution in patients with labile diabetes receiving insulin or oral antidiabetic drugs. Selective β_1-blockers are safer in this respect, because they are less likely to delay recovery from hypoglycaemia. All β-blockers mask the important warning sign tachycardia, which is typically seen in patient with hypoglycaemia. β-blockers rarely impair insulin release, though β-agonists potentiate insulin secretion.

- **Miscellaneous effects:** β-blockers antagonize (block) essential tremors induced by catecholamines. They also inhibit catecholamine induced facilitation of platelet aggregation and inhibition of mast cell degranulation (to release histamine and other autacoids).

Clinical Uses (Indications) of β-blockers

These are given as follows:

- **Cardiovascular conditions (diseases):**
  - **Essential (primary) hypertension:** Propranolol, atenolol, nebivolol or metoprolol is used either alone or with a diuretic or a vasodilator in mild to moderate hypertension. Labetalol or dilevatol or carvidilol is used in severe hypertension.
  - **Angina pectoris:** Propranolol, atenolol or nebivolol is used for chronic prophylaxis of angina pectoris (except variant angina) and acts by inhibiting sympathetic support to the heart. In variant (vasospastic/Prinzmetal's) angina β-blocker is

contraindicated due to unopposed α-effect (α$_1$-mediated vasoconstriction) leading to worsening of the condition.

– **Cardiac arrhythmias:** Propranolol, atenolol, nebivolol, celiprolol or esmolol is used to control both atrial and ventricular tachyarrhythmias.

– **Myocardial infarction (MI) without CCF:** Propranolol, atenolol, celiprolol or esmolol is used in early phase of myocardial infarction to prevent rupture of myocardium, to reduce infarct size and to prevent reinfraction and occurrence of cardiac arrhythmias including ventricular fibrillation.

– **Portal hypertension:** Propranolol can be used to reduce the heart rate, cardiac output and splenchnic blood flow. It reduce portal pressure, blood flow through azygous system and bleeding from oesophageal varices (hemetemeris) in subjects of portal cirrhosis.

– **Hypertrophic obstructive (subaortic) cardiomyopathy:** Propranolol, atenolol or metoprolol is used to decrease ventricular outflow resistance.

– **Dissecting aortic aneurysm:** Propranolol, atenolol or metoprolol is used to reduce myocardial contractile force and aortic regurgitation.

• **Noncardiovascular conditions**

– **Thyrotoxicosis and thyroid crisis:** Propranolol is useful to control the symptoms and signs (palpitation, tremors, chest pain and raised BMR) and acts by inhibiting peripheral conversion of T$_4$ to T$_3$.

– **Pheochromocytoma:** Propranolol along with an α-blocker or labetalol alone is used to control severe BP before surgical removal of the tumour. In pheochromocytoma there is excessive release of catecholamines (NA and AD) which act on cardiac and vascular receptors to raise BP. When β-blockers are used alone there will be severe rise of BP as the released catecholamines which stimulate the α-receptors causing an increase in peripheral resistance. This overrides β-receptors blocked action in blood vessels, causing rise in BP.

– **Migraine:** Propranolol or timolol is used for chronic prophylaxis of migraine.

– **Chronic simple (open angle) glaucoma:** Timolol or betaxolol is used as eye drops to reduce secretion of aqueous humour by choroid plexus.

– **Essential tremors:** Propranolol or timolol is used to control muscle tremors mediated through β$_2$ receptors and not tremors due to parkinsonism.

– **Anxiety state:** Propranolol or timolol is used to relieve panic state in public meeting or conference and acts by reducing somatic manifestations of anxiety (palpitation, tremors and nervousness).

– **Alcohol withdrawal syndrome:** Propranolol or timolol is used to control symptoms and signs of alcohol withdrawal.

Contraindications of β-blockers

• Bronchial asthma and COPD—as it aggravates these conditions by causing bronchoconstriction.

• Myocardial insufficiency—as it precipitates congestive cardial failure (CCF) by blocking sympathetic support to the heart.

• Left ventricular failure (LVF) and cor pulmonale as it blocks sympathetic supports to the heart.

• Variant (Prinzmetals) angina—as it aggravates the condition.

• Heart (AV) block—as it converts partial block to complete block.

• Insulin dependent diabetes receiving insulin or oral hypoglycaemic drugs—as it produces hypoglycaemia unresponsiveness.

• Peripheral arteriosclerotic or diabetic arterial disease as it worsen the condition.

• With other cardiac depressant drugs, e.g. verapamil, quinidine, halothane, etc.—as it produces further myocardial depression.

Adverse Reactions of β-blockers

These are given as follows:

- **CVS effects:** They produce bradycardia. In patients with heart (AV) block, they may cause life-threatening bradyarrhythmias. They produce hypotension and cold extremities (due to reduction of peripheral blood flow by vasospasm). They may exacerbate CCF in susceptible patients by blocking β₁ receptors in heart, because sympathetic nervous system provides support for cardiac performance in those patients with impaired myocardial function. They can cause cold extremities Raynaud's phenomenon by peripheral vasoconstriction due to blocking of β₂-receptor action. Abrupt withdrawal of β-blockers after long-term treatment produces rebound phenomenon manifested as hypertension, severe angina, acute myocardial infarction or even sudden death of patients with ischaemic heart disease. This may be due to supersensitivity of β receptors to endogenous catecholamines in patients due to long term reduction of agonist stimulation of these receptors. So β-blockers should be withdrawn gradually in tapering dosage.

- **Respiratory effects:** They can produce bronchospasm by blocking β₂ receptors in the bronchial smooth muscle. They may cause life-threatening bronchoconstriction in patients with bronchospastic diseases like bronchial asthma and COPD. Selective β₁-blockers produce less bronchospasm in these patients.

- **CNS effects:** β-blockers which are highly lipid-soluble, e.g. propranolol, timolol, metoprolol and labetalol can easily cross BBB and produce CNS side effects like muscular weakness, fatigue, lethargy, insomnia, nightmares, muscle cramps and mental depression.

- **Metabolic effects:** They are capable of altering the carbohydrate and lipid metabolism. They blunt recognition of hypoglycaemia in diabetic patients by masking the cardinal sign, tachycardia. They also delay recovery from insulin or other drug induced hypoglycaemia. They should be used with caution in patients of diabetes, who are prone to hypoglycaemic reactions. Selective β₁-blockers are preferable for these patients. They produce alteration of lipid profile of blood. They cause rise of serum triglyceride and low density lipoprotein (LDL) cholesterol levels and decrease the serum concentration of high density lipoprotein (HDL) cholesterol. Due to rise in ratio of LDL and HDL in blood, there is chance of coronary atherosclerosis.

- **Miscellaneous effects:** They may rarely cause constipation, diarrhoea or indigestion, skin rashes and fever. They may produce sexual dysfunction (impotence) in male with hypertension. They can be safely used during pregnancy.

Acute Interval Toxicity (due to Overdose) β-blockers

It is manifested as severe bradycardia, cardiac failure and hypotension. In ECG, prolonged (AV conduction time) and widened QRS complex are found.

Treatment

Severe bradycardia is treated by administration of atropine sulphate or isoprenaline sulphate. A cardiac pacemaker may have to be instilled if heart (AV) block occurs. Hypotension is treated by administration of an α-adrenergic agonist (e.g. noradrenaline or phenylephrine) in large doses.

Drug Interactions

These are given as follows:

- Aluminium salts, cholestyramine resin and cholestipol may decrease absorption of β-blockers by binding with them.
- Cimetidine and hydralazine increase bioavailability of β-blockers by increasing hepatic circulation.
- Microsomal enzyme inducers like phenytoin, rifampicin and phenobarbitone increase metabolism of β-blockers in liver leading to decreased plasma concentrations and therapeutic effects of β-blockers.

- Calcium channel blockers and antihypertensive drugs have additive effects with β-blockers on cardiac conduction and BP respectively.

- Indomethacin and phenylbutazone decrease the antihypertensive effects of β-blockers.

DISCUSSION OF SOME β-BLOCKERS

Propranolol

It is a nonselective β-blocker. It has no intrinsic sympathomimetic activity (β-agonist action). It has membrane stabilizing action. It is highly lipid-soluble (lipophilic). It is completely absorbed after oral administration but it undergoes high first pass metabolism in the liver during its passage through portal circulation and only 25% of it reaches the systemic circulation (low bioavailability). It can easily cross BBB and enters CNS. It is highly plasma protein bound (about 90%). It is metabolized in the liver and is excreted in urine mainly as metabolites. One of its active metabolites is 4-hydroxypropranolol. It has a plasma half-life of about 4 hours but its antihypertensive effect is sufficiently long lived. It has high interindividual variability in plasma concentrations due to genetically determined difference in the rate of metabolism in the liver.

Clinical Uses

It is mainly used in the treatment of hypertension, angina pectoris and cardiac arrhythmias.

Preparations and Dosage

- Propranolol hydrochloride (Inderal) tablet (10, 40 and 80 mg)—10 to 40 mg twice daily and gradually increased up to 180 mg twice daily.
- Propranolol hydrochloride injection (1 mg/ml)—1 to 3 mg IV slowly.

Adverse Reactions

Discussed previously.

Atenolol

It is a selective β_1 (cardioselective) blocker. It is devoid of intrinsic sympathomimetic activity and membrane stabilizing action. It is highly water-soluble (hydrophilic). It is incompletely absorbed (about 50%) after oral administration, but most of the absorbed drugs reach the systemic circulation (high bioavailability). It cannot easily cross BBB and has little CNS effects. It is moderately (about 50%) plasma protein bound. It is little metabolized in the liver and is excreted in urine largely as unchanged form. It has a plasma half-life of about 8 hours. It has little interindividual variability in plasma concentrations in comparison to propranolol. It is accumulated in the tissues in patients with renal failure due to slow excretion.

Clinical Uses

It has uses like propranolol. It can be used safely in patients of insulin-dependent diabetes mellitus, bronchial asthma and COPD.

Preparation and Dosage

Atenolol (Atend, Teholol) tablet (50 and 100 mg)— 50 to 100 mg once daily.

Adverse Reactions

Discussed previously.

Metoprolol

It is a selective β_1-blocker like atenolol. It is devoid of intrinsic sympathomimetic activity but has membrane stabilizing action. It is highly lipid-soluble. It is almost completely absorbed after oral administration but it undergoes high first pass metabolism in the liver, giving a bioavailability of about 40%. It is metabolized in the liver and excreted in urine mainly as metabolites (90%). It has high interindividual variability of plasma concentrations like propranolol. It has a plasma half-life t½ of about 4 hours.

Clinical Uses

It has uses like propranolol and atenolol.

Preparations and Dosage

- Metoprolol tartrate (Lopressor) tablet (50 and 100 mg)— 50 to 100 mg twice daily.
- Metoprolol tartrate injection (5 mg/ml)— 5 to 10 mg IV slowly.

Adverse Reactions

Discussed previously.

Esmolol

It is a selective β_1-blocker with very short duration of action (ultrashort-acting). It is devoid of intrinsic sympathomimetic activity and membrane stabilizing action. Its plasma t½ is about 9 minutes. It is water-soluble. It is used when β-blockade of short duration is desired or in critically ill patients, as in patient with acute myocardial infarction, in whom severe bradycardia, heart failure or hypotension may necessitate rapid withdrawal of the drug.

Preparation and Dosage

Esmolol hydrochloride (Esocard) injection (5 mg/ml)—50 to 100 mg/min IV slowly.

Adverse Reactions

Discussed previously.

Labetalol

It is a non-selective β-blocker with additional α_1-blocking activity. It has intrinsic sympathomimetic activity and membrane stabilizing action. It is lipid-soluble and well-absorbed orally. It has a plasma half-life of 8 hours.

Clinical Uses

It is used in severe hypertension and hypertensive crisis (as in pheochromocytomas and after withdrawal of clonidine).

Preparations and Dosage

- Labetalol hydrochloride (Normadate) tablet (100 mg)— 100 mg once daily.
- Labetalol hydrochloride injection (100 mg/ml)—100 mg IV slowly.

Adverse Reactions

Discussed previously.

Timolol

It is a nonselective β-blocker like propranolol. It has no intrinsic sympathomimetic activity and membrane stabilizing action. It is used orally as timolol maleate (Glucomol) tablet (10, 20 mg) in the dose of 10 to 20 mg twice daily.

Topically (as eye drops—0.25 to 0.5% soln) It is used in the treatment of wide (open) angle glaucoma to reduce intraocular tension. It decreases cAMP formation and reduces formation of aqueous humour like propranolol. It has no effect on pupillary size. It has less side effects than propranolol.

Other b-blockers like—Nebivolol (Nebicard) tablet (2.5, 5 mg), carvedilol (cardivas) tablet (12.5, 25 mg), bisoprolol (Corbis) tablet (5, 10 mg) celiprolol (celipres) tablet (100, 200 mg), and sotalol (sotagard) tablet (40, 60 mg), are now available for clinical uses in cardiac disorders.

Section III

AUTACOID PHARMACOLOGY

17

Histamine and Histamine Antagonists

INTRODUCTION

The term autacoid is derived from two Greek words, *viz. autos* means self and *akos* means medicinal agent or remedy. Autacoids are biologically active substances produced by wide variety of cells in the body and not by endocrine glands. They generally act locally at the site of synthesis and release and so they are called local hormones. They have brief life time (short duration of action). They are involved in a number of physiological and pathological processes and even serve as transmitters or modulators in the nervous system. They usually exert their action at the site of inflammatory lesion or injury. A number of useful drugs, which mimic or antagonize the actions or alter synthesis and metabolism of autacoids have been developed for clinical use.

Classification of Autacoids

These are of three groups:
1. Amines, e.g. histamine and 5-hydroxy-tryptamine.
2. Peptides, e.g. angiotensin and kinins (bradykinin and kallidin).
3. Lipids, e.g. eicosanoids (prostaglandins and leukotrienes) and platelet-activating factor (PAF).

Histamine

It is derived from the Greek word Histos meaning tissue. Chemically it is 2-(1H-imidazol-4-yl ethylamine (as shown in **Fig. 17.1).**

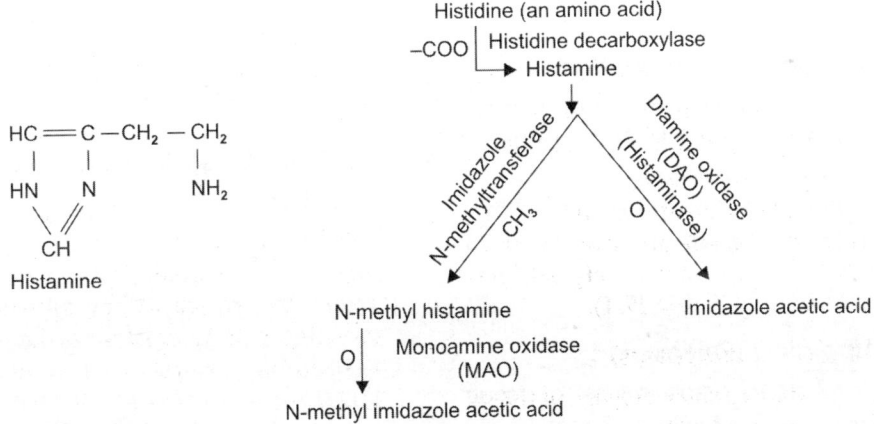

Fig. 17.1: Chemistry, synthesis and degradation of histamine

Source

It is present in almost all mammalian tissues, in some wasp and bee venoms and in some plants. Tissues rich in histamine are lungs, liver, gastrointestinal tract, placenta and skin. In tissues it is present in mast cells, basophils of blood and neurons of CNS. Rupture of mast cells releases free histamine into the circulation. It was first isolated from ergot by Barger and Dale in 1910. Its pharmacological actions were described by Dale and Laidlaw in 1911.

Synthesis, Storage and Degradation

In the mammals, it is formed by decarboxylation of the amino acid, histidine. This reaction is catalyzed by the enzyme, histidine decarboxylase (as shown in **Fig. 17.1**). It is also synthesized by the microflora in the gastrointestinal tract from dietary histidine, but a very little amount of it reaches the circulation as most of it is destroyed in the intestinal wall and the liver.

Histamine is stored in the granules of mast cells along with heparin and 5-HT. When present in the cells it is inert but when released it becomes active and produces a number of biological actions. Nonmast cell histamine is present in brain, epidermis, blood, body secretions, venoms and pathological fluids. After release from the cells, histamine is rapidly degraded by methylation and oxidation (as shown in **Fig. 17.1)** and excreted in urine as metabolites (N-methyl imidazole acetic acid and imidazole acetic acid). It cannot cross BBB.

Functions of Endogenous Histamine

- Plays a central role in immediate hypersensitivity reaction and allergic responses.
- Regulates gastric acid secretion.
- Functions as a neurotransmitter in the CNS.

Histamine receptors: There are three types of histamine receptors, *viz.* H_1, H_2 and H_3 receptors (as shown in **Table 17.1**).

Histamine Liberators (Releasers)

A number of substances cause release of tissue histamine from the mast cells and may cause histamine reactions. These are as follows:

- Proteolytic enzymes, e.g. trypsin, certain venoms, stings and food product alike crabs, lobsters and certain fish.
- Drugs causing allergy, e.g. morphine, pethidine, codeine, amphetamine, d-tubocurarine, hydralazine, tolazoline, chlortetracyline, polymyxin-B, vancomycin, dextran and polyvinyl pyrrolidone.
- Drugs causing anaphylaxis (antigen antibody reaction), e.g. penicillins, cephalosporins, procaine, ATS, ADS and ACS.
- Trauma due to cold and chemical, thermal or radiant energy.

Pharmacological Actions of Histamine

Mechanism of Action

Histamine combines with its specific receptors (H_1, H_2 and H_3) producing effects. All histamine receptors are G-protein coupled receptors. H_1 receptors are coupled to phospholipase-C and their activation leads to formation of inositol triphosphate (IP_3) and diacylglycerol (DAG) from phospholipids in the cell membrane. It causes rapid release of Ca^{2+} from the endoplasmic reticulum membrane. DAG activates protein kinase-C and Ca^{2+} activates Ca^{2+}/calmodulin dependent protein kinase-C and phospholipase-A_2 in the target cell to generate the characteristic response. H_2 receptors are linked to the stimulation of the adenylcyclase and thus to the activation of cAMP dependent protein kinases in the target cells. H_3 receptors are linked to inhibition of adenylcyclase and thus to inhibition of cAMP dependent protein kinases in the target cells.

Histamine Produces Following Effects

- **CVS Effects:**
  - **On blood vessels:** It causes marked dilatation of smaller blood vessels like arterioles, precapillary sphincter and venules but it contracts large blood vessels like arteries and veins. Vasodilatation is due to stimulation of H_1-receptors in the endothelial cells leading to local formation of EDRF. As a result of

Table 17.1: Histamine receptors

	H_1 receptor	H_2 receptor	H_3 receptor
• Location (sites)	Blood vessels, intestines, bronchi, uterus, nerve endings, ganglion cells and brain	Gastric glands, blood vessels, heart, uterus and brain.	Brain (presynaptically), some blood vessels, intestine and bronchi.
• Functions	Dilatation of small blood vessels but contraction of large blood vessels, contraction of nonvascular smooth muscles, stimulation of ganglion cells and nerve endings, transmitter role in brain.	Secretion of gastric glands, dilatation of small blood vessels but contraction of large blood vessels, stimulation of heart and relaxation of uterus, transmitter role in brain.	Inhibition of histamine release in brain nerve endings, inhibition of release of noradrenaline in some blood vessels leading to vasodilation, inhibition of release of acetylcholine in intestine and bronchoconstriction.
• Selective agonists	2-methyl histamine, β-histine	4-methyl histamine, betazole	α-methyl histamine, imidil.
• Selective antagonists	Chlorpheniramine, mepyramine, etc.	Cimetidine, ranitidine, etc.	Thioperamide, impromidine, etc.

dilatation of blood vessels, excess blood enters the capillaries (which do not contain smooth muscles) leading to increased capillary permeability and oedema formation and decreased plasma volume and venous return to heart.

– **On BP:** It produces fall of BP (hypotension) by dilatation of arterioles. It causes fall of both systolic and diastolic BPs. In large dose or in anaphylaxis, it may produce severe fall of BP called histamine shock. It produces a fall of pulmonary artery pressure by dilatation of pulmonary vessels. By causing dilatation of cranial blood vessels, it causes throbbing headache, which is accompanied by palpable temporal pulsations and a transient increase in the cerebrospinal fluid pressure. Histamine induced headache is due to stretching of sensory nerve endings around the cranial arteries.

– **On heart:** It increases the sinus rate (positive chronotropic action), increases the amplitude of venticular contraction (positive inotropic action) and slows down AV conduction. It increases coronary blood flow and at high concentration produces ventricular arrhythmias like ventricular fibrillation. In intact animal, due to hypotension it produces reflex tachycardia.

• **Triple response of Lewis:** Intradermal injection of histamine (10 to 20 µg) in man produces a characteristic effect called triple response (described by Lewis). It consists of:

i. Development of a red spot within a minute at the site of injection, which is called 'flush'. The spot then gradually becomes a bluish discolouration. It is due to local dilatation of capillaries and venules.

ii. Development of a bright red area called flare which is irregular in outline and extending to 5 cm beyond the flush. It is due to dilatation of arterioles produced by axon reflex.

iii. Development of localized oedema called whear, which reaches maximum within 10 minutes. It is due to increased capillary permeability leading to exudation of plasma proteins and fluid from the capillaries into the extracellular spaces. The triple response/urticaria is accompained by itching.

- **Effects on nonvascular smooth muscles:** It causes direct stimulation of the smooth muscle of various organs. The bronchial and uterine smooth muscles are highly sensitive to its action producing contraction. It produces severe bronchospasm in guinea pigs and patients with bronchial asthma or allergic disorder. Histamine induced bronchospasm can be effectively antagonized by adrenaline, isoprenaline and aminophyline but not by antihistaminic or atropine. The gastrointestinal and the ureteral smooth muscles respond moderately to histamine by contraction. Human uterus is not much affected by histamine. Guinea pig uterus is contracted, while rat uterus is relaxed. Visceral smooth muscle contraction is a H_1 response and relaxation is a H_2 response.
- **Effects on exocrine glands:** It causes marked increase in gastric secretion by the parietal cells, which is mediated by H_2 receptors. It has variable effects on other exocrine secretions, which are mediated by H_1 receptors.
- **CNS effects:** When administered systemically (SC, IM or IV) it cannot cross and does not produce CNS effects. It is formed locally in the brain and its physiological role is not clear.
- **Miscellaneous effects:** It stimulates autonomic ganglia and adrenal medulla leading to release of catecholamines. It stimulates sensory nerve ending producing itching.

Uses of histamine: It has no clinical use. It is used for diagnostic purposes such as:

- To test gastric acid secretion capacity (now replaced by the use of pentagastrin).
- To test bronchial hypersensitivity, in patients of bronchial asthma or allergic disorder.
- To test integrity of sensory nerves in leprosy (where intradermal injection fails

to elicit the flare in the affected region due to loss of axon reflex).

- To test BP rise due to release of catecholamines from the tumour pheochromocytoma, but this is a provocative and dangerous test as severe rise of BP may occur leading to cerebral haemorrhage and so phentolamine must be at hand during administration of histamine.

Preparation of histamine: Histamine acid phosphate injection (0.5 to 1 mg/ml).

Histamine like substances (histamine receptor agonists): These are β-histine, 2-methyl histamine, betazole, 4-methyl histamine, α-methyl histamine and imedil. Of these drugs, only β-histine is used clinically.

β-histine

It is H_1-selective histamine analogue. It is orally effective. It is used to control episodes of vertigo in some patients of Menier's syndrome. It causes vasodilatation and improves blood flow to the labyrinth and brain stem.

Preparation and Dosage

β-histine hydrochloride (Vertin) tablet (8 mg)—8 to 16 mg thrice daily after meals.

Adverse Reactions

It can produce GIT upset. It may aggravate peptic ulcer and bronchial asthma and so contraindicated in these conditions.

Histamine Receptor Antagonists

These are drugs that competitively antagonize the actions of histamine by occupying histamine receptors in the effector cells. These are of three groups:

- H_1-receptor antagonists (H_1-blockers), e.g. chlorpheniramine, diphenhydramine and promethazine.
- H_2-receptor antagonists (H_2-blockers), e.g. cimetidine, ranitidine and famotidine.
- H_3-receptor antagonists (H_3-blockers), e.g. thioperamide and impromidine.

Histamine receptor antagonists (classical/conventional antihistamines). These drugs block the actions of histamine by acting on H_1 receptors.

Classification

These can be classified either chemically or clinically.

Chemical classification: These are of two groups:

1. First generation drugs

- Ethanolamines, e.g. diphenhydramine, dimenhydrinate and carbinoxamine.
- Ethylene diamines, e.g. mepyramine, antazoline and tripelenamine.
- Alkylamines, e.g. chlorpheniramine, brompeniramine, pheniramine and triprolidine.
- Piperazines, e.g. cyclizine, buclizine, meclizine, cinnarizine and hydroxyzine.
- Phenothiazines, e.g. promethazine, methdilazine and trimeprazine.
- Piperidines, e.g. orphenadrine, cyproheptadine, mebhydrolin, dimethindene.

2. Second generation drugs

- Alkylamines, e.g. acrivastine
- Piperazines, e.g. cetrizine and levocetrizine
- Piperidines, e.g. loratodine, terfenadine, fexofenidine, astimizole and levocabusttine.
- Phthalazinones, e.g. azelastine

Clinical classification: These are of four groups:

- Highly sedative drugs, e.g. diphenhydramine, dimenhydrinate, promethazine and hydroxyzine.
- Moderately sedative drugs, e.g. pheniramine, trimeprazine, antazoline, buclizine, meclizine dimethindene and cyproheptadine.
- Mild sedative drugs, e.g. chlorpheniramine, methdilazine, mepyramine, triprolidine, mebhydroline, cyclizine and clemastine.
- Nonsedative drugs (newer antihistaminics), e.g. terfenadine, loratadine, acrivastine, azelastine, fexofenadine, cetrizine, astemizole, etc.

Chemistry

These are heterogeneous compounds with different chemical groups.

The general structure of antihistaminics and chemical structures of some antihistaminics are shown in **Fig. 17.2.**

Pharmacokinetics

These durgs are well-absorbed from the GIT. Following oral administration, peak plasma concentrations are reached in 2 to 3 hours and effects usually last for 4 to 6 hours. However, second generation compounds are longer-acting. As majority of antihistamines are lipid-soluble, so they are distributed throughout the body and readily enter the CNS. Some are localized in the lungs. They are metabolized in the liver by oxidative enzymes and excreted in urine as metabolites and partly as unchanged form. Cetrizine is an active metabolite of hydroxyzine.

Pharmacological Actions

Mechanism of Action

They are reversible competitive antagonists of histamine at H_1-receptor sites. They produce following effects:

- **On smooth muscles:** They effectively inhibit the response of smooth muscle to histamine on blood vessels and various organs. They inhibit the vasoconstrictor effect of histamine on large blood vessels and vasodilator effect on smaller blood vessels by blocking H_1 receptors. They prevent histamine induced bronchoconstriction and contraction of intestinal and other smooth muscles.
- **On capillary permeability:** They strongly block the action of histamine that results in increased capillary permeability and leakage of plasma proteins and fluid from the capillaries into the extracellular spaces. They suppress triple response, especially oedema and wheal formation.
- **On nerve endings:** They block the action of histamine on nerve endings which cause flare and itching (pruritus) by axon reflex.

- **On exocrine glands:** They do not block gastric acid secretion, which is mediated by H_2 receptors. They can inhibit other exocrine secretions such as salivary, bronchial and lacrimal glands. Some of them have anticho-linergic activity like atropine, which causes dryness of mouth and respiratory tract.

- **On immediate hypersensitivity reactions (anaphylaxis) and allergy:** They suppress many manifestations (utricaria, itching and angioedema) of type I (immediate hyper-sensitivity) reactions. They can partially prevent anaphylactic fall of BP. They cannot control bronchoconstriction, where adrenaline is useful.

- **CNS effects:** They can bind to H_1 receptors in the CNS and cause depression (commonly occurs) or stimulation (rarely occurs). They produce variable degree of CNS depression causing sedation, drowsiness and sleep. They also potentiate the effects of CNS depressants. Triprolidine and phenindamine can produce CNS stimulation causing restlessness, excitement, and insomnia. Antihistamines like promethazine, diphenhydramine, cyclizine and meclizine are effective in preventing motion sickness and vomiting due to vestibular disturbances. Antihistamines like promethazine, diphenhydramine and orphenadrine have antiparkinsonism effect due to central anticholinergic action.

- **Local anaesthetic effect:** Antihistamines like promethazine, mepyramine and antazoline have local anaesthetic activity (by membrane stabilizing property). But they are not used clinically as local anaesthetics, because they cause local irritation when injected subcutaneously.

Clinical Uses (Indications) of Antihistamines

- **Allergic disorders:** Antihistamines are most useful in acute exudative type of allergic disorders like rhinitis, conjunctivitis, hay fever, pollinosis and urticaria. They relieve the sneezing, rhinorrhoea and itching of eyes, nose and throat in hay fever and pollinosis. They effectively counter the urticaria and pruritus in atopic and contact dermatitis and that induced by various drugs, chemicals and vegetables. They partially control pruritus of eczema. They can control to some extent the pain and itch due to bee or wasp stings. Their antipruritic action is probably nonspecific with regard

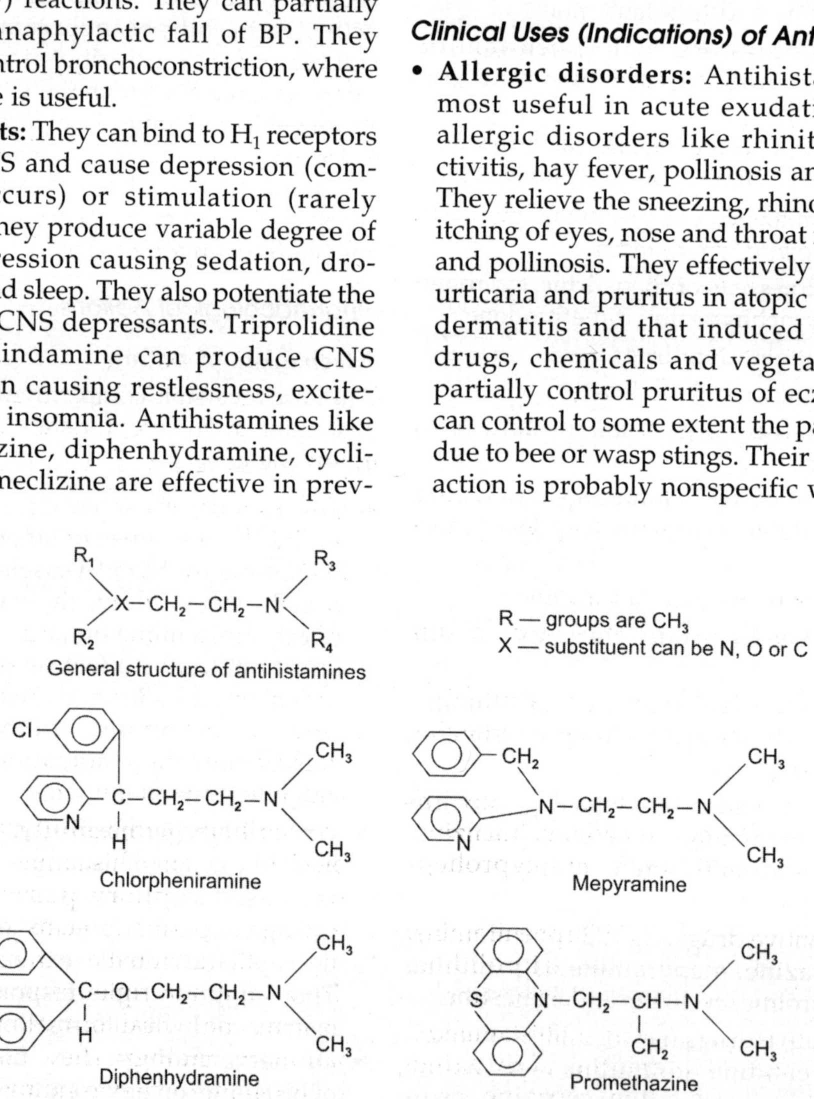

General structure of antihistamines

R — groups are CH_3
X — substituent can be N, O or C

Chlorpheniramine

Mepyramine

Diphenhydramine

Promethazine

Fig. 17.2: Chemical structures of antihistamines

to their effect on the mechanism of itch. This is probably related to their central sedative action. Their topical use, however, is not recommended due to the risk of sensitization and a marked tendency to cause eczematous reactions. They are not effective in bronchial asthma where PAF, PGs and leukotrienes are involved. They can produce symptomatic relief of common cold reducing rhinorrhoea and sneezing. They are of some values in controlling mild blood transfusion reactions but not pyrexia and haemolysis.

- **Motion sickness and vomiting:** Antihistamines like promethazine, diphenhydramine, dimenhydrinate, cyclizine and meclizine can be used in milder cases of motion sickness, though scopolamine is the drug of choice in motion sickness. They have prophylactic value and should be taken an hour before the journey. Promethazine is also used as an antiemetic in morning sickness, radiation sickness, postoperative vomiting and drug induced vomiting.

- **Vertigo:** Antihistamines like cinnarizine, diphenhydramine, dimenhydrinate, cyclizine and promethazine are used in the treatment of vertigo. Cinnarizine is the preferred drug which has calcium channel blocking activity in addition to antihistaminic, anticholinergic and anti-5-HT activities. It is a vasodilator and sedative. It produces benefit by producing vasodilation in the internal ear.

- **Parkinsonism:** Antihistamines like diphenhydramine, promethazine and orphenadrine are used in the treatment of drug induced parkinsonism due to their central anticholinergic action. They relieve rigidity but not tremor.

- **Acute muscular dystonia** of antipsychotic drugs and metoclopramide—though anticholinergic drugs are the preferred drugs in this condition but antihistamines like promethazine and diphenhydramine can be used parenterally (IM or IV) due to their prominent anticholinergic activity.

- **Cough:** Antihistamines like diphenhydramine, promethazine, chlorpheniramine and chlorcyclizine are useful antitussives to relieve dry irritating cough. They do not have any effect on cough centre. They may reduce secretions by antiallergic actions. Some relief of cough is due to their sedative and anticholinergic actions.

- **As sedative hypnotics:** Antihistamines like promethazine, diphenhydramine and chlorpheniramine are used as sedative hypnotics.

  In children, as they do not depress respiratory centre (RC), they can be used as preanaesthetic medication in children because of their sedative and anticholinergic actions.

Some Preparations and Dosage

- Diphenhydramine hydrochloride (Benadryl) capsule (25, 50 mg)—25 to 50 mg, syrup (12.5 mg/5 ml)—5 mg/kg/day, injection (10 mg/ml)—10 mg IM.
- Dimenhydrinate (Dramamine) tablet (50 mg)—50 to 100 mg, syrup (15.5 mg/5 ml)—5 mg/kg/day, injection (50 mg/ml)—50 mg IM.
- Mepyramine maleate (Anthisan) tablet 25 mg)—25 to 50 mg, syrup (12.5 mg/5 ml)—5 mg/kg/day, injection (25 mg/ml)—25 mg IM.
- Chlorpheniramine maleate (Zeet) tablet (4 mg)—4 to 12 mg, syrup (2 mg/5 ml)— 0.35 mg/kg/day, injection (10 mg/ml)— 10 mg IM.
- Pheniramine maleate (Avil) tablet (25, 50 mg)—25 to 50 mg, syrup (15 mg/5 ml)— 5 mg/kg/day, injection (25 mg/ml)—25 mg IM.
- Hydroxyzine hydrochloride (Atarax) tablet (10, 25 mg)—10–25 mg b.d.
- Promethazine hydrochloride (Phenergan) tablet (10, 25 mg)—10 to 25 mg, syrup (5 mg/5 ml)—1 mg/kg/day, injection (25 mg/ml)—25 mg IM.
- Terfenadine (Terfed) tablet (60, 120 mg)—60 to 120 mg once daily, syrup (30 mg/5 ml)—15 to 30 mg twice daily.

- Fexofenadine (Allegra) tablet (120, 180 mg) o.d.
- Astemizole (Astelong) tablet (10 mg)— 10 mg once daily, syrup (5 mg/5 ml)—2 to 5 mg twice daily.
- Cetrizine (Alday) tablet (10 mg)—10 mg once daily, syrup (5 mg/5 ml)—2 to 5 mg twice daily.
- Levocetrizine (xyzel) tablet (5 mg)—5 to 10 mg o.d.
- Loratadine (Lorfast) tablet (10 mg)—10 mg once daily, syrup (5 mg/5 ml)—2 to 5 mg twice daily.
- Cinnarizine (Vertigon) tablet (25 mg)— 25 to 75 mg.
- Cyclizine hydrochloride (Marzine) tablet (50 mg)—50 to 100 mg.
- Meclizine hydrochloride (Ancolan) tablet (25 mg)—25 to 50 mg.
- Dimethindene (Foristal) tablet (1 mg)— 1 to 3 mg.
- Cyproheptadine (Periactin) tablet (4 mg)— 4 to 20 mg, syrup (2 mg/5 ml)—0.5–1 mg/kg/day.

Adverse Reactions

The most common side effect of antihistamines is sedation, characterized by drowsiness, lack of mental concentration, dizziness, motor incoordination and tendency to sleep (ataxia). Marked sedation is produced by ethanolamines and phenothiazines. Triprolidine and phenindamine are less sedatives and may produce CNS stimulation. They should not be used during driving of motor vehicles or operating machines which require constant attentions. Many antihistamines produce anticholinergic side effects like dryness of mouth, blurring of vision, tremors, tachycardia, nervousness, irritability, insomnia, urinary retention, constipation and rarely impotence. Gastrointestinal side effects of antihistamines are anorexia, nausea, vomiting and epigastric distress (common with ethylenediamines). Antihistamines may rarely cause hypotension, a sense of tightness in the chest, agranulocytosis, leucopenia and thrombocytopenia on prolonged use. They can produce contact dermatitis after topical application, though they are antiallergic drugs. Cyclizine and meclizine produce teratogenic effects in animals and should not be used in pregnant women.

Acute antihistamine poisoning due to overdose may occur. It is characterized by marked CNS stimulation. It resembles belladonna poisoning and manifested as dryness of mouth and respiratory tract, mydriasis, pyrexia, hallucinations, delirium and convulsions. BP and respiration are usually well-maintained. Death may occur due to CNS depression leading to coma and cardiorespiratory failure. The treatment is symptomatic and supportive. Diazepam may be used to control convulsions.

Drug Interactions

Barbiturates, benzodiazepines, alcohol or tricyclic antidepressants enhance (potentiate) the sedative action of antihistamines.

Newer antihistamines (second generation antihistamines): These compounds are longer-acting (12 to 24 hours). They do not significantly cross the blood-brain barrier and so produce minimum sedative action. They are more specific for H_1 receptors and have no anticholinergic side effects. They do not produce sleepiness, dryness of mouth and impairment of psychomotor performance. Cycling or driving can be performed and children can attend school with same concentration so they have no subjective effects. They do not potentiate CNS depressant drugs. They are useful only in allergic conditions such as allergic rhinitis, conjunctivitis, hay fever, pollinosis, urticaria, atopic eczema, and acute allergic reactions to drugs and foods.

They have minimum adverse effects in comparison to older antihistamines.

Histamine H_2-receptor antagonists—these drugs are discussed in GIT—Pharmacology.

Histamine H_3-receptor antagonists—these drugs have no clinical use.

18

5-Hydroxytryptamine and 5-HT Antagonists

5-Hydroxytryptamine (Serotonin/Enteramine)

Source and Distribution

It is a biogenic amine widely distributed in animal tissues and plants. It is present largely in enterochromaffin cells of the intestinal wall, mast cells, platelets and pineal gland. It is called serotonin as it was first isolated from the serum of clotted blood (by Rapport in 1948). It is also called enteramine as it was isolated from enterochromaffin cells of intestine (by Erspamar in 1948). The body content of 5-HT is an adult male is about 10 mg, of which 96% is present in the enterochromaffin cells of the intestinal wall. It is present in high concentration in the pineal gland, where it serves as a precursor for the synthesis of the hormone, melatonin. It is also present in the venoms of bees and wasps. Fruits like pineapple, pear, banana, tomato, plum and nut contain considerable amounts of 5-HT.

Chemistry

It is an indole alkylamine. Chemically it is β-aminoethyl-5-hydroxyindole (as shown in **Fig. 18.1**).

Synthesis, Storage and Degradation

It is synthesized in the body from the amino acid, tryptophan by hydroxylation and decarboxylation (as shown in **Fig. 18.1**). Hydroxylation of tryptophan by the enzyme, tryptophan-5-hydroxylase produces 5-hydroxytryptophan (5-HTP). Decarboxylation of 5-HTP by the enzyme, 5-HTP decarboxylase

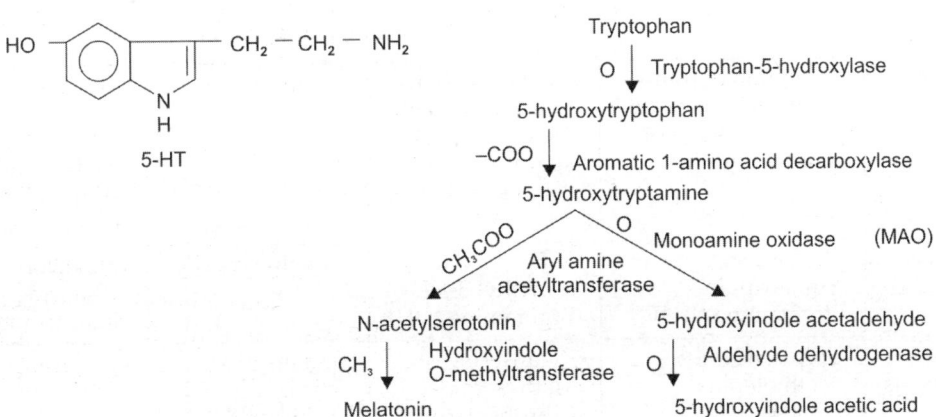

Fig. 18.1: Chemistry, synthesis and degradation of 5-HT

produces 5-hydroxytryptamine (5-HT) within the CNS and GIT. 5-HT is stored in cellular cytoplasmic granules similar to the chromaffin granules that store catecholamines. Platelets cannot synthesize 5-HT, but they have the capacity for its uptake and storage. Some amount of 5-HT is converted to melatonin in the pineal gland. 5-HT is degraded in the body by the enzymes, monoamine oxidase (MAO) and aldehyde dehydrogenase and excreted in urine as 5-hydroxyindole acetic acid (5-HIAA).

5-HT is not significantly absorbed from GIT after oral administration as it is rapidly degraded in the gut wall. It cannot cross BBB like catecholamines. It is actively taken up by an amine pump, which operates at the membrane of platelets and serotonergic nerve endings.

Functions of Endogenous 5-HT

- Neurohumoral transmission: It is a central neurotransmitter released by tryptaminergic neurons in the brain.
- Regulation of psychic functions (behaviour, mood, emotion and memory).
- Control of release of pituitary hormones through hypothalamic neurons.

- Control of gastrointestinal motility (peristalsis) through enteric nervous system (ENS).
- Involvement in producing migraine, nausea and vomiting, carcinoid tumour of small intestine, inflammation, hypertension, variant angina and Raynaud's phenomenon.
- 5-HT receptors: Types and subtypes (as shown in **Table 18.1).** There are four types of 5-HT receptors, some of which have different subtypes.

Pharmacological Actions

Mechanism of Action

5-HT combines with its specific types or subtypes of receptors producing effects. All 5-HT receptors are G-protein coupled receptors. $5\text{-}HT_1$ receptor subtypes are linked to inhibition of adenylcyclase (AC) with decrease of intracellular concentration of cAMR $5\text{-}HT_2$ receptor subtypes are linked to activation of phospholipase-C (PLC) with the formation of the second messengers DAG (which activates protein kinase-C) and IP_3 (which releases intracellular stores of Ca^{2+}).

Table 18.1: 5-HT receptors and subtypes

	$5HT_1$	$5HT_2$	$5HT_3$	$5HT_4$
Sybtypes	$5HT_{1A-1D}$	$5HT_{2A-2C}$	—	—
Distribution	Mainly in CNS, intestines, blood vessels, neurons and stomach plexus.	CNS, smooth muscles and platelets	PNS, nociceptive sensory neurons and dorsal horn of spinal cord.	Nerve endings of cholinergic and motor neurons.
Functions	Inhibition of transmitter release of CNS and contraction of smooth muscles	Excitatory to neurons and smooth muscles, platelet aggregation and behavioural effects	Excitatory	Stimulation produces increased release of acetylcholine and stimulation of GIT motility.
Specific agonists	Buspirone, Sumatriptan Ergotamine/DHE	LSD α-methyl 5-HT Ergotamine/DHE	2-methyl 5-HT	Metoclopramide Cisapride Renzapride
Specific antagonists	Spipirone, Methiotepine	Ketanserin, Methysergide, Ciproheptadine, Pizotifen, etc.	Ondansetron Granisetron Tropisetron	Tropisetron Dolasetron

5-HT$_3$ receptor functions as a ligand operated ion channel and 5-HT$_4$ receptor is linked to activation of adenylcyclase with increase of intracellular concentrations of cAMP. 5-HT produces following effects:

- **CVS effects:** It causes constriction of many blood vessels including veins, except coronaries, skeletal muscle blood vessels and capillaries of skin, which are dilated. On IV injection in anaesthetized animals (cats/dogs) it produces triphasic response on BP characterized by initial sharp fall in BP (due to coronary chemoreflex/Bezold-Jarisch reflex), intermediate brief rise in BP (due to vasoconstriction and increased cardiac output) and later on prolonged fall in BP (due to arteriolar dilatation and extravasation of fluid). It has a mild stimulant action on isolated heart of animals, acting both directly and by release of noradrenaline from nerve endings. In intact heart of animals it produces bradycardia through action on receptors in the coronary bed and producing hypotension and apnoea.

- **Effect on nonvascular smooth muscles:** It is a potent stimulator of GIT both by direct action as well as through enteric plexus. It increases peristalsis and can cause diarrhoea. It constricts bronchi, but less potent than histamine. Its effects on other smooth muscles in man are feeble and inconsistent.

- **Effects on respiration:** It produces brief stimulation of respiration (mostly by reflex from bronchial afferents) and can produce hyperventilation, but large doses can cause transient apnoea through coronary chemoreflex.

- **Effects on exocrine glands:** It inhibits gastric secretion of acid and pepsin, but increases mucus secretion. It has thus ulcer-protective activity. Its effects on other secretions are not significant.

- **CNS effects:** It has both excitatory and inhibitory effects. When it is injected directly into the brain by intraventricular canulation, it causes sleepiness, changes in body temperature and some behavioural effects.

- **Effects on nerve endings:** It stimulates afferent nerve endings producing tingling, pricking sensation and pain.

- **Miscellaneous effects:** It is an aggregator of platelets by causing change in shape of platelets. It releases catecholamines from adrenal medulla but less potent than histamine.

Uses of 5-HT: It has no clinical use. It is used as an experimental stool. Preparation of 5-HT: 5-HT creatinine phosphate injection (0.5, 1 mg/ml).

5-HT like substances (5-HT receptor agonists): These are lysergic acid diethylamide (LSD), 5-Hydroxydipropyl-amino-tetramine (5-OH-DPAL), *m*-chlorophenyl piperazine (MCPP), sumatriptan metoclopramide and cisapride. LSD is nonselective 5-HT agonist (stimulates 5-HT$_{2A}$, 5-HT$_{2C}$ and 5-HT$_{3C}$ receptors). It is a hallucinogen (produces hallucinations). 5-OH-DPAL is a selective 5-HT$_{1A}$ agonist while MCPP is a nonselective 5-HT agonist (stimulates 5 HT$_{1B}$, 5HT$_{2A}$ and 5HT$_{2C}$ receptors). Sumatriptan (Sumitrex, Sumin, Migratan) is a selective 5-HT$_{1D}$ agonist used in acute attack of migraine. Cisapride (Cisawal) is a selective 5-HT$_4$ agonist used as antiemetic (prokinetic agent). Sumatriptan is available as tablet (50, 100 mg) and used in dosage of 50 to 100 mg once or twice daily. Cisapride is available as tablet (10 mg) and used in dosage of 10 mg thrice daily.

- **5-HT receptor antagonists:** These are methylsergide (5-HT$_{2A}$ and 5-HT$_{2C}$ blockers) used in migraine, carcinoid syndrome and postgastrectomy dumping syndrome; ketanserin (5-HT$_{2A}$, 5-HT$_{2C}$ and 5-HT$_{3C}$ blockers) used in Raynaud's syndrome and hypertension.

Cyproheptadine (5-HT$_{2A}$ and histamine H$_1$ blockers) used in allergic disorders, carcinoid syndrome and postgastrectomy dumping syndrome and as an appetizer.

Pizotifen (5-HT$_{2A}$ and histamine H$_1$ blocker) used in migraine; Risperidone (5-HT$_{2A}$ and 5-HT$_{2C}$ blocker) used as antipsychotic.

Clozapine/Loxapine (5-HT'$_{2A}$ and 5-HT$_{2C}$ blockers) used as antipsychotic; Ondansetron/

Granisetron (5-HT$_3$ blockers) used as antiemetic in chemotherapy/cytotoxic drug induced vomiting. Tropisetron is also 5-HT$_4$ blocker.

Ergotamine (5-HT partial agonist) is used in migraine. Buspirone/Ipsaperone (5-HT$_{1A}$ partial agoinst) is used as anxiolytic.

- **5-HT synthesis inhibitors:** These are P-chlorophenylalanine (PCPA) and α-methyl-dopa.
- **5-HT transporter inhibitors:** These are fluoxetine/sertraline (specific inhibitors) and amitriptyline/protriptyline (non-specific inhibitors).

DISCUSSION OF SOME 5-HT ANTAGONISTS

Cyproheptadine

Chemically it resembles phenothiazines. It is a potent antagonist of 5-HT$_{2A}$ receptor. It has mild antihistaminic (H$_1$ receptor) and anticholinergic (muscarinic receptor) activities. It has also Ca^{2+} channel blocking activity. It is absorbed from the GIT. It is metabolized in the liver and excreted rapidly in urine and faeces. It stimulates appetite due to its anti-5-HT activity in the hypothalamus. It increases body weight during treatment. It is used in allergic disorders, diarrhoea of carcinoid tumour and postgastrectomy dumping syndrome. It is also used as an appetite stimulant and in prophylaxis and treatment of migraine.

Preparation and Dosage

Cyptoheptadine (Periactin) tablet (4 mg)—4 to 20 mg/day in divided doses, syrup (2 mg/5 ml).

Adverse Reactions

It can produce drowsiness, dryness of mouth, mental confusion, ataxia, dizziness, headache and visual hallucinations.

Methysergide

It is semisynthetic ergot alkaloid congener (derivative of LSD). Chemically it is l-methyl-d-lysergic acid butanolamide. It blocks the actions of 5-HT on a variety of smooth muscles. It has also independent mild vasoconstrictor and oxytoxic effects. It is a potent peripheral 5-HT$_2$ antagonist but acts centrally as a 5-HT$_2$ agonist. It is well-absorbed

from the GIT. It is little metabolized in the liver and excreted mostly unchanged in urine. It has a half-life of 10 hours. It is used for prophylaxis of migraine and for treatment of intestinal manifestation of carcinoid syndrome and postgastrectomy dumping syndrome.

Preparation and Dosage

Methysergide (Deseril) tablet (2 mg)—2 mg once or twice daily.

Adverse Reactions

It can cause nausea, vomiting, heart burn and diarrhoea (by GIT irritation), drowsiness, mental confusion, vertigo, nervousness insomonia, hallucinations and psychic disturbances (by CNS actions) and rarely retroperitoneal fibrosis and pleuropulmonary fibrosis (by inflammation). It should be avoided in patients with pregnancy, peptic ulcer, peripheral vascular diseases, renal diseases, coronary insufficiency and severe hypertension.

Ketanserin

It is a relatively selective 5-HT$_2$ receptor antagonist with little antagonistic effects on 5HT$_1$ and 5HT$_3$ receptors. It also acts as an antagonist for α_1-adrenergic, H$_1$-histaminergic and D$_1$-dopaminergic receptors. It inhibits 5-HT induced vasoconstriction, bronchoconstriction and platelet aggregation. It has hypotensive action by virtue of its 5-HT$_2$ and α_1-adrenergic receptors antagonistic activities. It is rapidly absorbed from GIT. It undergoes first pass metabolism in the gut wall and liver and has a bioavailability of 50%. It is metabolized in the liver and excreted in urine and faeces.

Clinical Uses

It is used in hypertension and Raynaud's syndrome.

Preparation and Dosage

Ketanserin tablet (40 mg)—40 to 80 mg daily.

Adverse Reactions

It can cause dryness of mouth, nausea, sedation, dizziness and headache. It should be used with caution in patients taking α-blockers, as severe hypotension may occur.

Table 18.2: Treatment of migraine according to stages

Stage of migraine	Clinical features	Treatment
Mild	Occasional throbbing headache. No major impairment of functioning.	Mild analgesic (aspirin/paracetamol/ codeine) or combination of analgesics ± Antiemetic (metoclopramide/ domperidone/cyclizine) if required.
Moderate	Moderate or severe throbbing headache. Some impairment of functioning. Nausea common.	Combination of analgesic and ergot-amine/sumatriptan + Antiemetic.
Severe	More than three severe throbbing headache in a month. Significant functional impairment. Marked nausea and/or vomiting.	Ergotamine/sumatriptan + Antiemetic Prophylactic drugs (β-blocker/ clonidine/calcium channel blocker/5-HT antagonist/tricyclic antidepressant)

Ondansetron

It is a selective 5-HT_3 antagonist used as antiemetic agent. It is well-absorbed from GIT, metabolized in the liver and excreted in urine.

Clinical Uses

It is very useful in the management of nausea and vomiting due to chemotherapeutic cytotoxic drugs.

Preparation and Dosage

Ondansetron hydrochloride (Zafer, Emeset) tablet (4, 8 mg)— 4 to 8 mg two hours before treatment, injection (2 mg/ml)—2–4 mg IV slowly one hour before treatment.

Adverse Reactions

It can cause headache, constipation and allergic reactions. It does not cause sedation and extrapyramidal effects.

Migraine and its Treatment

Migraine is a neurological syndrome manifested as throbbing headache (usually unilateral), nausea, photophobia, polyurea and sometimes diarrhoea. It is a vasospastic disorder, in which there is initially vasoconstriction of cerebral vessels (during prodromal phase), which is followed by vasodilatation of cerebral and extracerebral vessels (during headache phase). The exact cause of migraine is unknown. 5-HT is thought to be involved in the pathogenesis of migraine, because it is present in high concentration in plasma and excreted in large amount in urine during migraine attack. Moreover, drugs like reserpine and fenfluramine, which release 5-HT from tissue stores can precipitate migraine attack.

Treatment

Treatment of migraine is shown in **Table 18.2**. 5-HT receptor agonists are drugs of choice.

Prophylaxis of Migraine

Drugs used are given as follows:
- β-blockers (propranolol/metoprolol, atenolol, etc.).
- Adrenergic α_2-agonist (clonidine).
- Tricyclic antidepressants (amitriptyline/ nortriptyline, etc.)
- Calcium channel blockers (verapamil and flunarizine).
- 5-HT antagonists (methysergide, cyproheptadine and pizotifen).

General Advice to Patients of Migraine

- Identify and then avoid stress factors like alcohol (e.g. red wine), foods (e.g. chocolate, certain cheese, etc.), irregular sleep pattern and acute changes in stress levels.
- Attempt to manage environmental changes like time zone shift, high altitude and barometric pressure changes.
- Assess menstrual cycle relationship.

19

Renin-Angiotensin System and Kinins

RENIN-ANGIOTENSIN SYSTEM

It is a humoral system that modulates the homeostatic mechanism involved in regulation of hemodynamics, water and electrolyte balance and arterial blood pressure (as shown in **Fig. 19.1).** It consists of three substances, *viz.* renin, angiotensinogen and angiotensin.

Renin is a proteolytic enzyme, secreted by the granular juxtaglomerular cells (JG cells) of kidneys present in the walls of the afferent arterioles entering the glomeruli. Juxtaglomerular cells secrete renin directly into the renal arteriolar bloodstream. Decrease of plasma sodium concentration, renal perfusion pressure, blood volume or blood pressure tends to stimulate secretion of renin from the kidney through volume receptors and baroreceptors and by sympathetic stimulation. Renin stimulates synthesis of angiotensin from angiotensinogen within the kidney.

Angiotensinogen is a serum α-globulin, which acts as renin substrate. It is converted to angiotensin-I (an inactive decapeptide) in the bloodstream by the action of renin. Angiotensin-I during its passage through lungs is converted to angiotensin-II (an active octapeptide) by the action of another enzyme called angiotensin converting enzyme (ACE), dipeptidyl carboxypeptidase. Angiotensin-II is the most powerful direct vasoconstrictor agent effective in a very small dose of 0.1 µg/kg body weight. It also stimulates the synthesis and release of aldosterone from the zona glomerulosa cells of the adrenal cortex and thus regulates the extracellular fluid (ECF) volume. Angiotensin-II is converted to angiotensin-III (a heptapeptide) by the action of the enzyme, aminopeptidase. Angiotensin-III is as potent as angiotensin-II in its action on the adrenal cortex but is weaker in its other actions. It is broken down to peptide fragments by the action of the enzyme, angiotensinase. It has a plama t½ of about 1 minute.

Angiotensin Amide

It is a synthetic substance, which is chemically a minor structural variant of the naturally occurring angiotensin-II. It is ineffective orally as it is destroyed in GIT. It is administered by IV infusion.

Angiotensinogen

↓ ← Renin

Angiotensin-I

↓ ← ACE

Angiotensin-II

↓ ← Aminopeptidase

Angiotensin-III

↓ ← Angiotensinase

Peptide fragments

Fig. 19.1: Biosynthesis and degradation

146

Pharmacological Actions

It is a very potent vasoconstrictor agent. It is about 40 times more potent than nor-adrenaline as a vasoconstrictor. It directly stimulates the smooth muscle of blood vessels (by acting on angiotensin receptors AT_1 and AT_2) and increases the total peripheral resistance.

The precapillary blood vessels (arterioles) are constricted much more than the post capillary blood vessels (venules) and veins. The cutaneous, splanchnic and renal blood vessels are strongly constricted resulting in decreased blood flow to these regions. The cerebral coronary and skeletal blood vessels are only weakly constricted and so the blood flow to these regions increases following the rise of BP. Its effects on pulmonary blood vessels is negligible. It does not stimulate cardiac muscle. It does not produce tachyphylaxis. It may play an important role in the central control of the cardiovascular system. It acts on CNS sites to increase arterial BP, increase ADH secretion and stimulate thirst. It produces a prompt initial decrease in the quantitiy and electrolyte content of urine, followed by diuresis (due to inhibition of sodium reabsorption by distal tubule).

It can be used in the treatment of hypotension during anaesthesia with drugs that sensitize the heart to adrenergic arrhythmias (such as halothane, enflurane and isoflurane). It is not available commercially for clinical use.

Adverse Reactions

It can cause dizziness, headache, bradycardia, chest pain and cardiac arrhythmias.

Inhibitors of renin-angiotensin system— These are of three groups:

1. Inhibitors of renin release, e.g. β-adrenergic blockers (propranolol, metoprolol, etc.), adrenergic neuron blockers (guanethidine, bethanidine, etc.)
2. Angiotensin converting enzyme (ACE) inhibitors (prevent conversion of angiotensin-I to angiotensin-II), e.g. captopril, enalapril and lisinopril.
3. Angiotensin antagonists (block angiotensin receptors (AT_1 and AT_2), e.g. saralasin (a peptide analog of angiotensin).

Saralasin has high affinity for AT_2 receptor and low affinity for AT_1 receptor. Losartan has high affinity for AT_1 receptor and low affinity for AT_2 receptor.

All these drugs are used in the treatment of hypertension. They will be discussed with antihypertensive drugs in cardiovascular pharmacology.

Kinins (Bradykinin and Kallidin)

These are polypeptides, split off from a plasma globulin kininogen by the action of speciic enzyme kallikrein. Bradykinin is a non-apeptide (contains 9 amino acids, *viz.* Arg-Pro-Pro-Gly-Phen-Ser-Pro-Phe-Arg) and kallidin is a decapeptide (contains 10 amino acids, *viz.* Lys-Arg-Pro-Pro-Gly-Phen-Ser-Pro-Phen-Arg). Bradykinin is present in plasma and kallidin is present in plasma and tissues. Kallidin is produced by tissue, kallikrein and is converted to some extent in the plasma to bradykinin by the action of the enzyme, aminopeptidase.

Generation and Metabolism of Kinins

There are two types of kininogens (HMW and LMW), which are α_2 globulins present in plasma. Plasma also contains an inactive kininogenase called prekallikrein, which is activated to kallikrein by Hageman factor (factor XII of blood clotting) and plasmin (fibrinolysin). Kinins are also generated by trypsin, proteolytic enzymes in snake, bee and wasp venoms and kallikrein present in kidney, pancreas and other tissues. High moleuclar weight (HMW) kininogen yields bradykinin and low molecular weight (LMW) kininogen yields kallidin. Bradykinin is generated from kallidin on removal of lysin residue by the action of aminopeptidase. Kallikreins are normally present in their inactive forms. Physiologically only small amount of kinins are generated in plasma and tissues **(Fig. 19.2)**.

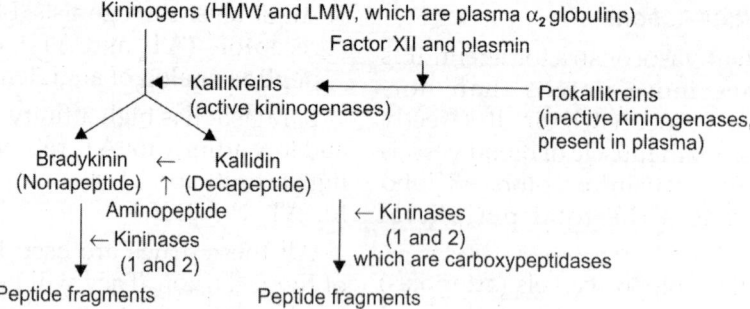

Fig. 19.2: Biosynthesis and degradation of kinins

Kinins are very rapidly degraded in the tissues (lungs, pancreas and other tissues) by the enzymes kininase-I (acts slowly) and kininase-II (acts rapidly) which are carboxypeptidases. The plasma half-life of kinins is < 1 minute.

Actions of Kinins

- **CVS actions:** They are more potent vasodilator (about 10 times) than acetylcholine and histamine. The vasodilatation is mediated through release of EDRF and involves mainly the arterioles in the heart, kidneys, liver, intestine and skeletal muscles. Larger arteries and most veins are constricted through action on the smooth muscle. They have no direct action on the heart. The vasodilatation is accompanied by a reflex increase in the heart rate, cardiac output and myocardial contractility. They also increase capillary permeability and venous pressure leading to oedema formation by passage of water and solutes into the extracellular space from the vascular compartment.

- **Actions at nonvascular smooth muscles:** They produce slow contraction of intestine (*brady* means slow and *kinin* means to move). They cause marked bronchoconstriction in asthmatic patients and in guinea pigs. Actions on other smooth muscles are not prominent, some may be relaxed.

- **Inflammatory action:** They can produce all the characteristic symptoms of inflammation. They strongly stimulate sensory nerve endings that carry the pain sensation from the skin and viscera and produce a burning sensation.

- **Other actions:** They can release catecholamines from the adrenal medulla and stimulate the sympathetic ganglia. They also release histamine from mast cells.

Kinin Receptors

These are β_1, β_2 and β_3 receptors. β_1 receptor mediates vasoconstriction in pathological states. β_2 receptor mediates all the classical actions of kinins including vasodilatation. The location and function of β_3 receptor is unknown.

Pathophysiological Roles of Kinins

They are involved in mediation of inflammation and pain, regulation of microcirculation, specially in kidney, clotting of blood, fibrinolysis, shock and carcinoid syndrome.

Clinical Uses

They have no clinical use as they have very short half-life (<1 min) and they produce unpleasant effects. Aprotinin (Trasylol) is obtained from parotid gland of sheep/cow. It is a trypsin inhibitor. It also inhibits kallikreins in tissues and thus reduces kinin synthesis. It is used in the treatment of acute pancreatitis and in controlling manifestations of carcinoid syndrome.

Preparation and Dosage

Aprotinin injection (1 lakh IU/ml)—1–2 lakhs IU IV.

20

Eicosanoids and Platelet Activating Factor

EICOSANOIDS

These are autacoids that are derived from cell membrane phospholipids, e.g. prostaglandins, prostacyclin, thromboxanes and leukotrienes. The term eicosanoid is derived from Greek words—*eicosa* meaning twenty (indicating a 20 C structure) and *enoic* meaning presence of double bonds. These are polyunsaturated essential fatty acids that are released from cell membrane phospholipids. They are present in almost every tissue and body fluid. They are formed from cell membrane phospholipids by the action of phospholipase-A_2. They are synthesized in the cells in response to a number of physical, chemical and hormonal stimuli including trauma, infection and inflammation. They produce a wide range of biological responses.

Synthesis of eicosanoids: Almost all cells of the body can synthesize the eicosanoids by following steps (as shown in **Fig. 20.1**).

Metabolism of eicosanoids: These are not stored in the cells and degraded very rapidly (very short half-life) in most tissues, especially in lungs and liver and the degraded products are excreted in urine.

DISCUSSION OF INDIVIDUAL EICOSANOIDS

Prostaglandins (PGs)

These are so-named because they were first obtained from the prostate gland in the extract of human seminal fluid by Kurzrok and Lieb in 1930 and confirmed by Von Euler in 1935. These are present more in genital tissues (like prostate, seminal vesicles and uterus) than in other tissues (like iris, lungs, pancreas, intestine, brain and kidneys). Chemically these are derivatives of prostanoic acid, which has a five-membered ring containing 20 carbons and two double bonds (as shown in **Fig. 20.2**). It is formed from arachidonic acid.

There are many series of prostaglandins which are designated as A, B, C, D, E, F, G, H and I depending on the ring structure and the substituents in it. Each series has members with subscripts 1, 2 and 3.

All prostaglandins contain two double bonds, the number of which is indicated by suffixing the number such as PGE_2, PGF_2 and PGD_2 which are primary prostaglandins (biologically important).

Physiologically natural PGs are synthesized locally at the site of action. There is no preformed stores of PGs. They are very active even in low concentration and are destroyed quickly. They have limited clinical use due to their instability, short duration of action and lack of tissue specificity. Synthetic PGs have been developed to overcome these difficulties.

Physiological/Pharmacological Actions of PGs

Prostaglandins produce following effects:

- **CVS effects:** PGE_2, $PGF_{2\alpha}$ and PGD_2 can increase the heart rate and the force of

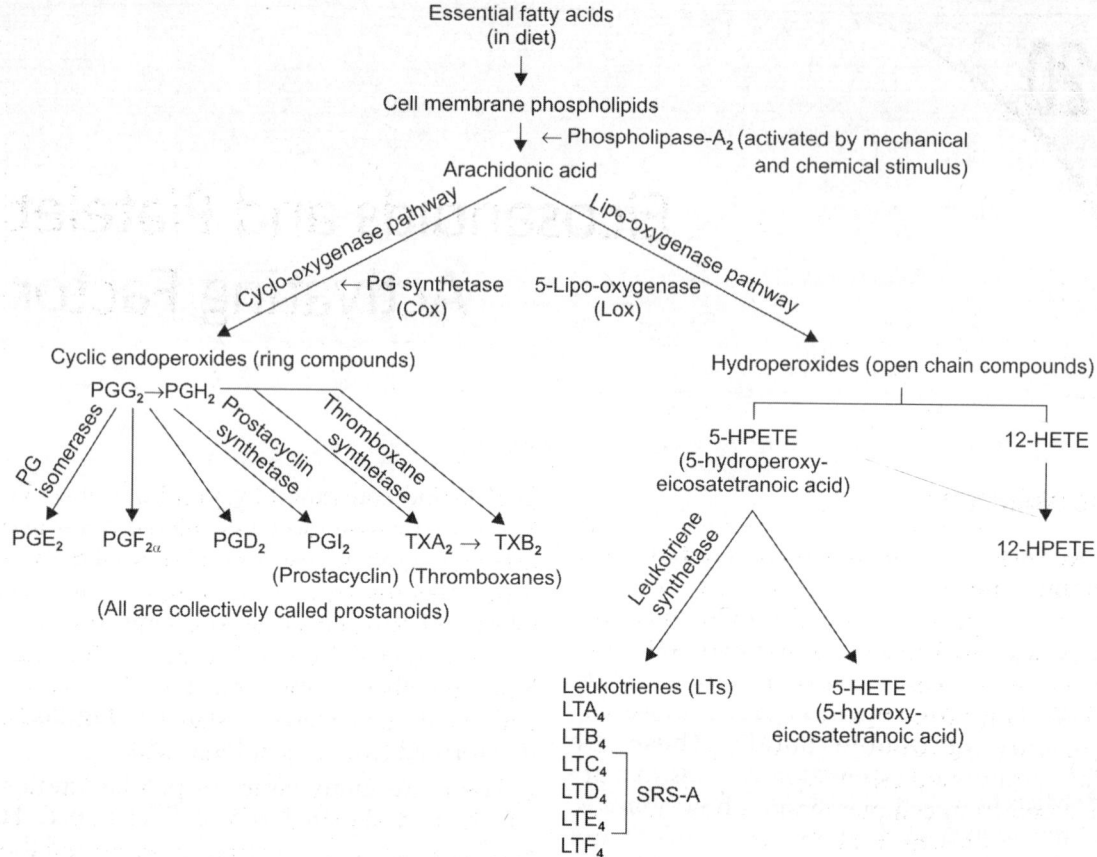

Fig. 20.1: Biosynthesis of eicosanoids

cardiac contraction. PGE_2 and PGA_2 produce peripheral vasodilation and can lower BP. They are potent natriuretic agents. $PGF_{2\alpha}$, however, constricts arterioles and veins. PGE_2 relaxes the smooth muscle of the ductus arteriosus and preserves the ductal patency in the foetus.

- **GIT effects:** PGE_2 increases the vascularity of the gastric mucosa and inhibits the gastric acid secretion and ulcer formation. It is, therefore, a cytoprotective agent in stomach against ulcer formation. Both PGE_2 and $PGF_{2\alpha}$ cause contraction of longitudinal muscle of the intestine and increase intestinal motility. They stimulate intestinal fluid secretion and cause diarrhoea when administered orally or parenterally in man.

- **Effects on reproductive system:** PGE_2 causes luteolysis, i.e. regression of corpus luteum of pregnancy around 12 weeks. PGE_2 and $PGF_{2\alpha}$ cause contraction of uterine muscle (myometrium). The sensitivity of the uterine muscle to PGs is more during pregnancy. The uterine cervix is soften and dilate easily with PGs at term. This facilitates the delivery of the foetus.
- **Respiratory tract effects:** PGE_2 inhibits the tone of tracheal and bronchial muscles and has a bronchodilator action.
- **CNS effects:** Prostaglandins produce many actions on CNS. Prostaglandin has been suggested as a central neurotransmitter. PGE_2 promotes the release of several anterior pituitary hormones. It has been implicated in the causation of fever and in the induction of normal sleep.

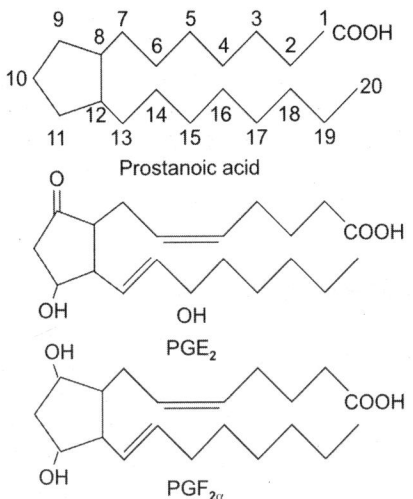

Fig. 20.2: Chemical structures of prostanoic acid, PGE$_2$ and PGF$_{2\alpha}$

- **Renal effects:** PGE$_2$ causes renal vasodilatation, increased renal blood flow and diuresis. It stimulates renin secretion from juxtaglomerular cells of kidneys.

- **Miscellaneous effects:** PGE$_1$ and PGE$_2$ block the lipolytic effect of adrenaline, ACTH and glucagon. They produce pain when applied to an exposed blister base. They also play role in the genesis of inflammation. PGE$_2$ causes bone resorption and hypercalcemia. The osteoporosis of rheumatoid arthritis may be due to oveproduction of PGE$_2$. Aspirin and indomethacin are potent inhibitors of the synthesis of prostaglandins and thus decrease biological actions of prostaglandins.

Prostanoid (PG) Receptors

These are present on the cell membrane of the target cells. There are five subtypes of PG receptors, *viz.* DP, EP, FP, IP and TP. Prostaglandins bind with their specific receptors leading to activation of cell membrane bound G proteins and generating second messengers (IP$_3$/DAG/cAMP) to produce biological actions.

Clinical Uses (Indications) of Prostaglandins

These are given as follows:

Obstetrical uses

- For induction of therapeutic abortion during first trimester (early weeks of pregnancy, i.e. 10 to 20 weeks), PGE$_2$ and PGF$_{2\alpha}$ are used.

- For induction of labour or medical termination of pregnancy (MTP), PGE$_2$ and PGF$_{2\alpha}$ are used.

- To expel the uterine contents in intra-uterine death of foetus by cervical priming, PGE$_2$ is applied in the cervical canal.

- To control pH due to uterine atony, 15-methyl PGF$_{2\alpha}$ (carboprost) is used if ergometrine or oxytocin fails.

Nonobstetrical uses

- To promote healing of peptic ulcer, especially drug induced (by NSAIDs)—synthetic stable analogue methyl PGE$_1$ (Misoprostol) or methyl PGE$_2$ (Enprostil) is used orally in high dosage.

- To maintain patency of ductus arteriosus in neonates with congenital heart defects until surgery is undertaken, PGE$_1$ (Alprostadil) is used. Apnoea occurs in few cases.

- For platelet storage and transfusion PGD$_2$ or PGI$_2$ is used to prevent damage of platelets.

- In peripheral vasospastic diseases, PGI$_2$ or PGE$_2$ is used.

Preparations and Dosage of Prostaglandins

- PGE$_2$ (Prostin E$_2$/Dinoprostone) vaginal tablet (3 mg)—one tablet is inserted into the posterior fornix, followed by another tablet if labour does not start within five hours. It is also available as vaginal gel and injection (for transamniotic administration).

- PGF$_{2\alpha}$ (Prostin F$_{2\alpha}$/Dinoprost) injection (5 mg/ml in 4 ml ampoule) for intra-amniotic injection. It is commonly used for induction of abortion/labour/MTP.

- 15-methyl PGF$_{2\alpha}$ (Carboprost/Prostolin) injection (0.25 mg/ml in 4 ml ampoule)—it is injected IM for mid-term abortion.

Adverse Reactions of Prostaglandins

These are GIT side effects (nausea, vomiting and diarrhoea), uterine cramps, severe uterine contractions, vaginal bleeding, flushing, shivering, fever, malaise, fall of BP, tachycardia and chest pain.

Prostaglandin Antagonists

Aspirin, indomethacin and other NSAIDs interfere with the synthesis of prostaglandins by inhibiting PG-synthetase (cyclo-oxygenase). Glucocorticoids inhibit the release of arachidonic acid from the cell membrane phospholipids by stimulating the production of a peptide lipocortin, which inhibits phosphorylase-A_2 and thus reduce the synthesis of prostaglandins.

Selective PG receptor blockers are polyphloretin phosphate and oxaprostanoic acid, which are under evaluation for clinical use.

Prostacyclin (PGI₂/Epoprostenol)

It is a derivative of prostanoic acid. It is a potent vasodilator and an inhibitor of platelet aggregation. It is produced by the vascular endothelium. It is also present in other tissues like brain, intestine, lung and kidney. It is formed from PG-endoperoxide by the action of the enzyme, prostacyclin synthetase. It inhibits platelet aggregation by stimulating the membrane enzyme adenylcyclase leading to increased formation of cAMP in the platelets. Its IV infusion may produce vasodilation causing hypotension, tachycardia, headache and flushing of face. It also causes renin release. It is very unstable and has a short half life (about three minutes). It is used for platelet storage and transfusion. It potentiates the effect of heparin and tranylcypromine (an antidepressant).

Thromboxanes (TXA₂ and TXB₂)

These are derivatives of prostanoic acid. TXA_2 is produced mainly by thrombocytes (platelets). It is a potent vasoconstrictor and promotes platelet aggregation. A balance between TXA_2 and PGI_2 formation regulates platelet cAMP *in vivo* and, therefore, platelet aggregability. TXA_2 is converted to TXB_2. Damage of the vascular endothelium reduces PGI_2 synthesis and increases the tendency for blood to clot because of the unopposed action of TXA_2. Aspirin in low dose blocks the synthesis of TXA_2 by inhibiting the enzymes thromboxane synthetase but not PGI_2 by inhibiting prostacyclin synthetase. So it is a prophylactic agent in thromboembolic diseases. Dazoxiben (a substituted imidazole) is a selective blocker (inhibitor) of TXA_2 synthesis.

Leukotrienes (LTs)

These are so-named as they were first obtained from leucocytes. These are derivatives of arachidonic acid. The parent compound is leukotriene A_4 (LTA_4), from which other leukotrienes (LTB_4, LTC_4, LTD_4 and LTE_4) are derived. LTC_4, LTD_4 and LTE_4 are collectively called slow reacting substances (SRS) which are sulphidopeptides. The enzymes involved in the synthesis of LTs are phospholipase A_2 and 5-lipo-oxygenase. 5-lipo-oxygenase is present only in neutrophils, eosinophils, monocytes, macrophages, mast cells, basophils and B lymphocytes. Leukotrienes exert their biological actions through specific LT-receptors. They play an important role in inflammatory process. LTA_4 and LTB_4 are potent neutrophil chemotactic agents and cause release of glucuronidase and lysosome from the neutrophils. They stimulate myelopoiesis and proliferation of T lymphocytes. They cause vasoconstriction and modulation of vascular (venular endothelial) permeability, leading to development of oedema. They constrict cutaneous blood vessels. They produce vigorous and sustained contraction of smooth muscle, specially of bronchial muscle. They increase mucus secretion in the airway. They also cause immune modulation. LTC_4 and LTD_4 have been implicated in the pathogenesis of anaphylactic shock, bronchial asthma and various inflammatory diseases like glomerulonephritis, rheumatoid arthritis, cystic fibrosis, psoriasis, inflammatory bowel disease and respiratory distress syndrome. LT-receptor antagonists, e.g. zafirlukast, pranlukast, cinaleukast, montelukast, etc. are in clinical trial in bronchial asthma. Leukotriene (LT) synthesis (5-lipo-oxygenase) inhibitors, e.g. Zileutin is in clinical trial in bronchial asthma. These are discussed in pharmacotherapy of bronchial asthma.

Platelet Activating Factor (PAF)

It is a cell membrane derived phospholipid with wide range of biological activities. It is released during mast cell degranulation and is implicated in the causation of pathophysiological states like allergic inflammation, bronchial asthma and anaphylactic shock. It is also produced by eosinophils, neutrophils, macrophages and vascular endothelium. Chemically it is acetylglyceryl etherphosphocholine (AGEPC). It is synthesized from the precursor phospholipid present in the cell membrane by the action of the enzymes phospholipase A_2 and PAF-acetyl transferase by following reactions:

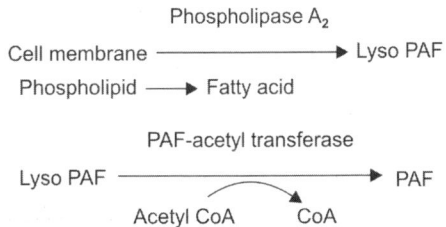

It is degraded rapidly by hydrolysis and acetylation.

Physiological/Pharmacological Actions

PAF produces following effects

- **CVS effects:** It is a potent vasodilator. It causes release of EDRF leading to fall of BP. It increases capillary permeability leading to oedema formation. Its effects on coronary blood vessels may differ.

- **Rspiratory tract effects:** Given by aerosol inhalation it causes dose dependent bronchoconstriction and inflammation of airways. It can produce oedema of airways. It also induces nonspecific bronchial hyperresponsiveness in nonasthmatic human subjects and in guinea pigs. It has a strong role in producing bronchial asthma.

- **Haematological effects:** It is a chemotactic (migration) factor for neutrophils, eosinophils and monocytes. It favours platelet aggregation and release of LTs from leucocytes. It produces IV thrombosis on IV injection.

- **GIT effects:** It is ulcerogenic to gastric mucosa. It causes contraction of smooth muscles of GIT and increases gut motility.

- **Miscellaneous effects:** It activates most inflammatory cells and plays important role in inflammation. It causes renal vasoconstriction and decreases urine output.

PAF Receptors

These are membrane bound G-protein receptors like eicosanoids. PAF acts through these specific receptors on the target cells. PAF receptor antagonists like Ginkgolides (A and B) obtained from the extracts of a Chinese plant Ginkgo biloba are in clinical trial in bronchial asthma and other allergic disorders.

Section IV

RESPIRATORY TRACT PHARMACOLOGY

21

Pharmacotherapy of Cough

PHYSIOLOGY OF COUGH

Cough is a useful physiological mechanism that serves to clear the respiratory passages of foreign materials and excess secretions. It should not be suppressed indiscriminately. When it annoys the patient or prevents rest or sleep, then it should be suppressed. Chronic cough can produce fatigue, specially in elderly patients. In such situations, drugs should be used to reduce the frequency or intensity of coughing. The cough reflex is complex involving the central and peripheral nervous systems, as well as the smooth muscles of the bronchial tree. Irritation of the bronchial mucosa causes bronchoconstriction which is turn stimulates cough receptors (special type of stretch receptors) located in the tracheo-bronchial tree. Afferent impulses from these receptors are carried by vagus nerve fibres to the cough centre, which is located in the upper part of medulla oblongata close to the respiratory, vomiting and vagal centres. Stimulation of cough centre initiates the act of coughing. The efferent impulses from the cough centre are carried by phrenic nerve fibres to the diaphragm, intercostal muscles and lungs. The act of coughing involves an initial deep inspiration followed by forced expiration against a temporarily closed glottis. Due to closure of glottis there is an increase in intrathoracic pressure as a result of relaxation of diaphragm, contraction of intercostal and abdominal wall muscles and

compression of lungs. This leads to opening of glottis and escapes of air from the lungs with a tremendous velocity and with a sound causing expulsion of mucus and unwanted materials (sputum) to the outside. Cough may be productive, when associated with a large amount of sputum and unproductive (dry), when without much sputum. Productive cough should not be suppressed, while unproductive cough should be suppressed. Environmental irritants may cause cough by irritating the respiratory tract. Smoking of cigarettes causes chronic persistent cough. Inhalation of allergens like dust, chemicals and pollen causes cough in asthmatics. Other important causes of cough are upper respiratory tract infections (rhinitis, sinusitis, tonsillitis, pharyngitis, adenoid infection, etc.), lower respiratory tract infections (bronchitis, bronchiectasis, asthma, tuberculosis, etc.), secondary to CCF and acute left ventricular failure and drug induced (produced by ACE inhibitors, β-blockers, amiodarone, Lugol's iodine, levodopa, nitrofurantoin, nebulized acetylcysteine and inhaled glucocorticoids and cromolyn sodium). Treatment of cough depends upon its cause. Thus, stoppage of smoking would correct chronic cough in heavy smokers. Cough caused by postnasal drip due to allergic rhinitis is relieved by antihistaminic therapy. Drug induced cough is benefitted by stoppage of the concerned drug or use of alternative drug. In case of productive cough, the patient should be

encouraged to cough voluntarily in appropriate posture from time to time. Simple steam inhalation produce beneficial effect in cough by liquefying respiratory tract secretions. For symptomatic treatment of cough following groups of drugs are used:
- Antitussives
- Expectorants
- Mucolytics.

Antitussives (Cough Suppressants)

These are drugs that act in the CNS to raise the threshold of cough centre or act peripherally in the respiratory tract to reduce tussal impulses or act by both of these actions. They are used only to suppress dry unproductive irritating cough.

Tussis is a Latin word meaning cough. Antitussives produce immediate symptomatic relief of cough.

Classification

These are of two groups:
1. Centrally acting antitussives (i.e. central cough suppressants).
   - Opioids, e.g. codeine, pholcodine, hydrocodone and morphine.
   - Nonopioids, e.g. noscapine, dextromethorphan, levopropoxyphane, carbetapentane, caramiphen, oxeladine, piperidone, chlophedianol, benzonatate and antihistaminics like diphenhydramine, chlorpheniramine and promethezine, etc.
2. Peripherally acting antitussives (i.e. peripheral cough suppressants).
   - Pharyngeal demulcents (prevent irritation of the sensory receptors of pharynx), e.g. syrups and linctuses containing glycerrhiza, lemon or candy sugar, lozenges and troches containing menthol.
   - Inhalation of steam (hot water vapour) or tincture benzoin compound in steam.

DISCUSSION OF DRUGS

Centrally Acting Antitussives

Of the opioids, morphine is an effective antitussive, but it is liable to produce respiratory depression and drug dependence and so not used as antitussive. Codeine is methylmorphine. It does not produce significant respiratory depression and has a low dependence liability. It is most commonly used as an antitussive. It is used as codeine phosphate linctus (12 mg/4 ml) in doses of 10 to 30 mg (4 to 12 ml) thrice daily. It can produce nausea, dizziness, palpitation, drowsiness, thickness of sputum and constipation. It decreases secretions in the bronchioles, which thickens the sputum and inhibits the mucociliary movement, thus reducing the clearance of thickened sputum. Pholcodine is a codeine derivative. It is as effective as codeine as an antitussive. It has a long half-life. It is administered once or twice daily. Hydrocodone, another derivative of codeine has antitussive action like codeine. Of the nonopioids, noscapine is a naturally occurring opium alkaloid of the benzyl isoquinoline group. It has no other CNS actions except antitussive action in therapeutic doses. It does not interfere with mucociliary movement. It has a smooth muscle relaxant action like papaverine. Its antitussive action is almost equal to that of codeine. It is used as noscapine linctus in doses of 15 to 30 mg 3 to 4 times a day. Its common side effect is nausea. In large dose it can cause bronchoconstriction and hypotension by releasing histamine from mast cells. Dextromethorphan is the d-isomer of the codeine analog levorphanol. As an antitussive, it is as effective as codeine and is probably safer than it. It has no other pharmacological actions and does not depress respiration in therapeutic doses. It is used as dextromethorphan hydrobromide linctus in doses of 10 to 30 mg 3 to 4 times a day. It produces fewer side effects than codeine. It does not inhibit ciliary activity. Its toxicity is low but in high dose it may produce CNS depression. Levopropoxyphene is the l-isomer of dextropropoxyphene. In doses of 50 to 100 mg orally, it suppresses cough to about the same doses as does 30 mg of dextromethorphan. Other centrally active antitussives like carbetapentane, caramiphen, oxeladine, piperidone and chlophedianol act like dextromethorphan as an antitussive (by raising the threshold of coughing). The mechanism of antitussive action of antihistaminics is unknown. Benzonatate is a long chain polyglycol derivative chemically related to procaine. It has local anaesthetic activity. It exerts its antitussive action on cough (stress) receptors in the lungs as well as by central mechanism like dextromethorphan. It is used in doses of 50 to 100 mg thrice daily. Centrally acting cough suppressants should not be used in presence of respiratory failure and in excessive respiratory secretion, as failure to expel it may lead to mechanical obstruction and atelectasis of lungs.

Peripherally Acting Antitussives

Pharyngeal demulcents act by producing protective coating on the sensory receptors (sensors) of cough in the pharynx and thus preventing irritation of the pharyngeal mucosa by irritant substances. They are used as lozenges, troches, or linctuses, which also increase salivary secretion producing protective and soothing effect. Their actual composition is not important. For soothing action in the tracheobronchial tree, where lozenges, troches or linctuses cannot reach, inhalation of hot water vapour (steam), often with some medication (tincture benzoin compound) is helpful.

Expectorants (Mucokinetics)

These are drugs which increase bronchial secretion or reduce its viscosity and facilitate its removal by coughing. Expectorant is derived from the Latin word *expectorare* meaning to drive from the chest. They are useful in productive cough such as in bronchitis, bronchiectasis, tuberculosis, emphysema and bronchial asthma.

Classification

These are of two groups:
1. Direct acting expectorants, e.g. sodium or potassium citrate/acetate, potassium iodide, guaicol, glycerylguaicol (guaiphensin), creosote, tolu syrup and terpene hydrate and volatile oils like eucalyptus oil, anise oil and lemon oil.
2. Reflex acting expectorants, e.g. ammonium chloride, ammonium bicarbonate, potassium iodide and ipecacuanha.

Mode of Action

Direct acting expectorants when taken orally are secreted via the bronchial gland and increase the bronchial gland secretion (including mucus) during their secretions. Reflexly acting expectorants when taken orally produce mild irritation of the gastric mucosa and increase bronchial gland secretion by stimulation of gastric reflexes. In large doses they may produce nausea and vomiting. Thus emetic drugs given in subemetic doses increase bronchial secretion producing a less tenacious sputum, which is easier to expectorate. Salts that produce such action are called saline expectorants, e.g. ammonium chloride, ammonium bicarbonate, potassium iodide and potassium citrate.

DISCUSSION OF SOME EXPECTORANTS

Ammonium Chloride

It is a reflex expectorant. It is given in a mixture form in a syrup base to mask the saline taste. It increases the respiratory secretion by stimulating gastric reflexes. Its dose is 100 to 200 mg (in 5 ml of cough mixture) twice daily. Its mixture is not pleasant to take and has smell of ammonia. It can cause nausea, vomiting and metabolic acidosis.

Ammonium Bicarbonate

It has properties like ammonium chloride except it does not produce metabolic acidosis.

Potassium Iodide

It is a both direct and reflex expectorant. It is given orally as cough mixture like ammonium chloride. It not only increases the respiratory secretion but also liquefy the thick and viscid sputum (by mucolytic action). Its dose is 200 to 300 mg (in 5 ml of cough mixture) thrice daily. Its mixture has a slightly bitter saline taste. Chronic administration of potassium iodide can cause symptoms of iodism, manifested as nasal catarrh, swelling of conjunctiva, oedema of eyelids, lacrimation swelling of salivary glands, increased respiratory tract secretion, oedema and ulcers of larynx, headache and skin rashes. It can occasionally cause goitre and hypothyroidism. It should not be used in children and pregnant women.

Potassium Citrate

It is a direct expectorant. It is much less effective than potassium iodide in increasing respiratory secretion. Its dose is 10 to 20 mg (in a teaspoonful of cough mixture) thrice daily. It does not produce goitre and hypothyroidism.

Ipecacuanha

It is a reflex expectorant. It is given as tincture in the dose of 1 ml twice daily. It increases the respiratory secretion as well as lower the viscosity of the sputum. It can produce nausea, vomiting and anorexia.

Sodium or Potassium Guaicol and Glycerylguaicol (Guaiphensin)

These are obtained from wood creosote. They are direct expectorants. They are given orally as cough mixture in the dose of 50 to 200 mg (in 5 ml) thrice daily. Glyceryl guaicol can interfere with haemostasis.

Terpene Hydrate

It is the active ingredient of cedar wood oil. It is a direct expectant. It is given orally as cough mixture in the dose of 5 to 10 mg (in 5 ml) thrice daily. It can also be added to steam inhalation and has similar effect of tincture benzoin compound (Friar's balsum) inhalation.

Mucolytics

These are drugs that make the thick and viscid sputum in the tracheobronchial tree to thin and less viscid sputum, so that it can be easily expectorated, e.g. bromhexine, ambroxol, acetylcysteine, carbocysteine, methylcysteine, pancreatic dornase, chymotrypsin, serratopeptidase, etc.

Mode of Action

Sputum (mucus) is chemically a high polymer of glycoprotein molecules. Mucolytics depolymerise (breakdown) the high polymer of glycoprotein into smaller molecules and thus make the sputum less viscid and thin.

DISCUSSION OF DRUGS

Bromhexine (Mucoline)

It is a synthetic derivative of an alkaloid vasicine obtained from the leaves of the plant *Adathoda vasica* (vasaka). Chemically it is a benzylamine compound. It possesses mucolytic, expectorant and bronchodilator properties. It causes thinning and fragmentation of mucopolysaccharide fibres of mucus of sputum and decreases viscosity of sputum. It is particularly useful when mucus plugs are present in the bronchioles. It can be given orally, parenterally and by inhalation. It is usually administered orally as tablet (8 mg) or syrup (4 mg/5 ml) in the doses of 8 to 16 mg thrice daily. It can cause nausea, rhinorrhoea and lacrimation as side effects. Ambroxol is better than bromhexine.

Acetylcysteine (Airborne)

It is a semisynthetic derivative of a naturally occurring amino acid l-cysteine. Chemically it is an amino acid. It is a mucolytic agent and acts by decreasing the viscosity of sputum by opening of disulphide bonds of glycoproteins of sputum. It is particularly useful in patients of cystic fibrosis of lungs and chronic bronchitis. It is rapidly metabolized in the body. It is administered by inhalation in the form of aerosol nebulizer (2 to 5 ml of 10% solution) into a face mask. Its onset of action is immediate and can be given every 8 hours for 5 to 10 days to liquefy viscid sputum. It is administered orally (as 5% solution) in paracetamol poisoning. It can cause fever, nausea, vomiting, stomatitis, rhinorrhoea as side effects. In patients with bronchial asthma, it may cause bronchospasm and so contraindicated. It reacts with most metals and with rubber. Carbocysteine and methylcysteine have similar properties of acetylcysteine.

Pancreatic Dornase

It is a deoxyribonuclease obtained from beef pancreas. It decreases the viscosity of sputum by degrading deoxyribonucleoprotein of sputum. It changes the thick and viscid sputum into thin milky material. It is administered by inhalation as aerosol (2 lakh units) twice daily. It can causes allergic reactions due to sensitivity to beef protein. Chymotrypsin and serratopeptidase are proteolytic enzymes that can be used orally as mucolytic agents but their clinical utility is disappointing.

22

Pharmacotherapy of Bronchial Asthma

INTRODUCTION

Bronchial asthma is a clinical syndrome characterized by paroxysmal dyspnoea and wheeze due to increased resistance to the flow of air through the narrowed bronchi. Narrowing of the bronchi is due to spasm of the bronchial smooth muscles, infiltration of inflammatory cells (eosinophil, lymphocyte, basophil and macrophage), oedema of bronchial mucosa and blocking of bronchial lumen by inspissated mucus. It can lead to COPD (chronic obstructive pulmonary disease).

Pathogenesis of Bronchial Asthma

It is predominantly an inflammatory disease. It has two characteristic features:

- Underlying inflammatory changes in the respiratory tract.
- Underlying bronchial hyperresponsiveness (abnormal sensitivity to stimuli). The development of allergic asthma involves exposure to genetically sensitive individuals to allergens. These cause activation of T lymphocytes, which in turn generate cytokines that promote activation of eosinophils, IgE production and release,

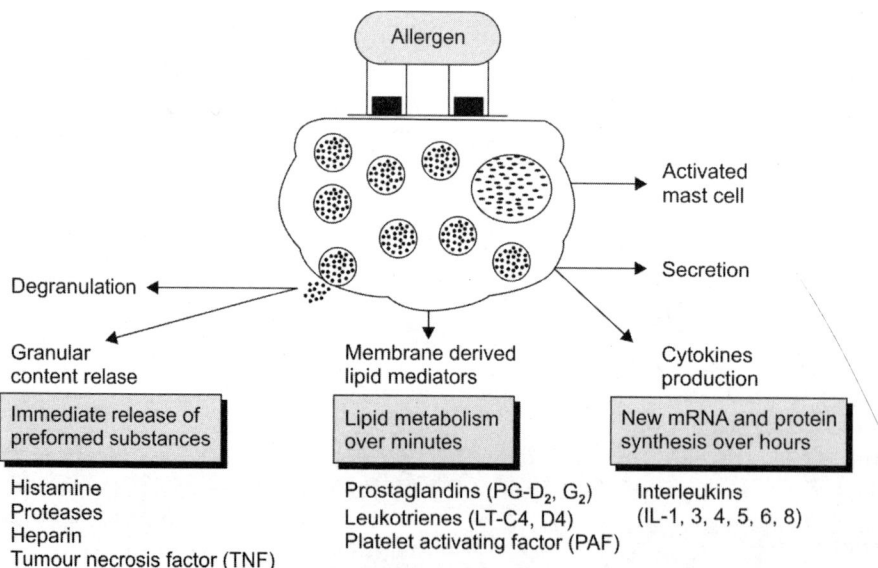

Fig. 22.1: Inflammatory mediators released by activated mast cell

and suppression of IgE receptors on mast cells and eosinophils. Inflammatory mediators released by activated mast cells in bronchial asthma are shown in **Fig. 22.1.**

In many subjects the asthmatic attack consists of two phases as follows:

- An immediate phase on exposure to eliciting agent (allergen/antigen) consisting mainly of bronchospasm. Common allergens are pollen grains, animal danders and feather particles.

- A late phase consisting of special type of inflammation comprising vasodilatation, oedema, mucus secretion and bronchospasm caused by inflammatory mediators released from eosinophils and T lymphocytes. Clinically there are three main forms of bronchial asthma:

  - **Episodic form:** Here the patient gets discrete, infrequent acute attacks, which are relieved by bronchodilator drugs, with no disability between the attacks. The acute attack is precipitated by allergy, an upper respiratory tract infection or psychological trauma.

  - **Status asthmaticus:** Here the acute attack is very severe and persistent and does not respond to routine treatment. It is accompanied by respiratory insufficiency or failure.

  - **Chronic form:** Here there is more or less persistent dyspnoea and wheeze of variable severity with acute attacks occurring from time to time. This is generally due to presence of inflammation and thickening of mucosa of the bronchioles, excessive mucus secretion, decreased elastic recoil of the lung tissue due to destructive changes in the alveolar walls and finally hyper-reactivity of the bronchi with bronchospasm. In such patients relief of bronchospasm by drugs may be incomplete. It can produce emphysema and COPD.

Classification

Classification of drugs used in bronchial asthma. There are of two groups:

1. **Bronchodilators:** These are as follows:
   - Sympathomimetics (adrenergic drugs).
     - Non-selective (both α and β agonists), e.g. adrenaline and ephedrine.
     - Selective β-agonists (both $β_1$ and $β_2$), e.g. isoprenaline and orciprenaline.
     - Selective $β_2$-agonists, e.g. salbutamol, terbutaline, salmeterol, pirbuterol, bitolterol, fenoterol, trimeterol and isoetharine.
   - Methylxanthines, e.g. theophylline, aminophylline, choline theophyllinate and etophyllin.
   - Anticholinergics, e.g. ipratropium bromide, tiotropium bromide, atropine methylnitrate (used as inhaler/aerosol).
   - Newer bronchodilators:
     - Cysteinyl leukotriene (LT) receptor antagonists, e.g. zafirlukast, pranlukast, cinalukast, montelukast, etc.
     - 5-lipo-oxygenase inhibitors, e.g. zileutin.

2. **Anti-inflammatory drugs:** These are suppressors of inflammation.
   - Glucocorticosteroids, e.g. beclomethasone dipropionate, budesonide, flunisolide, fluticasone propionate and triamcinolone acetonide (used as metered dose inhaler). Prednisone, prednisolone, betamethasone and dextramethasone (used as tablet or injection).
   - Mast cell stabilizers (cromolyn-like drugs), e.g. cromolyn sodium, nedocromil sodium (used as metered dose inhaler or nebulized solution) and kitotifen (used as tablet).

DISCUSSION OF INDIVIDUAL GROUPS OF DRUGS

Bronchodilators

Sympathomimetics (adrenergic drugs): Adrenaline is a nonselective adrenergic agonist. It is a potent bronchodilator drug. It also relieves pulmonary congestion by constricting the pulmonary arteries. It produces dramatic relief of acute attack of bronchial asthma. It is administered subcutaneously in a dose of 0.2 to 0.5 ml of a 1:1000 aqueous solution. It is injected slowly and no further injection is made if the attack subsides. It is effective within a few minutes. To be maximally effective, it must be injected early in an attack. It can cause unpleasant palpitation and tremulousness. It should not be injected into a vein, as serious cardiac arrhythmias and cerebrovascular accident can occur due to high rise of BP. Its use is dangerous in patients with cardiac asthma, hypertension, myocardial disease, hyperthyroidism, hypoxic patients in status asthmaticus, patients receiving tricyclic antidepressant drugs and soon after isoprenaline inhalation (may cause sudden death). Prolonged use of adrenaline in bronchial asthma may cause adrenaline resistance.

Ephedrine is a nonselective adrenergic agonist. It is a mixed acting adrenergic drug. It is useful in preventing nocturnal asthmatic attacks, where it is given orally in the dose of 30 mg (per tablet) at bed time. Patient who gets daytime attacks need 60 mg on waking and 30 mg at mid-day. It can cause insomnia, palpitation and difficulty in passing urine, specially in elderly patients. It also raises BP in patients receiving antihypertensive drugs. Tolerance to it develops after several weeks of continuous therapy but it is reversible after stopping the drug for a few days.

Isoprenaline (Isoproterenol) is a selective β-adrenergic drug (blocks both β_1 and β_2 receptors). It causes bronchodilatation as well as cardiac stimulation producing tachycardia, palpitation and cardiac arrhythmias. It is administered sublingually as tablet in the dose of 5 to 10 mg 3–4 times daily. It can be administered as inhaler (1:100 and 1:200 solutions in normal saline).

Orciprenaline (Metoproterenol) is a derivative of isoprenaline. It stimulates β_2 receptors more than β_1 receptors. It has longer duration of action than isoprenaline. It is administered orally, parenterally and by inhalation. Its oral dose is 20 mg (per tablet) 3 to 4 times daily

and parenteral dose is 0.5 to 1 mg IM or SC. It has less cardiac stimulant action than isoprenaline. When used by inhalation, it is approximately as effective as isoprenaline.

Salbutamol is a selective β_2-receptor agonist. It is chemically related to isoprenaline. It has a prominent bronchodilator action. It has poor cardiac stimulant action in comparison to isoprenaline. Hence, it causes less tachycardia and palpitation or a rise of BP in therapeutic dose. It is resistant to inactivation by COMT and, therefore, has a longer duration of action (about 4 to 6 hours). It is more rapidly effective by inhalation than by oral administration.

Preparations and Dosage of Salbutamol (Ventorlin)

- Tablet or syrup (2, 4 mg)—tablet 8 to 4 mg thrice daily, syrup (per 5 ml).
- Metered dose inhaler (90 µg/puff)—2 puffs every 4 to 6 hours.
- Rota caps, powder inhaler (200 µg/capsule)—1 to 2 capsules every 4 to 6 hours.
- Nebulized solution (6 mg/ml)—2.5 mg 3 to 4 times daily.

Adverse Reactions

It can cause muscle tremor of hands, nervousness and headache.

Terbutaline is a selective β_2 receptor agonist. It has similar properties like salbutamol but less potent.

Preparations and Dosage of Terbutaline (Bricaryl)

- Tablet (2.5, 5 mg)—2.5 to 5 mg thrice daily.
- Metered dose inhaler (200 µg/puff)—2 puffs every 4 to 6 hours.
  Adverse reactions are similar to salbutamol.

Salmeterol, pibuterol, bitolterol, fenoterol, rimeterol and isoetharine are other selective β_2-receptor agonists with similar properties as salbutamol and terbutaline.

Methylxanthines

Theophylline and its derivatives are used as bronchodilators in bronchial asthma. They act directly on the bronchial smooth muscles by inhibiting the phosphodiesterase enzyme and thus preventing degradation of cAMP to 5' AMP. The increased intracellular cAMP concentration leads to bronchodilatation. They also block adenosine receptors in producing bronchodilation (adenosine is a bronchoconstrictor.). Aminophylline (theophylline ethylene diamine), a water-soluble salt is available as injection (250 mg/10 ml ampoule) and tablet (100, 200 mg). In acute attack of bronchial asthma, it is administered by slow intravenous infusion with 5% dextrose solution in a dose of 5 mg/kg over 15 to 30 minutes, followed by 0.5 to 1 mg/kg/hour for several hours. IM injection is very painful and so not given. It is injected IV slowly to avoid sudden cardiac stimulation causing cardiac arrhythmias, cardiac arrest or anaphylactoid shock (due to sudden fall of BP). It is safer than adrenaline or isoprenaline in hypoxic subjects, in status asthmaticus and in patients with concomitant heart disease. It is especially helpful when one cannot decide whether a given attack is of bronchial asthma or cardiac asthma (left ventricular failure). Oral tablet of aminophylline in the doses of 100 to 200 mg thrice daily can be used in mild to moderate cases of bronchial asthma. Extended/slow release capsule of theophylline (Theolong 100, 200 mg) is available and used in the dosage of 200 to 300 mg, twice daily. Deriphylline (etophylline + theophylline) is available as tablet, syrup and injection. Choline theophyllinate is available as syrup.

Adverse reactions of theophylline and its derivatives in high doses include nausea, vomiting, headache, tremors, anxiety, tachycardia, hypertension, cardiac arrhythmias, convulsions and collapse.

Anticholinergics

They cause bronchodilatation by blocking cholinergic M_3 receptors. They reduce the concentration of cGMP in the bronchial muscles (which is increased by acetylcholine) and thus produce bronchodilatation. They are less effective than adrenergic drugs and produce slower response. They act predominantly in larger bronchi. They reduce and thicken (dry) bronchial secretion producing mucus plugs, which may cause respiratory obstruction (as difficult to expectorate). Atropine is now not used in bronchial asthma due to low efficacy and frequent side effects like dryness of mouth, mydriasis, tachycardia and retention of urine. Atropine methylnitrate can be given by inhalation as aerosol for selective action on M_3 receptors of bronchial muscles. Ipratropium bromide, a synthetic quaternary ammonium compound is preferred than atropine in the treatment of bronchial asthma. It is administered by inhalation as aerosol (Ipravent) in the dose of 1 to 2 puffs (40 to 80 µg) thrice daily. It acts locally on M_3 receptors of bronchial muscles and gives complete protection of bronchospasm. It does not interfere with (inhibits) mucociliary movement and removal of bronchial secretion (as it does not reduce and dry bronchial secretion). Its effect is seen after 30 minutes and lasts for 3 to 5 hours. It is useful in bronchial asthma and COPD. It is devoid of systemic side effects of atropine. It produces additive effects with a β-adrenergic agonist. Triotropium bromide is a congener of ipratropium. It is administered by inhalation as aerosol like ipratrupium) twice daily.

Corticosteroids (Glucocorticoids)

These are steroidal anti-inflammatory agents. When acute attacks of bronchial asthma are frequent and are not easily relieved by the bronchodilators and interfere with daily activities and sleep, then corticosteroids are used prophylactically on a regular basis. They act by decreasing bronchial hyperactivity and mucosal oedema in the late inflammatory phase of bronchial asthma when used continuously. The traditional route of administration is oral route, but it produces many adverse reactions after systemic administration. Now inhaled corticosteroids are preferred than systemic corticosteroids as they are devoid of systemic hazards due to little absorption in systemic circulation. Moreover, the concentration of the drug in the bronchial mucosa is high when inhalation route is used. Asthmatic patients maintained on inhaled corticosteroids show improvement (within one week) in symptoms and lowered requirement for β_2 agonists. Systemic corticosteroids are used in acute exacerbations of bronchial asthma and in chronic severe asthma for short-term therapy in patients not improving with bronchodilators. They are life-saving drugs in cases of severe acute attacks of bronchial asthma and in status asthmaticus, which cannot be controlled by bronchodilators alone.

Preparations and Dosage

- Beclomethasone dipropionate (Beclate)—metered dose inhaler (50 µg/puff)—2 to 4 puffs 3 to 4 times daily.

- Budesonide (Pulmicort)—metered dose inhaler (50 µg/puff)—2 to 4 puffs 3 to 4 times daily.

- Flunisolide (Aerobid)—metered dose inhaler (250 µg/puff)—2 to 4 puffs twice daily.

- Fluticasone propionate (Flonase)—metered dose inhaler (250 (µg/puff)—2 to 4 puffs twice daily.

- Triamcinolone acetonide (Azmacort)—metered dose inhaler (100 mg/puff)—2 to 4 puffs twice daily.

- Prednisone/Prednisolone (Wysolone)—oral tablet (5, 10 mg)—up to 50 mg/day in 3 divided doses for 5 to 14 days.

- Betamethasone (Betnelan/Betnesol)—oral tablet (0.5/1 mg)—up to 5 mg/day in three divided doses. Injection (4 mg/ml as sodium phosphate in ampoule)—4 to 20 mg IM or slow IV and repeated as required.

- Dexamethasone (Decadron)—oral tablet (0.5 mg)—up to 10 mg/day in three divided doses. Injection (4 mg/ml in vial) (as sodium phosphate)—4 to 20 mg IM or slow IV and repeated as required.

Adverse Reactions

Inhaled corticosteroids can produce oropharyngeal candidiasis and dysphonia, which can be reduced by saline gargle after every inhalation. Adverse reactions of systemic corticosteroids will be discussed in respective chapter.

Mast Cell Stabilizers

These are cromone (benzopyrone) derivatives.

Cromolyn Sodium (Disodium Chromoglycate)

It is a synthetic drug. It has no bronchodilator activity. It is an anti-inflammatory drug like corticosteroids. It acts by stabilizing the mast cell membrane and inhibiting release of inflammatory mediators like histamine, 5-HT, PGS and LTS from mast cells by degranulation in response to a variety of stimuli, including the interaction between cell bound IgE and specific antigen. As a result of this action, allergic inflammatory changes of the bronchial tree and subsequent bronchospasm are prevented. It also presents eosinophilic and neutrophilic chemotaxis and subsequent local inflammation. It thus ultimately reduces the hyperactivity of the bronchial tree. It is poorly absorbed after oral administration. It is administered by inhalation, when about 10% is absorbed. The absorbed drug is rapidly excreted unchanged in urine and bile. It is not effective in acute attacks of bronchial asthma. It is effective only as a prophylactic agent in allergic bronchial asthma, allergic alveolitis and allergic rhinitis. It has also been used in the treatment of aphthous stomatitis, ulcerative colitis and food allergy.

Nedocromil sodium has properties like cromolyn sodium.

Preparations and Dosage

- Cromolyn sodium (Ifiral/Intal)—Spinhaler, powder (20 mg/capsule)—1 capsule 3 to 4 times daily. Metered dose inhaler (800 µg/puff)—2 to 4 puffs 3 to 4 times daily. Nebulized solution (10 mg/ml)—20 mg 3 to 4 times daily.

- Nedocromil sodium (Tilade)—Metered dose inhaler (175 µg/puff)— 2 to 3 puffs 3 to 4 times daily.

Adverse Reactions

These are rare, because absorption into the systemic circulation after inhalation is small. When powder form is inhaled, bronchospasm can occur. Anaphylaxis can develop very rarely.

Ketotifen (Ketasma)

It is a cromolyn analogue. It is a potent antihistamine (H_1-blocker). It is a mast cell stabilizer and prevents mast cell degranulation and release of inflammatory mediators from mast cells. It also antagonizes the actions of histamine and PAF on bronchial smooth muscles. It has prophylatic uses like cromolyn sodium. It is effective orally.

Preparation and Dosage

Ketotifen tablet (1 mg)—1 to 2 mg twice daily. It is not recommended for children below two years. It can cause sedation and drowsiness.

Newer Bronchodilators and their Role in Bronchial Asthma

Several cysteinyl leukotriene (cyst LT) receptor antagonists, e.g. zafirlukast, pranlukast, cinalukast, montelukast, etc. are now used prophylactically in bronchial asthma. They do not allow the leukotrienes to produce actions (bronchospasm, increased vascular permeability and recruitment of eosinophils. They have high affinity for LTB_4, LTC_4 and LTD_4 receptors acting as competitive antagonists. They are well absorbed orally and have high bioavailability. They are highly plasma protein bound, metabolized in the liver and excreted in urine. They prevent aspirin sensitive asthma as well as antigen induced and exercise induced bronchospasm and relax the airways in mild to moderate asthma. They can be used as alternatives to inhaled glucocorticoids though their efficacy is lower. They are not effective to abort an attack of bronchial asthma. Zafirlukast has one-third of bronchodilator activity of salbutamol and its effects are additive with β-receptor agonists, 5-lipo-oxygenase (5-Lox) inhibitors, e.g. zileutin blocks synthesis of LTB_4, LTC_4 and LTD_4 and can be used in bronchial asthma but it has hepatotoxic potential and so has restricted use in bronchial asthma.

Leukotriene receptor antagonists can block antigen induced and exercise induced bronchospasm and may inhibit or reduce later phase of inflammation. They are given orally. Montelukast (Montair) tablet (10 mg o.d.) and zafirlukast (20 mg b.d.) are usually used in bronchial asthma. They are very safe drugs and produce a few side effects like headache and rashes. Eosinophilia and neuropathy occur rarely.

Management of bronchial asthma shown in **Table 22.1**.

Table 22.1: Stepwise management of bronchial asthma

Severity of disease	Clinical characteristics	Treatment	Outcome
Mild asthma	Intermittent, brief (< 1 hour) symptoms, 2 times/week. Asymptomatic between exacerbations. Brief (< ½ hour) symptoms with activity. Infrequent (< 2 times/month) nocturnal symptoms.	Inhaled β_2-adrenergic agonist (as needed), 1 or 2 puffs daily and/or cromolyn sodium before exposure to exercise, allergen or other stimuli. β_2-adrenergic agonist orally (as needed).	Prevents symptoms (wheeze/cough/dyspnoea/tightness). Controls symptoms. Normal activity. No nocturnal cough/wheeze. Normal lung function.
Moderate asthma	Symptoms > 1 or 2 times per week. Exacerbations may last few days. Requires occasional emergency care.	Inhaled β_2-adrenergic agonist (as needed), 1 or 2 puffs 2 to 3 times daily and inhaled cromolyn sodium/nedocromil sodium. If symptoms persist inhaled steroid is used. theoral theophylline or β-adrenergic agonist can be considered.	Same as above plus decreases need of β_2-adrenergic agonist. Decreases frequency of exacerbations. No emergency care requires.
Severe/acute asthma	Continuous symptoms. Limited activity. Frequent exacerbations. Frequent nocturnal symptoms. Occasional hospitalization and emergency care.	Inhaled β_2-adrenergic agonist (as needed), 1 or 2 puffs 3 to 4 times daily and inhaled steroid with or without inhaled cromolyn sodium or nedocromil sodium, oral theophylline and/or oral β_2-agonist and oral steroid may be considered.	Improves pulmonary function. Near normal activity. Decreases frequency of nocturnal symptoms and exacerbations. Decreases need for β_2-adrenergic agonist, oral steroid and emergency care.
Acute attack of asthma	Continuous symptoms. Limited activity. Needs hospitalization and emergency care.	Aminophylline IV or adrenaline SC and then inhaled β_2-adrenergic agonist in sufficient doses.	Same as above
Status asthmaticus	A serious form of acute attack. A medical emergency requiring urgent hospitalization and vigorous treatment.	Glucocorticoid in large doses (e.g. hydrocortisone hemisuccinate injection —100 to 200 mg IV followed by IV infusion). Inhaled β_2-adrenergic agonist in sufficient doses. Humidified O_2 inhalation (2 L/min by nasal cannula). Administration of antibiotic. Correction of dehydration and hypokalemia.	Same as above

Treatment of acute bronchial asthma: see page 174–177

1. Correction of dehydration and acidosis with normal saline, sodium bicarbonate or lactate preparation by IV infusion.
2. Inhalation of moist oxygen (humidified oxygen)—2 to 3 litres/minute.
3. Antibiotic prophylaxis.
4. Chest X-ray to exclude pneumothorax.
5. Avoidance of exposure to allergic substance (allergens) and environment.
6. Prophylactic use of mast cell stabilizers or leukotriene inhibitors.

Section V

GASTROINTESTINAL TRACT PHARMACOLOGY

23

Drug Therapy of Peptic Ulcer

INTRODUCTION

Peptic ulcer is an ulcer of GIT due to acid-pepsin digestion of the mucosa. It occurs at the area exposed to acid-pepsin mixture. Important sites are stomach (mostly in the lesser curvature), duodenum (in the proximal part), oesophagus (as a result of gastroeso-phageal reflux), Meckel's diverticulum and jejunum (after gastrojejunal anastomosis). The ratio between duodenal and gastric ulcer is about 4:1. It may be acute or chronic ulcer (common). Both penetrate the muscularis mucosae but the acute ulcer shows no fibrosis. Gastric mucosa contains parietal cells and peptic cells. Gastric acid (dilute HCl) is secreted from gastric parietal cells (as shown in **Fig. 23.1**) by a proton pump (H⁺, K⁺-ATPase). Endogenous secretagogues for gastric acid are histamine, acetylcholine and gastrin. Pepsin is secreted by gastric peptic cells. It digests protein only when the gastric pH is sufficiently low (below 3.5). At higher pH pepsin becomes inactive and cannot digest protein. PGE_2 and PGI_2 inhibit gastric acid secretion and stimulate mucus and bicarbonate secretion. The genesis of peptic ulcer involves the imbalance between aggressive factors (mucosal damaging factors) like gastric acid (dil. HCl), pepsin and *Helicobacter pylori*

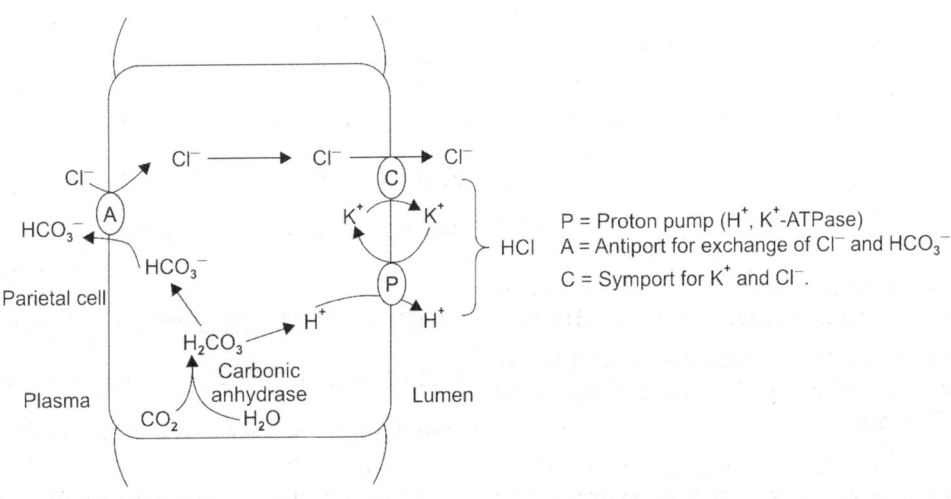

Fig. 23.1. Secretion of gastric acid (dil. HCl) by the parietal cells

infection and mucosal protective factors (defensive factors) like secretion of mucus, bicarbonate and locally synthesized PGE_2 and PGI_2. Increase in acid-pepsin secretion and decrease in mucosal resistance is the basic cause of peptic ulcer. Gastric ulcer is mainly due to defective mucosal resistance, whereas duodenal ulcer is mainly due to increase in acid-pepsin secretion. Drugs producing peptic ulcer (ulcerogenic drugs) include NSAIDs (aspirin, phenyl butazone, indomethacin, ibuprofen, etc.), theophylline, aminophylline, glucocorticoids, reserpine, serotonin, histamine, etc.

Classification of Drugs Used in Peptic Ulcer

These are of two groups:

1. **Drugs reducing aggressive factors (mucosal damaging factors)**
   - Antacids, e.g. aluminium hydroxide gel, magnesium trisilicate, magnesium hydroxide and calcium carbonate. They neutralize gastric acid that is already secreted.
   - Antisecretory drugs: They decrease secretion of gastric acid.
     - H_2-receptor antagonists (blockers), e.g. ranitidine, famotidine and roxatidine.
     - Proton pump inhibitors, e.g. omeprazole, lansoprazole, pantoprazole and rabeprazole.
     - Anticholinergics (muscarinic M_1 antagonists), e.g. pirenzepine, telenzepine, etc.
     - Somatostatin analogue: Octreotide.
   - Anti-*Helicobacter pylori* drugs (for complete eradication of *H. pylori*), e.g. metronidazole/tinidazole and amoxycillin/tetracycline/clarithromycin.
2. **Drugs strengthening mucosal defences/ protective factors (cytoprotective drugs)**
   - Ulcer protective drugs (coating agents), e.g. sucralfate and colloidal bismuth subcitrate.
   - Ulcer healing drugs (mucus secretion stimulants), e.g. carbenoxolone and deglycerrhized liquorice.

- Prostaglandin analogs, e.g. misoprostol and rioprostil (congeners of PGE_1), enprostil and arbaprostil (congeners of PGE_2).

DISCUSSION OF DRUGS USED IN PEPTIC ULCER

Gastric Antacids

These drugs by neutralizing the gastric acid (dil. HCl) secreted by gastric parietal cells. They are compared qualitatively in terms of their acid neutralizing capacity, i.e. the quantity of 1N HCl (expressed in milliequivalent) which can be brought to pH 3.5 in 15 min, e.g. acid neutralizing capacity of aluminium hydroxide gel, magnesium trisilicate, magnesium hydroxide and magaldrate are 25, 24, 14 and 30 mEq per tablet or ml gel respectively.

Classification

These are of two types:

1. Non-systemic (non-absorbable) antacids, e.g. aluminium hydroxide gel, magnesium trisilicate, magnesium hydroxide, magaldrate, calcium carbonate, etc. They are commonly used.

2. Systemic (absorbable) antacids, e.g. sodium bicarbonate, sodium citrate, etc.

Mechanism of Action

Antacids react with the gastric acid (dil. HCl) to form chlorides, H_2O and CO_2 by neutralizing HCl by the following reactions:

$$Al(OH)_3 + 3HCl \xrightarrow{slow} AlCl_3 + 3H_2O$$

$$Mg_2Si_3O_3 \cdot n\,H_2O + 4HCl \xrightarrow{slow/moderate} MgCl_2 + 3SiO_2 + (n+2)H_2O$$

$$Mg(OH)_2 + 2HCl \xrightarrow{slow/moderate} MgCl_2 + 2H_2O$$

$$CaCO_3 + 2HCl \xrightarrow{fast} CaCl_2 + H_2O + CO_2$$

$$NaHCO_3 + HCl \xrightarrow{fast} NaCl + H_2O + CO_2$$

Aluminium and magnesium salts are called buffer antacids as they do not permit the rise of pH of gastric contents above 3.5 and do not impair pepsin digestion of protein food. On the other hand, calcium carbonate and sodium bicarbonate are nonbuffer antacids as they permit the rise of pH of gastric contents above 3.5 and impair pepsin digestion of protein food. The hydroxides of aluminium and magnesium are relatively insoluble and so OH^- does not accumulate to corrosive level. $Mg(OH)_2$ reacts relatively rapidly with HCl. $MgCO_3$ though more soluble than $Mg(OH)_2$, but reacts more slowly with HCl owing to its crystal structure. $Al(OH)_3$ acts relatively slowly and can provide sustained acid neutralizing capacity. Thus, combination of aluminium hydroxide and magnesium trisilicate or hydroxide provides relatively fast and sustained acid neutralizing capacity. Magnesium trisilicate forms hydrated silicondioxide gel, which forms protective coating over ulcer surface. Magaldrate is a hydroxymagnesium aluminium complex, which is rapidly converted by HCl to magnesium and aluminium hydroxides, which are poorly absorbed and thus provides a fast and sustained antacid effect with balanced effects on intestinal motility (magnesium salt produces laxative effect and aluminium salt produces constipating effect).

Calcium carbonate and sodium bicarbonate are rapidly acting antacids but raise the pH of the gastric contents above 5 and impair protein digestion of food by pepsin.

Clinical Uses

Antacids are mainly used to produce prompt relief of pain of peptic ulcer by reducing acid irritation of the ulcer. They are also used in gastroesophageal reflux disease (GERD) along with simethicone (methylpolysilxone/MPS) and as preanaesthetic medication prior to general anaesthesia to avoid regurgitation of gastric contents into lungs producing pneumonitis or pneumonia.

Some Preparations of Antacids

- Dried aluminium hydroxide gel tablet (840 mg)/gel (610 mg/5 ml) (Aludrox).

- Dried aluminium hydroxide gel (400 mg) and magnesium trisilicate tablet (400 mg) gel (in 5 ml) (Gelusil).
- Dried aluminium hydroxide gel (400 mg) + Magnesium hydroxide (400 mg) + Simethicone × (30 mg) tablet/gel (in 5 ml) (Gelusil MPS).
- Magnesium hydroxide gel (containing 390 mg of $Mg(OH)_2$/5 ml) (milk of magnesia).
- Megaldrate (1080 mg) and simethicone (30 mg) tablet/gel (in 5 ml) (Rolac plus).

Adverse Reactions

Aluminium salts produce constipation, phosphate depletion (hypophosphatemia) by binding with phosphate on prolonged use and aluminium encephalopathy in presence of renal failure. Magnesium salts produce diarrhoea, hypermagnesaemia in presence of renal failure on prolonged use. Combination of aluminium and magnesium salts counteract each others' side effects. Calcium carbonate stimulates secretion of gastrin and HCl, producing rebound acidity and produces constipation, hypercalcaemia (in renal failure) and milk alkali syndrome (when administered with milk). Sodium bicarbonate causes systemic alkalosis, liberates CO_2, which can cause gastric distension and belching with acid reflux, stimulates secretion of gastrin and HCl producing rebound acidity and can produce sodium overload in circulation.

Drug Interactions

By altering gastric and urinary pH, antacids may alter the rates of dissolution and elimination of a number of drugs. Aluminium and magnesium compounds alter gastric motility and therefore alter the rate at which drugs reach the absorptive surface of the small intestine. Aluminium compounds adsorb drugs and form insoluble complexes that are not absorbed. In general, concurrent administration of antacids and drugs intended for systemic absorption should be avoided. Most drug interactions can be avoided by taking antacids two hours before or after ingestion of other drugs.

H₂-Receptor Antagonists (Blockers)

These drugs competitively inhibit the inter-action of histamine with H_2 receptors present in the parietal cells of stomach and decrease gastric acid secretion produced by histamine, gastrin and to some extent by acetylcholine and other muscarinic agonists. They inhibit basal (fasting) and nocturnal acid secretion in the stomach. They also decrease acid secretion stimulated by food and other chemical agents. They reduce both the volume of gastric juice secreted and its H^+ concentration. They also reduce secretion of pepsin by the chief cells of the gastric glands. They do not interfere with the gastrointestinal motility.

They are rapidly well-absorbed after oral administration. Their peak concentration in plasma are attained in 1 or 2 hours. They have bioavailability of about 50%, except nizatidine, which has bioavailability of about 90%. They are metabolized in the liver to some extent and a larger part is excreted in urine in unchanged form. Thus renal impairment requires a reduction in the doses of these drugs. Hepatic impairment also prolongs their duration of action or plasma half-life.

Clinical Uses

They are popular drugs used in duodenal and gastric ulcers. About 80% of duodenal ulcers heal with them within 4 to 6 weeks. Gastric ulcers require longer time to heal (i.e. 8 to 12 weeks). They are used as preanaesthetic medication to prevent gastroesophageal reflux leading to aspiration of gastric contents into lungs producing pneumonitis or pneumonia. They are also used in Zollinger-Ellison syndrome (ZES), peptic oesophagitis, NSAID induced ulcers and gastroduodenal bleeding due to severe burn and trauma (stress ulcers). Zollinger-Ellison syndrome is the peptic and esophageal ulceration associated with gastrin producing tumors (gastrinomas).

Preparations and Dosage

- Cimetidine (Tagamet) tablet (200 mg)—200 to 400 mg thrice daily after meals and at bed time.
- Ranitidine (Zinetac) tablet (150, 300 mg)—150 mg twice daily after meals or 300 mg at bed time.
- Ranitidine hydrochloride (Zinetac) injection (50 mg/2 ml)—50 mg IV twice daily.
- Famotidine (Famocid) tablet (20, 40 mg)—20 mg twice daily after meals or 40 mg at bed time.
- Roxatidine (Rotane) tablet (150, 300 mg)—150 mg twice daily after meals or 300 mg at bed time.
- Nizatidine (Axid) tablet (150, 300 mg)—As above.

After 4 to 6 weeks treatment, they are used in maintenance dose (1/2 of the initial dose), taken at bed time.

Adverse Reactions

Cimetidine can cause skin rashes, headache, dizziness, nausea, diarrhoea, muscle pain and bradycardia. It can cross BBB to some extent and produces some CNS symptoms like somnolence, drowsiness and mental con-fusion especially in elderly patients and in those with renal failure. It has an anti-androgenic action on prolonged use. It displaces dihydrotestosterone from its cytoplasmic receptors and produces gynaeco-mastia, loss of libido, impotence and tem-porary decrease of sperm count in males. It increases prolactin secretion and produces altered lactation in females. It also inhibits degradation of oestradiol in liver by inhibiting hepatic microsomal enzyme system. Ranitidine and other H_2-receptor blockers are relatively free from these adverse effects.

Drug Interactions

Cimetidine is a hepatic microsomal enzyme (cytochrome P_{450}) system inhibitor. It decreases the metabolism of many drugs by oxidation (by mixed function oxidases), e.g. phenobarbitone, phenytoin, propranolol, warfarin, diazepam, oestradiol, theophylline, lignocaine, quinidine and imipramine and so these drugs are accumulated in the body to toxic levels. It also decreases absorption of ketoconazole and increases hepatotoxicity produced by isoniazid and paracetamol. Ranitidine and other H_2-receptor blockers do not produce these drug interactions.

Proton Pump Inhibitors (PPI)

The ultimate mediator of gastric acid secretion is H^+, K^+-ATPase (proton pump) of the apical membrane of the gastric parietal cells. Proton pump inhibitors contain a sulphinyl group in a bridge between substituted benzimidazole and pyridine rings. At neutral pH, they are chemically stable, lipid-soluble and neutral weak bases that are devoid of inhibitory activity become active in acidic pH (<5). They reach the parietal cells from blood and diffuse into the secretory canaliculi, where they become protonated and thereby trapped. The protonated agent forms sulphenic acid and sulphemide by rearrangement. The sulphemide interacts covalently with sulphydryl groups at critical sites in the extracellular (luminal) domain of the parietal cell membrane by inhibiting H^+, K^+-ATPase. Full inhibition occurs when 2 molecules of the inhibitor is bound with 1 molecule to the enzyme. Due to inhibition of the enzyme H^+, K^+-ATPase, exchange of H^+ (proton) ions for K^+ ions in the canaliculi of parietal cells (where H^+ ion unites with Cl^- ion to form HCl) cannot occur and so no HCl (gastric acid) will be formed.

Proton pump inhibitors produce marked inhibition of basal, nocturnal and food stimulated gastric acid secretion. They are better than H_2-receptor blockers as they can cause 100% inhibition of gastric acid secretion. They are prodrugs and absorbed after oral administration. They have oral bioavailability of 70 to 80%. They are metabolized in the liver and converted to active drugs. They are highly plasma protein bound (about 90%). They are excreted in urine mainly as metabolites. They have plasma half-life of 1 to 1.5 hours.

Clinical Uses

They are used in both gastric and duodenal ulcers to promote healing of ulcers. They are especially useful where H_2-receptor blockers have failed as in Zollinger-Ellison syndrome (ZES). They are also used in reflux oesophagitis and NSAID induced peptic ulcers.

Preparations and Dosage

- Omeprazole (Omez) capsule (10, 20 mg)— 10 to 20 mg once daily for 4 to 6 weeks.
- Lansoprazole (Lanzap) capsule (15, 30 mg)—15 to 30 mg once daily for 4 to 6 weeks.
- Pantoprazole (Pantocid) tablet (20, 40 mg)— 20–40 mg once daily for 4 to 6 weeks.
- Rabeprazole (Aciless) tablet (20, 40 mg) as pantoprazole.

Adverse Reactions

They are generally well-tolerated. They can cause GIT side effects like nausea, diarrhoea and abdominal colic and CNS side effects like headache, dizziness and somnolence. They can also produce skin rashes and transient rise of the plasma activities of hepatic aminotransferases.

Drug Interactions

They can inhibit hepatic microsomal enzyme (cytochrome P_{450}) system leading to inhibition of metabolism of certain drugs like phenytoin, diazepam and warfarin and so increase their toxicity due to accumulation in the body.

Anticholinergics (Muscarinic Receptor Antagonists)

They can reduce volume (basal secretion) of gastric acid by 40 to 50%. Food stimulated gastric secretion is inhibited to a lesser extent. Selective M_1 receptor antagonists (e.g. pirenzepine and telenzepine) are as effective as nonselective muscarinic antagonists (e.g. atropine and scopolamine) but produce less adverse effects (e.g. dry mouth, blurred vision and tachycardia) which are characteristics of cholinergic blockade. They have low affinity for M_2 and M_3 receptors. They may also inhibit the secretion of gastrin, mucus and bicarbonate. Although they are less effective than H_2-receptor antagonists in reducing gastric acid secretion, but they produce comparable rates of healing of duodenal and gastric ulcers. They are hydrophilic and penetrate BBB poorly.

Clinical Uses

They are used to reduce gastric acid secretion and pain in duodenal and gastric ulcers. Their response is better in duodenal ulcer than in gastric ulcer.

Preparations and Dosage

- Pirenzepine tablet (50 mg)—50 mg 2 or 3 times daily for 4 to 6 weeks.
- Telenzepine tablet (3 mg)—3 mg once daily for 4 to 6 weeks (more potent).

Adverse Reactions

They can cause dry mouth, blurred vision and constipation as side effects.

Somatostatin Analogue

Octreotide: It is a synthetic long-acting somatostatin analogue with antigastrin activity. Somatostatin receptors are present in the gastric parietal cells. Somatostatin inhibits gastric acid secretion by binding with somatostatin receptors. Octreotide inhibits gastric acid secretion as well as pancreatic secretion. It is used mainly in Zollinger-Ellison syndrome (ZES). It is also used in portal hypertension (to reduce pressure) and bleeding from portal varices. It is available as octride injection. It is administered parenterally (0.5 mg/1 ml SC/day).

Anti-*Helicobacter pylori* Drugs

These are used for eradication of *H. pylori*, the causative organism of peptic ulcer diseases. *H. pylori* is a gram-negative bacillus (rod-like) that colonizes in the mucus on the luminal surface of the gastric epithelium. It causes an inflammatory gastritis, peptic ulcer diseases, gastric lymphoma and adenocarcinoma. Eradication of *H. pylori* by drugs concurrently with the use of H_2-receptor antagonists or proton pump inhibitors enhances the rate of ulcer healing than the use of later drugs alone.

Single drug therapy of *H. pylori* is relatively ineffective *in vivo* and produces emergence of resistant strains of *H. pylori* to drugs, especially to metronidazole and tinidazole (via a mutant nitroreductase activity). Amoxycillin, clarithromycin or tetracycline is effective in some patients. Due to development of resistant strains of *H. pylori* multiple drug therapy is needed in some patients. Resistance is less problematic when metronidazole/tinidazole is combined with a bismuth compound (colloidal bismuth subcitrate) and an antibiotic (amoxicillin/tetracycline). The triple drug therapy with metronidazole (400 mg thrice daily), colloidal bismuth subcitrate (120 mg 4 times daily) and amoxycillin (500 mg thrice daily) or tetracycline (500 mg 4 times daily) produces eradication of about 90% of *H. pylori*. In treating peptic ulcer, the triple drug therapy is added to an antisecretory medication (H_2-blocker/proton pump inhibitor), which may be used for about six weeks or prophylactically. Limitations of triple drug therapy are:

- Less patient compliance
- Combined cost is high
- Frequent side effects like nausea, diarrhoea and dizziness
- Cannot be used in infirm elderly patients.

Combination of an antisecretory drug (ranitidine or omeprazole) with an antibiotic (amoxycillin or clarithromycin) and metronidazole or tinidazole is available as kit for eradication of *H. pylori*.

Ulcer Protective Drugs

Sucralfate

It is a complex formed from sucrose octasulphate and polyaluminium hydroxide. In a strong acid medium (pH <4), it polymerizes and forms sticky viscid yellow white gel, which adheres to the epithelial cells and ulcer craters and forms a protective coating, which prevents diffusion of H^+ and pepsin. It binds with pepsin and inhibits pepsin mediated protein hydrolysis. It also binds with bile salts and prevents irritation of ulcer craters by bile acids. If the gastric pH is high (>5) then it is ineffective. The coating formed by it on ulcer craters stays about 12 hours. It is not absorbed. It should not be used with antacids (e.g. aluminium hydroxide), H_2-blockers (e.g. ranitidine) or proton pump inhibitors (e.g. omeprazole), because it is effective only in acid medium.

Clinical Uses

It is used in gastric and duodenal ulcers and chronic gastritis. It promotes healing of gastric and duodenal ulcers approximately as effectively as H_2-blockers.

Preparation and Dosage

Sucralfate (Sucral) tablet (1 g) suspension (1 g/5 ml)—1 g to be taken one hour before meals and at bed time for 4 to 8 weeks.

Adverse Reactions

It can produce nausea, constipation, dyspepsia, headache and hypophosphataemia (by binding with phosphate in the intestine).

Drug Interactions

It decreases the absorption of digoxin, phenytoin and warfarin. It is ineffective with antacids, H_2-blockers or proton pump inhibitors.

Colloidal Bismuth Subcitrate (CBS)

Chemically it is tripotassium dicitrato-bismuthate. It has no substantial capacity to neutralize gastric acid. It has cytoprotective action (by increasing secretion of bicarbonate arid mucus), pepsin inhibition activity, capacity to accumulate in the ulcer craters and anti-*Helicobacter pylori* activity in the gastroduodenal mucosa. In acidic pH, it chelates with proteins in the ulcer base and forms a protective barrier against acid diffusion and peptic digestion.

Clinical Uses

It is used in gastric and duodenal ulcers and chronic gastritis **(Table 23.1)**. It promotes healing of gastric and duodenal ulcers as effectively as H_2-blockers. It prevents ulcer recurrence. It is an important component of triple drug regimen for eradication of *H. pylori*. It is also used in gastroesophageal reflux disease (GERD).

Preparation and Dosage

Colloidal bismuth subcitrate (Trymo) tablet / suspension (120 mg/5 ml)—240 mg to be taken 30 minutes before meals twice daily for 4 to 8 weeks.

Adverse Reactions

It can cause black tongue and black stool. Prolonged use can lead to encephalopathy and osteodystrophy.

Ulcer Healing Drugs
Carbenoxolone

It is an oleandane derivative of glycyrrhizic acid, obtained from liquorice root. It alters the composition and quantity of mucus, thereby producing a mucosal barrier to HCl. Its mechanism of action is not clear. It is a steroid congener and exhibits significant mineralocorticoid aldosterone activity. Thus sodium and fluid retention, hypertension, hypokalemia and impaired glucose tolerance are commonly observed with it. For these adverse effects, it is now less used in gastric and duodenal ulcers. Deglycerrhized liquorice has similar properties of carbenoxolone. They are available as tablets (100 and 400 mg respectively) and administered thrice daily for 4 to 6 weeks.

Prostaglandin Analogs

Gastric and intestinal mucosa synthesize a large amount of PGE_2 and PGI_2 which inhibit the secretion of gastric acid and stimulate the secretion of mucus and bicarbonate to promote cytoprotection. A number of slowly metabolized PG-analogs have been developed for the treatment of peptic ulcer, e.g. misoprostol (15-methyl PGE_1, enprostil (dehydro PGE_2), etc.

Clinical Uses

They are moderately effective in treating duodenal and gastric ulcers. They promote

Table 23.1: Treatment of gastroduodenal ulcers

Triple therapy	Quadruple therapy
1. A proton pump inhibitor (PPI), *viz.* omeprazole (20 mg), rabeprazole (20 mg), lansoprazole (30 mg) or pantoprazole (40 mg) is administered twice before breakfast and supper for 4 weeks or H_2-blocker, *viz.* ranitidine (300 mg), or famotidine (40 mg) is administered twice daily after meal for 3 weeks.	1. A proton pump inhibitor (PPI), *viz.* omeprazole (20 mg), Rabeprazole (20 mg), lansoprazole (30 mg) or pantoprazole (40 mg) is administered twice daily before breakfast and supper for 3 weeks.
2. An antibiotic, *viz.* amoxicillin (500 mg) or tetracycline (500 mg) or clarithromycin (500 mg) is administered twice daily for 7 days.	2. An antibiotic, *viz.* amoxycillin (500 mg), tetracycline (500 mg) or clarithromycin (500 mg) is administered thrice daily for 7 days.
3. A nitromidazole, *viz.* metronidazole (400 mg) or tinidazole (300 m g) is administered thrice daily for 7 days.	3. A colloidal bismuth salt, *viz.* bismuth sub-citrate or bismuth subsalicylate is administered 4 times daily for 3 weeks.
	4. A nitronidazole, *viz.* metronidazole (400 mg) or tinidazole (300 mg) is administered thrice daily for 7 days.

ulcer healing by inhibiting food and drug induced gastric acid secretion and increasing secretions of mucus and bicarbonate, thus producing cytoprotection. They are valuable as cytoprotective agents in patients who require NSAIDs for treatment of arthritis or other diseases.

Preparation and Dosage

Misoprostol (Cytotec) tablet (300 mg)—300 µg 3 times daily with food.

Adverse Reactions

They can cause diarrhoea, abdominal cramps and abortion (in pregnant woman).

24

Emetics and Antiemetics

PHYSIOLOGY OF VOMITING (EMESIS)

Nausea is urge to vomit and vomiting is the forceful expulsion of gastric content to the exterior via oral cavity. The act of vomiting is accompanied by a complex series of movements, which are controlled by the vomiting centre in the medulla oblongata. This centre receives input from the chemoreceptor trigger zone (CTZ) situated in the lateral border of the area, prostema of the medulla oblongata at the floor of the 4th ventricle. The CTZ is in direct contact with the circulating blood and is outside the BBB. It is a purely sensory relay station and is incapable of initiating vomiting in the absence of vomiting centre. A variety of chemicals including drugs like morphine, apomorphine, cholinomi-metics, cytotoxic drugs, ipecac, *l*-dopa, bromo-criptine and digitalis glycosides stimulate CTZ, while phenothiazines and certain antihi-staminics depress it. Vomiting of vestibular origin is mediated through CTZ as follows— vestibular apparatus in internal ear → vestibular nuclei → cerebellum → CTZ → vomiting centre. Besides CTZ, vomiting centre receives afferent impulses from the periphery (GIT and other viscera) and cerebral cortex (higher centres) as shown in **Fig. 24.1**.

Following stimulation of the vomiting centre, efferent impulses are carried by vagus, phrenic and spinal nerves to the diaphragm, abdominal muscles, GIT sphincters and muscles. Pyloric region of the stomach contracts, while upper portion of the stomach

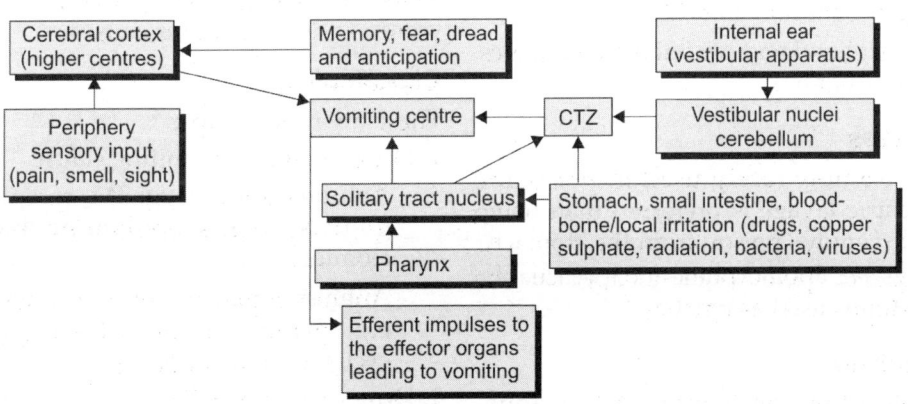

Fig. 24.1: Reflex pathway of vomiting

179

and LES (lower oesophageal sphincter) relax. Intra-abdominal pressure rises as the diaphragm descends and anterior abdominal muscles contract. The stomach is subjected to high pressure and its content escapes *via* oesophagus and expelled outside. A reverse peristalsis in the stomach and oesophagus helps in vomiting. All these motor effects occur due to neuronal discharges from the vomiting centre. Vomiting is also under the volitional control and can be induced voluntarily.

The vomiting centre mainly contains cholinergic and muscarinic (M_1) receptors, while CTZ contains dopaminergic (D_2), histaminergic (H_1), muscarinic (M_1) and serotonergic (5-HT_3) receptors. Dopaminergic receptors in the stomach mediate the inhibition of gastric motility that occurs during nausea and vomiting and are the site of action of antiemetic dopamine receptor antagonists.

Emetics

These are drugs that induce vomiting and can be used in poisoning cases.

Classification

These are of three groups:
- Centrally acting emetics: They act by direct stimulation of CTZ, e.g. apomorphine, morphine and hydergine.
- Peripherally acting emetics: They act by GIT irritation leading to stimulation of CTZ, e.g. mustard powder, antimony and potassium tartrate (tartar emetic) and hypertonic sodium chloride.
- Both peripheral and central acting emetics, e.g. ipecacuanha.

Clinical Uses

Emetics are now rarely used in poisoning cases. Gastric lavage is preferred than using emetics to remove poison from the stomach. Two drugs, *viz.* apomorphine and ipecacuanha are sometimes used as emetics.

Apomorphine

It is a morphine derivative. It is a dopaminergic (D_2) receptor agonist, that stimulates

CTZ. It causes vomiting within 15 minutes. It is administred SC or IM but not orally in poisoning cases.

Preparation and Dosage

Apomorphine hydrochloride injection (1 mg / ml)—1 to 2 mg SC or IM.

Adverse Reactions

It can produce respiratory depression, restlessness, tremors, convulsions, hypotension, syncope and coma in large doses. It can be treated by nalorphine (5 to 10 mg IV).

Ipecacuanha

It contains the alkaloid emetine, which is a safe emetic especially in children. It acts both by gastric irritation and stimulation of CTZ.

Preparation and Dosage

Ipecacuanha syrup—15 ml orally and may be repeated after 20 minutes if the individual fails to vomit.

Adverse Reactions

It is safer than apomorphine.

Contraindications of Emetics

Emetics should be avoided in children and elderly persons, pregnant women and patients with cardiac decompensation, hypertension, hernia, peptic ulcer and pulmonary tuberculosis.

Antiemetics

These are drugs that prevent or relieve vomiting due to various causes.

Classification

These are four groups:
1. Drugs acting on vomiting centre
   - Antimuscarinic drugs (M_1-receptor antagonists), e.g. scopolamine and dicyclomine.
   - Antihistaminics (H_1-receptor antagonists), e.g. promethazine, dimenhydrinate, cyclizine, and cinarizine.
2. Drugs acting on CTZ
   - D_2-receptor antagonists:

- Phenothiazines, e.g. chlorpromazine, perphenazine, prochlorperazine and triflupromazine.
- Butyrophenones, e.g. haloperidol and droperidol.
- Benzimidazole derivative domperidone.
- Substituted benzamides, e.g. metoclopramide and trimethobenzamide.
  - 5-HT_3 receptor antagonists—e.g. ondansetron, granisetron and dolasetron
3. Drugs acting peripherally (at GIT) (D_2-receptor antagonists/M_1-receptor agonists). Prokinetic agents, e.g. metoclopramide, domperidone, cisapride, itopride and mosapride.
4. Miscellaneous drugs
  - Corticosteroids, e.g. dexamethasone and methylprednisolone.
  - Cannabinoids, e.g. dronabinol and nabilone.
  - Benzodiazepines, e.g. lorazepam and alprazolam.

Of these drugs, those are effective in severe vomiting are metoclopramide and ondansetron or other 5-HT_3 antagonists; and those are effective in mild to moderate vomiting are domperidone, cisapride, chlorpromazine or other D_2 antagonists, corticosteroids and cannabinoids. Improved (increased) antiemetic effect can be produced by combination of antiemetics, e.g. 5-HT_3 antagonist + Corticosteroid/phenothiazine/butyrophenone. Substituted benzamide + Corticosteroid + M_1 or H_1 antagonist. Phenothiazine/ Butyrophenone + Corticosteroid. Cannabinoid + Corticosteroid. Corticosteroid + Benzodiazepine.

DISCUSSION OF INDIVIDUAL GROUP OF ANTIEMETICS

Antimuscarinic Drugs (M_1-antagonists)

Scopolamine (Hyoscine) is the most effective drug for the prevention of motion sickness. It acts by blocking the afferent impulses from the vestibular apparatus of internal ear to the vomiting centre (blocking cholinergic M_1-receptors). Its sedative effect also contributes to antiemetic action. It is suitable for short brisk journeys. It should be given 1 hour before journey, because if vomiting starts it becomes difficult to control. It is available as hyoscine hydrobromide tablet (0.2 mg), injection (0.2 mg/ml) and transdermal patch (1.5 mg of hyoscine to be delivered in 3 days and applied behind the pinna). It is injected SC or IM.

Adverse Reactions

It can produce sedation, drowsiness, dryness of mouth and blurring of vision.

Dicyclomine is another M_1-antagonist used for prevention of motion sickness and acts like scopolamine. It is administered orally as tablet in the dose of 10 to 20 mg. It can produce dryness of mouth and blurring of vision as side effects.

Antihistaminic Drugs (H_1-antagonists)

Promethazine, dimenhydrinate, cyclizine, and cinnarizine are antihistaminic drugs with prominent anticholinergic properties. They act by antimuscarinic action (blocking M_1-receptors) on vomiting centre as well as sedative action. They are used to prevent vomiting due to motion sickness and morning sickness. Promethazinetheoclate (Avomine) tablet (25 mg) is commonly used in the dose of 25 to 50 mg orally. It can also be used as syrup (25 mg/ml) or injection (25 mg/ml in 2 ml ampoule). Promethazine hydrochloride (Phenergan) is also available as tablet, syrup and injection in similar strengths. Dimenhydrinate (Dramamine) and cinnarizine (Vertigon) tablets are used in vertigo and Meniere's syndrome. These drugs can produce sedation and antimuscarinic side effects.

D_2-Receptor Antagonists

Some neuroleptic drugs (e.g. phenothiazines and butyrophenones) in relatively low doses can act as antiemetic by virtue of their capacity to antagonize the interaction of dopamine with D_2-receptors. Chlorpromazine is a potent and selective antiemetic drug useful in controlling vomiting associated with a variety of diseases, radiation and moderately emetogenic cancer chemotherapy. The antimuscarinic and antihistaminic effects of chlorpromazine and other phenothiazines also contribute to their antiemetic effects. Their antiemetic effects increase with dose, but produce many side effects like hypotension, sedation and extrapyramidal movement disorders, which limit their use as antiemetic. Prochlorperazine produces high incidence of muscular dystonias, especially when administered IM and should be used with caution. Butyrophenones also act as competitive antagonists of dopamine at D_2 receptors. They are useful antiemetics for patients receiving cancer chemotherapy. They are administered IM. They are moderately effective antiemetics. They cause less sedation and hypotension than phenothiazines.

Benzimidazole derivative domperidone has D_2-receptor antagonist activity, prokinetic activity and antiemetic action. Benzamide derivatives cisapride and mosapride have D_2-receptor antagonist activity and cholinomimetic (M_1-receptor agonist in GIT) activity.

Substituted Benzamides

Metoclopramide and trimethobenzamide are D_2-receptor antagonists and potent antiemetics. At higher concentrations, metoclopamide also blocks $5-HT_3$ receptors, which also contributes to its antiemetic effect. They also exert prokinetic effects on the intestine by increasing the action of Ach at muscarinic receptor (M_1) in the intestine (M_1-receptor agonist).

$5-HT_3$-Receptor Antagonists

Ondansetron is a potent $5-HT_3$-antagonist, can prevent vomiting due to high doses of the potent emitogencisplatin and that due to radiation. It is effective orally and has an oral bioavailability of about 60%. Its effective blood levels appear within 30 to 60 minutes of its administration. It is extensively metabolized by the liver and excreted in urine mainly as metabolites. It has a plasma half-life of 3 to 4 hours.

Preparations and Dosage

- Ondansetron hydrochloride (Emeset/Ondemn) tablet (4, 8 mg)—4 to 8 mg twice daily.

- Ondansetron hydrochloride injection (2 mg/ml in 2 ml ampoule)—4 to 8 mg by slow IV injection immediately prior to chemotherapy.

Adverse Reactions

It can cause headache, dizziness and constipation. It does not produce extrapyramidal effects.

Granisetron has similar properties of ondansetron. It is useful in preventing nausea and vomiting induced by cisplatin and other emetogenic cancer therapy. It is less potent than ondansetron. It is administered orally (as tablet) and parenterally (as IV injection). It can cause headache, somnolence, diarrhoea or constipation. Dolasetron is a new drug.

Corticosteroids

Dexamethasone and methyl prednisolone have antiemetic effect but the mechanism of antiemetic action is unknown. When administered IV (120 mg of dexamethasone or 150 mg of methylprednisolone), they are effective against moderately emetogenic chemotherapy. They also enhance the antiemetic effect of other antiemetics and can reduce the severity of their adverse effects. They may exacerbate hyperglycaemia in diabetic patients and should be used with caution in patients with a history of psychiatric illness, in whom psychiatric reactions may occur.

Cannabinoids

Tetrahydrocanabinol and its derivatives (Dronabinol and Nabilone) can reduce vomiting due to moderately emetogenic chemotherapy. They are used in patients refractory to or intolerant to other antiemetic drugs, but they can produce CNS adverse effects like dysphoria, hallucination, disorientation and vertigo. Prochlorperazine can reduce the incidence of dysphoria produced by them.

Benzodiazepines

Lorazepam, alprazolam and other benzodiazepines can produce antiemetic effects by virtue of their sedative, anxiolytic and amnesic properties. They can enhance antiemetic effect of corticosteroids.

Prokinetic Agents (*Pro* Meaning Front and *Kinesia* Meaning Movement)

These are gastric hurrying drugs that increase the motility of smooth muscle from the oesophagus to the proximal part of small intestine and accelerate gastric emptying and the transit of intestinal contents from the duodenum to the ileocaecal valve. They increase the tone of lower oesophageal sphincter (LES), relaxes upper part of stomach, increases contraction of pyloric antrum and increases persistalsis of proximal part of small intestine. They are used in gastrointestinal disorders manifested as nausea, vomiting, heart burn, postprandial discomfort, indigestion and gastroesophageal reflux due to gastric hypermotility with delayed emptying of gastric contents.

Metoclopramide (Reglan) is a D_2- and $5HT_3$-receptors antagonist and cholinomimetic (M_1-receptor agonist). It is rapidly and completely absorbed after oral administration but hepatic first pass metabolism reduces its bioavailability to 70%. It is distributed rapidly in most tissues and readily crosses BBB and placental barrier. It is metabolized in the liver and about 30% is excreted unchanged in urine. It is administered orally as tablet (10 mg) or syrup (10 mg/5 ml) in the dose of 10 mg twice daily. It is also available as injection (5 mg/ml in 2 ml ampoule) and administered IM once or twice daily.

Adverse Reactions

It can cause extrapyramidal side effects like Parkinsonism, anxiety, depression, sedation, drowsiness, diarrhoea and hyperprolactinemia (which can lead to galactorrhoea, breast tenderness and menstrual irregularities in women) especially in high doses. These symptoms can be prevented by administration of antihistaminic drugs like promethazine or diphenhydramine.

Domperidone (Domstal) is a D_2-receptor antagonist. As it does not cross BBB, so it does not produce central effects like parkinsonism and sedation.

However, it can reach the CTZ (which is outside the BBB) and exerts its D_2-receptor antagonist effects on CTZ. It is rapidly absorbed after oral administration but its oral bioavailabity is low (only 15%). Most of the drugs and their metabolites are excreted in faeces. It has uses like metoclopramide. It is available as tablet (10 mg) and suspension (1 mg/ml in 30 ml phial) and administered in doses of 10 to 20 mg 3 to 4 times daily.

Adverse Reactions

It is well-tolerated. It can cause headache, dry mouth, loose stool and skin rash.

Cisapride (Syspride) is a benzamide derivative. It has no D_2-receptor antagonist activity. It has cholinomimetic (M_1-receptor agonist activity) and $5-HT_3$-receptor antagonist activity. Its effects on the motility of the stomach and small intestine closely resemble those of metoclopramide and domperidone but unlike these drugs it also increases colonic motility and can cause diarrhoea and colicky pain in abdomen. Its GIT effects can be blocked by atropine. It is used in gastroesophageal reflux (GER) and chronic constipation. It is not an effective antiemetic. It does not produce extrapyramidal side effects (parkinsonism) and hyperprolactinemia. It is well-absorbed orally and has a bioavailability of about 40%. It is metabolized in the liver and excreted in urine. It is available as tablet (10 mg) for oral administration twice daily. Mosapride (Moza) is available as 2.5 mg tablet and administered twice daily. It is better tolerated than cisapride. If antifungal or macrolide antibiotics are taken concurrently with metoclopramide, dangerous cardiac arrhythmia can develop. Itopride (150 mg) is administered along with rabeprazole (20 mg) once daily as capsule (Aciflux).

25

Purgatives and Antidiarrhoeals

GENERAL CONSIDERATIONS

Drugs causing diarrhoea are purgatives, cholinergic drugs, adrenergic neuron blockers (reserpine, guanethidine, etc.), cisapride, quinidine, antimicrobials (sulphonamides, tetracyclines, chloramphenicol, ampicillin, amoxycillin, etc.), bile acids, fatty acids and autacoids (prostaglandins, 5-HT, substance P, vasoactive intestinal peptides, etc.).

Drugs causing constipation are antidiarrhoeals, anticholinergic drugs, antacids (containing, calcium carbonate or aluminium hydroxide), iron salts, heavy metals (especially lead), propranolol, clonidine, verapamil, lithium, octreotide, opioids, phenothiazines (anticholinergic effect), MAO inhibitors, antihistamines (anticholinergic effect), tricyclic antidepressants (anticholinergic effect), NSAIDs, corticosteroids, diuretics that cause hypokalemia, ganglionic blocking drugs, muscle relaxants, barium sulphate and polystyrene resins. Purgatives and antidiarrhoeals will be discussed here.

Purgatives (Laxatives)

These are drugs that promote defecation and used in constipation.

Classification

These are of three groups:

1. **Drugs causing softening of faeces** (act in 1 to 3 days). These are given as follows:

- Bulk forming laxatives, e.g. methylcellulose, sodium carboxymethylcellulose, gumkaraya, psyllium ispaghula (isapgol) preparation (husks), bran, agar and calcium polycarbophil.
- Surfactant laxatives, e.g. docusate and poloxamers.
- Emollient laxative, e.g. liquid paraffin.

2. **Drugs causing soft or semifluid stool** (act in 6 to 8 hours). These are stimulant laxatives:

   - Diphenyl methane derivatives, e.g. phenolphthalein and bisacodyl.
   - Anthraquinone derivatives, e.g. senna, cascara segrada and danthron.

3. **Drugs causing watery evacuations** (act in 1 to 3 hours). These are given as follows:

- Osmotic laxatives:

  - Saline laxatives, e.g. magnesium sulphate, magnesium hydroxide, magnesium citrate, sodium phosphate and sodium potassium tartrate.
  - Non-saline laxatives, e.g. lactulose, glycerine, sorbitol and mannitol.

- Fixed oil, e.g. castor oil.

Uses of Purgatives

- Bulk forming laxatives are used to supplement the nonpharmacological measures (fibre-rich diet, adequate fluid intake, appropriate physical activity, etc.) for the prevention and treatment of constipation. They are used before and after surgery to maintain soft faeces in patients with haemorrhoids or other anorectal disorders. They are also used in the management of diverticular disease of the colon and irritable bowel syndrome.

- Stimulant laxatives are used only in refractory cases of constipation.
- Osmotic (saline) laxatives in cathartic (high) doses are frequently used prior to radiological examination of GIT, kidneys or other abdominal or retroperitoneal structures and prior to elective bowel surgery. They are used after anthelmintic therapy. They have replaced enemas for emptying the large bowel prior to endoscopy or proctological examination. In the treatment of oral drug poisoning, they may be administered in cathartic doses to remove the poison from the intestine. Stimulant laxatives must be avoided in oral drug poisoning.
- Faecal softners and liquid paraffin are used in painful anal conditions like haemorrhoids (piles) and anal fissures.
- Lactulose is used in hepatic coma (encephalopathy due to liver failure) and in food or drug poisoning. Castor oil is now rarely used as purgative, though it is a safe purgative for all ages.

  In cases of drug induced constipation correlation by readjustment of drug doses or use of alternative drugs should be attempted before starting the use of a laxative. Valid uses of laxatives include maintenance of soft faeces, prevention of straining at the stool (especially in the elderly persons and in patients with cardiac disease or hernia) and evacuation of the bowel prior to diagnostic or surgical procedures.

Contraindications of Purgatives

These are given as follows:
- Inflammatory bowel diseases (peptic ulcer, ulcerative colitis, etc.).
- Patients with abdominal cramps, colic, nausea and vomiting.

- Undiagnosed acute abdominal pain (appendicitis, peritonitis, intestinal obstruction, etc.).
- Colonic atony and impacted rectal faecal mass.
- Bed ridden patients due to acute myocardial infarction (AMI), cerebral stroke, fractures of bones, etc.

Abuses of Purgatives

Purgatives should not be used for prolonged period because it is unhealthy due to following reasons:
- They may flare up the inflammatory intestinal conditions like appendicitis, diverticulitis, enteritis and colitis.
- They can produce fluid and electrolytes imbalance due to loss of excessive fluid and electrolytes (Na^+, K^+, Cl^-, etc.).
- They can produce nutritional deficiency of proteins, fats, vitamins, and minerals leading to steatorrhoea, malabsorption syndrome, protein losing enteropathy, hypocalcaemia, hypokalemia, osteomalacia, etc.
- They can produce nausea, vomiting, dyspepsia and spastic (cathartic) colon.

DISCUSSION OF INDIVIDUAL GROUP OF PURGATIVES

Bulk Forming Laxatives

These substances contain vegetable fibres and hydrophilic colloids including cellulose, hemicellulose, pectin, lignin, wax, resin and some glycoproteins. They are not digested by the intestinal enzymes. They bind with water and ions in the colonic lumen and cause softening of faeces and increase the bulk. This stresses the Auerbach's (myenteric) plexus and Meissner's plexus in enteric nervous system (ENS) leading to stimulation of peristalsis and evacuation of bowel. They are taken at night with sufficient water and produce evacuation of soft and formed stools within 1 to 3 days without producing irritation or griping.

Clinical Uses

They are used in habitual constipation, before and after surgery, painful anal conditions (piles and fissures), diverticulitis and irritable bowel syndrome.

Preparations and Dosage

- Isapgol husks (Isogel/Naturolax)—5 to 15 g mixed with sufficient amount of water taken at bed time.
- Methylcellulose/sodium carboxymethyl-cellulose granules—1 to 1.5 g mixed with sufficient amount of water 2 to 3 times daily.
- Gum karaya and cortex frangulae granules (kanormal)—1 to 1.5 g mixed with sufficient amount of water twice daily.

Adverse Reactions

They have few side effects. Flatulence and borborygmi occur occasionally. Allergic reactions may occur with the use of plant gums. Cellulose can bind and reduce the intestinal absorption of many drugs including digitalis glycosides, salicylates and nitrofurantoin. Psyllium may bind coumarin derivatives and bile acids, reducing their intestinal reabsorption and promoting their excretion. Intestinal obstruction and impaction may occur after their administration, especially in patients with pre-existing gastrointestinal disease. Patients with stenosis, ulceration or adhesion should avoid these agents. Oesophageal and intestinal obstruction can occur when these substances are taken without sufficient water.

Surfactant Laxatives

These are docusate and poloxamers. They act primarily as stool wetting and softening agents, allowing the mixing of water, lipids and other faecal materials. Docusate (Dioctyl sodium sulphosuccinate) is a typical stool softner. It acts by its physical property of lowering surface tension of water in the gut lumen and so water can easily enter the stool in the colon more freely leading to softening of stool. It does not stimulate intestinal peristalsis. Poloxamers, e.g. polyoxyethylene polymer and polyoxypropylene polymer are other agents acting like docusate. They have uses like bulk forming laxatives.

Preparations and Dosage

- Docusate sodium (Laxicon) tablet (100 mg) — 1 to 3 tablet at bed time.
- Docusate sodium (Laxicon) enema (0.25% soln, 50 ml)—The content of the container is squeezed into rectum.

Adverse Reactions

They can cause abdominal cramps and diarrhoea. They should not be used with liquid paraffin as they may increase the absorption of the later.

Emollient Laxative

Liquid paraffin: It is a mineral oil, which is neither digested nor absorbed. It acts as a laxative by causing lubrication of stool, softening the stool and increasing the bulk of intestinal content by reducing water absorption in the intestine. It takes 1 to 2 days to act. It produces soft and formed stool.

Clinical Uses

It has uses like bulk forming laxatives.

Preparation and Dosage

- Liquid paraffin—10 to 30 ml at bed time.

Adverse Reactions

It interferes with the absorption of fat-soluble vitamins (A, D, E and K). It can leak out of anal sphincter and cause discomfort. It may be refluxed into the oesophagus when the patient is sleeping and aspirated into lung producing lipoid pneumonia. Its chronic little absorption from intestine can cause paraffinoma in intestinal submucosa. For these reasons it should not be freely used.

Stimulant Laxatives

They promote accumulation of water and electrolytes in the intestinal lumen and stimulate intestinal motility (peristalsis). Concentration of these drugs that reduce net absorption of water and electrolytes also increase the permeability of the mucosa, possibly by making tight junctions leaky. They may inhibit intestinal Na^+, K^+-ATPase leading to laxative effect. Some of them also increase the synthesis of PCs and cAMP,which may contribute to increased secretion of water and electrolytes. Diphenyl methane derivatives are phenolphthalein and bisacodyl. They act primarily on the colon. They are also called contact laxatives. Their laxative effects usually are not produced in less than 6 hours after oral administration. They are taken at bed time to produce their effect in the next morning. They produce soft or semifluid stools.

Pharmacokinetics

About 15% of the therapeutic dose of phenolphthalein is absorbed and excreted in urine, mostly as conjugated form. The colour of urine becomes pink or red if the urine is alkaline. Some amount of the absorbed drug is excreted in bile. It undergoes enterohepatic recycling, which prolongs its duration of laxative effect. Bisacodyl is rapidly converted by intestinal and bacterial enzymes to its active desacetyl metabolite. Only 5% of the orally administered drug is absorbed and excreted in urine as glucuronide.

Clinical Uses

They are used prior to radiological exam-ination of GIT, kidneys or other abdominal or retroperitoneal structures and prior to endoscopy, colonoscopy or elective surgery of the gut. They are also used in refractory cases of constipation.

Preparations and Dosage

- Phenolphthalein (Modane) tablet (50 mg)—50 to 200 mg at bed time.
- Bisacodyl (Dulcolax) tablet (5 mg)—10 to 15 mg at bed time.

Adverse Reactions

They can produce fluid and electrolyte deficits by causing excessive laxative effect. They can damage enterocytes and can produce an inflammatory response in the colonic mucosa. In large doses they can produce abdominal cramps, griping and fluid stools. Phenol-pthalein can produce allergic reactions and pink colour of urine and faeces. Bisacodyl should not be taken within one hour of drinking milk or taking antacid preparation. To avoid gastric irritation, patients should swallow tablets without chewing or crushing.

Anthraquinone laxatives include dihydroxy-anthraquinone (Danthron) and its glycoside derivatives, which are contained in senna and cascara segrada. Senna is obtained from the dried leaflets or pods of *Cassia acutifolia* or *Cassia angustifolia*. Cascara segrada is obtained from the bark of the buck thorn tree *Rhamnus purshiana*. They act as laxatives by increasing colonic motility as a result of irritation of intestinal mucosa and enteric nervous system. Their laxative effects depend on their anthraquinone (Emodin) content and ease of liberation of the active constituents from their precursor glycosides by the colonic microflora. They must reach the colon to be activated. Their effects are limited mainly in the large intestine and occur 6 hours or more after oral administration.They are prodrugs. They are poorly absorbed from the small intestine. Removal of sugar (glucose or rhamnose) from them and reduction to anthol occur in the colon by the bacteria releasing the active constituents, which are absorbed to a moderate degree. The absorbed materials are excreted in the bile to the small intestine causing irritation of intestinal mucosa and enteric nervous system (ENS). They produce soft formed stools in 8 to 10 hours. They are also excreted to some extent in saliva, breast milk and urine.

Clinical Uses

They have uses like bulk purgatives.

Preparations and Dosage

- Senna tablet (0.5 g)—0.5 to 2 g at bed time.
- Senna liquid extract—2 to 5 ml at bed time.
- Cascara segrada tablet (0.3 g)—0.3 to 1 g at bed time.
- Cascara segrada liquid extract—2 to 3 ml at bed time.

Adverse Reactions

They can produce excessive purgation (leading to water and electrolyte loss) and colic or griping in large doses. Their chronic use leads to benign melanolic pigmentation of colonic mucosa.

Osmotic Laxatives

Saline laxatives are magnesium sulphate, magnesium hydroxide, magnesium citrate, sodium phosphate and sodium potassium tartrate. They are poorly and slowly absorbed from the intestine. They act as laxatives by their osmotic action on the intestinal luminal fluid. They retain water in the intestine due to increased intraluminal osmolarity. Saturated solutions of these salts have high osmotic pressure, which prevents absorption of water from the intestine and also draws water from the intestinal wall leading to increased volume of intestinal contents and stressing of pressor receptors in the intestinal wall causing increased motility (peristalsis) and evacuation of bowel. They also increase secretion of cholecytokinin in the duodenum, which stimulates intestinal fluid secretion and gut motility leading to prompt evacuation of bowel.

Clinical Uses

They are used prior to endoscopy, colonoscopy or radiological examination of the gut, after anthelmintic therapy and in food and drug poisoning.

Preparations and Dosage

- Saturated solution (s.s) of magnesium sulphate (30 g of magnesium sulphate containing 7 molecules of water of crystallization is mixed with 45 ml of water to produce 60 ml)—30 ml to be taken in the morning in empty stomach.
- Milk of magnesia (7 to 8.5% aqueous solution of magnesium hydroxide)—20 ml twice daily in empty stomach.

Adverse Reactions

They can produce dehydration and electrolyte imbalance. Magnesium salts can produce hypermagnesemia after systemic absorption in renal failure leading to toxicity. Sodium salts should not be used in patients of CCF or renal disease. Phosphate salts can cause hyperphosphataemia and a reduction in plasma Ca^{2+} level.

Non-saline laxatives are unabsorbed carbohydrates like lactulose, glycerine, sorbitol and mannitol. They are resistant to digestion in the small intestine. They are osmotic laxatives. Lactulose is commonly used and others are occasionally used.

Lactulose

It is a semisynthetic disaccharide and composed of galactose and lactose. It is not acted by the disaccharide splitting enzymes of the small intestine and so it enters large intestine, where it is broken down to lactose and galactose and then to lactate, acetate and formate by the colonic bacteria. These are only partially absorbed and so increase osmotic pressure of intestinal contents. Lactate can bind ammonia in the gut and decreases its absorption. Concomitant reduction in luminal pH also increases intestinal motility and secretion causing moderate accumulation of fluid in the gut. It causes passage of soft, formed stools in 1 to 3 days.

Clinical Uses

It is used as an osmotic lactative in the treatment of constipation and in hepatic encephalopathy (manifested as coma), where it decreases blood ammonia concentration (due to reduced production and increased utilization of ammonia by intestinal bacteria and increased faecal excretion of ammonia by binding with lactic acid in the gut).

Preparation and Dose

Lactulose (Livoluk) syrup (3.5 g/5 ml)—10 to 20 ml twice daily.

Adverse Reactions

It can cause flatulence, cramps, abdominal discomfort, nausea and vomiting. In high doses it can cause diarrhoea, loss of fluid and K^+, hypernatraemia and exacerbation of hepatic encephalopathy.

Glycerine, sorbitol and mannitol are administered rectally (as suppository or concentrated solution) to produce laxative effect by osmotic action. They soften and lubricate the dried up stool and stimulate rectal contractions leading to evacuation of bowel.

Fixed Oil

Castor oil: It is obtained from the castor seeds (*Ricinous communis* Linn). It is a triglyceride of ricinoleic acid, an unsaturated hydroxy fatty acid. It is a bland (non-irritant) oil having emollient property on the skin and mucous membrane. It may be used as a soothing drops after removal of foreign body from the eye. When administered orally it is acted upon by the pancreatic lipase (bile salts activate it) in the intestine and hydrolyzed into ricinoleic acid, isoricinoleic acid and glycerol. These acids are converted into sodium ricinolate and sodium isoricinolate by the alkaline intestinal juice and irritate the intestinal mucosa and enteric nervous system (ENS). This increases intestinal motility (peristalsis) leading to evacuation of bowel. It also reduces absorption of water and electrolytes from the intestine and increases intestinal secretion. It takes 2 to 3 hours to act and produces few copious fluid stools. It is a safe purgative for all ages as the amount of lipase to hydrolyze it is limited.

Clinical Uses

It can be used in habitual constipation.

Preparations and Dosage

- Castor oil—5 to 10 ml in the morning in empty stomach.
- Castor oil emulsion—30 ml in the morning in empty stomach.

Adverse Reactions

It can cause griping, pelvic congestion, dehydration (due to excessive fluid loss) and after constipation (due to complete evacuation of bowel). It can stimulate uterine contraction in pregnant women. Its chronic use can produce nutritional deficiency by interfering with the absorption of various nutrients in the intestine.

Antidiarrhoeal Agents

These are drugs used in the treatment of diarrhoea. A knowledge of the types of diarrhoea can help the physician to know when to use specific antidiarrhoeals and when to use non-specific antidiarrhoeals. In diarrhoea there is frequent passing of profuse liquid stools with or without mucus or blood. Diarrhoea may be infectious diarrhoea or non-infectious diarrhoea. Non-infectious diarrhoea are inflammatory diarrhoea, osmotic diarrhoea, malabsorption diarrhoea and secretory diarrhoea. Treatment of infectious diarrhoea is done by the use of specific antimicrobials, e.g. ampicillin, amoxycillin, tetracyclines, chloramphenicol, metronidazole, tinidazole, cotrimoxazole, quinolones, aminoglycosides, etc.

Treatment of non-infectious diarrhoea is done according to cause. Diarrhoea due to chronic inflammatory bowel diseases (ulcerative colitis and Crohn's disease) is treated by anti-inflammatory drugs, e.g. sulphasalazine, mesalazine, prednisolone, betamethasone, etc.

Osmotic diarrhoea due to high osmotic tension of gut contents as in lactose indigestion (which is poorly absorbable and osmotically active) is treated initially by avoiding the offending osmotic agent, e.g. lactose in lactose intolerance and then administering the appropriate enzyme, e.g. lactase in lactose intolerence. Malabsorption diarrhoea as in malabsorption syndrome is treated by correcting the underlying malabsorption process, e.g. pancreatic enzymes for pancreatic insufficiency or gluten-free diet for gluten-sensitive enteropathy. Secretory diarrhoea as in cholera, *E. coli* diarrhoea, carcinoid syndrome, vasoactive intestinal peptide (VIP) secreting tumour or AID related diarrhoea is treated by somatostatin analog (octreotide).

The excessive faecal loss of fluid and electrolytes that characterizes diarrhoea is an important aspect of many infectious and noninfectious diarrhoea and requires administration of fluid and electrolytes for correction of dehydration. For this oral rehydration therapy (ORT) or parenteral (IV) fluid therapy is done according to severity of diarrhoea.

Acute onset of diarrhoea is most often of infectious origin and requires specific chemotherapy (as mentioned before). Chronic onset of diarrhoea is mostly noninfectious and treated by nonspecific antidiarrhoeals.

Classification of Nonspecific Antidiarrhoeals

These are of five groups:

1. Opioids, e.g. diphenoxylate, difenoxin and loperamide.
2. Bismuth compounds, e.g. bismuth subcarbonate and bismuth subsalicylate.
3. Adsorbents, e.g. kaolin, pectin, chalk and activated charcoal.
4. Absorbents, e.g. psyllium, polycarbophil and carboxymethylcellulose.
5. Other agents, e.g. octreotide, lactobacilli, berberine, donidine and muscarinic antagonists (atropine, scopolamine, etc.).

DISCUSSION OF INDIVIDUAL GROUP OF DRUGS

Opioids

Opioid agonists can affect GIT function by both central and peripheral sites of action. Although codeine and aqueous alcoholic solution of opium powder (tincture of opium/paregoric) have been used for many years to treat diarrhoea but the synthetic opioids (e.g. diphenoxylate, difenoxin and loperamide) are now preferred because they penetrate poorly into the CNS and can produce antidiarrhoeal effects at doses that produce a few central effects. Opioid agonists act at μ and δ receptors in the GIT to reduce both motility and secretion. Activation of both receptors may lead to increased absorption of sodium chloride and water. Some of their effects occur

via receptors on enteric neurons and by direct effects on intestinal epithelial cells and smooth muscle cells. Thus opioid agonists produce intestinal transit (permitting more time for absorption), reduce intestinal secretion and stimulate intestinal absorption. The net effect is a reduction in the quantity of fluid presented to the large intestine from the small intestine.

Clinical Uses

They are used in moderate to severe diarrhoea. They should not used in patients with chronic ulcerative colitis or acute bacillary or amoebic dysentery as they potentiate ulcerating process in the colon and can produce toxic megacolon. Diphenoxylate is a piperidine opioid that is structurally related to meperidine. It can produce systemic effects when used in doses greater than those required for treatment of diarrhoea. Dipenoxin (Motofen) is related to diphenoxylate and has similar action. Loperamide is another piperidine opioid which acts predominently on μ receptors in the GIT. It is 40 to 50 times more potent than morphine as an antidiarrhoeal agent. For controlling diarrhoea it is superior to other opioids. It does not require concurrent administration of atropine. It is very useful in traveller's diarrhoea, when combined with antimicrobial drugs like cotrimoxazole or a fluroquinolone.

Preparations and Dosage

• Diphenoxylate hydrochloride (2.5 mg) with atropine sulphate (2.5 μg) (Lomotil) tablet—1 to 2 tablets every 4 to 6 hours.
• Loperamide hydrochloride (Lopamide, Imodium) tablet (2 mg)—2 to 4 mg thrice daily.

Adverse Reactions

They have some adverse effects like morphine and codeine. With excessive use or overdose, they can produce exaggerated GIT effects including constipation and development of toxic megacolon. In higher doses, they can cause CNS and anticholinergic effects (drowsiness, dryness of mouth and abdominal discomfort).

Bismuth Compounds

Bismuth subcarbonate or bimuth subsalicylate has an astringent, protective and adsorbent effect. It binds with bacterial toxins (produced by *V. cholerae* and *E. coli*) and prevents their action and absorption. Salicylic acid liberated from bismuth subsalicylate inhibits the synthesis of prostaglandins and thus prevents intestinal inflammation and hypermotility. It may also exert an antisecretory action and stimulates absorption of fluid and electrolytes by the intestinal mucosa.

Clinical Uses

Bismuth salts are used in the treatment of mild to moderate traveller's (infectious) diarrhoea.

Preparations and Dosage

- Bismuth subcarbonate suspension—0.6 g (in 30 ml) 3 to 4 times daily.
- Bismuth subsalicylate tablet (520 mg) or suspension (520 mg/30 ml)—520 mg 6 hourly.

Adverse Reactions

They are water-insoluble and nonabsorbable salts. They produce little adverse effects on oral administration. They are expensive.

Adsorbents

Kaolin, pectin, prepared chalk (a native form of calcium carbonate) and activated wood charcoal were previously used as adsorbents and protective agents (form protective coating over the intestinal mucosa) in the treatment of diarrhoea, but they have little or no value in the treatment of acute infectious diarrhoea and so they are now less used.

Absorbents

Fibre supplements (e.g. psyllium, polycarbophil and carboxymethyl cellulose) used in constipation can increase the viscosity of faeces in diarrhoea but these are not useful in the treatment of acute diarrhoea and so less used.

Other Agents

Octreotide is a stable analog of somatostatin. It can suppress secretory effects of many gastrointestinal hormones. It is useful in the parenteral treatment of diarrhoea of myriad origin including diarrhoea of carcinoid syndrome and high output diarrhoea (as in *Cholera* or *E. coli* infection), which is refractory to other drug therapy. It is also used in acromegaly.

Lactobacilli *(Lactobacillus acidophillus)* preparation is available as oral tablets and is used in the treatment of certain chronic diarrhoeas to promote the growth of saccharolytic intestinal flora and alter the intestinal pH, so that the growth of pathogenic bacteria in the intestine is inhibited. Curd or buttermilk is the cheaper substitute for such tablets.

Berberine is an alkaloid obtained from the plant *Berberis aristata*. It is effective in the treatment of certain bacterial diarrhoeas (e.g. *Cholera* and *E. coli* due to liberation of toxins). It reduces inflammation and acts as an antagonist, of intestinal hormone motilin. It is administered orally in the dose of 150 mg thrice daily. Clonidine is a synthetic α_2-adrenergic agonist. It can reduce intestinal smooth muscle tone and secretory activity. It is useful in the treatment of diabetic diarrhoea. Muscarinic antagonists (e.g. atropine, propantheline and hyoscine butyl bromide) can be used in diarrhoea associated with intestinal colics/cramps. They are antimotility and antisecretory drugs.

Oral Rehydration Therapy (ORT)

The major risk of diarrhoea is dehydration. It can be prevented or treated by providing readily absorbed sugars and amino acids, that increase the absorption of water and electrolytes by the small intestine. Oral rehydration solution (ORS) containing sodium chloride (3.5 g), potassium chloride (1.5 g), trisodium citrate dehydrated (2.9 g) or sodium bicarbonate (2.5 g), glucose (20 g) and water (1 litre) is useful in mild to moderate acute diarrhoea due to various cases but IV fluid therapy containing water, electrolytes and glucose (e.g. 5% dextrose saline, molar lactate solution etc.) is required in severe diarrhoea, especially in patients who are unable to take fluids by mouth (due to vomiting). Patients with severe dehydration can be treated with ORS containing glucose, once the initial hypovolaemia is corrected by 2–4 litres of intravenous fluid replacement. Moderate dehydration and acidosis can be corrected in 3 to 6 hours by repeated administration of ORS alone. Glucose helps in absorption of sodium and water in the small intestine. Amino acids like glycine and alanine can also be added to increase absorption of sodium and water. ORS is less expensive than IV fluids and can be easily prepared with the components on the spot.

26

Miscellaneous Drugs

Carminatives

These are drugs which help expulsion of gas from stomach (by eructation) and colon (as flatus), e.g. sodium bicarbonate (1 to 1.5 g) aromatic spirit of ammonia (1 to 2 ml), compound cardamom tincture (1 to 2 ml), ginger tincture (1 to 2 ml), oil of peppermint or dil (0.1 to 0.2 ml) and dimethyl polysiloxane/dimethicon (50 to 100 mg). Carminative mixture contains sodium bicarbonate (1 g), compound cardamom tincture (2 ml), aromatic spirit of ammonia (1 ml) and water (added up to 30 ml). Compound cardamom tincture contains cardamom oil, cinnamon oil, caraway oil, cochineal/amaranath, glycerine, alcohol and water. Aromatic spirit of ammonia contains ammonium bicarbonate, strong solution of ammonia, lemon oil, nutmeg oil, alcohol and water.

Mode of Action

Sodium bicarbonate reacts with gastric HCl and evolves CO_2, which distends stomach and relaxes lower esophageal sphincter (LES) and pyloric sphincter. Aromatic compounds contain volatile oils, which cause mild irritation of stomach and intestine, relax LES and pyloric sphincter and increase gastrointestinal motility. Dimethyl polysiloxone (DMPS) is a silicon polymer. It is usually used in combination with antacids. It lowers surface tension of the fluid and collapses bubbles in the froth. Thus it acts as a defoaming agent. It

is not absorbed from GIT. It is pharmacologically inert. It relieves flatulence; coats and protects ulcer surface and prevents gastroesophageal reflux. It is a modern carminative.

Digestants

These are drugs which help in digestion of food, e.g. dilute HCl (10%) and digestive enzymes like pepsin, papain, diastase, pancreatin and pancrelipase.

Dilute HCl (10%) is used in hypochlorhydria or achlorhydria produced in pernicious anaemia, atrophic gastritis or gastric carcinoma. It is administered orally in the dose of 5 to 10 ml diluted with 100 to 200 ml of water and sipped with straw (to prevent corrosion of teeth) during meals.

Pepsin is a proteolytic enzyme obtained from glandular layer of fresh stomach of pig or ox. It helps in protein digestion when used in the dose of 50 to 100 mg (1 or 2 tablets) twice daily after meals.

Papain is a proteolytic enzyme obtained from the juice of carica papaya. It helps in protein digestion when used in the dose of 50 to 100 mg (1 or 2 tablets) twice daily after meals. Diastase is an amylolytic enzyme obtained from the fungus *Aspergillus oryzae* grown in wheat bran or from malt. Fungal diastase is more potent than malt diastase. It helps in carbohydrate digestion in the dose of 150 to 500 mg (as tablets) twice daily after meals. Pancreatic enzymes are pancreatin and pancrelipase. They contain amylase, proteases and lipase. Pancreatin is obtained from the pancreas of pig or ox and pancrelipase is obtained from the pancreas of pig. Pancrelipase has relatively more lipase activity than does pancreatin. They are used in the treatment of conditions in which secretion of pancreatic juice is deficient as in chronic pancreatitis and pancreatic insufficiency. Relatively large quantities of enzymes are required due to inactivation by gastric acid and pepsin. Enteric coated tablets provide better effects and used in doses of 100 to 200 mg twice daily after meals. They reduce faecal fat and nitrogen content.

In large doses they can cause nausea, headache, diarrhoea and hyperuricaemia.

Appetizers (Appetite Stimulants)

These are drugs which improve appetite in anorexia, produced in debilitating illness and in anorexia nervosa, e.g. bitters, cyproheptadine dilute alcohol, vitamin B_{12} and anabolic steroids. Bitters like chirata, gentian, kalmegh and neem are used as tincture, liquid extract or capsule in empty stomach. They increase gastric secretion reflexly and improve appetite. Cyproheptadine stimulates appetite by blocking the 5-HT dependent lateral hypothalamic satiety centre. It is used as tablet (4 mg) or syrup (2 mg/5 ml) in the dose of 2 to 4 mg twice daily before meals. It can produce drowsiness, dryness of mouth and mental confusion. Dilute alcohol (7 to 12%) stimulates appetite by increasing gastric secretion reflexly (by stimulation of taste buds) and also directly (by stimulation of gastric glands). It is taken before meals in the dose of 15 to 30 ml. It is a constituent of various tonics. In high concentrations it can cause gastritis and anorexia. Other drugs like vitamin B_{12} and anabolic steroids also improve appetite by unknown mechanism. Insulin and sulphonylureas induce hunger by causing hypoglycaemia.

Hepatoprotective Agents

These are drugs which protect the liver cells in hepatotoxicity or jaundice produced by drugs or hepatitis viruses, e.g. tricholine citrate, sorbitol, methionine, choline, sodium phosphate, sodium benzoate, and bile salts. These are available as tablets and syrups and used in doses of 2 tablets/2 teaspoonful twice daily before meals.

Choleretics

These are drugs which increase bile secretion by stimulating liver cells, e.g. bile acids and salts. These are used in hepatic insufficiency, fatty infiltration of liver and chronic hepatitis.

Bile Acids and Salts

Normally about 1000 ml of bile is secreted by the liver cells per day. Cholecystokinin (a polypeptide hormone) secreted by the duodenal mucosa is the main chemical stimulant for biliary secretion but it is not available for therapeutic use. Bile acids and their salts are essential components of bile. They increase the flow as well as the concentration of bile. They also facilitate the dispersion and absorption of lipids and fat-soluble vitamins. Bile acids are water-soluble products of cholesterol metabolism. They solubilize cholesterol in bile and promote intestinal cholesterol excretion. The primary bile acids are cholic acid and chenodeoxycholic acid. Bacterial metabolism of these primary bile acids in the colon forms secondary bile acids like deoxycholic acid, lithocholic acid and ursodeoxycholic acid. These secondary bile acids are absorbed in the colon and cycle with primary bile acids. Bile acids exist largely as glycine and taurine conjugates, the salts of which are called bile salts (glycocholate and taurocholate). Once secreted, bile acids are largely reabsorbed in the ileum and recycled *via* enterohepatic cycle. Small amounts of bile acids are excreted in faeces. Excess bile acids by reaching colon can reduce net water absorption and cause diarrhoea. Normal functioning of GIT depends on the appropriate synthesis and enterohepatic circulation of bile acids.

Clinical Uses

Chenodeoxycholic acid (Chenodiol) and ursodeoxycholic acid (Ursodiol) are used for gallstones dissolution and for preventing their recurrence. They reduce biliary cholesterol concentration by depressing hepatic cholesterol synthesis and secretion. Chenodeoxycholic acid increases the secretion of bile acids in some patients but ursodeoxycholic acid does not increase the secretion of bile acids into bile. They dissolve radiolucent (cholesterol) gallstones but cannot dissolve radioopaque (bilirubin or calcium salt) gallstones. They produce poor responses in the presence of a nonfunctioning gallbladder, in very obese persons and in persons with high dietary cholesterol intake.

Preparations and Dosage

- Chenodeoxycholic acid (Chenofalk) capsule (0.5g)—14 to 16mg/kg/day (0.5 g thrice daily).

- Ursodeoxycholic acid (Udca) tablet (150 mg)—8 to 10 mg/kg/day (300 mg thrice daily).

The treatment is continued for 3 to 24 months, depending on the size of the stone. Complete dissolution may be obtained only in 10–15% of patients.

Adverse Reactions

Chenodeoxycholic acid can produce diarrhoea, increase in plasma transaminase activity and increase in low density lipoprotein fraction of cholesterol. Ursodeoxycholic acid causes less frequent diarrhoea and does not alter serum cholesterol and plasma transaminase activities.

Cholagogues

These are drugs which cause evacuation of gallbladder by causing its contraction, e.g. magnesium sulphate (33% solution) and olive oil.

Section VI

HAEMATOLOGIC PHARMACOLOGY

27

Haematinics and Haematopoietic Growth Factors

Haematinics are drugs that help in formation and maturation of red blood cells (RBCs) and used in the prevention and treatment of anaemias.

Classification

These are of two groups:

1. Essential haematinics, e.g. iron salts, vitamin B_{12} and folic acid.
2. Accessory haematinics, e.g. vitamin C, pyridoxine, riboflavin, copper, manganese, cobalt, erythropoietin and thyroxine. Haematopoietic growth factors help in haematopoiesis, which is a process of formation of mature blood cells in the bone marrow and other sites. The short lifespan of mature blood cells requires their continuous replacement by haematopoiesis. Red blood cell production can be more than 5 folds in response to anaemia or hypoxia. White blood cell production increases dramatically in response to systemic infection. Platelet production can increase several folds when the platelet destruction results in thrombocytopenia. The regulation of haematopoiesis is complex and involves cell to cell interaction in the bone marrow and haematopoietic growth factors like erythropoietin, myeloid growth factors and thrombopoietin. It also requires adequate supplies of minerals like iron, copper, manganese, cobalt and vitamins like vitamin B_{12}, folic acid, pyridoxine, vitamin C and riboflavin. Deficiency of these minerals and vitamins results in characteristic anaemias and a general failure of haematopoiesis.

HAEMATOPOIETIC GROWTH FACTORS

These are given as follows:

Erythropoietin

It is a glycoprotein produced primarily by the peritubular cells in the renal cortex. It is also synthesized in the liver to a small extent. Renal synthesis and secretion of erythropoietin is increased to about 100 folds in anaemia or hypoxemia. It is essential for normal erythropoiesis. In the absence of erythropoietin severe anaemia may occur. Erythropoietin acts by binding with a specific receptor on the surface of erythroid precursor cells.

Clinical Uses

Erythropoietin is highly effective in the treatment of a number of anaemias, especially those associated with a poor erythropoietic response. It is used in the treatment of patients with anaemia of chronic renal origin.

Preparation and Dosage

Recombinant human erythropoietin injection 200 to 400 units given IV or SC three times a week for 3 to 4 months.

Adverse Reactions

It can produce local skin reactions and arthralgia but no allergic reactions.

Myeloid Growth Factors

These are glycoproteins that stimulate the proliferation and differentiation of one more myeloid cell lines. They also enhance the function of granulocytes and monocytes. They are produced naturally by fibroblasts, endothelial cells, macrophages and T-cells. They are active in very low concentrations, e.g. granulocyte-colony stimulating factor (G-CSF). It stimulates the proliferation, differentiation and function of the granulocyte linkage. Granulocyte/macrophage-colony stimulating factor (GM-CSF). It stimulates the proliferation, differentiation and function of a number of the myeloid cell lines.

Clinical Uses

G-CSF (Filgrastim) is effective in the treatment of severe neutropenia following autogenous bone marrow transplantation and high dose myelosuppressive chemotherapy and severe congenital neutropenias. It is also effective in neutropenia of AIDS patients receiving zidovudine, GM-CSF (Molgrastim) is under clinical trial. It has similar uses of G-CSF.

Preparation and Dosage

Recombinant human G-CSF (Filgrastim/ Neupogen) injection—5 to 20 µg/kg/day by SC or rapid IV infusion till recovery.

Adverse Reactions

It can cause bone pain, local skin reactions and rarely a cutaneous necrotizing vasculitis.

Thrombopoietin

It is a glycoprotein that selectively stimulates megakaryocytopoiesis.

Clinical Uses

It can be used in severe thrombocytopenia to increase rapidly the platelet count and to reduce multiple platelet transfusions.

Preparation

Recombinant human thrombopoietin (a cytokine) is under clinical trial. It can be combined with erythropoietin and G-CSF to correct anaemia, neutropenia and thrombocytopenia, associated with high dose chemotherapy.

DRUGS USED IN IRON DEFICIENCY (MICROCYTIC HYPOCHROMIC) ANAEMIA

These are iron salts, vitamin C, copper, manganese, pyridoxine and riboflavin.

Iron and Iron Salts

Iron is vital for life. It is an important inorganic constituent present in every cells of the body. In an adult man about 3.5 g of iron is present in the body. It is more in male (50 mg/kg) than in female (38 mg/kg). It is present in the body as iron containing compounds, e.g. haemoglobin (66%) and myoglobin (3%), iron stores, e.g. ferritin and haemosiderin (25%) and parenchymal iron (6%) in haeme enzymes (cytochromes, catalase and peroxidase) and metaloflavoprotein enzymes (xanthine oxidase and mitochondrial enzyme α-glycerophosphate oxidase). Iron is essential for haemoglobin synthesis. Haemoglobin is made of haeme (a protoporphyrin) and globin (a protein) and present in red blood corpuscles (RBS). Each molecule of haemoglobin contains 4 iron containing haeme residues having 0.33% iron. Myoglobulin is the haemeprotein present in muscles. The prominent site of storage of iron (ferritin and haemosiderin) are reticuloendothelial cells (in liver, spleen and bone marrow), hepatocytes and muscle cells. In circulation, iron binds to its transport protein transferrin (a β-glycoprotein).

Transferrin bound iron through its cell surface receptor is utilized by erythron for haemoglobin synthesis. In the erythroblast iron is incorporated into protoporphyrin for haemoglobin synthesis.

Iron Deficiency

Iron deficiency anaemia results from an inadequate dietary intake of iron to meet normal requirements (nutritional iron deficiency), blood loss either from GIT or uterus (in female) or some interference in iron absorption as in partial gastrectomy or malabsorption in the small intestine. When severe, it results in a characteristic microcytic hypochromic anaemia. Clinically, it is manifested as weakness, tiredness, breathlessness, dizziness, headache, insomnia, dyspepsia, atrophy of skin, glossitis, brittle nails and koilonychia (spoon nail). Iron deficiency can affect metabolism in muscle independent of the effect of anaemia or oxygen delivery. It may well reflect a reduction in the activity of iron dependent mitochondrial enzymes. Iron deficiency can produce behavioural and learning problems in children. So early detection of iron deficiency and its prevention must be done.

Dietary Sources of Iron

Rich sources of iron are liver, egg yolk, oyster, pulses, beans, fruits and yeast. Medium sources are meat, chicken, fish, spinach, banana and apple. Poor sources are milk and its products and root vegetables.

Daily Requirement of Iron

- Adult male—0.5 to 1 mg.
- Adult female—1 to 2 mg (to compensate menstrual loss).
- Pregnant woman—3 to 5 mg (for foetal demand).
- Children—30 μg/kg.
- Infants—60 μg/kg.

Absorption, Distribution, Storage and Excretion of Iron (Pharmacokinetics)

Iron is normally ingested in the form of food. Iron from animal foods is generally better absorbed than that from vegetable foods. Haeme iron is present in animal foods and absorbed better than nonhaeme iron present in vegetable foods. It is directly absorbed into the intestinal mucosa. Inorganic iron remains mostly in the ferric form and is absorbed by active transport process. It needs to be reduced to ferrous form before absorption can take place (as shown in **Fig. 27.1**). Absorption of iron can occur from any part of gastrointestinal tract but maximum iron absorption occurs in the duodenum (in an acidic pH).

Factors Influencing Iron Absorption

Gastric HCl and reducing substances like vitamin C and amino acids containing SH group (present in meat and fats) increase iron absorption by reducing ferric iron to ferrous iron. On the other hand, antacids, phosphates, phytates (present in maize and wheat) and tetracyclines (by complexing with iron) decrease iron absorption. When body iron reserves are increased, then iron absorption is decreased and vice versa.

Mechanism of Iron Absorption

Iron present in normal diet is absorbed by active transport process involving carrier protein (enzyme) and expenditure of energy (ATP). Iron combines with the protein apoferritin in the villous epithelial cells to form ferritin. The absorption of iron is controlled

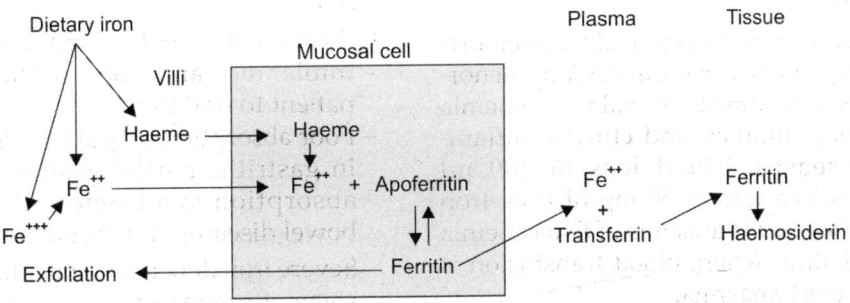

Fig. 27.1: Iron absorption, transport, storage and excretion

by the availability of apoferritin in the mucosal cells. If it is fully saturated to ferritin, then no more iron is absorbed (mucosal block theory). Thus, the body is protected from excessive absorption of iron. However, the low serum iron and the anoxemia due to anaemia can increase the breakdown of ferritin and make more apoferritin available for increasing absorption of iron. At the vascular surface of the mucosal cells, the iron of ferritin is reduced to ferrous iron and apoferritin is released. Ferrous iron then binds with the plasma carrier protein transferrin and is transferred to iron stores in tissues like liver, spleen and bone marrow to remain as ferritin and haemo-siderin (aggregated ferritin). Apoferritin released from ferritin in the mucosal cells then acts as a transporter of more iron. Passive diffusion of iron in combination with amino acids such as glycine and serine can occur when the dosage of iron exceeds those in a normal diet. The body iron is regulated mostly by regulation of iron absorption by the GIT. The total daily iron excretion is only 0.5 to 1 mg (more during menstruation). The channels of iron excretion are—faeces with exfoliation of villous cells, bile, sweat, urine, desqua-mation of skin and hair, menstrual bleeding and milk (during lactation).

Uses of Iron

Iron salts are used for prevention and treatment of iron deficiency anaemia.

Prophylactic uses: In pregnancy, infancy, childhood, menstruating women, chronic illness, gastrointestinal abnormalities pro-fessional blood donors and after partial gastrectomy.

Therapeutic uses: In peptic ulcer, haemorr-hoids (piles), hookworm infestation, menor-rhagia, repeated attacks of malaria, anaemia of pregnancy/infancy and chronic inflam-matory diseases. Blood loss of 100 ml corresponds to a loss of 50 mg of iron. Iron should not be used in anaemia of thalassaemia and renal failure where blood transfusion is given to correct anaemia.

Preparations and Dosage of Iron

- Oral preparations (contain 30 to 33% elemental iron) except ferrous gluconate (contains 12% only), e.g.
  - Dried ferrous sulphate (Fersolate) tablet (200 mg)—600 mg/day.
  - Ferrous sulphate syrup (60 mg/5 ml)— 300 mg/day.
  - Ferrous gluconate (Fergon) tablet (300 mg)—900 mg/day.
  - Ferrous fumerate (Autrin) capsule (200 mg)—600 mg/day.
  - Ferrous succinate (Hematrin) capsule (200 mg)—400 mg/day.
  - Ferric ammonium citrate mixture (2 g/ 30 ml)—6 g/day (a scale preparation of iron, soluble in water).

Various other iron preparations such as ferroglycine sulphate, ferric choline citrate, ferrous calcium citrate, ferric hydroxide, ferric hydroxypolymaltose, ferric aminoate and ferric glycerophosphate are also available for oral use, but they do not offer remarkable advantages over the preparations described before.

They may be better absorbed but more costly.

- Parenteral preparations (contain 50 mg of elemental iron/ml), e.g.
  - Iron-dextran (Imferon) injection (2 ml ampoule)—2 ml IM daily. It can be given IV as infusion.
  - Iron-sorbitol citric acid complex (Jectofer) injection (1.5 ml ampoule)— 1.5 ml IM daily.
  - Iron-carbohydrate complex (Uniferon) injection (2 ml ampoule) (contains iron, dextran, sorbitol and citric acid)—2 ml IM daily.

Indication of parenteral iron therapy:

- Intolerance and noncompliance of the patient to oral iron,
- Poor absorption of oral iron from GIT as in gastritis, partial gastrectomy, mal-absorption syndrome, inflammatory bowel diseases and rheumatoid arthritis.
- Severe iron deficiency anaemia in the late stage of pregnancy.

– Severe iron deficiency anaemia due to chronic blood loss as in pepticular piles, menorrhagia and hookwarm infestation.

– Severe iron deficiency anaemia in the late stage of pregnancy.

– Along with erythropoietin in severe iron deficiency anaemia.

Calculation of total dose of iron for parenteral therapy: The following formula is used:

Total dose of iron (mg) =

4.4 × body weight (kg) × haemoglobin deficit (g/dl).

The average oral dose of iron for the treatment of iron deficiency anaemia is about 200 mg of iron/day (2 to 3 mg/kg) given in 2 equal doses of 60 mg. Children weighing 15 to 30 kg can take half the average adult dose, while small children and infants can tolerate relatively large doses of iron, e.g. 5 mg/kg.

Orally administered ferrous sulphate, the least expensive of iron preparations is the treatment of choice for iron deficiency anaemia. Ferrous salts are absorbed about three times more than the ferric salts. Variations in the particular ferrous salt have relatively little effect on bioavailability and the sulphate, fumarate, succinate, gluconate and other ferrous salts are absorbed approximately to the same extent.

Adverse Reactions of Iron

Oral preparations of iron can produce intolerance. Heart burn, nausea, epigastric discomfort or pain, constipation or diarrhoea are common side effects. Constipation and diarrhoea are due to iron induced changes in the intestinal bacterial flow. Blackening of teeth and faeces due to formation of iron sulphide can also occur. Parenteral preparations of iron can cause pain at the site of injection, pigmentation of skin, sterile abscess, fever, headache, chest pain, dyspnoea, joint pain, flushing, tachycardia, vomiting, lymphadenopathy and allergic reactions.

Acute toxicity (poisoning) occurs mostly in children due to ingestion of large amounts of iron tablets, confusing them with candy. The fatal doses of iron range from 2 to 10 g. The signs and symptoms of severe poisoning may occur within 30 minutes or may be delayed for several hours after ingestion. They consist of abdominal pain, vomiting, diarrhoea, pallor or cyanosis, lassitude, drowsiness, hyperventilation (due to acidosis) and cardiovascular collapse. Death may occur in 12 to 24 hours. The corrosive injury in the stomach may result in pyloric stenosis or gastric scarring. Haemorrhagic gastroenteritis and hepatic damage are prominent findings in autopsy.

Treatment

• Gastric lavage with sodium bicarbonate or sodium phosphate solution is done to render iron insoluble and to remove it by stomach tube.

• Administration of milk or egg yolk orally is done to form insoluble iron complex.

• Administration of iron chelating agent desferrioxamine mesylate (Desferol) orally 5 to 10 g 100 ml of normal and parenterally (1 to 2 g IM or slow IV infusion 6 hourly) in 5 to 10 ml normal saline after gastric lavage is done, to remove iron from the body by forming stable, water-soluble and poorly absorbable chelate complex with iron. Conventional supportive measures to combat shock, dehydration and acid–base imbalance are taken. Dimercaprol (BAL) is not used in iron poisoning, because it forms toxic complex with iron. With the early effective treatment, the motility from iron poisoning can be greatly reduced.

Chronic toxicity (poisoning) can occur due to long continued administration of iron producing iron overload (hemochromatosis) especially in individuals with underlying genetic disorders causing excessive absorption of iron. Desferrioxamine is useful in the prevention and treatment of haemochromatosis 10 to 15 mg/kg is administered by continuous IV infusion. Adjuvant drugs used in iron deficiency anaemia are vitamin C (increases iron absorption), copper and manganese (help in iron absorption and its release from storage sites) and pyridoxine and riboflavin (utilize iron in erythropoiesis). Their deficiency can cause microcytic hypochromic anaemias.

DRUGS USED IN MEGALOBLASTIC ANAEMIAS

These are vitamin B_{12} and folic acid. Vitamin B_{12} and folic acid are dietary essentials. They take part in nucleic acids synthesis in the cell. A deficiency of either vitamin results in defective synthesis of DNA in any cell in which chromosomal replication and division are taking place. They are incorporated in red blood cells during erythropoiesis. Since tissues with the greater rate of cell turnover show the most dramatic changes, the haemopoietic system is specially sensitive to deficiencies of these vitamins producing macrocytic hyperchromic anaemia. Abnormal macrocytic RBCs are present in peripheral blood, which are haemolyzed early and the patient becomes anaemic. Pernicious anaemia is a serious form of megaloblastic anaemia (megloblasts in bone marrow) due to abnormal haematopoiesis.

Vitamin B_{12}

It is a cobalt containing vitamin existing as cyanocobalamin or hydroxycobalamin in the diet. It occurs as water-soluble, thermostable red crystals. It is synthesized solely by microorganisms in soil, water and animal intestine (colon). It is almost entirely absent from plant products.

Dietary Sources

Muscle, liver, kidney, oysters, cheese, fish and egg yolk are rich in vitamin B_{12}. Milk and milk products contain small amounts of vitamin B_{12}.

Commercial source of vitamin B_{12} is *Streptomyces griseus* as a by-product of steptomycin industry.

Daily Requirement

- Adults—1 to 3 µg/day.
- During pregnancy and lactation—3 to 5 µg/ day.
- Children and infants—0.3 to 0.15 µg/day.

Absorption, Distribution and Excretion of Vitamin B_{12}

It is absorbed from GIT by active transport process with the help of intrinsic factor, secreted by the parietal cells of the stomach. It (extrinsic factor) combines with the intrinsic factor forming haematinic principle which is absorbed in the small intestine. In the absence of intrinsic factor, the absorption of vitamin B_{12} in intestine is not possible and so deficiency of vitmin B_{12} occurs. When a large amount of vitamin B_{12} is taken orally, then small amount of vitamin B_{12} is absorbed by passive diffusion (without intrinsic factor). Absorbed vitamin B_{12} is transported in the plasma by binding with a β_2 globulin called transcobalamin-II. Only 1 to 5% circulates in blood as free form. The major form of vitamin B_{12} in the plasma is methylcobalamin attached to a globulin. It is specially taken up by liver cells and stored there. The total body stores of vitamin B_{12} is about 2 to 5 mg, of which about 50 to 80% is present in the liver. It is not degraded in the body. It is excreted mainly in bile but most of it is reabsorbed and undergoes enterohepatic circulation. Its turnover rate is very slow and only 0.2 to 0.3% of the total vitamin B_{12} contained in the body is excreted per day in faeces and urine. It is completely absorbed after IM or deep SC injection and a large amount is excreted in urine.

Metabolic Functions of Vitamin B_{12}

The active co-enzymes of vitamin B_{12} are methylcobalamine and 5-deoxyadenosylcobalamin (DAB_{12}). These are essential for cell growth and replication (division). Methylcobalamin is required for the formation of methionine and its derivatives S-adenosylmethionine from homocysteine by the above reaction **(Fig. 27.2)**.

In addition, when concentrations of vitamin B_{12} are inadequate, folate (THF) becomes trapped as methyl tetrahydrofolate to cause a functional deficiency of other required intracellular forms of folic acid. The haematological abnormalities that are observed in vitamin B_{12} deficiency are the result of this process. 5-

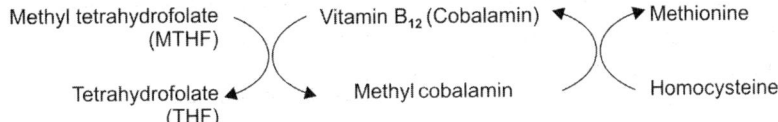

Fig. 27.2: Relationship between vitamin B_{12} and folic acid

deoxyadenosyl cobalamin is required for the isomerization of L-methylmalonic CoA to succinyl CoA. This reaction does not require folate but is responsible for demyelination (as seen in vitamin B_{12} deficiency) leading to neurological damage.

Vitamin B_{12} Deficiency

It produces following problems:
- Haematological disorders like megaloblastic anaemia (bone marrow contains megaloblasts, which are abnormally large, nucleated red blood cell precursors) and macrocytic hyperchromic anaemia (peripheral blood contains abnormal cells called macrocytes, which are large red blood cells showing fully haemoglobinized and undergo early haemolysis (short lifespan).
- Neurological complications like peripheral neuritis (manifested as paresthesia of hands and feet and diminution of vibration and position senses), optic atrophy and subacute combined degeneration of spinal cord and in late stages confusion, moodiness, loss of memory, loss of central vision, delusions, hallucinations and psychosis.

Uses of Vitamin B_{12}

It is used in the treatment of megaloblastic macrocytic hyperchromic anaemias such as Addisonian pernicious anaemia (requires lifelong treatment), tropical nutritional anaemia, pregnancy anaemia and anaemia due to fish tapeworm (*D. latus*) or abnormal flora in intestine (blind loop syndrome). It is also used in neuropathies, tobacco amblyopia, cutaneous sarcoid and psychiatric disorders and as a general tonic.

Preparations and Dosage
- Cyanocobalamin (Macrabin) injection (100 ng/ml)—100 µg IM daily (never IV) till improvement.
  Maintenance dose—100 µg IM monthly.
- Hydroxycobalamin (Macrabin-H) injection (100 µg/ml)—same as above.

Adverse Reactions

It is quite safe even in large doses. Its injections are painless. It may rarely produce allergic reactions. Its IV injection may produce anaphylactoid reactions and so contraindicated.

Folic Acid

It is so-called as it is present in green leaves (folia). Chemically it is petroyl glutamic acid (PGA) consisting of pteridine, PABA and glutamic acid.

Dietary Sources

Green leafy vegetables, some fruits, liver, yeast, egg, meat and milk. Prolonged boiling during cooking destroys most of the folic acid.

Daily Requirement
- Adults—50 µg/day.
- Children and infants —25 µg/day.
- During pregnancy and lactation—100 to 200 µg/day.

Absorption, Distribution and Excretion of Folic Acid

It is mainly absorbed from small intestine as methyl tetrahydrofolate by active transport process. When administered orally in large doses, a fraction of it is absorbed by passive diffusion. It is distributed in all tissues. It is stored mainly in the liver. Total body stores of folic acid is 5 to 10 mg. Its exact metabolism and degradation in the body is not known. It is excreted in bile and urine.

Metabolic Functions of Folic Acid

It is involved in following intracellular metabolic reactions:

- Conversion of homocysteine to methionine. This reaction requires methyl tetrahydrofolate as a methyl donor and utilizes vitamin B_{12} as a cofactor.
- Conversion of serine to glycine. This reaction requires tetrahydrofolate as an acceptor of methylene group from serine and utilizes pyridoxal phosphate as a cofactor. It results in the formation of 5, 10-methylene tetrahydrofolate (an essential coenzyme for the synthesis of thymidylate) by donating a methylene group.
- Metabolism of histidine to glutamic acid. Methyl tetrahydrofolate acts as an acceptor of a formimino group in the conversion of formiminoglutamic acid to glutamic acid.
- Synthesis of purine and pyrimidine nucleotides.
- Incorporation of formate into the purine ring.

These reactions are necessary for the synthesis of nucleic acids.

Folic Acid Deficiency

It can produce macrocytic (megaloblastic) anaemias like tropical nutritional anaemia, anaemia of pregnancy and anaemia of infancy (due to impaired absorption/utilization/increased requirements of folic acid) and certain other anaemias (due to liver disease, chronic alcoholism, malabsorption syndrome or antiepileptic drug therapy).

Clinical Uses

It is used in the treatment of macrocytic megaloblastic anaemias due to folic acid deficiency (as mentioned above). It is also used prophylactically along with iron in anaemia of pregnancy.

Contraindications

- Leukaemias, anaemia with malignancy, haemolytic anaemia and chronic infections, where active cell proliferation due to nucleic acid synthesis can lead to aggravation (worsening) of the conditions.
- Pernicious anaemia without using vitamin B_{12}—if folic acid is used alone in pernicious anaemia, it may correct the haematological abnormality but it precipitates or worsens the neurological complications. This is because folic acid accelerates the utilization of the meagre vitamin B_{12} stores in an already deficient subject for haematopoiesis and may thus produce further deficiency of vitamin B_{12}, which is essential for maintaining the integrity of the CNS and the peripheral nerves.

Folinic Acid

It is N5 formyl tetrahydrofolic acid. It was originally found in the liver cell. It was demonstrated to have a growth-promoting effect on the organism called *Leuconostoc citrovorum* and so it is known as citrovorum factor. It is used in methotrexate toxicity as folic acid cannot be used in it.

Preparations and Dosage

- Folic acid (Folvite) tablet (5 mg)—5 to 10 mg daily. It is also available as injection (1 mg/ml in ampoule).
- Folinic acid (Leucovorin) injection (3 mg/ml in ampoule)—3 to 6 mg IM daily.

It is used in methotrexate toxicity which cannot be treated by folic acid as methotrexate is a folic acid antagonist (inhibits dihydrofolate reductase) and so conversion of folic acid to folinic acid cannot occur.

Adverse Reactions

Folic acid is almost nontoxic in man. It may rarely produce allergic reactions.

28

Coagulants and Anticoagulants

Drugs used in coagulation disorders are coagulants and anticoagulants.

Mechanism of Blood Coagulation

Blood coagulation means the conversion of fluid blood to a solid gel or clot. The main event is the conversion of soluble fibrinogen to insoluble strands of fibrin (the last step in a complex enzyme cascade). The components (factors) are present in blood as inactive precursors (zymogens) of proteolytic enzymes and cofactors. They are activated by proteolysis, the active forms being designated by the suffix 'a'. Factors IIa (thrombin), IXa, Xa, XIa and XIIa are serine proteases. The activation of a small amount of one factor catalyzes the formation of larger amount of the next factor, which catalyzes the formation of still larger amount of the next factor, and so on. Thus, the cascade provides a mechanism of amplification. There are two main pathways of fibrin formation, *viz.* intrinsic pathway (because all the factors are present in blood) and extrinsic pathway (because some factors come from outside the blood). The intrinsic pathway is activated

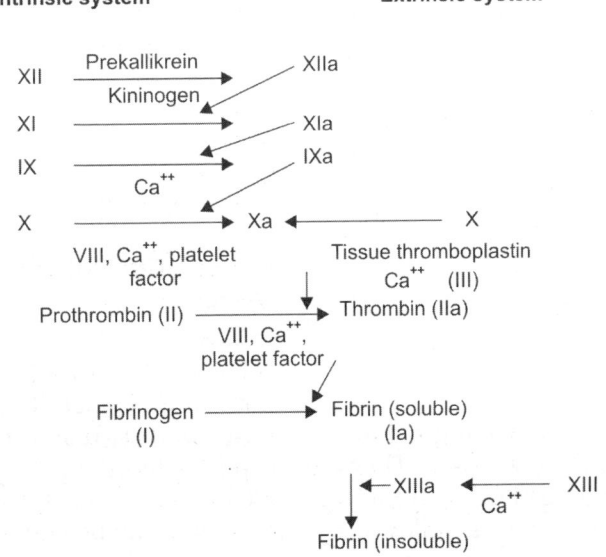

Fig. 28.1: Steps in coagulation of blood

when the shed blood comes into contact with an artificial surface such as glass and the extrinsic pathway is important in controlling blood coagulation in the body. Steps in coagulation of blood is shown in **Fig. 28.1**.

Blood clotting factors are 16 in numbers, *viz.* fibrinogen (I), prothrombin (II), thromboplastin (III), ionic calcium (IV), proaccelerin (V), accelerin (VI), proconvertin (VII), antihaemophilic globulin (VIII), plasma thromboplastin component/Christmas factor (IX), Stuart-Prower factor (X), plasma thromboplastin antecedent (XI), Hageman factor (XII), fibrin stabilizing factor (XIII), prekallikrein (XIV), kallikrein (XV) and platelet factor (XVI).

Coagulants

These are drugs that promote coagulation (clotting) of blood and used to control bleeding in haemorrhagic states. Fresh whole blood or plasma provides all clotting factors and acts immediately in controlling bleeding. These are haemostatics.

Classification

These are of two groups:

1. Local coagulants (agents acting locally), e.g. thrombin, thromboplastin, fibrin, gel foam, oxidized cellulose, microfibrillar collagen haemostat and certain snake venoms (Russel's viper venom and copper head snake venom).
2. Systemic coagulants (agents acting systematically), e.g. fibrinogen, antihaemophilic globulin, adrenochrome monosemicarbazone, ethamsylate, vitamin K, vitamin C, vitamin P (Rutin).

DISCUSSION OF INDIVIDUAL GROUP OF DRUGS

Local Coagulants

These are effective in controlling oozing of blood from superficial blood vessels. They are not effective in controlling bleeding from large blood vessels. They are given as follows:

Thrombin

It is obtained from bovine plasma. It is stable as a dry powder stored between 2° and 8°C. It is applied locally in oozing of blood. It can be used mixed with plasma to anchor the skin grafts in place.

Thromboplastin

It is a powder prepared from acetone extracted brain and lung tissues of freshly killed rabbits. It is used as a local haemostatic in surgery. It is also used for determination of prothrombin time.

Fibrin

It is obtained from human plasma. It is used in the dehydrated form as sheet, from which portion of desired size is cut and placed on bleeding surface.

Gelfoam

It is a porous, pressed form of gelatin sponge used along with thrombin to control oozing of blood from surface wounds. It is moistened with normal saline before use. It is completely absorbed within 4 to 6 weeks and so it is left in place after suturing of a surgical wound.

Oxidized Cellulose (Oxycel)

It is a surgical gauze treated with nitrogen dioxide. It promotes clotting of blood by a reaction between haemoglobin and cellulosic acid. When wet with tissue juice, it becomes sticky and gummy, and stimulates formation of artificial clot over the surface of the wound. It is completely absorbed within 5 to 10 days.

Microfibrillar Collagen Haemostat (Avitene)

It is prepared from purified bovine corium collagen. When applied to a bleeding surface, it forms a platelet plug, which is followed by natural clot. It is effective in controlling capillary bleeding due to any cause. It is non-allerginic. It is inactivated by autoclaving and so should not be sterilized.

Snake Venoms

Russel's viper venom and copper head snake venom enhance coagulation of blood by acting as thromboplastin (stimulating thrombokinase). They are used locally or parenterally to control severe bleeding of haemophilia.

Systemic Coagulants

These are effective in controlling bleeding from deep blood vessels when administered systematically. They are:

Fibrinogen (Fibrinal)

It is obtained from human plasma. It is transformed into fibrin by addition of thrombin. It is used to control bleeding in haemophilia and afibrinogenemia or hypofibrinogenemia. It is also used in disseminated intravascular coagulation. It is available as fibrinogen solution (0.5 g/bottle) for IV infusion.

Antihaemophilic Globulin (AHG)

It is obtained from human plasma as a dry powder. It is used in patients with haemophilia and antihaemophilic globulin deficiency, who are susceptible to bleeding. It is available as fibrinal-H solution (containing 150 units of AHG and 0.5 g of fibrinogen/bottle) for IV infusion. Its action is short-lasting (1 to 2 days).

Adrenochrome Monosemicarbazone (Chromostat)

Adrenochrome is the degradation product of adrenaline on exposure to light or heat. It reduces capillary fragility and controls capillary bleeding. It is used in epistaxis, haemoptysis, haematuria, retinal haemorrhage and haemorrhage from wounds.

It is available as tablet (0.5, 1 mg) and injection (1.5 mg/2 ml ampoule) and administered in dosage of 1 to 5 mg orally or IM.

Ethamsylate (Dicyanine, Cosklot, Hemsyl)

It is a synthetic drug. It reduces capillary bleeding in the presence of normal number of platelets. It does not act by fibrin stabilization but probably by correcting abnormal platelet adhesion. It is used in menorrhagia, metrorrhagia, epistaxis, haemoptysis, haematuria, haematemesis, malena and after abortion. It is available as tablet (250, 500 mg) and injection (250 mg/ml) and administered in dosage of 250 to 500 mg twice or thrice daily. It can cause nausea, headache and skin rashes.

Vitamin K

It is a fat-soluble vitamin. It is a naphthoquinone compound. It is called coagulation vitamin.

Dietary Sources

Green leafy vegetables like cabbage, cauliflower, spinach, alfalfa, soyabean, seafish, liver and cheese. Daily requirement—50 to 100 µg/day (in adult).

Types of Vitamin K

These are of three types:
1. Vitamin K_1 (from plants, fat-soluble)— phytomenadione (Mephytoin).
2. Vitamin K_2 (produced by bacteria, fat soluble)— Menaquinone.
3. Vitamin K_3 (produced synthetically):
    – Fat-soluble, e.g. menadione, acetomenadione/acetomenaphthone (Kapilin).
    – Water-soluble, e.g. menadione sodium bisulphite (Cadisper), menadione sodium diphosphate (Synkavite).

Physiological Functions

It is essential for the biosynthesis of prothrombin (factor II) and factors VII, IX and X in the liver. In the absence of vitamin K (or in the presence of oral anticoagulants), these factors are biologically inactive. Vitamin K functions as an essential cofactor for the microsomal enzyme system that activates these precursors by carboxylation of glutamic acid residues of these proteins in the final stage of their synthesis. It is also involved in electron transport and oxidative phosphorylation in cells.

Pharmacokinetics

Fat-soluble K vitamins are absorbed from intestine via lymph in presence of bile salts. Water-soluble K vitamins are absorbed directly into portal blood, even in absence of bile salts. Both fat- and water-soluble K vitamins are absorbed satisfactorily after parenteral administration. The metabolic fate of vitamin K is not known. It is excreted in bile and urine.

Clinical Uses

It is used in vitamin K deficiency in adults (produced by malabsorption syndrome or obstructive jaundice) and infants (during acute diarrhoea), haemorrhagic disease of neonate and bleeding states during salicylate or oral anticoagulant therapy.

Preparations and Dosage

- Vitamin K_1 tablet (10 mg) and injection (10 mg/ml)—10–20 mg orally IM or IV. In neonate—1–2 mg in umbilical vein.
- Acetomendione tablet (5 mg)—5 to 10 mg daily.
- Menadione sodium diphosphate injection (5–10 mg/ml)—5–15 mg SC, IM or IV.

Adverse Reactions

Vitamin K_1 may produce flushing, cyanosis, breathlessness, fall of BP and hypersensitivity reactions on IV injection. Menadione and its water soluble salts can produce haemolytic anaemia, hyperbilirubinemia and kernicterus (jaundice) in neonates in large doses.

Vitamin C (Limcee)

It is a water-soluble vitamin. It is effective in controlling bleeding due to vitamin C deficiency as in scurvy. It is administered in the dosage of 500 mg twice daily.

Vitamin P (Rutin)

It is a plant glycoside. It is used in the treatment of increased capillary erythroper-meability. It is less effective if there is an accompanying vitamin C deficiency. So it is administered along with vitamin C in the dosage of 20 mg of rutin and 100 mg of vitamin C (Kalpastin) three to four times daily.

Other Haemostatics Used to Control Bleeding

- Vasoconstrictors, e.g. octeotide, diosmin, vasopressin/desmopressin. These are used to control bleeding of oesophageal varices and piles. Adrenaline (1% solution used locally soaked in cotton swab).
- Astringents, e.g. tannic acid (20%) in glycerine (used in gum bleeding).
- Sclerosing agents, e.g. phenol (5% in almond oil)—2 to 3 ml injected. Quinine (12.5%) in urethane (25%) solution—2 to 3 ml injected. Ethanolamine oleate (5%) solution—2 to 5 ml injected.

These are irritant substances and cause inflammation, coagulation and ultimately fibrosis when injected into haemorrhoids (piles) or varicose veins. They are injected once in a week for 4 to 6 weeks. They can cause allergic reactions. Diosmin (Daflon) tablet (500 mg) thrice daily is used in acute haemorrhoids to stop bleeding.

Anticoagulants

These are drugs that reduce coagulability of blood and used in thromboembolic disorders.

Classification

These are of two groups:

1. Fast-acting anticoagulants (acting both *in vivo* and *in vitro*), e.g. heparin and hirudin.
2. Slow-acting anticoagulants (acting only *in vivo*).
   - Coumarin derivatives, e.g. bishydroxy-coumarin (dicoumarol), warfarin sodium, acenocoumarol, nicoumalone, ethyl biscoumacetate and phenprocoumon.
   - Indandione derivatives, e.g. phenindine, anisindione, bromindione and diphenadione.

Laboratory anticoagulants used in blood in glass vials for haematological investigations are calcium complexing (precipitating) agents, e.g. sodium citrate (38 mg/ml of blood), sodium oxalate (10 mg/ml of blood) and sodium edetate (2 mg/ml of blood).

CPD (citrate-phosphate-dextrose) solution or CPDA (citrate-phosphate-dextrose-adenine) solution is used for preservation (storage) of blood in fluid state for blood transfusion.

DISCUSSION OF INDIVIDUAL GROUP OF DRUGS

Fast-acting anticoagulants/parenteral anticoagulants.

Heparin

Discovery

It was discovered in 1916 by McLean, a medical student. While preparing thromboplastin extracts from liver and lungs he observed that they contain a powerful anticoagulant. Howell and Holt in 1918 isolated heparin from liver and named it heparin. It was used clinically in 1937, when it was purified.

Source

It is present in all tissues containing mast cells. It is present in high concentrations in liver, lungs and intestinal mucosa. Commercial sources of heparin are bovine lungs and porcine intestinal mucosa. Purified heparin preparations obtained from different animals have different activities.

Chemistry

It is a sulphated mucopolysaccharide (glycosaminoglycan) composed of an unknown number of alternating D-glucuronic acid and N-acetyl-D-glucosamine units linked through an oxygen bridge. The content of esterified sulphuric acid is very high and this makes heparin a strongly electronegative compound. It is thus the strongest organic acid in the body. Its anticoagulant activity is due to strong electronegative charge. It is used as the sodium salt. It has a molecular weight of about 40,000. Low molecular weight (LMW) heparins are prepared from standard heparins by gel filtration, chromatography or differential precipitation with ethanol. They have molecular weight varying from 4000 to 6500.

Physiological Functions of Heparin

It is the naturally occurring anticoagulant responsible for fluidity of blood in the intact vasculature. It occurs intracellularly in tissues that contain mast cells. Its functions within the secretory granules of mast cells are unknown. When released from mast cells, it is ingested rapidly and destroyed by macrophages. It cannot be detected in plasma under normal circumstances. Its molecules on the surface of vascular endothelial cells or in the subendothelial extracellular matrix interact with the circulating antithrombin to provide a natural antithrombotic mechanism.

Pharmacological Actions

These are given as follows:

- **Anticoagulant action:** It acts by binding and activating antithrombin-III (a heparin cofactor) in the plasma. Antithrombin is a glycosylated polypeptide (α_2-globulin) synthesized in the liver and circulates in plasma. It rapidly inhibits thrombin only in the presence of heparin. It also inhibits other activated coagulation factors (Xa, IXa, XIa, XIIa and kallikrein), but it has little activity against factor VIIa. It is a suicide substrate for these proteases. Heparin increases the rate of thrombin and antithrombin reactions at least a thousand folds by serving as a catalytic template to which both the inhibitor and the protease bind. Once thrombin has become bound to antithrombin the heparin molecule is released from the complex.

- **Antiplatelet action:** High doses of heparin can inhibit platelet aggregation and thereby prolong the bleeding time.

- **Lipemia clearing action (antichylomicronemic action):** It clears turbid postprandial lipemic plasma *in vivo* by causing the release of lipoprotein lipase from the vessel wall and tissues into the circulation. Lipoprotein lipase hydrolyzes triglycerides to glycerol and free fatty acids. The clearing of lipemic plasma occurs at lower concentration of heparin than that required for anticoagulant action. It does not occur *in* *vitro*, when heparin is added to turbid plasma.

- **Miscellaneous actions:** It is claimed to exert some anti-inflammatory activity. It may inhibit aldosterone secretion.

Pharmacokinetics

It is not effective orally, because it has a large, highly ionized molecule. It is well-absorbed after SC or IM injection. It is stored in mast cells after absorption. It is metabolized mainly by a liver enzyme called heparinase and fragments are excreted in urine. It does not cross the placental barrier and is not secreted in milk. The anticoagulant action of heparin after IV dose is almost immediate and reaches peak within 5 to 10 minutes. The prolonged clotting time returns to normal within 2 to 4 hours. It does not effect bleeding time.

Clinical Uses of Heparin

These are given as follows:
- Prevention and treatment of deep vein thrombosis and pulmonary embolism.
- Treatment of myocardial infarction (to reduce thromboembolic complications).
- Treatment of rheumatic heart disease (if embolism occurs).
- During cardiovascular surgery (heparin is a must during cardiac bypass surgery and in placing artificial heart valves to prevent emboli).
- Prevention of postoperative thrombosis and embolism.
- Treatment of peripheral arterial (e.g. retinal vessel) embolism.
- Treatment of disseminated intravascular coagulation.

Contraindications of Heparin Therapy

- Cerebrovascular haemorrhage (increases bleeding).
- Subacute bacterial endocarditis (chances of detachment of the bacterial vegetations from the damaged valves into the general circulation).
- Haemorrhagic tendency and blood dyscrasias (e.g. purpura, haemophilia, etc.).

- Benign or malignant ulcers, e.g. peptic ulcer, ulcerative colitis, diverticulitis and cancer colon.
- Threatened abortion and injury to brain and spinal cord.
- Severe hepatic or renal impairment.
- Malignant hypertension.

Unit of Heparin

One unit of heparin is the amount of heparin that will prevent 1 ml of citrated sheep plasma from clotting for 1 hour after the addition of 0.2 ml of $CaCl_2$ solution. 1 mg of heparin sodium has 120 to 140 units of activity. Thus 1unit = 0.8 µg.

Preparations and Dosage

- Heparin sodium (Beparin) injection (1000, 5000 units/ml in 5 ml vial)—10,000 units initially IV (loading/bolus dose) followed by 5,000 units IV every 4 to 6 hours (IV intermittent regimen) or 5,000 units into the tubing of infusion initially followed by 1000 units/hour in isotonic saline (IV infusion regimen) or 10,000 units SC every hourly (subcutaneous regimen), IM injection is painful and so not used. Monitoring of heparin therapy is done by clotting time (should be kept at 2 to 3 times of the normal value) or activated partial thromboplastin time (APTT) (should be kept at 1 to 2 times of the normal value).
- Low molecular weight (LMW) heparins, e.g. Enoxaparin (Clexane) injection (5000 units/ml) and Dalteparin (Fragmin) injection (5000 units/ml). They are administered SC in dosage of 5000 units twice or thrice daily. They differ from standard (conventional) heparin in pharmacokinetic properties and mechanism of action.

They are preferred than standard (conventional) heparin due to following advantages:

– They are absorbed more completely than standard heparin after SC administration.

– They have longer duration of action than standard heparin.

– They bind less avidly to heparin binding proteins than standard heparin and so their response is predictable.
– They interact relatively less with platelets than standard heparin and so produce less bleeding episodes.

- They do not require repeated monitoring of blood sample.
- LMW heparin antithrombin III complex inactivates factor Xa selectively and has minimum action against thrombin.
- They have prophylactic, and therapeutic uses in thromboembolic disorders.

Adverse Reactions of Heparin

These include following adverse reactions:

- Allergic and anaphylactoid reactions like asthma, urticaria, rhinitis and fever. It is advisable to give a trial dose of 1000 units of heparin SC, though these reactions rarely occur.
- Bleeding from various sites, e.g. peptic ulcer, ulcerative colitis, kidneys (haematuria), haemorrhoids, haemarthrosis and wound haematoma.
- Thrombocytopenia (mild or severe) due to platelet aggregation or formation of anti-platelet antibodies.
- Transient alopecia (after prolonged therapy).
- Osteoporosis (on long-term use in high doses).

Heparin Antagonists

These are strongly basic compounds, which rapidly antagonize the anticoagulant effect of heparin (a strongly acidic compound), e.g. protamine sulphate and toludine blue.

Protamine sulphate: It is the commonly used heparin antagonist. It is a simple protein with low molecular weight and obtained from sperms of certain fish. It is available as 1% solution. It is administered IV slowly (not more than 50 mg in 10 minutes). One mg of protamine sulphate neutralizes the anti-coagulant effect of 80 to 100 units of heparin activity. If more than 30 minutes have elapsed after heparin administration, then half of the dosage of protamine is required. It is used only in severe bleeding due to heparin. Its dosage should not exceed 100 mg, because it possesses anticoagulant activity (in high dose). Its rapid IV injection can cause sudden fall of BP, bradycardia, dyspnoea, flushing and feeling of warmth. Toluidine blue can be used if protamine sulphate is not available.

Hirudin

It is a powerful and specific thrombin inhibitor obtained from leech buccal cavity. It is now prepared by recombinant DNA technology. Its action is independent of antithrombin-III, which means it can reach and inactivate fibrin bound thrombin in thrombi. It has little effect on platelets and the bleeding tissue. It is administered parenterally like heparin. It is under clinical trial.

SLOW-ACTING ANTICOAGULANTS/ORAL ANTICOAGULANTS

These are effective by mouth and slowly acting synthetic drugs:

Coumarin Derivatives

Bishydroxycoumarin (Dicoumarol) is the first coumarin derivative isolated from spoilt sweet clover in 1943, after an outbreak of a haemorrhagic disease in cattle in North America due to feeding of spoilt sweet clover. The disease caused by prothrombin deficiency was cured by feeding alpha, alpha grass, containing vitamin K. Later on many cogeners of dicoumarol were synthesized for clinical use. Warfarin sodium is the most commonly used anticoagulant.

Pharmacological Actions

These are given as follows:

- **Anticoagulant action:** They act as anti-coagulant only *in vivo* and not *in vitro*. This is because they act indirectly by interfering with the synthesis of vitamin K dependent clotting factors, *viz.* prothrombin (factor II) and factors VII, IX and X by the liver, by competitive inhibition of carboxylation of the glutamic acid residues by vitamin K in the liver (vitamin K hydroquinone is converted to vitamin K epoxide by the microsomal epoxidase in the liver during carboxylation reaction, vitamin K epoxide is converted back to vitamin K hydroquinone by epoxide reductase. The regeneration of vitamin K hydroquinone is essential for sustained carboxylation and synthesis of these clotting factors). They may increase plasma antithromobin level. Their anticoagulant effect takes 1 to 3 days to develop. Monitoring of coumarin therapy is done by estimation of prothrombin time of blood. They do not alter bleeding time.

- **Antimetastatic action:** They reduce the incidence of spontaneous metastasis from malignant neoplasms. This action runs parallel with the depression of prothrombin activity of blood.
- **Uricosuric action:** They can produce uricosuric effect, by interfering with the renal tubular reabsorption of urate.

Pharmacokinetics

They are slowly and incompletely absorbed from GIT. They are highly plasma protein bound (90 to 98%) and slowly metabolized in the liver. There is considerable variation (as much as 14 folds) in the rate of metabolism in different individuals. They cross the placental barrier and are also secreted in milk. They are slowly excreted in urine.

Clinical Uses

They have clinical uses like heparin but they cannot be used in emergency.

Preparations and Dosage

- Warfarin sodium (Uniwarfin) tablet (5 mg) and injection (15 mg/ml)—15 to 30 mg initially (loading dose) orally, IM or IV followed by 5 to 10 mg daily (maintenance dose) orally.
- Ethylbiscoumacetate (Tromexan) tablet (300 mg)—600 to 900 mg initially (loading dose) orally followed by 300 mg daily (maintenance dose) orally.

Adverse Reactions

These include following adverse reactions:
- Bleeding from various sites (like heparin).
- GIT side effects (nausea, vomiting, anorexia and diarrhoea).
- Foetal toxicity: They can cross the placental barrier and may cause teratogenic effect and severe haemorrhage in foetus.
- Cutaneous toxicity: They can produce dermatitis, alopecia, ecchymoses, haemorrhagic bullae and necrosis/gangrene of skin.
- Allergic reactions: They rarely produce skin rash, urticaria, fever, hepatitis, nephropathy and agranulocytosis.

Treatment of Bleeding by Oral Anticoagulants

- Withdrawal of the drug.
- Administration of vitamin K_1 (specific antidote)— 10 to 20 mg IM or IV.
- Fresh whole blood or frozen plasma transfusion (to supply clotting factors and to replenish lost blood) produces immediate control of bleeding.

Indandione Derivatives

These are synthetic oral anticoagulants. Phenindione is commonly used. They have pharmacokinetics, pharmacological effects therapeutic uses and adverse reactions like coumarin derivatives. They have limited use due to toxicity. They are only used in patients who cannot tolerate warfarin.

Preparation and Dosage

Phenindione (Dindevan) tablet (50 mg)— Initially 200 mg (as loading dose) orally, followed by 50 mg daily (maintenance dose) orally.

Drug Interactions of Oral Anticoagulants

Decreased effect of oral anticoagulants occurs due to:
- Reduced absorption of the anticoagulant by binding to cholestyramine resin.
- Increased metabolism of the anticoagulant in the liver due to induction of hepatic

microsomal enzyme system by barbiturates, rifampicin, phenytoin, carbamazepine, griseofulvin or chronic ingestion of ethanol. These drugs shorten prothrombin time (PT). Increased effect of oral anticoagulants leading to haemorrhagic tendency occurs due to:

– Displacement of the anticoagulant from plasma protein binding sites by aspirin, phenyl butazone, indomethacin, sulphinpyrazone, metronidazole, disulphiram, allopurinol, cimetidine, amiodarone, probenecid, sulphamethoxazole or acute intake of ethanol.

– Decreased metabolism of the anticoagulant in the liver by inhibiting hepatic microsomal enzyme system, e.g. chloramphenicol, cimetidine, metronidazole or disulphiram.

All these drugs increase prothrombin time (PT).

29

Antithrombotic and Thrombolytic Drugs

ANTITHROMBOTIC DRUGS (ANTIPLATELET DRUGS)

These are drugs which interfere with platelet function and used for prophylaxis of thrombo-embolic disorders like myocardial infarction. Haemostasis is cessation of blood loss from a damaged blood vessel (artery or vein). Platelets first stick to the damaged wall of blood vessel and then they aggregate (stick to each other) and release ADP and thromboxane A_2 (TXA$_2$), which promote further aggregation of platelets producing a haemostatic plug at the site of vascular injury. Prostacyclin (PGI$_2$) synthesized in the intima of blood vessels is a strong inhibitor of platelet aggregation. A balance between thromboxane A_2 (released from platelets) and PGI$_2$ (released from vascular endothelium) controls intravascular thrombus formation. Platelets also play a role in atherosclerosis and pathological thrombosis.

Antagonists of platelet function are used to prevent thrombosis and to alter the natural process of atherosclerotic vascular disease. These drugs are aspirin, dipyridamole and clopidogrel, ticlopidine.

Aspirin

It is acetyl salicylic acid. In low dose (100 mg/day) it acts as an antithrombotic (antiplatelet) drug. In platelets the major cyclo-oxygenase product is thromboxane-A_2, which is an inducer of platelet aggregation and a potent vasoconstrictor. Aspirin blocks production of thromboxane-A_2 by covalently acetylating a serine residue near the active site of cyclo-oxygenase, the enzyme that produces the cyclic endoperoxide precursor of thromboxane-A_2. Since platelets do not synthesize new proteins, so the action of aspirin on platelet cyclo-oxygenase is permanent, lasting for the life of the platelet (7 to 10 days). Thus repeated doses of aspirin produces a cumulative effect on platelet function. Complete inhibition of platelet cyclo-oxygenase is achieved when 100 mg of aspirin is taken daily. Thus aspirin produces antithrombotic effect when taken in lower dosage than that required to produce other effects (like analgesic and anti-inflammatory actions). At higher dosage it is less effective as anti-thrombotic drug, because it then inhibits synthesis of prostacyclin (PGI$_2$) by the vascular endothelium, which is a vasodilator and inhibitor of platelet aggregation and also increases toxicity especially bleeding. In lower dosage it blocks the synthesis of thromboxane-A_2 without blocking the synthesis of PGI$_2$.

Preparation and Dosage

Aspirin (Loprine, Ecosprin) tablet (50, 100 mg)—50 to 100 mg daily.

Dipyridamole

It is a coronary dilator. It dilates coronary resistance vessels (unlike nitrates which dilate coronary conductance vessels). Though it increases coronary blood flow in experimental

216

animals but it is disappointing in the treatment of angina pectoris as it produces coronary steal phenomenon. It has also a weak platelet inhibiting action. It blocks platelet aggregation and acts as an antithrombotic drug. Used in combination with aspirin it reduces thrombosis in patients with thrombotic diseases. It increases cAMP concentration in platelets and so causes inhibition of release of ADP and no platelet aggregation. This action is mediated by inhibition of cyclic nucleotide phosphodiesterase and/or by blockade of uptake of adenosine, which acts at A_2 receptors for adenosine to stimulate platelet adenylate cyclase.

Preparation and Dosage

Dipyridamole (75 mg) with aspirin (60 mg) tablet (Dynasprin)—1 tablet daily.

Ticlopidine

It is a thienopyridine. It acts as an anti-thrombotic drug by inhibiting platelet function and producing a thrombasthenia state. It is used in patients who are intolerant to aspirin. Unlike aspirin, it does not inhibit PG synthesis. It inhibits platelet aggregation by selectively inhibiting the binding of ADP to its platelet receptor and subsequent ADP mediated activation of glycoprotein (GPIIa/IIIa) complex. It is about 50% absorbed from GIT, metabolized in the liver and excreted in urine.

It is used as a prophylactic drug in cerebrovascular and coronary thromboembolic diseases.

Preparation and Dosage

Ticlopidine (Ticlid, Ticlop) tablet (250 mg)—250 mg twice daily.

Adverse Reactions

It can cause diarrhoea, vomiting, headache, bleeding, agranulocytosis, thrombocytopenia and skin rashes.

It is a newer congener of ticlopidine. It selectively inhibits the binding of ADP to its platelet receptor and the subsequent ADP mediated activation of the glycoprotein (GPIIa

and IIIa) complex, thereby inhibiting platelet aggregation. It does not inhibit phosphodiesterase activity. It is 50% absorbed orally and metabolized in the liver. It has uses like ticlopidine. It is available as 75 mg tablet (Deplatt, Clopiet) and administered once daily. It is better tolerated than ticlopidine. It rarely produces agranulocytosis and thrombocytopenia. It can produce diarrhoea, epigastric pain and skin rashes.

Other drugs like sulphinpyrazone and clofibrate, which inhibit platelet function are no longer used as antithrombotic drug due to toxicity.

Thrombolytic (Fibrinolytic) Drugs

These are drugs used to lyse (dissolve) thrombi (clots) in blood vessels (mainly coronary arteries) in order to recanalyse the occluded vessels. They are curative, rather than prophylactic. They act by activating the natural fibrinolytic system.

The fibrinolytic system dissolves intra-vascular clots as a result of the action of plasmin, an enzyme that digests fibrin plasminogen, an inactive precursor of plasmin is a single chain glycoprotein containing 791 amino acid residues. It is converted to plasmin by cleavage of a single peptide bond.

Plasminogen → Plasmin   → Fibrin digestion
(Profibrinolysin) (Fibrinolysin)   and clot dissolution

Plasmin is a nonspecific active protease, which digests fibrin clots and other plasma proteins, including several coagulation factors. Therapy with thrombolytic drugs tends to dissolve both pathological thrombi and fibrin deposits at sites of vascular injury. Therefore, these drugs can cause haemorrhage (bleeding) as side effect. Plasminogen activators, e.g. streptokinase, urokinase and recombinant tissue plasminogen activator (rTPA) (Alteplase) are used as thrombolytic drugs.

Streptokinase

It is a protease (enzyme) produced by β-haemolytic Streptococci. It has no intrinsic enzyme activity, but it forms a stable, non-covalent 1:1 complex with plasminogen. It forms plasmin by conformational change. It is metabolized in the liver. It has a half-life of 40 to 80 minutes. It is used in acute myocardial infarction (MI) (for coronary thrombolysis), pulmonary embolism, deep vein thrombosis and acute peripheral arterial occlusion (by clots).

Preparation and Dosage

Streptokinase (Streptase) injection (freeze dried powder in a vial containing 2.5 lakh units)—initially 2.5 lakh units (2.5 mg) by IV infusion with normal saline in 30 minutes (loading dose), followed by 1 lakh units by IV infusion every hour for 24 to 72 hours.

Adverse Reactions

It can cause bleeding and allergic reactions (as it is antigenic) and rarely anaphylaxis and fever. Epsilon aminocaproic acid is the specific antidote of streptokinase.

Due to antibody formation, it cannot be used within one year. It is least expensive than other thrombolytic drugs.

Streptokinase Plasminogen Complex (Antistreplase/Eminase)

It is a plasminogen complex in which lyse plasminogen is acylated at its catalytic site serine. It is used for coronary thrombolysis. The acyl group is hydrolyzed *in vivo*, allowing the complex to bind to fibrin prior to activation. This modification confers some specificity towards clots on the fibrinolytic process. However, marked systemic fibrinolysis occurs when the drug is administered as a bolus injection at a dosage of 30 units for coronary thrombolysis.

Urokinase (Abokinase)

It is a protease (enzyme) originally isolated from human urine, is now obtained from cultured human kidney cells. It is a direct potent plasminogen activator. Unlike strepto-kinase, it is nonantigenic and nonpyrogenic and does not cause allergic reactions. It has a half-life of 15 to 30 minutes. It is metabolized in the liver. It is the treatment of choice in massive acute myocardial infarction or acute pulmonary embolism.

Preparation and Dosage

Urokinase injection (freeze dried powder in a vial containing 2.5 lakh units)—initially 2.5 lakh units by IV infusion with normal saline in 10 minutes (bolus injection) followed by continuous infusion of the same dose per hour for 12 to 24 hours.

Adverse Reactions

It is less toxic than streptokinase. It can produce haemorrhage like streptokinase. It is more expensive than streptokinase.

Recombinant Tissue Plasminogen Activator (rt-PA/Alteplase)

It is a serine protease (enzyme) occurring in human tissue. It is now prepared by recombinant DNA technology from human tissue culture. It is a poor plasminogen activator in the absence of fibrin. It binds to fibrin and activates plasminogen already bound to fibrin. It has little action on plasminogen in the circulation. It is rapidly metabolized in the liver and has a half-life of 3 to 4 minutes. It is the drug of choice in cerebral stroke.

Preparation and Dosage

Alteplase injection (100 mg/vial)—initially 15 mg IV bolus injection followed by IV infusion of 0.75 mg/kg of body weight over 30 minutes (not exceeding 50 mg) and then 0.5 mg/kg (up to 30 mg) for 2 to 3 hours.

Adverse Reactions

It is less toxic than streptokinase. It can produce haemorrhage like streptokinase. It is very expensive.

Treatment of Haemorrhage

Antithrombolytic (antifibrinolytic) drug used is epsilon-amino caproic acid (Amicar, Hemocid): It is a lysine analog that binds to lysine binding sites on plasminogen and plasmin, thus blocking the binding of plasmin to target fibrin. It is a potent inhibitor of fibrinolysis and can reverse states that are associated with fibrinolysis. It is used to control bleeding due to thrombolytic therapy after prostatic surgery or after tooth extractions in hemophilics. It is rapidly absorbed after oral administration and is partly metabolized in the liver. About 50% of the drug is excreted unchanged in urine within 12 hours.

Preparation and Dosage

Epsilon-aminocaproic acid (Hamostat) tablet (0.5 g) and injection (5 g/20 ml vial): Initial loading dose of 5 g orally or IV slowly, followed by 1 g every hour till bleeding IV stops (maximum 30 g in 24 hours).

Adverse Reactions

It can rarely cause myopathy and muscle necrosis.

Plasma Expanders

Plasma expanders are high molecular weight compounds, given IV and exert colloidal osmotic pressure to retain fluid in the intramuscular compartments. They are used as plama substitutes where there is loss of plasma as in severe burn and hypovolemic shock. Due to high molecular weight they cannot leave the vascular compartment to escape into tissue fluid easily. They cannot be filtered easily by the kidney. They cannot be quickly metabolized in the body. They should not be precipitated in the capillaries. They should be pharmacologically inert. Commonly used plasma expanders are human albumin, dextran 40, hetastarch (a synthetic high polymer, less antigenic than dextran) and degraded gelatin polymer (polygeline which is not antigenic). Human plasma albumin transfusion unlike plasma transfusion does not carry the risk of viral hepatitis and does not cause hypersensitivity reactions on repeatition of transfusion. It can also be used to replenish albumin in albumin deficient states like cirrhosis of liver and malnutritional oedema.

Dextran 40 (mol. wt 40 kDa) is a good plasma expander but it has some antigenicity and can cause hypernsensitivy reactivity. In some coses it can increase bleeding time.

Section VII

CARDIOVASCULAR PHARMACOLOGY

30

Drug Therapy of Congestive Cardiac Failure

CARDIAC GLYCOSIDES

Introduction

These are drugs obtained from digitalis and other plants and used in the treatment of congestive cardiac failure (CCF) characterized by raised jugular venous pressure, tachycardia, oedema and dyspnoea.

History: Crude plant products containing cardiac glycosides were used in the treatment of cardiac oedema (dropsy) for long time. William Withering, a Burmingham physician observed the diuretic effect of digitails in 1785. Cardiac effects of digitalis were demonstrated by James Meckenzie and Cushney in 1911. Harry Gold standardized the preparation of digitoxin in 1938. It was found to be much safer and more reliable than the older crude preparations and introduced for clinical uses.

Source: These are obtained from the leaf or seed of certain plants (as shown in **Table 30.1**).

Chemistry

They are steroidal glycosides containing a steroid nucleus (cyclopentanoperhydrophenanthrene ring, CPP ring). In the plants they remain as precursor glycosides (purpurea glycosides A and B; lanatosides A, B and C), which on mild alkaline and enzymatic hydrolysis liberate the active glycosides. The seeds of *Strophanthus gratus* or *kombe*, however, do not contain such precursors and liberate the glycosides directly. Each glycoside is made up of an aglycone (genin) and a sugar. If the sugar is glucose, the glycoside is called as a glucoside, e.g. strophanthin G or K. The sugar of digitalis glycoside is digitoxose. The pharmacological activity of the glycoside is contained in the aglycone, which has a less potent and more transient action than the parent glycoside. The sugar portion confers increased water solubility, cell permeability and potency on the aglycone. A cardiac

Table 30.1: Important cardiac glycosides	
Source	*Active glycosides*
Digitalis purpurea (leaf)	Digitoxin, Gitoxin, Gitalin
Digitalis lanata (leaf)	Digitoxin, Gitoxin, Digoxin
Strophanthus gratus (seed)	Strophanthin-G (Ouabain)
Strophanthus kombe (seed)	Strophanthin-K

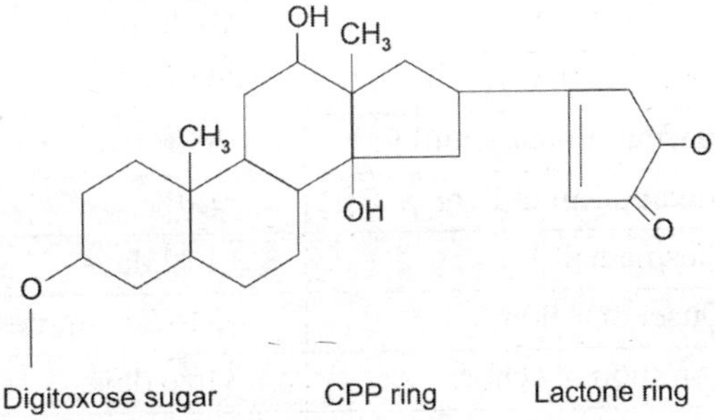

Fig. 30.1: Chemical structure of digoxin

glycoside molecule basically consists of three moities, *viz.* a sugar, a CPP ring and a lactone ring (as shown in **Fig. 30.1**).

Pharmacokinetics

They differ from each other in their pharmacokinetic properties (as shown in **Table 30.2**).

They are administered orally or IV, but not SC or I M, because their absorption from these sites are irregular (unreliable) and may produce pain, swelling and abscess formation.

They are excreted in bile (undergo enterohepatic recycling) and urine. They are filtered by the glomeruli and secreted by renal tubules. The body eliminates per day not a fixed quantity of a cardiac glycoside but a fixed proportion of the drug that is present in the body at the beginning of the day (exponential elimination). This is 30% in case of digoxin and 10% in case of digitoxin. Thus, on repeated daily administration, a digitalis glycoside will accumulate in the body producing cumulative toxicity, if its dose is not properly adjusted.

Digoxin

It is the commonly used cardiac glycoside. It is discussed as a prototype drug.

Pharmacological Actions of Digoxin

It is a cardiotonic drug, i.e. it increases myocardial contractility without increasing oxygen consumption of the heart (unlike cardiac stimulant like adrenaline). It has cardiac and extrala cardiac effects.

Cardiac effects: These are on:
- **Cardiac contractility:** It has a positive inotropic action on the heart. It increases the force of cardiac contraction by acting directly on the myocardium. It shortens the duration of systole and prolongs the duration of diastole. This gives greater time for both ventricular feeling and rest to the heart. The diastolic size of the heart is reduced. The more forceful contraction of the heart during systole results in more complete ventricular emptying with an increase in stroke volume and cardiac output. There is also an increased capacity to propel blood against increased peripheral resistance. By cardiotonic action it increases ventricular performance in the failing heart (CCF). In individual with normal heart, though it increases the force of cardiac contraction, but it does not increase cardiac output, because normal heart empties nearly completely during systole.

Mechanism of Action

The positive inotropic action of digoxin on the heart is due to binding and inhibition of the membrane bound enzyme Na$^+$, K$^+$-ATPase (sodium pump) which is responsible for Na$^+$ and K$^+$ transports across the myocardial cell membrane during phase 3 of action potential. As a result there is accumulation of intracellular Na$^+$ and loss of K$^+$ from the cell. Increased concentration of intracellular Na$^+$ increases the transport of Ca^{++} from ECF into

Table 30.2: Pharmacokinetic properties of some cardiac glycosides

Property	Digoxin	Digitoxin	Ouabain
Lipid solubility	Medium	High	Low
Intestinal absorption	40 to 60%	90 to 100%	< 5%
Plasma protein binding	25 to 30%	90 to 95%	0%
Metabolism in liver	< 30%	> 80%	< 5%
Plasma half-life	1 to 2 days	5 to 7 days	15 to 20 hours
Onset of action	15 to 30 minutes	2 to 3 hours	5 to 10 minutes
Duration of action	3 to 6 days	2 to 3 weeks	1 to 2 days
Route of administration	Oral, IV	Oral, IV	Oral

the cell across the cell membrane by Na^+/Ca^{++} exchange mechanism. One molecule of extracellular Ca^{++} is exchanged for 3 molecules of intracellular Na^+. Increased concentration of intracellular Ca^{++} triggers the release of large amount of Ca^{++} from the internal stores of sarcoplasmic reticulum (SR) into the cytoplasm of the cell through Ca^{++} channels. This Ca^{++} interacts with troponin-C of myofilaments and stimulates the reaction between actin and myosin forming actomycin, which is the contractile protein responsible for contraction of myocardial cell. Normally an energy dependent calcium pump (Ca^{++}-ATPase) in the sarcoplasmic reticulum actively pumps back Ca^{++} from the cytoplasm and decreases the concentration of Ca^{++} around the myofilaments.

The mechanism of positive inotropic action of digoxin is shown in **Fig. 30.2.**

- **Heart rate:** It has a negative chronotropic action on the heart. It decreases heart rate by both vagal and extravagal actions. It is a vagotonic drug in small dosage. It increases vagal tone by directly stimulating the vagal centre in medulla and reflexly through stimulation of no dose ganglia of vagus nerves and sensitization of carotid baroreceptors. By vagal action it reduces sinus (SA node) activity, decreases AV conduction velocity and prolongs refractory period of AV node but shortens atrial refractory period. This vagal action can be abolished by atropine, exercise or sectioning of the vagus nerves. In large dosage, it decreases the heart rate by a extravagal action, i.e. by a direct depressant action on the heart especially on SA and AV nodes. This action cannot be abolished by atropine or exercise. In an individual with CCF, the sympathetic activity is increased as a compensatory phenomenon. This leads to tachycardia. Digoxin decreases sympathetic tone by improving circulation and thus reduces heart rate.

Refractory period: It has varying actions on the refractory period of different cardiac tissues. It causes shortening of the atrial refractory period in small dosage (by vagal action) and prolongation of the refractory period in larger dosage (by direct action). It prolongs the refractory period of the AV node by both vagal and direct actions. This leads to a decrease in the transmission of the number of stimuli arising from the SA node to the ventricle. It also shortens the ventricular refractory period by a direct action.

Conduction velocity: In small dosage, it slightly increases the conduction velocity in the atria and ventricles (by vagal action) but in larger dosage it depresses their conduction velocity (by direct action). It depresses conduction velocity of AV node by both vagal and direct actions. It also

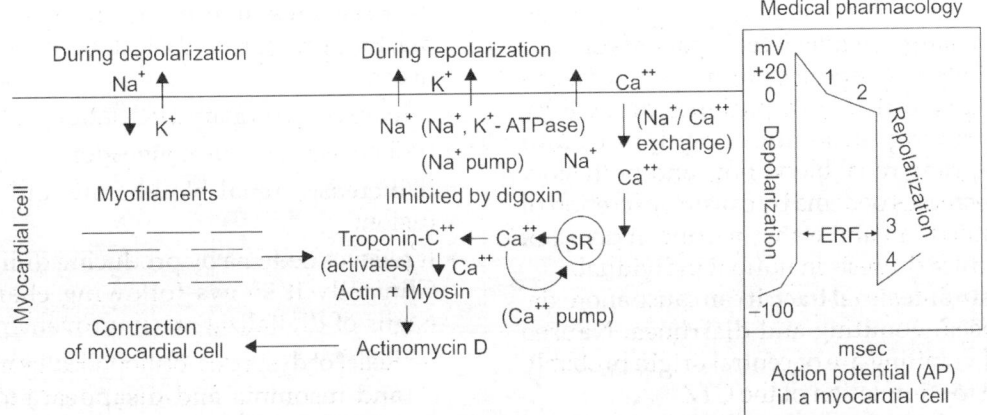

Fig. 30.2: Mechanism of myocardial cell contraction by digoxin

depresses conduction through the Purkinje fibre system of the ventricles by a direct action.

- **Automaticity:** It increases the ability of the Purkinje cells and the ventricular muscle to initiate impulses. This leads to the development of ventricular extra systoles, pulses bigeminy and even ventricular fibrillation (if accompanied by depression of the conduction velocity).
- **Coronary circulation:** It has no direct action on coronary vessels. It improves coronary circulation by increasing cardiac output and slowing the heart rate.
- **Electrocardiogram (ECG):** It prolongs P-R interval (due to slowing of AV conduction) and shortens Q-T interval (due to shortening of ventricular systole). In large dosage, it depresses ST segment and produces inversion of the first portion of the T wave (due to interference with repolarization). It can cause extra systoles, various degrees of AV block and ventricular fibrillation at the terminal event.

Extracardiac Effects

These are on:

- **Blood vessels:** It has a mild vasoconstrictor action on blood vessels (arterioles and venules), but this action in counteracted by increased cardiac output and decreased sympathetic activity. So there is little change in BP. It decreases raised venous pressure and relieves venous congestion such as engorged neck veins, pulmonary congestion and enlarged tender liver in patients of CCF.
- **Kidneys:** It produces diuresis (increased urinary output) in patients of CCF by improving systemic circulation and increasing renal blood flow and perfusion. It decreases oedema by causing excretion of retained salt and water in urine. It does not produce diuresis in normal individual.
- **Gastrointestinal tract:** It can cause anorexia, nausea, vomiting and diarrhoea. Nausea and vomiting are of central origin probably due to stimulation of the CTZ.
- **Central nervous system:** It can cause visual disturbances, mental confusion and disorientation. Visual disturbances are blurring of vision, photophobia, impairment of colour vision (especially green or yellow) and dark spot (halos or ring) in the centre of vision.

Clinical Uses (Indications) of Digoxin

It is used in chronic congestive cardiac failure, left ventricular failure and cardiac tachyarrhythmias of atrial origin with congestive cardiac failure.

a. **Congestive cardiac failure (CCF):** It is useful in the treatment of low output cardiac failure due to systolic dysfunction (pump failure) as in myocardial ischaemia, valvular defects, hypertension and congenital heart diseases, where it is capable of restoring cardiac function by positive inotropic action. It is of limited value in cardiac failure due to cor pulmonale (of lung cause) and cardiac myopathy (inflammatory or degenerative myocardial damage).

It is ineffective in high output cardiac failure as in severe anaemia, thyrotoxicosis, beriberi, arteriovenous fistula or pulmonary emphysema.

It improves cardiac function in failing heart by following ways:

- It increases the force of cardiac contraction (positive inotropic action).
- It decreases heart rate (negative chronotropic action).
- It increases cardiac output, which decreases residual blood in heart, end diastolic pressure and diastolic size of the heart.
- It increases coronary circulation.
- It decreases venous congestion.
- It increases renal blood flow and perfusion.
- It relieves oedema by producing diuresis. Clinically it shows following changes (signs of digitalization/improvement):
  - Relief of dyspnoea, orthopnoea, cyanosis and insomnia and disappearance of basal rales (by decreasing pulmonary congestion).

– Relief of tachycardia and ventricular gallop (by decreasing heart rate).
– Relief of venous congestion (engorged neck veins, pulmonary congestion and enlarged tender liver).
– Relief of oedema (by increasing urinary output).
– Change of dry and paper-like skin to normal moist and elastic skin (by increasing systemic circulation).

Congestive cardiac failure is treated by following measures:
- Bed rest (to limit physical activity).
- Restriction of dietary salt (NaCl) intake and promotion of sodium excretion by diuretics.
- Administration of digoxin or vasodilators.
- Use of ACE inhibitors to reduce neuro-humoral activation in CCF.
- Stopping of drugs that contribute to CCF, e.g. β-blockers, Ca^{++} channel blockers, NSAIDs and corticosteroids.

b. **Acute left ventricular failure:** It is used in the treatment of acute left ventricular failure in patients with hypertensive or ischaemic heart disease and aortic valve disease. It relieves dyspnoea and orthopnoea in these patients. If significant hypertension is present, it should be treated with an anti-hypertensive drug. Acute left ventricular failure with pulmonary oedema is treated by following measures:
- Upright (propped up) posture of the patient.
- Oxygen inhalation.
- IV morphine or frusemide and amino-phylline.
- IV digoxin in patients with atrial tachy-arrhythmias.
- Sublingual nitroglycerine or nifedipine.
- IV sodium nitropruside or nitroglycerine.
- Orally losartan (25 to 50 mg once daily to continue).

c. **Atrial tachyarrhythmias with CCF:** It is used in:
- **Paroxysmal supraventricular (atrial) tachycardia (PSVT):** In this condition, the atrial rate is 120 to 200/minute and atrial contractions are regular and synchronous (1:1 AV conduction). It improves this condition by vagal stimulant action causing slowing of AV conduction of impulses. It takes longer time to act and so less preferred than β-blockers or Ca^{++} channel blockers in this conditon.
- **Atrial flutter (AFl):** In this condition, the atrial rate is 200 to 350/minute and atrial contractions are regular and synchronous. Some degrees of AV block are produced here. It increases this AV block and thus decreases ventricular rate (by concealed conduction of impulses). It may convert atrial flutter to atrial fibrillation by decreasing atrial refractory period and making it inhomogeneous. In about 50% of patients, when digoxin is stopped after conversion to atrial fibrillation, then the fibrillation converts to normal sinus rhythm, as the cause of atrial inhomo-genicity is gone.
- **Atrial fibrillation (AF):** In this condition, the atrial rate is more than 350/minute and atrial contractions are irregular and asyn-chronous. It controls ventricular rate in AF with CCF by decreasing AV conduction of impulses and prolonging the refractory period of the conducting tissue (AV node and bundle of His) by vagal stimulant and direct myocardial depressant actions. It thus protects the ventricle from continuous bombardment of irregular impulses arising from the ectopic foci in the atrium.

Contraindications of Digoxin

These are given as follows:
- **Hypokalemia/hypercalcaemia:** It increases the binding of digoxin with Na^+, K^+-ATPase leading to increased toxicity of digoxin.
- **Elderly patients/severe hepatic or renal impairment:** These patients are more sensitive to digoxin.
- **Thyroid diseases:** Hyperthyroid patients are more prone to develop cardiac arrhy-thmias by digoxin, whereas hypothyroid patients are more sensitive to digoxin.

- **Heart (AV) block:** Partial heart block is converted to complete heart block by digoxin producing worsening of the condition.
- **Wolff-Parkinson-White (WPW) syndrome:** Digoxin causes rapid transmission of atrial impulses to the ventricle through accessory pathway (bypass tract) present in the heart by decreasing refractory period of the bypass tract in 1/3rd of patients leading to ventricular fibrillation.
- **Ventricular tachycardia:** Digoxin may precipitate ventricular fibrillation.
- **Recent myocardial infarction:** Digoxin may produce ventricular arrhythmias in this condition.
- **Acute myocarditis (diphtheritic/acute rheumatic carditis/toxic carditis/constrictive pericarditis/presence of tight mitral stenosis):** In it, response to digoxin is poor and can produce cardiac arrhythmias.

Preparations and Dosage of Cardiac Glycosides

- Digoxin (Lanoxin) tablet (0.125, 0.25 mg).
- Digoxin injection (0.25 mg/ml).
- Digitoxin (Crystodigin) tablet (0.1 mg).
- Lanatoside-C (Cedilanid) injection (0.25 mg/ml).
- Strophanthin-G (Ouabain) injection (0.25 mg/ml).

The method of administration of cardiac glycoside (digitalization) depends on the severity of CCF **(Table 30.3)**.

In mild or moderate CCF, slow digitalization is done. For this no initial loading dose is required.

Digoxin (0.25 mg) or digitoxin (0.1 mg) is administered orally once daily to digitalize the patient within a week. If there is no satisfactory improvement then the dose is gradually increased. If a stable clinical state is maintained for three months, then the drug is withdrawn.

In severe CCF, rapid digitalization is done. For this an initial loading dose orally is given followed by maintenance dose orally.

Digitoxin is not suitable for this purpose, because it has a slow onset of action.

Adverse Reactions (Toxicity) of Digoxin

These are given as follows:

- **Cardiac toxicity:** They produce cardiac arrhythmias due to disturbed impulse formation or disturbed impulse conduction or both. Disorders of impulse formation are due to ectopic pacemaker activity. The commonest manifestation are ventricular extrasystoles (ectopic beats), pulsus bigeminus (coupled beats) and partial or complete AV block. Less common manifestations are AV dissociation, paroxysmal atrial tachycardia, sinus bradycardia, SA arrest or exit block, ventricular tachycardia and ventricular fibrillation. Thus, they can

Table 30.3: Dosage of cardiac glycosides

	Loading dose	Maintenance dose
Digoxin or	0.5 to 0.75 mg 8 hourly (3 doses)	0.125 to 0.25 mg daily
Digitoxin	0.2 to 0.3 mg 12 hourly (2 doses)	0.05 to 0.1 mg daily

In very severe CCF (emergency), one of the following drugs is given IV rapidly followed by oral administration in maintenance dose daily.

Digoxin or	0.75 to 1.5 mg IV	
Ouabain or	0.5 to 1 mg IV	Action starts within 10 to 20 minutes and reaches a peak in 1 to 2 hours.
Lanatoside	0.75 to 1.5 mg IV	

produce almost every types of cardiac arrhythmias.

- **Extracardiac toxicity:** These are of following types:
  - **Gastrointestinal toxicity:** These are anorexia, nausea, vomiting, abdominal pain and diarrhoea.
  - **Neurological (CNS) toxicity:** These are mental confusion, disorientation, insomnia, restlessness, neuralgia, muscle weakness, nightmares, delirium and visual disturbances (as mentioned before).
  - **Miscellaneous toxicity:** These are skin rashes, eosinophilia and gynaecomastia (due to steroid nucleus of the glycoside).

Drug Interactions of Digoxin

- Drugs like quinidine, verapamil, methyldopa and indomethacin (NSAIDs) increase serum digoxin levels producing toxicity.
- Drugs like rifampicin (by induction of hepatic microsomal enzymes) and antacids, neomycin and kaolin pectin preparations (by reducing the bioavailability of digoxin) reduce serum digoxin levels decreasing therapeutic effects.

Important Symptoms and Signs of Digoxin Toxicity

- Anorexia, nausea and vomiting.
- Decrease in the pulse rate below 60 per minute, presence of extra systoles, pulsus bigeminus or any other arrhythmia.

Treatment of Digoxin Toxicity

- Digoxin is stopped.
- Diuretic if administered is stopped.
- Serum potassiun is estimated and potassium chloride is administered in the dosage of 1 to 2 g 6 hourly orally or by slow IV infusion with 5% dextrose solution to treat mild toxicity. It is contraindicated in AV block, hyperkalemia or severe renal insufficiency.
- Atropine sulphate is administered in the dosage of 0.6 to 1.2 mg IM twice daily to treat bradycardia and heart block.

- Propranolol is administered in the dosage of 40 to 80 mg orally in divided doses or 0.5 to 1 mg IV twice daily to treat supraventricular tachyarrhythmias. Verapamil is contraindicated here because it increases serum digoxin concentration.
- Phenytoin or lignocaine is administered IV to treat ventricular tachyarrhythmias specially ventricular fibrillation. Phenytoin is used in the dosage of 100 mg IV slowly every 5 minutes till arrhythmia is corrected. Lignocaine is used in the dosage of 1 to 2 mg per minute by slow IV infusion with 5% dextrose solution.
- Antidigoxin immunotherapy by using digoxin specific Fab antibodies (fragments) obtained from ovine antidigoxin antisera (sheep derived protein) is done in severe toxicity. It is rapidly acting, highly effective and safe in treating life-threatening digoxin toxicity, including cases of massive ingestion of digoxin for suicidal purpose. It is administered IV with normal saline solution in full neutralizing dose taking 30 to 60 minutes.

  It is an effective antidote in digoxin or digitoxin toxicities.

Other Drugs Used in Congestive Cardiac Failure

- **Diuretics,** e.g. hydrochlorothiazide, frusemide and amiloride. They act by reducing extracellular fluid volume and ventricular filling pressure (preload). They decrease oedema and also decrease afterload on the heart by arteriolar dilatation.
- **Vasodilators:** They may be arteriolar vasodilator, venous vasodilator or both. They are of following groups:
  - ACE inhibitors, e.g. captopril, enalapril and lisionopril. They act by decreasing both preload and afterload on the heart due to both arteriolar dilatation and venous dilatation.
  - Angiotensin receptor antagonist, e.g. Losartan. It is useful in left ventricular failure (LVF) and acts by decreasing ventricular preload.

– Nitrovasodilators, e.g. sodium nitroprusside, glyceryltrinitrate (nitroglycerine) and isosorbide dinitrate. They are useful in acute or chronic CCF. They act by decreasing ventricular filling pressure (preload), by decreasing venous return to the heart due to venous dilatation. Sodium nitroprusside also decreases afterload by arteriolar dilatation.

– Direct vasodilators, e.g. hydralazine and nicorandil. They act by decreasing afterload on the heart by arteriolar dilatation on the heart.

– Calcium (Ca^{++}) channel blockers, e.g. nifedipine and amlodipine. They act by decreasing afterload on the heart by arteriolar dilatation. They can also decrease ventricular preload by venodilatation, causing venous pooling.

– Phosphodiesterase-III inhibitors (Inodilators), e.g. amrinone, milrinone and vesnarinone.

These are synthetic bipyridines. They produce positive inotropic action on the heart and direct vasodilation (dilate both arterioles and veins). They increase cAMP concentration in myocardial cells. They are useful in CCF and left ventricular failure (LVF). They are administered by IV infusion with 5% dextrose solution. Dose of Amrinone (Cardiotone is 5 to 10 mg/kg/minute. They can produce cardiac arrhythmias, thrombocytopenia and hepatic damage.

• Adrenergic receptor antagonists, e.g. prazosin, phentolamine, labetalol and carvedilol. They act by decreasing both preload and afterload on the heart.

• β-adrenergic receptor agonists, e.g. dobutamine and prenalterol. They act by positive inotropic action with little chronotropic action on the heart. They increase myocardial cAMP concentration by activating adenylate enzyme. They tend to increase myocardial O_2 consumption and so less preferred in CCF.

Commonly used vasodilators in CCF

• Captopril (12.5 to 25 mg twice daily) or enalapril (10 to 20 mg once daily) or lisinopril (2.5 to 10 mg twice daily).

• Isosorbide dinitrate (20–40 mg orally or 5 to 10 mg sublingually 6 hourly) or glyceryl trinitrate IV (0.2 to 10 µg/kg/min) or as ointment (5 to 6 mg transdermally).

• Nifedipine (10 to 30 mg thrice daily) or amlodipine (2.5 to 10 mg once daily).

• Losartan (25 to 50 mg twice daily)

• Amrinone (5 to 10 µg/kg/min IV)

• Hydralazine (50 to 100 mg 8 hourly)

• Prazosin (1 to 5 mg 6 hourly).

31

Drug Therapy of Angina Pectoris

INTRODUCTION

The primary symptom of ischaemic heart disease is angina pectoris, caused by transient episodes of myocardial ischaemia. These episodes of ischaemia are due to an imbalance in the myocardial oxygen supply demand relationship and may be caused by an increase in myocardial oxygen demand (determined by heart rate, ventricular wall tension and ventricular contractility) or by a decrease in myocardial oxygen supply (determined by coronary blood flow, radiating to the left shoulder and flexor aspect of left arm. Angina may occur in a stable pattern over many years or may become unstable, increasing in frequency or severity and even occurring at rest. In typical stable angina, there is fixed atherosclerotic narrowing of an epicardial coronary artery, upon which exertion,

emotional stress, etc. superimpose an increase in mycocardial oxygen consumption. In variant angina, focal or diffuse coronary vasospasm episodically reduces coronary blood flow. In aortic pressure and oxygen carrying capacity of blood) or by both (**Fig. 31.1**).

There are three types of angina

1. Typical (classical/exertional/effort) angina.
2. Variant (Prinzmetal's/vasospastic) angina.
3. Unstable (crescendo/preinfarction) angina.

Both typical and variant angina are commonly experienced as a heavy, pressing, substernal discomfort (complaint by the patient as pain), often the majority of patients with unstable angina, rupture of an atherosclerotic plaque with consequent platelet adhesion and aggregation decreases coronary blood flow severely. They experience pain frequently, even with minimum exertion. It is

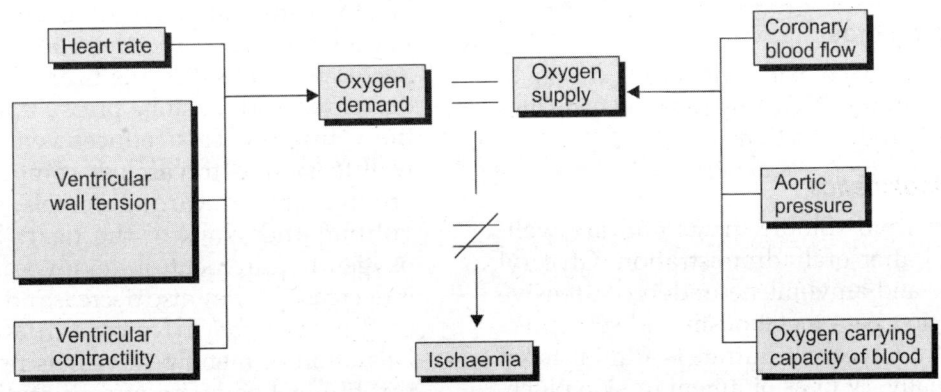

Fig. 31.1: Mechanism of myocardial ischaemia

a serious condition as it leads to myocardial infarction if immediate surgery is not done. In it coronary angioplasty or coronary artery bypass grafting (bypass surgery) is done. In atherosclerosis, there is deposition of fatty material in the subendothelial layer of coronary arteries. Usually bigger arteries (epicardial arteries) are affected but not the arterioles of the coronary system. As a result of atherosclerotic deposition (plaque), the overlying intima is elevated and the arterial lumen is narrowed leading to stenosis of coronary blood vessels.

Classification of Antianginal Drugs

These are of five groups:

1. Organic nitrates, e.g. glyceryl trinitrate (nitroglycerine), isosorbide dinitrate and isosorbide 5-mononitrate. First two are used sublingually in acute attack of angina pectoris. Other drugs are used orally for prophylaxis.
2. Calcium channel blockers, e.g. verapamil, nifedipine, diltiazem, nicardipine and felodipine.
3. β-adrenergic receptor antagonists, e.g. propranolol, atenolol, metoprolol and acebutolol.
4. Potassium channel openers, e.g. nicorandil, pinacidil and cromakalin.
5. Miscellaneous drugs, e.g. dipyridamole trimatazidine, oxyfedrine, cyclandelate, etc.

DISCUSSION OF INDIVIDUAL GROUP OF DRUGS

Organic Nitrates

They are nitrogen oxide containing drugs. In the body nitrates (NO_3^-) are reduced to nitrites (NO_2^-) to produce action.

Pharmacokinetics

They are lipid-soluble drugs and are well-absorbed after oral administration. Glyceryl trinitrate and amyl nitrite undergo extensive hepatic first pass metabolism and so ineffective orally. Glyceryl trinitrate is administered sublingually, IV or as ointment or skin patch, where it bypasses hepatic metabolism and also acts rapidly. Amyl nitrite is administered as inhalation. Other nitrates are administered orally or sublingually. They are metabolized in the liver by the enzyme glutathione reductase and excreted in urine and through lungs (especially amyl nitrite).

Pharmacological Actions

Mechanism of Action

They act by forming reactive free radical nitric oxide (NO) by the action of NO synthetase in the smooth muscle cell. This nitric oxide interacts with and activates the membrane enzyme guanyl cyclase leading to increased synthesis of cGMP from GTP in the smooth muscle cell. cGMP activates (stimulates) a protein kinase (PK), which produces dephosphorylation of the light chain of myosin leading to relaxation of the smooth muscle. Normally, phosphorylation of myosin light chain regulates the maintenance of the contractile state of the smooth muscle through calcium calmodulin (a protein) complex by promoting interaction between actin and myosin. Endothelial derived relaxing factor (EDRF) is probably the free radical nitric oxide (NO).

Nitrates produce following effects:

- **Cardiovascular effects:** These are as follows:
  - **Systemic blood vessels:** They are predominantly venodilators. In larger doses they also dilate arterioles. Due to generalized vasodilatation, they cause pooling of blood in veins leading to decreased venous return to the heart and decreased preload to the heart. There is decreased end diastolic pressure in both the ventricles. This reduces ventricular wall tension, extravascular compression around subendocardial vessels, stroke volume and work of the heart. Thus, oxygen requirement of the myocardium is decreased. They also decrease afterload of the heart by arteriolar dilatation. Dilatation of meningeal vessels produce throbbing headache and dilatation of

cutaneous vessels of face and neck producing flushing of face and neck. They produce fall of BP by decreasing total peripheral resistance.

– **Coronary blood vessels:** They dilate normal coronary vessels but they cannot adequately dilate atherosclerotic coronary vessels. This is because they selectively dilate large epicardial vessels and help in redistribution of blood from blood vessels in nonischaemic area to ischaemic subendocardial vessels by opening of collateral vessels. They do not increase coronary blood flow.

– **Heart:** They cause relief of angina by improving coronary circulation due to opening of collateral vessels. They increase exercise tolerance in most patients without increasing their angina index (= heart rate × aortic pressure × ejection time). Angina index signifies myocardial oxygen consumuption. Nitrates decrease angina index and so the duration of exercise by the patient is increased.

• **Effects on nonvascular smooth muscles**

They can relax almost all types of smooth muscle. Bronchial smooth muscle is relaxed irrespective of the cause of the pre-existing tone. The muscles of the biliary tract, including those of the gallbladder, biliary duct and sphincter of Oddi are effectively relaxed. Smooth muscles of GIT including that of the oesophagus can be relaxed and its spontaneous motility is decreased. Similarly, urethral and uterine smooth muscles are relaxed but these effects are somewhat unpredictable. They can antagonize the spasmogenic action of opioids and other drugs.

Clinical Uses of Nitrates

These are given as follows:

• **Angina pectoris:** They are used in all types of angina pectoris for treatment and prevention. To relieve pain of acute attack of angina pectoris, glyceryl trinitrate or isosorbide dinitrate is used sublingually.

For prevention of acute attack of angina pectoris, isosorbide dinitrate, isosorbide mononitrate or erythrityl tetranitrate is used orally or glyceryl trinitrate is applied as transdermal ointment or skin patch.

• **Acute left ventricular failure:** Glyceryl trinitrate produces dramatic relief in paroxysmal nocturnal dyspnoea of left ventricular failure (LVF). It decreases pulmonary congestion (oedema) by causing peripheral vasodilation, pooling of blood in the veins and decreasing venous return to heart. It decreases both afterload and preload to the heart. Other drugs that are used in this condition are morphine, frusemide and aminophylline.

• **Congestive cardiac failure (CCF):** Glyceryl trinitrate and isosorbide dinitrate are useful in the management of acute or chronic congestive cardiac failure due to ischaemic heart disease.

• **Acute myocardial infarction (AMI):** Glyceryl trinitrate may be used to produce vasodilation and to reduce infarct size. It should be done in intensive coronary care unit under supervision of a specialist.

• **Biliary colic and oesophageal spasm:** Glyceryl trinitrate or isosorbide dinitrate is used to relieve muscle spasm by spasmolytic action.

• **Cyanide poisoning:** Amyl nitrite by inhalation or sodium nitrite by IV administration (10 ml of 3% solution) is used in the treatment of sodium or potassium cyanide poisoning. The lethal action of cyanide (CN⁻) ion is due to tissue anoxia caused by chelation of ferric part of the respiratory enzyme cytochrome oxidase. The specific treatment is to use the chelating agent, cobalt edetate which chelates cyanide ion. Alternative drug is sodium nitrite, which converts haemoglobin to methaemoglobin and methaemoglobin competes with cytochrome oxidase for the cyanide ion. Combination of methaemoglobin with cyanide ion forms cyanomethaemoglobin. It is converted to methaemoglobin and sodium thiocyanate by sodium thiosulphate

(50 ml of 25% soln IV). Sodium thiocyanate is excreted in urine.

Preparations and Dosage

- Glyceryl trinitrate (Angised) tablet (0.5 mg)—0.5 mg sublingually and repeated every five minutes for three doses till relief of pain occurs. When the pain is relieved, the tablet is spit out from the mouth to avoid side effects.
- Glyceryl trinitrate sustained release (Nitro-retard) capsule (2.5 mg)—2.5 mg orally twice daily.
- Glyceryl trinitrate (GTN) injection (1 mg/ml)—5 to 10 µg/min by IV infusion with normal saline.
- Glyceryl trinitrate (Nitrobid) transdermal ointment (2%) or skin patch (15 mg per inch)—to be applied on the skin of area over the chest every four hourly and without rubbing.
- Glyceryl trinitrate (Nitrolingual) lingual aerosol (0.4 mg/metered dose)—one metered dose every five minutes for three doses.
- Isosorbide dinitrate (Sorbitrate) sublingual tablet (5 mg)—5 to 10 mg sublingually.
- Isosorbide dinitrate (Sorbitrate) oral tablet (10 mg)—10 to 20 mg orally thrice daily.
- Isosorbide dinitrate (Sorbitrate) sustained release tablet (40 mg)—40 to 80 mg once or twice daily.
- Isosorbide 5-mononitrate (Monotrat, Imdur, Ismo) tablet (10, 30 mg)—10 to 30 mg orally twice daily.
- Amyl nitrite pearl (0.3 ml)—one pearl is broken in handkerchief and then inhaled.

Adverse Reactions of Nitrates

These are given as follows:

- **Headache and dizziness:** Nitrates produce throbbing headache and dizziness due to dilatation of meningeal and retinal vessels. It decreases gradually on repeated administration (due to development of tolerance) and can be controlled by aspirin or paracetamol. Factory workers, who manufacture explosives from nitroglycerine (GTN) are continously exposed to high concentration of nitrate. These workers find that on starting their work on Monday, they suffer from headache and dizziness. After one or two days, these symptoms disappear due to development of tolerance. At the end of week, i.e. on Sunday, as the factory is closed, so exposure to nitrate does not occur and tolerance disappears. On Monday, due to re-exposure to nitrate, headache and dizziness appear. This is called Monday sickness.
- **Flushing of face and neck:** It occurs due to dilatation of superficial blood vessels in face and neck.
- **Postural hypotension leading to syncope:** It occurs due to generalized vasodilatation. Cold sweats, nausea, vomiting and involuntary passage of urine and faeces may accompany postural hypotension. Head low position of the patient to increase venous return to the heart and administration of oxygen to prevent anoxia quickly correct the nitrate syncope. Marked hypotension may occur when nitrates are used with vasodilators, β-blockers or alcoholic beverages.
- **Skin rashes:** This intolerance occurs occasionally with nitrates.
- **Tolerance:** It develops within 24 hours after administration of nitrates. Headache, dizziness, flushing and postural hypotension disappear after repeated administration of nitrates (probably by causing exhaustion of the –SH groups). Tolerance is rare with sublingual nitrate, because of the intermittent exposure to the nitrate.

Sodium nitrate → Cyanide → Sodium thiosulphate

Haemoglobin ⟶ Methaemoglobin ⟶ Cyanomethaemoglobin ⟶ Methaemoglobin + Sodium thiosulphate excreted in urine

Contraindications of Nitrates

- Pregnancy
- Severe anaemia
- Hypertrophic obstructive cardiomyopathy.

Calcium (Ca⁺⁺) Channel Blockers

Calcium (Ca^{++}) ions enter the cell *via* Ca^{++} channels. There are three types of voltage sensitive Ca^{++} channels, *viz.* L, T and N. Most well-known channels are L-channels (voltage dependent slow Ca^{++} channels), through which Ca^{++} ions enter the intracellular fluid (ICF) from the extracellular fluid (ECF). Calcium channel blockers block the L-channels and thus inhibits Ca^{++} influx. Calcium ions which enter the ICF serve two major functions, *viz.* (1) cause development of action potential (AP) and (2) cause muscle contraction. Calcium channel blockers are coronary vessel dilators and effective in reducing or preventing the acute attacks of all types of angina pectoris. They are primarily arteriolar dilators (i.e. they reduce peripheral vascular resistance) and so decrease afterload on the heart. They reduce BP, work of the heart and myocardial oxygen consumption during rest and exercise. They increase coronary blood flow and exercise tolerance. They also cause relaxation of the medium sized arteries, e.g. epicardial arteries. For this reason, they are very effective in variant (vasospastic/Prinzmetal) angina, where β-blockers are contraindicated.

Preparations and Dosage of Commonly Used Drugs

- Verapamil (Isoptin) tablet (40, 80 mg)— 40 to 80 mg twice daily.
- Verapamil (Isoptin) injection (5 mg/2 ml)—5 mg IV in acute coronary arterial spasm under ECG monitoring.
- Nifedipine (Calcigard) capsule (5, 10 mg)—5 to 10 mg thrice daily.
- Nifedipine sustained release (Calcigurd retard) tablet (20 mg)—20 mg once daily.
- Diltiazem (Dilzem) tablet (30, 60 mg)— 30 to 60 mg 3 to 4 times daily.

- Amlodipine (Amlogard) tablet (2.5, 5, 10 mg)—2.5 to 10 mg once daily.

Adverse Reactions

Constipation and bradycardia are common side effects of verapamil. These are less with other calcium channel blockers. These drugs are discussed in detail with antihypertensive drugs.

β-adrenergic Receptor Antagonists (Blockers)

These are effective in reducing or preventing the acute attacks of angina pectoris except variant (Prinzmetal/vasospastic) angina, where they may worsen the condition. They have cardioprotective effects by blocking $β_1$ receptor in the heart. They decrease myocardial oxygen consumption during rest and exercise. They increase exercise tolerance by decreasing cardiac response (tachycardia) to adrenergic activity during exercise. They increase blood flow to the ischaemic area by coronary vasodilation. They decrease afterload of the heart by producing arteriolar dilatation. They reduce BP by various mechanisms (discussed in ANS Pharmacology).

Preparations and Dosage of Commonly Used Drugs

- Propranolol hydrochloride (Inderal) tablet (10, 40 mg)—10 to 40 mg thrice daily.
- Atenolol (Aten) tablet (50, 100 mg)—50 to 100 mg once daily.
- Metoprolol (Metolar) tablet (100 mg)—100 to 200 mg twice daily.

Adverse Reactions

Their common side effects are bradycardia, bronchospasm, headache, insomnia, nightmares, muscle weakness, fatigue and cold extremities.

These drugs are discussed in detail in ANS Pharmacology.

Potassium (K⁺) Channel Openers (Activators)

These are newer antianginal drugs for prophylaxis of angina pectoris. Nicorandil (Nikoran) tablet (5, 10 mg) is used twice daily.

MISCELLANEOUS DRUGS

Dipyridamole

It is a coronary dilator, but unlike nitrates, which dilate coronary conductance vessels (venules), it dilates coronary resistance vessels (arterioles). It acts as coronary dilator by increasing plasma adenosine level due to inhibition of the uptake of adenosine into RBCs and other tissues and thus allowing it to produce dilatation of coronary vessels. It also inhibits phosphodiesterase enzyme leading to accumulation of cAMP in the cell. By dilating the arterioles in the nonischaemic area, it diverts the blood flow from the ischaemic area (where the blood flow is already reduced) to the non-ischaemic area. This produces the phenomenon called coronary steal. It has also a weak platelet inhibiting action and can be used as anti-thrombotic drug. It has only prophylactic value in angina pectoris. Along with aspirin it can be used to prevent acute myocardial infarction in unstable angina (hydrallazine also produces coronary steal phenomenon).

Preparations and Dosage
- Dipyridamole (Persantin) tablet (50 mg)—50 to 100 mg twice or thrice daily.
- Dipyramole (75 mg) with aspirin (150 mg) tablet (Dynasorin)—one tablet daily.

Trimatazidine

It is a new calcium channel blocker. It is claimed to exert a cytoprotective effect on myocardial metabolism in the presence of ischaemia. It has no effect in the presence of normal oxygen supply to the myocardium. It maintains normal left ventricular function without exerting any haemodynamic effect. It relieves angina of effort in patients with stable angina. It is used as tablet (20 mg) twice daily. Other drugs like oxyfedrine, cyclandelate, lidoflazine, perhexiline maleate, nicotic acid, nicotinylxanthenate and papaverine were used in the past in angina pectoris, but they are now obsolete, due to availability of better drugs.

32

Drug Therapy of Hypertension

INTRODUCTION

Blood pressure (BP) is the lateral pressure exerted by blood on the wall of the blood vessel (mainly arteriole) while flowing through it. It is the product of cardiac output and peripheral resistance (CO × PR). Systolic pressure is the maximum pressure during systole (contraction of the heart) and diastolic pressure is the minimum pressure during diastole (relaxation of the heart). Pulse pressure is the difference between systolic pressure and diastolic pressure (SP–DP). Mean pressure is the mean value of systolic pressure and diastolic pressure SP + DP/2. Normal BP in an adult is 110 to 130 mmHg of systolic pressure and 80 to 85 mmHg of diastolic pressure. It varies with age, state of health and conditions under which it is measured. BP is controlled mainly by two types of systems. One operates through the baroreceptors and autonomic nervous system. It is responsible for counteracting acute changes in BP. The second system is a humoral system (renin-angiotensin system), which has a slow response and is important in the long-term regulation of arterial pressure. This system is held responsible for the genesis of rapidly progressing hypertension *(Read angiotensin)*. When a person fails to adjust his BP on changing of posture (from lying down position to erect position) then BP falls. This is called postural or orthostatic hypotension.

When the BP is persistently high, i.e. more than 140/90 mmHg, then the condition is called hypertension. It is the most common cardiovascular disease. It causes pathological changes in blood vessels and produce hypertrophy of left ventricle. It is the principal cause of cerebral stroke, myocardial infarction due to disease of coronary arteries, left ventricular failure, dissecting aneurysm of aorta and renal insufficiency.

Causes of Hypertension

Hypertension may be primary (essential/ idiopathic) hypertension or secondary hypertension. In primary hypertension (about 90%) the underlying cause is unknown. In secondary hypertension (about 10%) the underlying cause is known, e.g. Cushing's syndrome (hypercorticism), thyrotoxicosis (hyperthyroidism), pheochromocytoma, acute or chronic glomerulonephritis, pyelonephritis, renal artery stenosis, polycystic kidney, coarctation of aorta, polycythemia vera, pregnancy, eclampsia or use of oral contraceptives. Primary hypertension is treated by antihypertensive drugs, while secondary hypertension is treated by removing the cause. If hypertension remains untreated for long time, it produces irrepairable damage to the vital organs like heart, kidneys, eyes and brain, as their normal functions depend on sufficient supply of blood. So hypertension should be treated properly if detected.

Diastolic pressure is the important index of BP. There are three grades of BP depending on diastolic pressure.

- **Mild hypertension**—diastolic pressure is 90 to 110 mmHg.
- **Moderate hypertension**—diastolic pressure is 111 to 130 mmHg.
- **Severe hypertension**—diastolic pressure is above 130 mmHg.

In moderate and severe hypertension there are also cardiac, renal and ocular changes (*see Medicine book*).

In malignant hypertension, the diastolic pressure is above 150 mmHg and there are papilloedema in eye, neurological changes in brain, cardiac abnormality and progressive reduction of renal function producing uraemia. Death may occur due to uraemia or cerebral haemorrhage. So emergency treatment is required.

Classification of Antihypertensive Drugs

These are of three groups (according to site or mechanism of action):

- **Diuretics**—these are given as follows:
  - Thiazides and related drugs, e.g. hydrochlorothiazide and chlorthalidone.
  - Loop diuretics, e.g. frusemide, bumetinide and ethacrynic acid.
  - Potassium sparing diuretics, e.g. amiloride, triamterene and spironolactone.
- **Sympatholytic drugs**—these are given as follows:
  - Centrally acting drugs, e.g. methyldopa, clonidine, guanabenz and guanfacine.
  - Autonomic ganglion blockers, e.g. trimethaphan camsylate.
  - Adrenergic neuron blockers, e.g. guanethidine, guanadrel and reserpine.
  - β-adrenergic antagonists, e.g. propranolol, atenolol, metoprolol and nebivolol.
  - α-adrenergic antagonists, e.g. prazosin, terazosin, doxazosin, phenoxybenzamine and phentolamine.
  - Mixed adrenergic antagonists, e.g. labetalol, dilevalol and carvedilol.
  - Catecholamine synthesis inhibitors, e.g. metyrosine.
- **Vasodilators**—these are of following types:
  - Directly acting vasodilators:
    - Arteriolar dilators, e.g. hydralazine, minoxidil and diazoxide.
    - Both arteriolar and venous dilators, e.g. sodium nitroprusside.
  - Indirectly acting vasodilators:
    - Ca^{++} channel blockers, e.g. verapamil, diltiazem, nifedipine, amlodipine, nicardipine, nimodipine, felodipine and isradipine.
    - ACE inhibitors, e.g. captopril, enalapril, lisinopril, perindopril and ramipril.
    - Angiotensin-II receptor antagonists, e.g. losartan, candesartan, etc.

Sites of action of antihypertensive drugs: They produce their actions by acting at different sites (as shown in **Fig. 32.1**).

DISCUSSION OF INDIVIDUAL GROUPS OF DRUGS

Diuretics

These are primary drugs in all grades (mild, moderate and severe) of hypertension. They lower BP by reducing extracellular fluid volume and cardiac output. In the initial stage, they increase excretion of sodium and water in urine. Subsequently, these effects return to normal by compensatory mechanisms in the body. On long-term therapy (about three weeks) they produce vasodilatation and reduction of total peripheral resistance by reducing Na^+ concentration in the smooth muscle of blood vessels, which decrease intracellular Ca^{++} concentration and thus makes the smooth muscle cells nonresponsive to endogenous noradrenaline and angiotensin-II to act on respective cell surface receptors. Thiazides and related diuretics are commonly used in hypertension. When a thiazide diuretic is used as a sole antihypertensive drug (monotherapy) it should be administered in a low dose (12.5 to 25 mg). When these

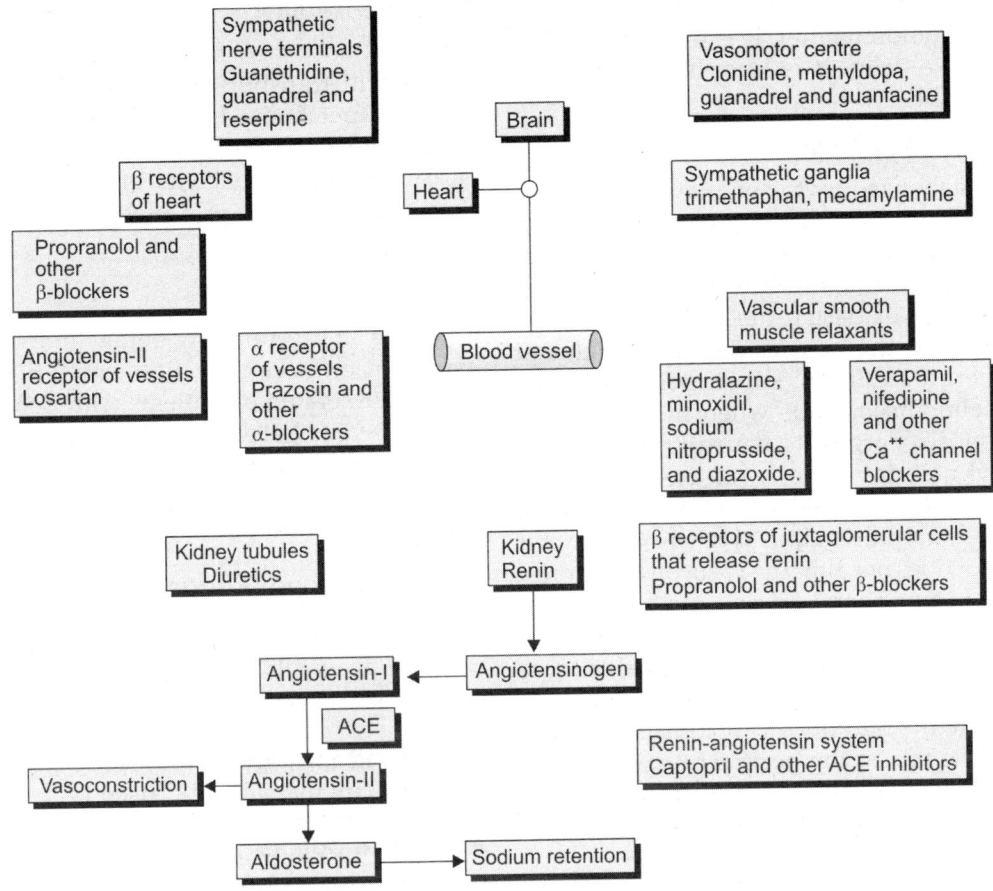

Fig. 32.1: Sites of action of antihypertensive drugs

diuretics are administered in the long-term treatment of hypertension, then they should be administered along with a K⁺ sparing diuretic like amiloride/triamterene to overcome the kaluretic effect of thiazides. In moderate and severe hypertension, thiazides are used in combination with vasodilators or some sympatholytic drugs. Common adverse effects of thiazides are sexual impotence, hypocalciuria, hypokalaemia, hyperuricemia leading to gout, muscle cramps, intolerance to carbohydrate (glucose) and alteration of plasma lipid profile (like β-blockers). Loop diuretics are less effective than thiazides as antihypertensive drugs in patients who have normal renal function. This is because they have short duration of effect. A single daily dose (20 to 40 mg) does not cause a significant net loss of Na⁺ for an entire 24 hours period. However, when these drugs are given twice daily, excessive diuresis is produced leading to more side effects than thiazides. They produce hypercalciuria, hypokalaemia, hyperuricemia leading to gout, glucose intolerance and alteration of plasma lipid profile (like thiazides). They are particularly useful in patients with azotemia and in patients with severe oedema associated with a vasodilator like minoxidil.

SYMPATHOLYTIC DRUGS

(i) Centrally Acting Drugs Methyldopa

It is the α-methyl analogue of dopa, which is a precursor of dopamine and noradrenaline. It is a prodrug, which exerts its antihypertensive action *via* an active metabolite (α-methyl noradrenaline). It is a potent antihypertensive drug. It is lipophilic and easily crosses BBB.

Mechanism of Action

It is metabolized by the enzyme dopa decarboxylase in the adrenergic neurons to α-methyl dopamine, which is then converted to α-methyl noradrenaline by the enzyme dopamine β-oxidase α-methyl noradrenaline is stored in the neurosecretory vesicles of adrenergic neurons, substituting for noradrenaline itself. Thus when the adrenergic neuron discharges its neurotransmitter, α-methyl noradrenaline is released instead of noradrenaline. α-methyl noradrenaline is as potent as noradrenaline as a vasoconstrictor and so it does not alter the vasoconstrictor response to peripheral adrenergic neurotransmission. Rather, it acts in the brain stem (VMC) to inhibit adrenergic neuronal outflow from the CNS (acting as an $α_2$-agonist) to attenuate the output of vasoconstrictor adrenergic signals to the peripheral sympathetic nervous system. This central effect is mainly responsible for its antihypertensive action.

Pharmacological Effects

It reduces vascular resistance without causing much change in cardiac output or heart rate in younger patients with uncomplicated hypertension. In older patients, cardiac output may be decreased as a result of decrease in heart rate and stroke volume. This is secondary to relaxation of veins and a reduction in preload on the heart. The fall of arterial BP is maximum in 6 to 8 hours after its administration. It produces less postural hypotension, as it does not completely block baroreceptor mediated vasoconstriction. It does not alter renal blood flow and GFR. It decreases renin secretion by the kidney but this is not necessary for its antihypertensive effect. It produces fluid retention on prolonged use, which blunts its antihypertensive effect. This is called pseudotolerance, which can be overcome by concurrent use of a diuretic.

Pharmacokinetics

It is well-absorbed from GIT by an active amino acid transport mechanism. It crosses BBB. It is metabolized in the liver by sulphate conjugation (about 60%). It is excreted in urine partly as sulphate conjugate and partly as unchanged form. It has a plasma t½ of 4 to 8 hours.

Clinical Uses

It is used in essential (moderate and severe) hypertension in combination with â diuretic. It is well-tolerated by patients with ischaemic heart disease, left ventricular hypertrophy, renal insufficiency, hyperthyroidism and during pregnancy and general anaesthesia. It is not indicated in pheochromocytoma.

Preparations and Dosage

- Methyldopa (Aldomet M-dopa) tablet (250 mg)—initially 250 mg twice daily and then gradually increased to 0.5 to 1 g twice daily.
- Methyldopa hydrochloride injection (50 mg/ml in 5 ml vial)—used IV.

Adverse Reactions

Its common side effects are sedation, drowsiness, headache, fatigue, lethargy, dryness of mouth, loss of libido, disturbed sleep, nightmares, bradycardia, constipation, nasal congestion, failure of ejaculation, peripheral oedema (due to fluid retention), Parkinsonism and hyperprolactinemia (causing gynaecomastia and galactorrhoea). Postural hypotension rarely occurs with it. It can also produce fever, hepatitis, leucopenia, thrombocytopenia, arthralgia, lupus erythematosus like syndrome, granulomatous skin eruptions, myocarditis, retroperitoneal fibrosis and pancreatitis (producing malabsorption and diarrhoea).

Clonidine

It is an imidazoline derivative. It is a potent antihypertensive drug. It is lipophilic and easily penetrates BBB.

Mechanism of Action

It is an α_2-adrenergic agonist like methyldopa. It acts by stimulating α_2-adrenergic receptors in the brain stem (VMC) resulting in a reduction in sympathetic outflow from the CNS. The decrease in plasma concentration of noradrenaline is responsible for hypotensive effect. Patients who have had a spinal cord transection above the level of the sympathetic outflow tracts do not produce hypotensive effect of clonidine. At doses higher than those required to stimulate central α_2-adrenergic receptors, they can activate α_2 receptors on vascular smooth muscle cells. This effect is responsible for initial vasoconstriction that occurs with overdose of clonidine, causing loss of therapeutic effect.

Pharmacological Effects

It lowers arterial BP by an effect on both cardiac output and peripheral resistance. In supine position, when the sympathetic tone of the blood vessel is low, it reduces both heart rate (by vagal stimulation) and stroke volume. In erect position, when the sympathetic outflow to the blood vessel is normally increased, that it reduces vascular resistance. It produces some degrees of postural hypotension due to reduction of venous return to the heart (secondary to systemic vasodilation). It produces partial inhibition (blunting) of sympathetic reflexes. It does not interfere with the haemodynamic response to exercise. So exercise induced hypotension is unusual. It decreases cardiac sympathetic tone leading to a reduction in myocardial contractility and heart rate. It does not alter renal blood flow and GFR. It often decreases the secretion of renin and so reduces plasma renin activity (PRA). It does not alter plasma lipid profile. It can decrease insulin secretion. On prolonged use it causes retention of sodium and development of tolerance to its antihypertensive effect. So a diuretic is to be used along with it.

Pharmacokinetics

It is a lipid-soluble drug and well-absorbed from GIT. It has a high volume of distribution.

It is partly metabolized in the liver and about one half of the drug is excreted unchanged in urine. It has a plasma t½ of about 12 hours and so it is administered twice daily.

Clinical Uses

It is used in moderate and severe hypertension in combination with a diuretic. It is also used in morphine, alcohol or nicotine withdrawal syndrome and menopausal hot flushes. It is used prophylactically in migraine.

Preparations and Dosage

- Clonidine hydrochloride (Catapress/Arkamin) tablet (0.1 mg)—0.1 to 0.2 mg twice daily.
- Clonidine hydrochloride transdermal patch—applied once a week.

Adverse Reactions

Its common side effects are drowsiness (central sedative action), lethargy (muscle weakness), vertigo, dizziness, dryness of mouth, nasal congestion, bradycardia, constipation, parotid pain and impotence (ejaculatory failure). It can also produce nausea, skin rashes, peripheral oedema (due to fluid retention), restlessness, hallucinations, insomnia, nightmares and mental depression. It potentiates insulin induced hypoglycaemia. In toxic dose it causes marked bradycardia, miosis and hypotension. It produces severe drowsiness when combined with propranolol. Clonidine should be withdrawn slowly after prolonged (chronic) use because sudden withdrawal of clonidine causes hyperirritability, tachycardia, headache, tremors, sweating and a dangerous rebound rise of BP. This is due to supersensitivity (upregulation) of α_1 receptors after prolonged inactivation or chronic suppression, allowing unopposed α_1-vasoconstriction by the high concentrations of circulating adrenaline and noradrenaline. Readministration of clonidine or use of labetalol or a combination of an alpha and a β-adrenergic blockers controls this withdrawal syndrome.

Guanabenz (Wytensin) and Guanfacine (Tenex)

These are newly introduced drugs acting like clonidine. They are available as tablets (2 mg and 1 mg respectively) and administered once daily. They have less adverse reactions than clonidine and methyldopa.

Autonomic Ganglion Blockers

These drugs are potent antihypertensive drugs but their use is limited to short term treatment of hypertension associated with dissecting aneurysm of aorta and in the production of controlled hypotension during surgery. The most useful drug for these purposes is trimethanphan camphor sulphonate/camsylate (Arfonad), which reduces arterial BP effectively by blocking sympathetic ganglia. It is administered by IV infusion at the rate of 0.3 to 5 mg/minute. The onset of hypotensive effect is within 5 minutes and the effect disappears with 15 minutes on discontinuation of the infusion. Tachyphylaxis to the antihypertensive effect develops after 24 to 48 hours. This is partly due to expansion of plasma volume and sensitivity can be restored by diuresis.

Adverse Reactions

It can produce paralytic ileus, constipation, bladder dysfunction, dryness of mouth, blurring of vision (by mydriasis and cycloplegia), postural hypotension and disturbances in sexual function (failure of ejaculation). In high dose, it can produce respiratory arrest.

Adrenergic Neuron Blockers Guanethidine

It is a guanidine containing compound. Guanidine group has a strongly basic nitrogen atom making the compound polar (ionized). It reaches its site of action by active transport into the neuron by the same transporter that is responsible for the uptake of noradrenaline. It is a potent antihypertensive drug.

Mechanism of Action

It inhibits the function of peripheral post-ganglionic adrenergic neurons. It is targeted uniquely to the peripheral adrenergic neurons, where it inhibits sympathetic function. In the neuron, it is concentrated within the neurosecretory vesicles, where it replaces noradrenaline. On prolonged use (chronic administration), it acts as a substitute neurotransmitter, i.e. it is stored in storage vesicles, depletes noradrenaline (normal neurotransmitter) and released by stimuli that normally release noradrenaline.

Pharmacological Effects

These are due to sympathetic blockade. It decreases cardiac and vascular sympathetic tone causing decrease in heart rate, cardiac output and peripheral vascular resistance. It does not decrease renin secretion by kidney and does not lower plasma renin activity. It decreases renal blood flow and GFR to some extent. It does not cross BBB and does not affect brain function.

Pharmacokinetics

It is incompletely (1/3rd) absorbed from the GIT. It is slowly metabolized in the liver and excreted in urine mainly as unchanged form. It has a plasma t½ of five days. It is accumulated in the body on prolonged administration producing cumulative toxicity.

Clinical Uses

It is used in moderate and severe hypertension with a diuretic and a vasodilator.

Preparation and Dosage

Guanethidine sulphate (Ismelin) tablet (25 mg)—25 to 50 mg once daily.

Adverse Reactions

It can produce postural hypotension, lightheadedness, dizziness, bradycardia, parotid pain, peripheral oedema, failure of ejaculation, nasal congestion, nausea, vomiting and troublesome diarrhoea. It may precipitate CCF due to fluid retention. Tricyclic antidepressants (Imipramine, etc.) inhibit the entry of guanethidine into the adrenergic neuron and can antagonize its antihypertensive action. It is contraindicated in pheochromocytoma as the sensitivity to pressor effects of adrenaline and noradrenaline is increased by guanethidine and it releases these catecholamines from the tumour.

Guanadrel (Hycor)

It is another guanidine containing adrenergic neuron blocker. It has pharmacological actions like guanethidine. It has more rapid onset and shorter duration of action than guanethidine. It is administered as tablet (10 mg) in the dosage of 10 to 30 mg once daily.

Reserpine

It is an alkaloid obtained from the root of the plant—*Rauwolfia serpentina (Sarpaganda).* It is a potent antihypertensive drug.

Mechanism of Action

It lowers arterial BP by both central and peripheral actions. Its peripheral action is more prominent than the central action. It binds strongly with storage granules in the adrenergic neurons and remains there for prolonged period of time. It slowly depletes catecholamines (noradrenaline, adrenaline and dopamine) and serotonin (5-HT) from the storage granules resulting in loss of neurotransmitters. Catecholamines that enter into the cytoplasm are destroyed by intraneuronal MAO and little or no active transmitter is released from nerve endings by nerve stimulation. This causes decrease in plasma concentration of noradrenaline leading to antihypertensive effect.

Pharmacological Actions

It decreases cardiac and vascular sympathetic tone leading to decrease in heart rate, cardiac output and peripheral vascular resistance. It decreases renin secretion by the kidney and lowers plasma renin activity. It does not alter renal blood flow and GFR. It produces pseudotolerance by causing fluid retention, which diminishes its antihypertensive effect. This can be overcome by concurrent use of a diuretic.

Pharmacokinetics

It is well-absorbed after oral administration. It is rapidly taken up by the lipid-rich tissues and easily reaches the CNS. It is metabolized in the liver and excreted slowly in urine mainly as metabolites. It can produce cumulative toxicity due to long plasma $t\frac{1}{2}$ and slow excretion in urine.

Clinical Uses

It is used in moderate and severe hypertension either alone or in combination with a diuretic and/or a vasodilator. In the past it was used as an antipsychotic drug but now obsolete.

Preparations and Dosage

- Reserpine hydrochloride (Serpasil) tablet (0.25 mg)—0.25 to 0.5 mg once daily.
- Reserpine hydrochloride injection (1.25 mg/ml)—1.25 mg IM.

Adverse Reactions

It can cause drowsiness (central sedative action), inability to concentrate, excessive salivation, nasal congestion, miosis, bradycardia, increased gastric secretion and diarrhoea due to parasympathetic predominance as a result of peripheral sympathetic blockade. It also produces postural hypotension, weight gain (due to increased appetite and retention of fluid), parkinsonism, endocrine disturbances (gynaecomastia and impotence in males and reduction in fertility in females), allergic reactions (thrombocytopenia and purpura) and mental depression with suicidal tendency.

β-adrenergic Antagonists

β-blockers like propranolol, atenolol and metoprolol are commonly used in hypertension (all grades) either alone or in combination with a diuretic and/or a vasodilator. Combination with a diuretic increases their antihypertensive effect and prevents development of tolerance after prolonged use. Combination with a vasodilator prevents reflex tachycardia of the vasodilator. They also reduce palpitation, angina and anxiety. Beta-blockers are discussed in detail in ANS Pharmacology.

α-adrenergic Antagonists

α-blockers like prazosin, terazosin, doxazosin, phenoxybenzamine and phentolamine are used in hypertension (all grades).

Prazosin (Minipress): It is a quinazoline derivative. It is a selective α-blocker. It blocks α_1 receptors in arterioles leading to a fall in BP. It is less likely to cause reflex tachycardia. It increases cardiac output and peripheral vascular resistance. It increases renin secretion by the kidney and plasma renin activity. It does not alter renal blood flow and GFR. It is used in mild to severe hypertension either alone or in combination with a diuretic, β-blocker or methyldopa. It is used orally as tablet (0.5 mg) in the dosage of 0.5 to 1 mg thrice daily. It is also used in CCF and benign prostatic hypertrophy (BPH). Its common side effects are 1st dose syncope, headache, dizziness, lethargy, constipation and peripheral oedema. The 1st dose effect (syncope) is due to severe fall of BP leading to fainting or syncopal attack on standing (postural hypotension). For this reason, the 1st dose of prazosin should be given at bed time. On long-term use this phenomenon disappears due to development of tolerance. Other α-blockers are discussed in ANS Pharmacology.

Mixed Adrenergic Antagonists

Combined α- and β-blockers like labetalol, dilevalol and carvedilol are used in pheochromocytoma before operation and hypertensive emergencies (crisis) to lower high BP by IV injection. Labetalol (Normodyne) is used IV in the rate of 2 mg/min to a maximum amount of 200 mg. It blocks all the effects of adrenaline and noradrenaline.

Catecholamines Synthesis Inhibitors

Metyrosine (Desmer): It is α-methyl para-tyrosine. It is an inhibitor of the enzyme-tyrosine hydroxylase, which converts tyrosine to dopa. It decreases catecholamines synthesis in about 50% of patients with pheochromocytoma. It is used for the preoperative treatment and long-term management of pheochromocytoma to lower BP. It is administered orally as capsule (250 mg) in the dosage of 250 to 500 mg thrice daily. It can produce postural hypotension, sedation, anxiety, tremors, gynaecomastia, sexual dysfunction and mental depression.

VASODILATORS

Directly Acting Vasodilators

Arteriolar Dilators

Hydralazine (Apresoline): It causes direct relaxation of arteriolar smooth muscle by an unknown mechanism. It lowers BP in normotensive and hypertensive subjects. Its effect on BP is slow in onset but prolonged. The fall of BP is accompanied by a decrease in total peripheral resistance and a compensatory increase in the heart rate (reflex tachycardia), stroke volume and cardiac output. It increases renal blood flow and GFR. It increases renin secretion by the kidney and plasma renin activity. It is used in moderate and severe hypertension in combination with a diuretic, β-blocker or reserpine. It is administered orally or parenterally (IM or IV) as tablet (25 mg) or injection (20 mg/ml) and the maximum dose is 100 mg/day in divided doses. It can produce nausea, vomiting, gastric hypersecretion, diarrhoea, postural hypotension, palpitation, tachycardia, anginal attack; headache, flushing, nasal congestion, tremors, dizziness, peripheral oedema and intolerance (fever, skin rash and polyneuritis). With high dose and prolonged use, a syndrome resembling acute rheumatoid arthritis or disseminated lupus erythematosus develops, which is treated by a corticosteroid for prolonged period.

Minoxidil (Mintop): It causes direct relaxation of arteriolar smooth muscle by acting as a K^+ channel opener. It activates ATPase-sensitive K^+ channels in the vascular smooth muscle and causes membrane hyperpolarization leading to relaxation of arteriolar smooth muscle. Its effects are similar to those of hydrallazine but it is more potent and more toxic than hydrallazine. It causes compensatory tachycardia, increased cardiac output and sodium retention. It is used in moderate and severe hypertension in combination with a β-blocker (to prevent tachycardia) or a diuretic (to prevent oedema). It is used orally as tablet (5 mg) in the dosage of 5 to 20 mg twice daily. It is also used as topical minoxidil lotion (2%) in male pattern baldness of head (applied twice daily for 3–6 months) to promote growth of hair. It can produce headache, lethargy, postural hypotension, tachycardia, anginal attack, pericardial effusion, pulmonary hypertension and hypertrichosis (growth of male type of hairs) on face, back, arms and legs (in females) on prolonged use.

Diazoxide (Hyperstat): It is another K+ channel opener which acts like minoxidil in causing direct relaxation of arteriolar smooth muscle. It has mechanism of action and pharmacological effects similar to minoxidil. Although it is well-absorbed orally but it is administered IV in severe hypertension and hypertensive emergencies (malignant hypertension). About 20 to 50% of the drug is excreted in urine as such and the rest is metabolized in the liver and is excreted as metabolites in urine. It has plasma t½ of 20 to 60 hours but its duration of action is 4 to 20 hours. It is administered by slow IV infusion at a rate of 15 to 30 mg/minute. Prior administration of a β-blocker increases its hypotensive effect. It should not be used in hypertension associated with coarctation of aorta or dissecting aneurysm of aorta, arteriovenous shunt, acute pulmonary oedema or ischaemic heart disease.

Adverse Reactions

It can produce peripheral oedema (by salt and water retention) and hyperglycaemia (due to inhibition of secretion of insulin from pancreatic β-cells). Retention of fluid can be avoided by restriction of salt and water. Use of a diuretic with diazoxide is not recommended as the patients with malignant hypertension are frequently volume depleted. It relaxes uterine muscle and may arrest labour when used to treat hypertensive crisis of eclampsia. Its rare side effects are nausea,

vomiting, flushing, local pain and inflammation after extravasation, excessive salivation and dyspnoea. Its long-term use can cause hypertrichosis like minoxidil.

Both Arteriolar and Venous Dilators

Sodium Nitroprusside: It is a short-acting nitrovenodilator. It is metabolized by smooth muscle cells to its active metabolite, nitricoxide (NO), which activates guanylate cyclase leading to the formation of cGMP producing vasodilatation. It is a non-selective vasodilator, dilating both arterioles and venules. It thus reduces arterial impedence and venous pooling. Due to its effect on venules, it produces greater hypotensive effect when the patient is upright (erect). It has little effect on regional distribution of blood. It does not alter renal blood flow and GFR. It increases renin secretion by the kidney and plasma renin activity. It causes moderate increase in heart rate in comparison to other vasodilators. It is used in hypertensive emergencies and in many situations when short-term reduction of cardiac preload and/or afterload is necessary as in dissecting aortic aneurysm (to lower BP), CCF (to increase cardiac output) and after myocardial infarction (to decrease myocardial oxygen demand). It is also used to produce controlled hypotension during anaesthesia (to reduce bleeding in surgical procedures). It should not be used in patients with COPD as it worsen arterial hypoxemia. It is available in vial containing 40 mg. The content of the vial is dissolved in 2 to 3 ml of 5% dextrose solution. This is added to 250 to 500 ml of 5% dextrose solution to produce a concentration of 50 to 100 µg/ml. The drug is administered as a controlled continuous infusion at a rate of 0.25 to 2.5 µg/kg/minute. Close monitoring of BP and cardiac conditions are necessary.

Adverse Reactions

It can produce severe hypotension (by excessive vasodilatation) and severe lactic acidosis (due to accumulation of cyanide in the body), if the infusion rate of it is greater than 5 µg/kg/minute. Accumulation of cyanide can be prevented by concomitant administration of sodium thiosulphate, which forms unstable thiocyanate for easy excretion in urine. Haemodialysis can be done in patients with renal failure to remove thiocyanate. Rarely excessive thiocyanate concentration can cause hypothyroidism by inhibiting iodine uptake by the thyroid gland.

Indirectly Acting Vasodilators
Ca⁺⁺ Channel Blockers (Calcium Antagonists)

These are an important group of drugs for the treatment of hypertension.

Classification

These are of following three groups according to chemical structure:

1. Phenylalkylamines, e.g. verapamil (hydrophilic).
2. Dihydropyridines, e.g. nifedipine, amlodipine, nicardipine, felodipine, nimodipine and isradipine (lipophilic).
3. Benzothiazepines, e.g. diltiazem (hydrophilic).

   Their use in hypertension comes from the understanding that fixed hypertension is the result of increased peripheral vascular resistance. As the contraction of vascular smooth muscle is dependent on the free intracellular Ca^{++} concentration, so inhibition of transmembrane movement of Ca^{++} decreases the total amount of Ca^{++} that reaches the intracellular sites.

Mechanism of Action

They produce inhibition of L-type voltage sensitive Ca^{++} channels in the vascular smooth muscle and thus lower BP by relaxing arteriolar smooth muscle and decreasing peripheral vascular resistance.

Pharmacological Effects

They lower BP and decrease both preload and afterload on the heart (i.e. reduces venous pooling and arterial impedence). By producing peripheral vascular resistance, they produce a reflex baroreceptor mediated sympathetic discharge. Mild to moderate tachycardia occurs with dihydropyridines due to stimulation of the SA node, whereas minimum or no tachycardia occurs with verapamil and diltiazem, because of the direct negative chronotropic effect of these two drugs. The increased adrenergic stimulation of the heart serves to counter the negative chronotropic effect of Ca^{++} channel blockers. The adrenergic reflex response to Ca^{++} channel blockers also acts to decrease the hypotensive effect of these drugs. Thus when the reflex vasoconstriction is diminished as in the elderly persons or during treatment with α-adrenergic receptor blockers, then their hypotensive effect is much increased. They increase renin secretion by the kidney and plasma renin activity. They do not alter renal blood flow and GFR. Unlike β-blockers, they do not alter exercise tolerance and plasma concentrations of lipids, uric acid or electrolytes. They inhibit release of insulin from pancreatic β-cells. They have antianginal and antiarrhythmic effects (discussed in respective chapters).

Pharmacokinetics

They are well-absorbed orally but their bioavailability is low (20% with verapamil and diltiazem) due to extensive hepatic first pass metabolism. They are highly plasma protein bound (80 to 90%). They are metabolized in the liver and excreted in urine and faeces. They have plasma t½ of 3 to 6 hours. Nifedipine is highly lipid-soluble and can be administered sublingually in hypertensive crisis.

Clinical Uses

They are used in the treatment of all grades of hypertension. They are especially valuable in low renin hypertension compared with other groups of antihypertensive drugs. They produce greater control of BP when used alone (monotherapy). They can be combined with β-blockers, ACE inhibitors or diuretics to increase their efficacy. They can be safely used in hypertensive patients with bronchial asthma, hyperlipidaemia, diabetes mellitus and renal dysfunction.

Contraindications

They should not be used in patients with SA or AV nodal abnormalities or in patients with overt CCF.

Commonly used Preparations and Dosage

- Nifedipine (Nicardia) capsule (5, 10 mg)— 5 to 10 mg thrice daily and gradually increased to 20 mg thrice daily.
- Nifedipine SR (Retard) tablet (10, 20 mg)— 10 to 20 mg twice daily.
- Amlodipine (Amlosun) tablet (2.5, 5 mg)— 2.5 to 10 mg once daily.
- Diltiazem (Dilzem) tablet (30 mg)—30 to 60 mg 2 to 3 times daily.
- Diltiazem retard tablet (90 mg)—90 mg once daily.
- Verapamil (Isoptin) tablet (40 mg)—40 to 80 mg 3 to 4 times daily.
- Verapamil retard tablet (240 mg)—240 mg once daily.
- Felodipine (Felogard) tablet (5 mg)—5 to 10 mg once daily.
- Nimodipine (Nimodip) tablet (30 mg) and injection (10 mg/5ml) twice daily.

Adverse Reactions

They can cause gastroesophageal reflux by inhibiting contraction of the lower oesophageal sphincter. Constipation is the common side effect of verapamil but occurs less frequently with other Ca^{++} channel blockers. Inhibition of SA node function by verapamil and diltiazem can produce bradycardia and even SA node arrest, particularly in patients with SA node dysfunction. This effect is increased by concomitant administration of a β-blocker. Dihydropyridines (nifedipine, etc.) cause more vascular side effects like headache, flushing, dizziness, reflex tachycardia and peripheral oedema than other groups of Ca^{++} channel blockers.

Drug Interactions

- Verapamil can increase plasma concentration of digoxin.
- When used with quinidine, Ca^{++} channel blockers may cause excessive hypotension, particularly in patients with idiopathic hypertrophic subaortic stenosis.

ACE Inhibitors (Angiotensin Converting Enzyme Inhibitors)

These drugs inhibit conversion of angiotensin-I to angiotensin-II, which is an important regulator of cardiovascular system. These are important group of antihypertensive drugs. They are very useful in the treatment of hypertension due to their efficacy and relatively less side effects. They offer a special advantage in the treatment of hypertensive patients with diabetes mellitus, as they slow the development of diabetic granulopathy. They are also effective in slowing the progress of other forms of chronic renal disease such as glomerulosclerosis as many of these patients have hypertension. They are the preferred drugs for the initial treatment of hypertensive patients with left ventricular hypertrophy. They are also used in hypertensive patients with ischaemic heart disease, including the immediate post- myocardial infarction period.

Pharmacological Effects

They produce some endocrine disturbances during treatment. They blunt the normal aldosterone response to Na^+ loss by diuretic. They increase the efficacy of diuretic drugs. They can produce slight rise of serum K^+ concentration, when used alone. In patients with renal insufficiency they can produce retention of K^+ leading to hyperkalaemia. This is also produced when they are used with K^+ sparing diuretics, NSAIDs, K^+ supplements and β-blockers.

They produce a little change in heart rate and cardiac output. They reduce both preload and afterload by inhibiting vasoconstrictor action of angiotensin-II and decreasing aldosterone secretion by the adrenal cortex. They do not increase renin secretion by the kidney and plasma renin activity. They do not alter renal blood flow and GFR.

Pharmacokinetics

They are well-absorbed orally. Their bio-availability varies from 40 to 80% depending on the compound. They are metabolized in the liver and excreted in urine mainly as meta-bolites. Enalapil is a prodrug and its active metabolite is enalaprilate. They have plasma t½ of 4 to 12 hours.

Clinical Uses

They are used in all grades of hypertension either alone (monotherapy) or in combination with diuretics (to increase their efficacy). They are used in both essential and renal hyper-tension. They are also used in left ventricular systolic dysfunction, myocardial infarction, progressive renal impairment (by both diabetes and hypertension) and scleroderma renal crisis.

Contraindications

They should not be used in pregnancy (as they produce foetal toxicity) and bilateral or unilateral renal artery stenosis or renal artery stenosis in single kidney (as they reduce or abolish glomerular filtration leading to progressive renal failure).

Commonly used Preparations and Dosage

- Captopril (Acetan/Angiopril) tablet (25 mg)—25 to 50 mg twice daily.
- Enalapril (Enam/Enace) tablet (2.5, 5 mg)—2.5 to 10 mg once daily.
- Lisinopril (Lispril/Cipril) tablet (2.5, 5 mg)—2.5 to 10 mg once daily.
- Perindopril (Coversl) tablet (2, 4 mg)—2 to 4 mg once daily.

Adverse Reactions

They can produce hypotension, chronic dry cough (mediated by accumulation of brady-kinin, substance P and/or prostaglandins in lungs), hyperkalaemia, skin rash, proteinuria, angioneurotic oedema, dysgeusia (alteration of taste sensation), neutropenia, glycosuria, hepatotoxicity, acute renal failure and teratogenicity (foetopathic potential like oligohydramnios, retardation of foetal growth and death of foetus occurs if used during 2nd and 3rd trimesters of pregnancy).

Drug Interactions

- Antacids reduce their absorption from gut and decrease bioavailability.
- NSAIDs reduce their antihypertensive effects.
- Potassium sparing diuretics or potassium supplements increase hyperkalaemia produced by them.
- They increase plasma levels of digoxin and lithium causing toxicity.
- They increase hypersensitivity reactions of allopurinol.

Angiotensin-II Receptor Antagonists

These are of two groups:

1. Peptide analog, e.g. saralasin.
2. Nonpeptide analogs, e.g. losartan, cande-sartan and irbesartan.

These are competitive antagonists of angio-tensin-II receptors, *viz.* AT_1 and AT_2. AT_1 receptor is present predominantly in vascular and myocardial tissue and also in brain, kidney and adrenal glomerular cells (which secrete aldosterone). AT_2 receptor is present in adrenal medulla and CNS.

Saralasin

It has high affinity for AT_2 receptor and low affinity for AT_1 receptor. It is ineffective orally and has to be administered IV. It has also partial agonist activity and may cause rise of BP. It is now not used in hypertension.

Losartan

It has high affinity for AT_1 receptor and low affinity for AT_2 receptor. It is a pure antagonist and has no partial agonist activity. It is effective orally. It is metabolized in the liver and excreted in urine mainly as metabolites. It produces vasodilatation by relaxation of vascular smooth muscle. It also increases renal salt and water excretion, decreases plasma volume and cellular hypertrophy. It has pharmacological effects like ACE inhibitors.

Clinical Uses

It is used in the treatment of hypertension (all grades) either alone or in combination with a diuretic (hydrochlorothiazide). It is also used in left ventricular failure (LVF).

Preparations and Dosage

- Losartan (Repace/Losacar) tablet (50 mg)— 50 to 100 mg daily in two divided doses.
- Losartan (50 mg) with hydrochlorothiazide (12.5 mg) tablet (Hyzaar)—1 to 2 tablets daily.

Adverse Reactions

It can produce dizziness, postural hypotension, diarrhoea, liver function abnormalities, myalgia, urticaria, pruritus and rarely skin rashes and angioedema. It does not produce chronic dry cough.

Contraindications

It should not be used during pregnancy (second and third trimesters, as it can produce foetal toxicity) and in lactating mother (as it is secreted in breast milk and may affect infants). Candesartan (Candesar) is a similar drug to iosartant. It is a available as tablet (4 mg) and used twice daily.

NON-PHARMACOLOGICAL THERAPY IN HYPERTENSION

Non-pharmacological approaches for the reduction of BP are generally advised to the hypertensive patients with mild hypertension (diastolic BP < 95 mmHg). These approaches will also increase the effectiveness of pharmacological therapy in patients with higher levels of BP. These include:

- **Reduction of body weight in obese persons:** Obesity and hypertension are closely associated. The degree of obesity is positively correlated with the incidence of hypertension. Obese hypertensives may lower their BP by losing weight. A combination of aerobic physical exercise and restriction of fat consumption can reduce obesity. Anorectic drugs like fenfluramine can be used to reduce food intake.

- **Restriction of salt consumption:** High salt (NaCl) diets are associated with a high prevalence of hypertension. Moderate restriction of salt (5 g NaCl containing 2 g Na^+) will lower BP by 12 mmHg systolic and 5 mmHg diastolic. The higher the initial BP the greater the response. An additional benefit of salt restriction is improved responsiveness to some antihypertensive drugs, e.g. diuretics.

- **Restriction of alcohol consumption:** Consumption of alcohol rises BP. Moderate restriction of alcohol (< 30 ml per day) reduces BP and improves the efficacy of antihypertensive drugs. Consumption of small amount of alcohol protects against the development of coronary artery disease but heavy consumption of alcohol increases the risk of cardiovascular accidents but not coronary heart disease.

- **Physical exercise and mental relaxation:** Regular isotonic exercise lowers both systolic and diastolic BPs in hypertensive patients. Lack of physical activity is associated with a higher incidence of hypertension. Increased physical activity lowers the rate of cardiovascular disease in men. Regular isotonic exercise reduces blood volume and plasma catecholamines. Stressful conditions cause rise of BP. Mental relaxation produces lowering of BP in some hypertensive patients. Reassurance of the hypertensive patients is also helpful in reducing BP to some extent.

- **Supplementation of potassium:** There is a positive correlation between total body Na^+ and BP and a negative correlation between total body K^+ and BP in hypertensive patients. Increased intake of K^+ can reduce BP by increasing excretion of Na^+, decreasing renin secretion by the kidney and causing arteriolar dilatation.

33

Drug Therapy of Cardiac Arrhythmias

INTRODUCTION

Individual cardiac cells undergo depolarization and repolarization to form cardiac action potential, about sixty times per minute. The shape and duration of each action potential are determined by the activity of ion channels on the surface of individual cells. Thus each heartbeat is the result of the highly integrated electrophysiological behaviour of multiple ion cells on multiple cardiac cells. Ion channel function can be deranged by certain factors such as acute myocardial ischaemia, sympathetic stimulation of the heart and myocardial scarring leading to abnormalities of cardiac rhythm (arrhythmias). Antiarrhythmic drugs generally suppress arrhythmias by blocking flow through specific ion channels or by altering autonomic function. They are used to terminate the ongoing arrhythmia or to prevent reoccurrence of arrhythmia. It has been found that antiarrhythmic drugs not only help to control arrhythmias but also can cause them, especially during long-term therapy. Thus before prescribing antiarrhythmic drugs, the precipitating factors must be excluded or minimized and a precise diagnosis of the type of arrhythmias must be made, so that the drug therapy will be beneficial and the risks of drug therapy is minimized.

Genesis of Cardiac Arrhythmias

SA node is the pacemaker of the heart, where the cardiac impulse is generated by spontaneous depolarization of the cells. From the SA node, the impulse is transmitted to AV node, from where conduction of impulse occurs through conducting tissue (His-Purkinje system), which includes bundle of His and its right and left branches and Purkinje fibres to reach the atrial or ventricular muscle cells. Normally SA node, AV node and His-Purkinje system have the ability to depolarize spontaneously (i.e. possess automaticity). Under abnormal conditions, myocardial cells acquire this property. In cardiac arrhythmias, impulses arise from ectopic foci in AV node, conducting tissue and atrial or ventricular muscle cells, when the activity of SA node is suppressed.

Failure of impulse initiation results in slowing of heart rate (bradyarrhythmias) and failure of impulse propagation from atrium to ventricle results in dropped beats or heart (AV) block (partial or complete) which usually reflects an abnormality in either the AV node or the His-Purkinje system. These abnormalities may be caused by drugs or structural heart diseases. Abnormally rapid heartbeat rhythms (tachyarrhythmias) caused by drugs or structural heart diseases are common clinical problems. These include supraventricular (atrial) tachycardia, atrial flutter, atrial fibrillation, ectopic beats (extrasystoles), idioventricular rhythm, ventricular tachycardia and ventricular fibrillation. Drugs like cardiac stimulants (adrenergic drugs, calcium salts and digitalis glycosides) produce tachyarrhythmias, whereas drugs like cardiac depressants (cholinergic drugs, potassium or magnesium salts, emetine, quinine and anti-arrhythmic drugs) produce bradyarrhythmias. Myocardial diseases like myocardial ischaemia, myocardial infarction, myocarditis, myocardial degeneration and myocardial injury can cause cardiac arrhythmias (tachyarrhythmias or bradyarrhythmias).

Mechanism of Cardiac Arrhythmias

There are three main mechanisms of cardiac arrhythmias:

1. Enhanced Automaticity

SA node has the highest automaticity which suppresses the automaticity of AV node and conducting tissue (His-Purkinje system). When the SA node is suppressed by any cause, then enhanced automaticity occurs in AV node and conducting tissue, atria or ventricle (ectopic pacemaker) producing a AV nodal rhythm, idioventricular rhythm or ectopic beats.

2. Triggered Activity (After Depolarization)

This is shown in **Fig. 33.1**. Normally, the resting membrane potential fluctuates a little, because the line which represents the membrane potential between two cardiac action potentials (APs) can show some small undulations. In cardiac abnormalities, instead of small undulations, there can be full-fledged APs, which are called after depolarization. They may be early after depolarization (EAD) or delayed after depolarization (DAD).

Triggered activity can be EAD or DAD, which may cause a single premature heartbeat or it can behave as a self-sustained ectopic focus in the conducting tissue producing paroxysmal ventricular tachycardia (PVT). Early after depolarization can develop in hypokalaemia and bradycardia whereas DAD develops during digitalis toxicity, adrenaline injection and hypercalcaemia.

3. Re-entry of Impulse (Re-entry Phenomenon)

It occurs in myocardial diseases (mentioned before). Normally, when a stimulus passes through a strip of Purkinje fibre (PF), it divides and passes through its two segments, PFO and PFT to reach the same strip of ventricular working myocardial cell (WMC). But when a portion of PFT is abnormal (block) due to myocardial disease, there develops delayed conductivity. Thus, the stimulus, passing through PFT becomes extinct and that passing through PFO proceeds on and reaches the WMC. This bifurcates again and so PFT gets a stimulus which comes from its opposite end (retrograde stimulus). Now as the block on PFT has disappeared, so the stimulus passes on and re-enters the PFO. It then passes through PFT and repeats the circus (circular) movement on and on, producing a sustained arrhythmia like ventricular tachycardia or fibrillation (as shown in **Fig. 33.2**).

The entire segment consisting of PFO-WMC-PFT continues to be excited by a selfsustaining stimulus, which does not extinguish and acts as an ectopic focus (pacemaker).

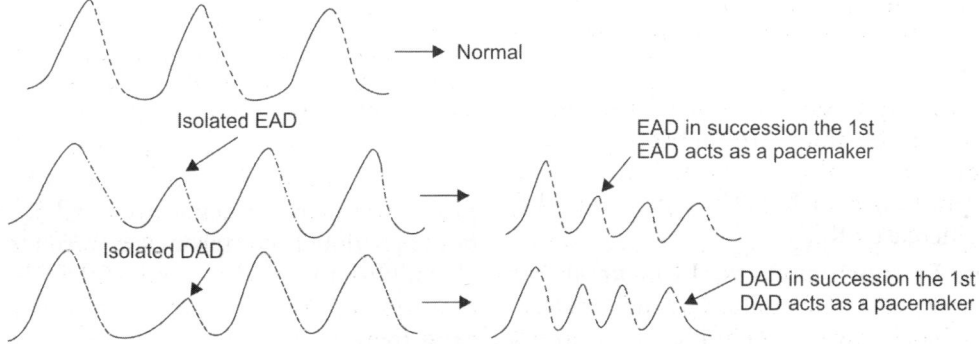

Fig. 33.1: Triggered activity (after depolarization)

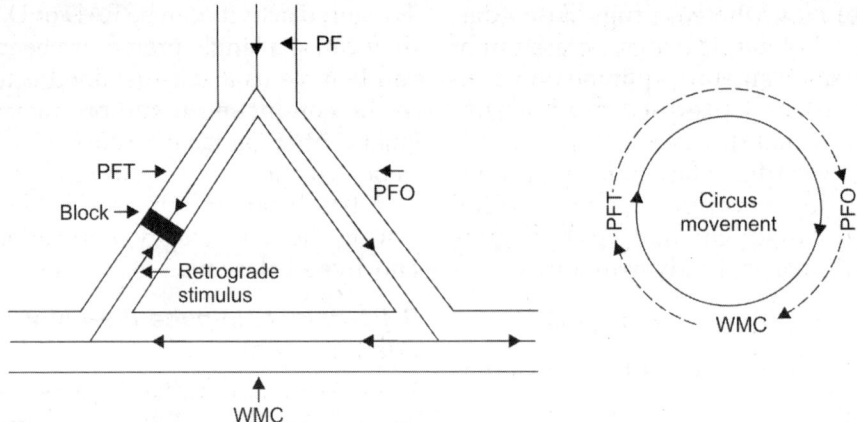

Fig. 33.2: Re-entry of impulse and circus movement

Classification of Antiarrhythmic Drugs

These are of five groups:

1. **Class I (sodium channel blockers):** They block inward sodium current (influx of Na^+). They are again three subclasses— class Ia, e.g. quinidine, procainamide and disopyramide. They prolong APD (action potential duration) and increase ERP (effective refractory period). Class Ib, e.g. Lignocaine, tocainide, mexiletine and phenytoin. They shorten APD and decrease ERP. Class Ic, e.g. propafenone, fecainide and encainide. They have no effect on APD and ERP.

2. **Class II (β-adrenergic receptor blockers):** For example, propranolol, esmalol, atenolol and metroprolol. They block β receptors in the heart. They suppress (flatten) diastolic depolarization (phase four of action potential), prolong repolarization (phase three of action potential) and decrease automaticity.

3. **Class III (potassium channel blockers):** For example, amiodarone, bretylium and sotalol. They block outward potassium current (efflux of K^+). They prolong APD and increase ERP.

4. **Class IV (calcium channel blockers):** For example, verapamil, diltiazem and biperidil. They block inward calcium current (influx

of Ca^{++}). They shorten APD and decline plateau (phase 2 of AP) and delay conduction at nodal tissue (AVN).

5. **Class V (miscellaneous drugs):** For example, digoxin, adenosine, magnesium sulphate, edrophonium and phenylephrine. They act by different mechanisms. The choice of antiarrhythmic drug in a specific arrhythmia depends on:

   - Correct diagnosis of arrhythmia
   - Urgency of treatment
   - Route of administration
   - Extent of cardiac damage
   - Risk-benefit ratio of the drug

All cardiac arrhythmias do not require the same aggressive drug therapy, e.g. sinus tachycardia and sinus bradycardia usually do not require any treatment other than that of the underlying cause. Cardiac arrhythmia precipitated by hypotension may be reversed by a vasopressor drug (mephenterine, methoxamine or phenylephrine restores normal BP). Only those cardiac arrhythmias which are lethal (ventricular fibrillation) produce dangerous rhythm (ventricular premature beats in acute myocardial infarction) or seriously compromised cardiac output (atrial fibrillation with rapid ventricular rate) requires rapid and effective antiarrhythmic drug therapy.

DISCUSSION OF INDIVIDUAL GROUPS OF DRUGS

Class IA

Quinidine

It is an alkaloid obtained from cinchona bark. It is the d-isomer of quinine. It is more potent than quinine as an antiarrhythmic drug. It is well-absorbed from GIT. It is highly plasma protein bound (80 to 90%). It is partly (1/3rd) metabolized in the liver by hydroxylation. It is slowly excreted in urine. It has a plasma t½ of 5 to 10 hours.

Pharmacological Actions

It is a Na$^+$ channel blocker. It has direct myocardial depressant action and anticholinergic (vagolytic) action. By direct depressant action on atria, AV node and ventricle, it decreases automaticity, excitability and myocardial contractility and slows AV conduction velocity. By slowing of depolarization, it increases ventricular AP duration and refractoriness (ERP) of AV node. By vagolytic action it tends to decrease refractoriness of AV node and increases automaticity, excitability and contractility of the myocardium and may produce paradoxical tachycardia. So it should better be used after using digoxin. It has also local anaesthetic action and a-receptor blocking action, which produces hypotension. It produces following ECG changes—increase in QT interval, depression of ST segment, prolongation of PR interval and widening of QRS complex.

Clinical Uses

It is a broad spectrum antiarrhythmic drug used in both atrial and ventricular tachyarrhythmias including Wolff-Parkinson-White (WPW) syndrome (in which there is presence of a bypass tract from atria to ventricle producing pre-excitation).

Preparations and Dosage

- Quinidine sulphate (Natcardine) tablet (200 mg)—200 to 400 mg thrice daily.
- Quinidine phenyl ethyl barbiturate tablet (100 mg)—100 to 200 mg twice or thrice daily.
- Quinidine gluconate injection (80 mg/ml)—80 to 160 mg IV or IM in emergency.

Adverse Reactions

It can produce GIT upset (nausea, vomiting abdominal discomfort and diarrhoea), CVS side effects (bradycardia, heart block, paradoxical tachycardia, torsades de pointes, hypotension, and heart failure, i.e. CCF), CNS side effects (cinchonism manifested as vertigo, tinnitus, deafness, blurring of vision, photophobia, headache, confusion and delirium), allergic reactions (skin rashes, fever, angiooedema, bronchial asthma, thrombocytopenia and haemolytic anaemia) and embolic phenomenon (in arterial fibrillation due to dislodgement of mural thrombi attached to the atrial appendages).

Contraindications

Heart block, previous history of embolism and 3rd trimester of pregnancy (can produce ecbolic action).

Procainamide

It is an amide of procaine. It has an amide bond in place of ester linkage of procaine, which protects it from enzymatic hydrolysis by esterases. It has no central stimulant action of procaine. It is well-absorbed from GIT. It is metabolized in the liver by acetylation and excreted in urine. Its pharmacological actions and uses are similar to quinidine but it is less potent. It has a weak local anaesthetic action and no α-receptor blocking action. It does not produce hypotension.

Preparations and Dosage

- Procainamide hydrochloride (Pronestyl) tablet (250 mg)—250 to 500 mg thrice daily.
- Procainamide hydrochloride injection (100 mg/ml)—100 to 200 mg IV or IM in emergency.

Adverse Reactions

It can produce GIT upset (nausea and vomiting), CVS side effects (like quinidine),

CNS side effects (weakness, confusion and hallucinations), allergic reactions (skin rashes, fever and angioedema) and on prolonged use agranulocytosis, arthritis and SLE (systemic lupus erythematosus).

Disopyramide

It is a synthetic antiarrhythmic drug. It is well-absorbed from GIT. It is metabolized in the liver and excreted in urine. It has pharmacological actions and uses like quinidine. It is used only in some forms of atrial and ventricular tachyarrhythmias, which are resistant to quinidine or procainamide. It is available as Norpace capsule (100 mg) and the dosage is 100 to 200 mg thrice daily. It can produce dryness of mouth, blurring of vision, photophobia, glaucoma and urinary retention due to anticholinergic action. It is contraindicated in heart failure (CCF).

Class IB
Lignocaine/Lidocaine

It is a synthetic local anaesthetic with antiarrhythmic action. It is a Na^+ channel blocker. It produces shortening of ventricular action potential duration (APD) and decreasing of refractoriness (ERP) of the AV node. It has no vagolytic (anticholinergic) action and α-receptor blocking action. It suppresses automaticity and excitability in ectopic foci and decreases AV conduction velocity. It is used in ventricular tachycardia or fibrillation induced by drugs (e.g. digoxin toxicity) after acute myocardial infarction or during cardiac surgery, as it has a rapid onset of action. It is ineffective in a trial tachyarrhythmias. It is administered IV because it undergoes extensive hepatic first pass metabolism when administered only.

Preparation and Dosage

Lignocaine (Xylocard) injection (100 mg/ ml)—50 to 100 mg IV rapidly (as bolus) and repeated after five minutes of necessary. It can produce drowsiness, confusion and convulsions as side effects. In high dose it can produce severe hypotension and heart failure (CCF).

Mexiletine and Tocainide

These drugs are analogue (congener) of lidocaine administered orally as tablet. Mexiletine is used in the dosage of 150 to 300 mg thrice daily.

It can cause nausea, vomiting and ataxia. Tocainide is used in the dosage of 400 to 800 mg thrice daily. It can cause tremors, diplopia and hallucinations.

Phenytoin Sodium

It is an antiepileptic drug with antiarrhythmic action. It has pharmacological actions and uses like lignocaine. It can be administered orally or IV. It is available as capsule (100 mg) and injection (100 mg/2 ml). It is administered in the dosage of 100 mg IV slowly and repeated every 10 minutes till arrhythmia is controlled and then 100 mg orally thrice daily. It can produce ataxia, vertigo, blurring of vision, hyperplasia of gum, nightmares and megaloblastic anaemia. Rapid IV injection of it can cause hypotension, heart block and cardiac arrest.

Class 1C
Propafenone

It is a sodium channel blocker. It has moderate depressant effects on AV conduction velocity and cardiac contractility. It slightly increases the ventricular APD and refractoriness (ERP) of AV node. It has a weak β-blocking activity. It is effective orally (as tablet). It is metabolized in the liver and excreted in urine. It has uses like quinidine. It can cause nausea, abnormal taste sensation, constipation, tremors and heart failure (CCF).

Flecainide

It is a fluorinated analogue of procainamide. It is well absorbed after oral administration. It is used as substitute of procainamide. It is administered as tablet (100 mg) in the dosage of 100 to 200 mg twice daily. It can also be given by slow IV injection.

Encainide

It has properties similar to flecainide and is effective orally. It has mild negative inotropic action. It is used as a substitute of quinidine.

Class II and Class IV

β-blockers and Ca^{++} channel blockers are used in supraventricular (atrial) tachyarrhythmias. They are discussed in respective chapters.

Class III

Amiodarone

It is a K$^+$ channel blocker. It can be used orally (tablet) and IV injection. It causes prolongation of ventricular APD and refractoriness (ERP) of the AV node, conducting tissue and ventricle. It reduces automaticity and conductivity of His-Purkinje system. It possesses antiadrenergic properties. It produces hypotension by vasodilation. It is used to treat refractory and life-threatening atrial and ventricular tachyarrhythmias. It is administered as capsule (100 mg) in the dosage of 100 to 200 mg thrice daily. It can cause anorexia, nausea, abdominal discomfort, tremors, hallucinations, peripheral neuropathy, hypotension, AV block, hypersensitivity pneumonitis and disorders of thyroid functions (as it contains iodine).

Bretylium Tosylate

It is an adrenergic neuron blocker with antiarrhythmic action. It is a K$^+$ channel blocker. It has actions like amiodarone. It has variable absorption after oral administration and so it is administered IV or IM. It is used in refractory and life-threatening atrial and ventricular tachyarrhythmias.

Sotalol

It is a nonselective β-blocker without membrane stabilizing action. It is a K$^+$ channel blocker. It prolongs atrial and ventricular APD and refractoriness (ERP) in all cardiac tissues, including AV node and His-Purkinje system. It is effective orally. It is metabolized in the liver and excreted in urine. It has a plasma t½ of 9 to 18 hours. It is used in supraventricular tachyarrhythmias, WPW syndrome (recurrent atrioventricular nodal tachycardia) and ventricular ectopic beats or tachycardia. Prophylactically, it is highly effective in suppressing inducible ventricular tachycardia and fibrillation.

Preparations and Dosage

- Sotalol hydrochloride (Betacardone) tablet (40, 80 mg)—40 to 80 mg thrice daily.
- Sotalol hydrochloride injection (10 mg/ml)—20 to 40 mg IV during emergency.

Adverse Reactions

It has low incidence of adverse effects than other antiarrhythmic drugs. It can produce hypokalaemia.

Class V

Digoxin

It is a digitalis glycoside with antiarrhythmic action. It is discussed in drug therapy of CCF. It is used only in supraventricular (atrial) tachyarrhythmias.

Adenosine

It is a naturally occurring purine nucleotide, which is released during myocardial ischaemia. It has local coronary dilator action. It is a K$^+$ channel opener. It acts by interacting with specific adenosine receptors on the cell membrane. It activates acetylcholine sensitive K$^+$ channels in the atria, SA node and AV node leading to fall of intracellular K$^+$ ion and hyperpolarization. It decreases automaticity, excitability and AV conduction.

ATP is the prodrug of adenosine. It is converted to adenosine in the body. Adenosine is used for the termination of paroxysmal supraventricular tachycardia (PSVT) involving the AV node. It is rarely used in ventricular tachycardia. It is contraindicated in the presence of sick sinus (SA) syndrome, AV block and bronchial asthma. It is available as Adenocor injection 30 mg/10 ml ampoule. It is administered IV in the dosage of 5 to 10 mg by rapid bolus injection. It has short lived action (< 1 min). Its plasma t½ is very short (few seconds). It is rapidly taken up by RBCs and endothelial cells, where it is converted to 5′AMP and inosine.

It can produce nausea, headache, flushing, transient asystole, bronchospasm and dyspnoea. Unlike verapamil it may be used after β-blocker.

Other drugs are discussed in respective chapters.

34

Drug Therapy of Plasma Hyperlipoproteinaemias

INTRODUCTION

Atherosclerosis, coronary heart disease and other diseases like xantholesma are strongly associated with disorder of lipid metabolism and plasma hyperlipoproteinaemias. Atherosclerosis is due to deposition of atheromatous plaque in the intima of blood vessels (medium- and large-sized arteries) leading to narrowing of the arterial lumen and causing distal ischaemia. The coronary and cerebral vessels are common sites of atherosclerosis. The cause of atherosclerosis is not known. It is common in persons with high levels of plasma lipids (cholesterol and triglycerides). A reduction of plasma lipids levels either by dietetic restriction of fats or by drugs may prevent the development of atherosclerosis or arrest its progress. The important lipids of plasma are cholesterol, triglycerides, phospholipids and free fatty acids. Their normal values are shown in **Table 34.1.**

The lipids as such are insoluble in plasma, but in combination with protein they are soluble in plasma. In the plasma they combine with a kind of protein called apolipoprotein, forming lipoproteins. There are several varieties of apolipoprotein (A, B and C). Lipoproteins are of several classes (as shown in **Table 34.2**). Lipoproteins differ from each other in density, lipid composition and apolipoprotein content. All lipids except free fatty acids take part in the formation of lipoproteins.

Table 34.1: Normal values of plasma lipids

Class	Values (mg/100 ml)
Cholesterol (total)	140 to 250
Triglycerides	30 to 150
Phospholipids	150 to 300
Free fatty acids	10 to 30
Total lipids	350 to 850

Lipids are transported in the blood as lipoproteins. High plasma levels of LDL-cholesterol and VLDL-cholesterol are considered as atherogenic while high HDL-cholesterol level has protective effect on blood vessels. There are five types of hyperlipoproteinaemia: Type I hyperlipoproteinaemia is due to hereditary deficiency of lipoprotein lipase and is produced by excessive fat intake, types II and III hyperlipoproteinaemias are hereditary and types IV and V hyperlipoproteinaemias are secondary (carbohydrate induced) and are associated with insulin resistance. The common hyperlipoproteinaemias (types II and IV) are secondary to dietary excess of fat, uncontrolled diabetes mellitus, obstructive liver disease, use of oral contraceptives, hypothyroidism, alcoholism, nephrotic syndrome and chronic renal failure (uremia). In these patients the risk of ischaemic heart disease is high.

Table 34.2: Plasma lipoproteins

Class	Composition	Common apoproteins
High density lipoprotein (HDL)	Protein (++), cholesterol (+), phospholipid (+), triglyceride very low	A_I and A_{II}
Low density lipoprotein (LDL)	Protein (+), cholesterol (+++), phospholipid (+), triglyceride low	B_{100}
Intermediate density lipoprotein (IDL)	Protein low, cholesterol (++), phospholipid (+), triglyceride (++)	B_{100}
Very low density lipoprotein (VLDL)	Protein low, cholesterol (++), phospholipid low triglyceride (++)	B_{100}, C
Chylomicron	Triglyceride (++), protein very low, cholesterol low	A_I B_{48}
Chylomicron remnant	Protein very low, cholesterol low	B_{48}

Metabolism of Lipoproteins

Food fat is converted into micelles in the intestinal lumen and absorbed forming chylomicrons, which contain triglycerides and some cholesterol. Chylomicrons are transported by the lymph duct and enter the blood vessels. While passing through the tissue capillaries they are acted upon by the endothelial bound lipoprotein lipase (LPL), which hydrolyzes triglycerides into free fatty acids (FFA) and glycerol. FFA thus formed is taken up by the muscles and utilized as energy and also by adipose tissue and stored as triglycerides. The chylomicron remnant containing mainly cholesterol ester is taken up by specific receptor mediated endocytosis into the hepatocyte (hepatic cell), where cholesterol ester is hydrolyzed to cholesterol. Cholesterol is either stored in the hepatocyte, excreted in bile as such, oxidized and excreted in bile as bile acids or secreted into plasma as newly synthesized VLDL and HDL. Liver secretes VLDL, which while passing through tissue capillaries is acted upon by the LPL forming VLDL remnant called IDL. IDL is either converted to LDL by losing triglycerides or is taken up by hepatocytes by LDL receptor mediated endocytosis. If the tissue contains sufficient amount of cholesterol, there is down-regulation of LDL receptors and decreased endocytosis. The reverse will occur, if there is more need for cholesterol. The cholesterol of LDL is mainly used for cell membrane synthesis. HDL secreted by the liver helps in the transport of excess cholesterol away from the peripheral tissues. It also supplies cholesterol to the adrenal gland for steroidogenesis.

Classification of Antihyperlipidemic Drugs

These are of four groups:
1. HMG CoA reductase inhibitors, e.g. lovastatin, simvastatin, pravastatin fluvastatin, mevastatin and atorvastatin.
2. Bile acid binding resins, e.g. cholestyramine and colestipol.
3. Fibric acid derivatives, e.g. clofibrate, gemfibrozil, bezafibrate and fenofibrate.
4. Miscellaneous drugs, e.g. nicotinic acid, probucol and gugulipid.

DISCUSSION OF INDIVIDUAL GROUPS OF DRUGS

HMG-CoA Reductase Inhibitors (Statins)
Lovastatin

It was isolated from cultures of aspergillus species. It is a potent inhibitor of the enzyme hydroxymethylglutaryl-coenzyme A reductase. HMG-CoA reductase in the liver catalyzes the conversion of hydroxymethyl-glutaryl-coenzyme A to mevalonate, an important rate limiting step in the biosynthesis of cholesterol. It blocks synthesis of cholesterol in the liver by competitively inhibiting HMG-CoA reductase activity. As a result of inhibition of cholesterol synthesis, the number of LDL receptors on the hepatocyte increases and more LDL is caught and degraded leading to decrease in serum LDL-cholesterol level (25 to 45%). It also lowers VLDL level in blood. It may rise HDL level and lower triglyceride level.

Pharmacokinetics

It is administered orally once or twice daily with the meal. It has 30% bioavailability due to high first pass metabolism in the liver. It is a prodrug, which is rapidly converted in the liver to active metabolite. It is excreted mainly in faeces and partly in urine.

Clinical Uses

- It is used to treat hyperlipidaemias.
- It is useful in lowering blood cholesterol levels in primary hypercholesterolemias (patients who are at high risk of myocardial infarction) and secondary hypercholesterolemias (associated with diabetes mellitus and nephrotic syndrome). It decreases progression of atherosclerotic lesions and occurrence of myocardial infarction and mortality in patients of ischaemic heart diseases.

Contraindications

Hepatic dysfunction and pregnancy.

Preparation and Dosage

Lovastatin (Recol, Rovacor) capsule (20, 40 mg)—20 to 40 mg once or twice daily with meals.

Adverse Reactions

It is well-tolerated. Its most important side effects are increase in hepatic transaminases (SGPT and SGOT) in serum and myopathy (myositis). It can also produce headache, nausea, insomnia, muscle tenderness and skin rashes.

Other statins: Simvastatin and pravastatin are analogues of lovastatin. Fluvastatin is a synthetic statin. They have similar properties of lovastatin. They differ from each other in hypolipidaemic potency, e.g. simvastatin is twice as potent as lovastatin. Pravastatin is as effective as lovastatin at lower doses but not at higher doses. Fluvastatin is half as potent as lovastatin. Mevastatin (the first statin isolated from cultures of penicillium species) is less potent than lovastatin. Their dosage are: simvastatin (10 mg), pravastatin (10 mg) and atorvastatin (Avasting)—10 mg with meals.

Bile Acid Binding Resins (Bile Acid Sequestrants)

Cholestyramine and colestipol are anion exchange resins. Normally up to 97% of bile acids are reabsorbed into the enterohepatic circulation and only a few percent are excreted in faeces. The anion exchange resins exchange chloride ion for negatively charged bile acids. As the resins are not absorbed, the net effect is to promote bile acid excretion. Inhibition of the return of bile acids to the liver results in an increase in conversion of cholesterol to bile acids. There is also a slight decrease in sterol reabsorption due to loss of bile acids. The loss of bile acids as well as neutral steroids, leads to a compensatory increase in the number of hepatic LDL receptors. So more LDL is caught and degraded leading to decrease in serum LDL-cholesterol level. Serum HDL-cholesterol level may slightly increase.

Clinical Uses

They are used in patients with type II hyperlipoproteinaemia with marked elevation of cholesterol level. They are also used to relieve pruritus associated with biliary cirrhosis and cholestatic jaundice.

Preparations and Dosage

- Cholestyramine resin—6 to 12 g twice daily with meals.
- Colestipol resin—5 to 10 g twice daily with meals.

Adverse Reactions

They can cause nausea, vomiting and constipation. In high dosage (over 30 g/day) they may interfere with absorption of fats and fat-soluble vitamins, causing steatorrhoea. They also interfere with the absorption of ingested thyroid hormones and organic acids like phenobarbitone, tetracycline, chlorothiazide and phenylbutazone.

Fibric Acid Derivatives

Gemfibrozil: It is the most popular drug of this group, as it is more effective and better tolerated than other drugs. It lowers the serum levels of VLDL and triglycerides to a greater extent (about 40%) than that of LDL and cholesterol (about 10%). It acts by increasing the activity of lipoprotein lipase (LPL) especially in the muscle. This leads to increased hydrolysis of VLDL triglyceride contents and an increased VLDL catabolism. It may alter the composition of VLDL by decreasing hepatic production of apo-C III, an inhibitor of LPL activity. It also decreases hepatic VLDL triglyceride synthesis, probably by inhibiting fatty acid synthesis and by promoting fatty acid oxidation.

Pharmacokinetics

It is completely absorbed after oral administration. It undergoes some enterohepatic circulation. It is metabolized in the liver and excreted as glucuronide in urine.

Clinical Uses

It is the drug of choice for the treatment of hyperlipidaemic subjects with high triglyceride level (hypertriglyceridemia). It reduces serum triglycerides in both genetic (types II and III hyperlipoproteinaemias) and secondary hypertriglyceridemias (types IV and V hyperlipoproteinaemias), who are at risk of pancreatitis.

Contraindications

Hepatic dysfunction and renal failure.

Preparation and Dosage

Gemfibrozil (Lopid, Normolip) capsule (300 mg)—300 mg twice daily 30 minutes before meals.

Adverse Reactions

It is well-tolerated. Side effects may occur in 5 to 10% of patients. GIT side effects (epigastric distress and diarrhoea) are common. Other side effects are infrequent and include skin rash, urticaria, hair loss, myalgia, fatigue, headache, impotence and anaemia. Minor increase in liver transaminases and decrease in alkaline phosphatase have been reported.

Clofibrate

It is the first fibric acid derivative introduced as hypolipidemic agent. It has pharmacological actions and adverse reactions like gemfibrozil. It is now rarely used because it increases lithogenicity of bile (cholelithiasis), which is less common with other drugs. It also potentiates the action of oral anticoagulants, in part by displacing them from their binding sites on albumin. It may be useful in patients with familial dysbetalipoproteinemias that do not respond to gemfibrozil.

Preparation and Dosage

Clofibrate (Atromid-S) capsule (500 mg)—1 g twice daily with meals.

Bizofibrate and Fenofibrate

Bizafibrate and fenofibrate are other fibric acid derivatives having similar pharmacological actions, uses and adverse reactions like gemfibrozil and may be used as alternative drugs.

Preparations and Dosage

- Bizafibrate (Bizalip) tablet (200 mg)—200 mg thrice daily with meals.
- Finofibrate (Lipantil) capsule (100 mg)—100 to 200 mg twice daily with meals.

  Bizafibrate can potentiate the action of oral anticoagulants like clofibrate and should be used cautiously with them.

MISCELLANEOUS DRUGS

Nicotinic Acid

It is a water-soluble B-complex vitamin and it functions in the body after conversion to nicotinamide adenine dinucleotide (NAD) and to nicotinamide adenine dinucleotide phosphate (NADP). Nicotinic acid has hypolipidemic properties but nicotinamide has no such activity. Nicotinic acid reduces the hepatic production of VLDL with consequent reduction in the serum levels of triglycerides, VLDL-cholesterol and LDL-cholesterol. It may rise HDL-cholesterol level during therapy.

Clinical Uses

It is useful in all types of hyperlipoproteinaemias except type I (which is due to hereditary deficiency of lipoprotein lipase). It is the drug of choice in type V hyperlipoproteinaemia with raised triglycerides and cholesterol levels and is helpful in preventing pancreatitis.

Preparation and Dosage

Nicotinic acid (Niacin) tablet (100 mg)—100 to 300 mg thrice daily with meals. The combination of nicotinic acid and cholestyramine resin is more effective than either drug alone in lowering plasma cholesterol levels in resistant cases.

Adverse Reactions

It can produce flushing and pruritus in face and upper part of the body. This can be minimized by starting with a small dose and gradually building it up to full dose. It produces GIT side effects (dyspepsia, vomiting and diarrhoea) which are less when given after meals. It can produce peptic ulcer disease, jaundice, hyperuricemia, hyperglycaemia and dry skin with hyperpigmentation on prolonged use.

Probucol

It is a cholesterol lowering agent. It is absorbed poorly and eratically from GIT. Presence of fat in the diet reduces its absorption. It is metabolized in the liver and excreted mainly in bile and faeces and slightly in urine. It increases the clearance of serum LDL by the liver through a receptor independent pathway. Thus, it reduces serum cholesterol levels without a reduction in serum triglyceride levels. It also reduces serum HDL levels.

Clinical Uses

It is used in patients with homozygous familial hypercholesterolemia, where it reduces tendon and plantar xanthomas.

Preparation and Dosage

Probucol (Lursel) tablet (500 mg)—500 mg twice daily with meals.

Adverse Reactions

It can produce GIT side effects (nausea, flatulence and diarrhoea), headache, dizziness, paraesthesias and eosinophilia. It should not be given in children, pregnant women and in patients with recent myocardial infarction.

Gugulipid

It is the steroidal fraction derived from the plant *Commiphora mukul*. It has anticholesterolemic activity. It is available as Guglip tablet (25 mg) and administered twice daily with meals. It is well-tolerated.

Nonpharmacological Measures in Hyperlipoproteinaemias

These are given as follows:
- Restriction of dietary fat (not more than 25% of the calories should come from fat and 50% of this fat must be vegetable oil or unsaturated fat)
- Reduction of obesity
- Physical exercise
- No smoking
- Reduction in alcohol consumption
- Increased consumption of vegetables, fresh fruits and sea fishes
- Restriction of cholesterol consumption (less than 300 mg/day, i.e. not more than three eggs/week).

Section VIII

RENAL PHARMACOLOGY

35

Urine Formation and Diuretics

URINE FORMATION

The basic urine forming unit of the kidney is the nephron which consists of a filtering apparatus called glomerulus, which is connected to a long tubular portion that reabsorbs and conditions the glomerular ultrafiltrate. Each human kidney is composed of approximately one million nephrons. Urine formation in nephron occurs by 3 processes (shown in **Fig. 35.1**) as follows:

Glomerular Filtration

Urine formation begins in the glomerular capillary tufts by the process of ultrafiltration.

A portion of plasma water flowing through the glomerular capillaries is forced through a filter composed of endothelial cells, basement membrane and visceral epithelial cells. Solutes of small size such as sodium chloride, sodium bicarbonate, glucose, urea, uric acid and creatinine flow with the filtered water into the Bowman's capsule (urinary space), whereas formed elements of blood and proteins (macromolecules) are retained by the filtration barrier. About 125 mL of glomerular ultra-filtrate is formed each minute (i.e. 180 L/day), but only 1 L/min (i.e. 1.5 L/day) of urine is produced. So more than 99% of glomerular

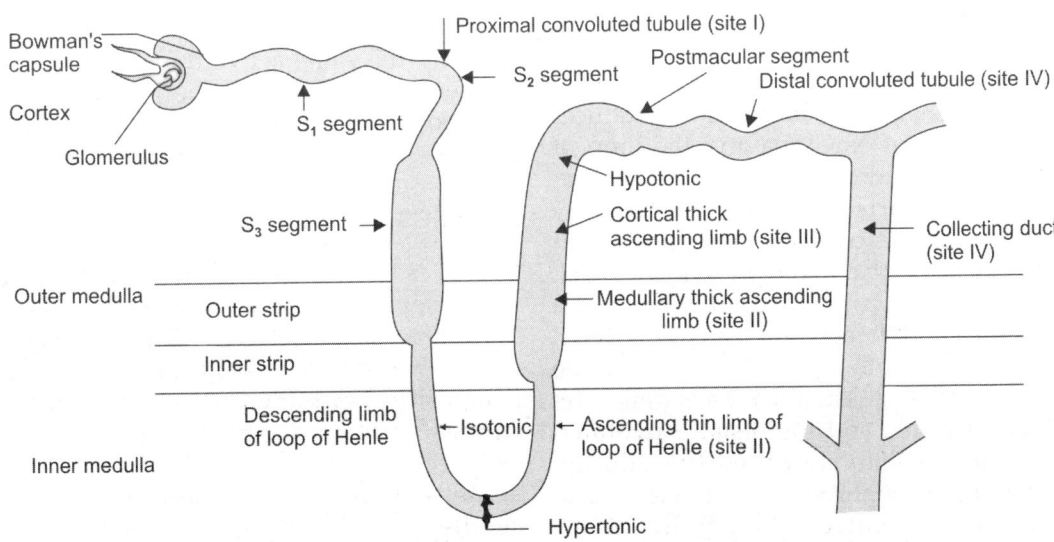

Fig. 35.1: Mammalian nephron and its divisions

263

ultrafiltrate is reabsorbed in the renal tubules. Many drugs are excreted in urine by glomerular filtration.

Tubular Reabsorption

The proximal tubule is contiguous with Bowman's capsule and takes a tortuous path in the renal cortex until finally forming a straight portion, that enters into the renal medulla. It is divided into 3 segments (S_1, S_2 and S_3) based on the morphology of epithelial cells lining the tubule. Normally, about 65% of filtered solutes are reabsorbed in the proximal tubule. As it is highly permeable to water, so reabsorption is essentially isotonic. Between the outer and inner strips of the outer medulla, the tubule becomes descending limb of loop of Henle, which enters the inner medulla and makes a hairpin bend and then forms the ascending thin limb of loop of Henle. At the junction between the inner and outer medulla, the tubule becomes thick ascending limb of loop of Henle, which is made up of three segments—a medullary segment, a cortical segment and a post-macular segment. The descending limb of loop of Henle is highly permeable to water but its permeability to NaCl and urea is low. In contrast, the ascending limb of loop of Henle is permeable to NaCl and urea but impermeable to water. The thick ascending limb passes between the afferent and efferent arterioles and makes contact with the afferent arteriole *via* a cluster of columnar epithelial cells called as macula densa. The macula densa produces concentration of NaCl leaving the loop of Henle by tuboglomerular feedback mechanism (countercurrent amplifier system). By this a condition is created in the thin limb of loop of Henle so that in the presence of ADH, urine becomes concentrated. The distal convoluted tubule actively transports NaCl and is permeable to water. As a result dilute urine is produced. The thick ascending limb of loop of Henle and the distal convoluted tubule are collectively called the diluting segment of the nephron. The tubular fluid in the distal convoluted tubule is hypotonic regardless of hydration state. But unlike the

thick ascending limb of loop of Henle, the distal convoluted tubule does not contribute to the countercurrent induced hypertonicity of the medullary interstitium.

The collecting duct controls the ultrafiltrate composition and volume. Here the final adjustments in electrolytes composition are made by the action of aldosterone (a mineralocorticoid). Moreover, ADH increases the permeability of this part of nephron to water. In the absence of ADH, the collecting duct is impermeable to water and a dilute urine is excreted. The hypertonicity of medullary interstitium plays a vital role in concentrating urine. Lipid-soluble drugs and weak acids or bases are reabsorbed in the distal renal tubules by passive diffusion.

Tubular Secretion

Some organic acids and bases are actively transported in the proximal renal tubules by two separate non-specific mechanisms and excreted in urine. Active transport of a drug across the tubules reduces concentration of its free form in the tubular vessels and promotes dissociation of protein bound drug, which again is secreted. Organic acid transport occurs for uric acid, penicillins, cephalosporins, probenecid, ethacrynic acid, salicylic acid, etc. Organic base transport occurs with histamine, serotonin, dopamine, chloroquine, quinine, quinidine, thiazides, etc. Drugs utilizing the same active transport compete with each other, e.g. probenecid blocks active transport of penicillin and uric acid and so decreases their excretion in urine.

DIURETICS

Diuretics are drugs that increase the rate, frequency and volume of urine formation. They increase the net loss of NaCl and H_2O in urine. They are used to adjust the volume and composition of body fluids in a variety of clinical conditions including hypertension (to reduce BP), acute or chronic heart failure, acute or chronic renal failure, nephrotic syndrome and cirrhosis of liver (to reduce edema).

Classification

These drugs can be classified in three ways:

1. According to mechanism of action: These are of seven groups:

a. Inhibitors of Na^+–Cl^- symport (symport means cotransport): These are as follows:

- Thiazides, e.g. hydrochlorothiazide, thiazide, bendroflumethiazide, benzthiazide, polythiazide, cyclopenthiazide, etc.

- Thiazide-like drugs, e.g. Chlorthalidone, indapamide, xipamide, metolazone, quinethiazone, etc.

b. Inhibitors of Na^+–K^+–$2Cl^-$ symport (high ceiling diuretics), e.g. frusemide, mefruside, bumetanide, piretanide, torsemide, tripamide and ethacrynic acid.

c. Inhibitors of renal epithelial Na^+ channels (K^+ sparing diuretics)—e.g. triamterene and amiloride.

d. Antagonists of mineralocorticoid receptors (aldosterone antagonists)—they are also K^+ sparing diuretics, e.g. spironolactone and potassium conreonate.

e. Inhibitors of carbonic anhydrase, e.g. acetazolamide, dichlorophenamide and methazolamide.

f. Osmotic diuretics, e.g. mannitol, glycerol, isosorbide and urea.

g. Miscellaneous diuretics, e.g. ammonium chloride (acidifying diuretic), theophylline (xanthine diuretic), mersalyl (mercurial diuretic) and carbacrylamine resin (cation exchange resin).

2. According to potency: These are of three groups:

a. High efficacy diuretics, e.g. high ceiling diuretics and organic mercurial diuretics.

b. Medium efficacy diuretics, e.g. thiazides and thiazide-like diuretics.

c. Weak efficacy (adjunctive) diuretics, e.g. K^+ sparing diuretics, carbonic anhydrase inhibitor diuretics, osmotic diuretics and miscellaneous diuretics.

3. According to site of action: These are of four groups:

a. Acting on site I (proximal convoluted tubule), e.g. osmotic diuretics, carbonic anhydrase inhibitors and xanthine diuretics.

b. Acting on site II (medullary thick segment of ascending limb of loop of Henle), e.g. high ceiling diuretics, mercurial diuretics and osmotic diuretics.

c. Acting on site III (cortical thick segment of ascending limb of loop of Henle and early distal convoluted tubule, e.g. thiazides and thiazide-like diuretics.

d. Acting on site IV (late part of distal convoluted tubule and collecting duct), e.g. K^+ sparing diuretics.

DISCUSSION OF INDIVIDUAL GROUPS OF DIURETICS

Inhibitors of Na^+–Cl^- Symport (Thiazides and Thiazide-like Diuretics)

They are sulphonamide derivatives. They have a sulphanilamide nucleus, to which a heterocyclic ring is attached. They have similar mechanism of action. They differ from each other in potency and duration of action.

Pharmacological Action

Mechanism of action: They cause inhibition of Na^+–Cl^- symporter (enzyme protein) in the site III of nephron (i.e. cortical thick segment of the ascending limb of loop of Henle and early part of distal convoluted tubule) leading to excretion of Na^+ and Cl^- in urine. In this site, transport of Na^+ is powered by Na^+ pump in the basolateral membrane. The energy in the electrochemical gradient for Na^+ is supplied by a Na^+–Cl^- symporter in the luminal membrane, which moves Cl^- ions into the epithelial cells against its electrochemical gradient. Cl^- ions then passively enter the basolateral membrane *via* a Cl^- channel. These drugs inhibit the Na^+–Cl^- symporter probably by competing for the Cl^- binding site. They produce following effects:

Renal Effects

- **Effects on serum electrolytes and urinary excretion:** They increase the excretion of electrolytes Na$^+$ and Cl$^-$ in urine. They are moderately efficacious diuretics (i.e. maximum excretion of filtered load of Na$^+$ is only 5 to 10%), since about 90% of the filtered load of Na$^+$ is reabsorbed before it reaches the site III. Some of them are also weak inhibitors of carbonic anhydrase in the proximal convoluted tubule and so increase excretion of HCO$_3^-$ and PO$_4^{2-}$ in urine. They increase the excretion of K$^+$ and H$^+$ (titrable acid) due to increased delivery of Na$^+$ to the distal renal tubule. On acute administration they increase the excretion of uric acid but on chronic administration they decrease the excretion of uric acid. They also decrease excretion of Ca^{++}, probably by increasing Ca^{++} reabsorption in the distal convoluted tubule. They may cause a mild magnesuria leading to magnesium deficiency on long-term use, especially in elderly persons. By inhibiting Na$^+$–Cl$^-$ transport in the cortical diluting segment they attenuate the ability of the kidney to excrete dilute urine during water diuresis. They do not alter the kidney's ability to concentrate urine during hydropenia.

- **Effect on renal haemodynamics:** They do not affect renal blood flow (RBF). They may variably reduce GFR due to increase in intratubular pressure. They have little effect on TGF (tuboglomerular feedback). They decrease urinary volume in patients with diabetes insipidus, especially the nephro-genic type, on prolonged administration.

Other Effects
- **Effects on blood vessels and BP:** They produce a mild hypotensive effect partly due to their action on sodium metabolism and partly due to their direct action on blood vessels (discussed with antihypertensive drugs).
- **Metabolic effects:** They can cause hyperglycaemia, hyperuricaemia, hypercalcaemia and hyperlipidaemia. They can unmask or aggravate the pre-existing diabetes mellitus. The mechanism by which they cause hyperglycaemia is not known. It may

be due to catecholamine release, secondary to volume depletion, a direct inhibition of insulin release and hypokalaemia. They cause hyperuricaemia by decreasing excretion of uric acid. This is usually asymptomatic, but occasionally acute attack of gouty arthritis may be precipitated. They cause hypercalcaemia by decreasing calcium excretion in urine. They produce slight rise of serum cholesterol and triglycerides levels on prolonged administration. They may inhibit phosphodiesterase, mitochondrial respiration (O$_2$ consumption) and renal uptake of fatty acids.

Pharmacokinetics

They are well-absorbed from GIT and the effect starts within 1 hour of oral administration. Their action is variable depending on water or lipid solubility and plasma protein binding. Water-soluble thiazides like hydrochlorothiazide, chlorothiazide, hydroflumethiazide and cyclopenthiazide have short duration of action (6 to 12 hours); while lipid-soluble thiazides like polythiazide, benzthiazide, bendroflumethiazide and trichloromethiazide have long duration of action (12 to 24 hours). Chlorthalidone has longest duration of action (about 72 hours). They are distributed throughout the extracellular fluid (i.e. they have large volume of distribution). They are relatively concentrated in the kidney. They can cross the BBB and placental barrier. They are little metabolized in the liver and are excreted as such in urine by being secreted in the proximal renal tubule like other organic acids.

Clinical Uses

These are given as follows:
- **As diuretics:** They are used in the treatment of oedema associated with sodium retention as in cardiac oedema (CCF), hepatic oedema (cirrhosis of liver) and renal oedema (nephrotic syndrome, acute glomerulonephritis and chronic renal failure). They are also used in pulmonary or cerebral oedema, oedema of pregnancy, drug induced oedema (caused by cortico-

steroids, NSAIDs, carbenoxolone, etc.) and idiopathic oedema. With the exceptions of metolazone and indapamide, most thiazide diuretics are ineffective in oedema when GFR is less than 30 mL/minute.

- **As antihypertensives:** They are widely used in the treatment of hypertension, either alone or in combination with other antihypertensive drugs.
- **In diabetes insipidus:** They are used for the treatment of both central and nephrogenic diabetes insipidus. By causing natriuresis, they deplete the plasma volume, which consequently reduce the urine output in diabetes insipidus.
- **In the prevention of recurrent renal calculi (idiopathic calcium nephrolithiasis):** Hydrochlorothiazide (50 mg twice daily) reduces the frequency of calcium stone formation in the kidney in patients with essential hypercalciuria.
- **In the prevention and treatment of osteoporosis:** Hydrochlorothiazide is usually used in osteoporosis to reduce calcium excretion in urine.

Some commonly used preparations and dosage:

- Hydrochlorothiazide (Esidrex) tablet (25, 50 mg)—25 to 200 mg daily.
- Chlorothiazide (Diuril) tablet (250, 500 mg)—250 to 1000 mg daily.
- Hydroflumethiazide (Naclex) tablet (50 mg)—25 to 200 mg daily.
- Bendroflumethiazide (Neo-Naclex) tablet (2.5, 5 mg)—2.5 to 5 mg daily.
- Polythiazide (Nephril) tablet (1, 2 mg)— 1 to 4 mg daily.
- Chlorthalidone (Hygroton/Hythalton) tablet (100 mg)—50 to 200 mg daily.
- Xipamide (Xipamid) tablet (20 mg)—20 to 40 mg daily.
- Clopamide (Brinaldix) tablet (20 mg)—20 to 80 mg daily.

Adverse Reactions

They can rarely cause CNS side effects (vertigo, headache, paraesthesia and weakness), GIT side effects (anorexia, nausea, vomiting, abdominal cramps and diarrhoea/constipation), sexual disorders (impotence and decreased libido), skin disorders (skin rashes and photosensitivity) and blood disorders (dyscrasias) Their most serious adverse effects are related to abnormalities of fluid and electrolyte balance producing extracellular fluid volume depletion, hypotension, dilutional, hyponatraemia, hypokalaemia, hypochloraemia, metabolic alkalosis, hypomagnesaemia, hypercalcaemia, and hyperuricaemia. They also decrease glucose tolerance and can produce hyperglycaemia. Latent diabetes mellitus may be unmasked by them. They may increase plasma levels of LDL cholesterol, total cholesterol and total triglycerides.

Contraindications

- In individuals who are hypersensitive to sulphonamides.
- With digitalis they may increase digitalis toxicity by producing hypokalaemia, where potassium supplements must be given.
- With quinidine they may produce ventricular tachycardia due to prolongation of Q-T interval by quinidine.
- In patients of hepatic insufficiency, as they may precipitate hepatic encephalopathy by decreasing renal excretion of NH_3.
- With corticosteroids and amphotericin-B, as they increase the risk of hypokalaemia produced by thiazides.

Inhibitors of Na⁺-K⁺-2Cl⁻ Symport (High Ceiling/Loop Diuretics)

Chemically these are:
- Sulphonamide derivatives, e.g. frusemide, mefruside, bumetanide and piretanide.
- Sulphonyl urea derivatives, e.g. torsemide and tripamide.
- Phenyl acetic acid derivative, e.g. ethacrynic acid.

They are called high ceiling diuretics because they have high efficacy as diuretics. They are called loop diuretics as they act on the thick ascending limb of the loop of Henle (in renal medulla). Their high efficacy is due to following two factors:

- About 25% of the filtered solute load normally is reabsorbed by the medullary thick ascending limb of loop of Henle.
- Nephron segments pass the thick ascending limb possess little reabsorptive capacity for the filtered solutes. The special features are:
  - Highly effective diuretics
  - Act on loop of Henle
  - Can produce action in acid–base imbalance (acidosis/alkalosis)
  - Can be administered orally or parenterally.
  - Ototoxic.

Pharmacological Actions

Mechanism of action: They cause inhibition of $Na^+- K^+- 2Cl^-$ symporter (enzyme protein) in the site II of nephron (medullary thick segment of ascending limb of loop of Henle), leading to excretion of Na^+, K^+ and Cl^- in urine. Frusemide and mefruside can also act on sites I and III (except at distal site, where Na^+ is exchanged for K^+). They have no effect on carbonic anhydrase at site I. In the medullary thick ascending limb of loop of Henle, fluxes of Na^+, K^+ and Cl^- from the lumen into the epithelial cell is mediated by a $Na^+- K^+- 2Cl^-$ symporter. This symporter captures the energy in the Na^+ electrochemical gradient established by the Na^+ pump in the basolateral membrane and supplies it for uphill transport of K^+ and Cl^- into the cell. K^+ channels in the luminal membrane provide a conductive pathway for the apical recycling of this cation and basolateral Cl^- channels provide a basolateral exit mechanism of Cl^-. In addition, a $Na^+- Cl^-$ symporter in the basolateral membrane permits cotransport of Cl^- down the electrochemical gradient with concomitant transport of Na^+ against an electrochemical gradient. These diuretics bind with $Na^+- K^+- 2Cl^-$ symporter and block its function to transport salt across the medullary thick segment of ascending limb of the loop

of Henle. They may produce this action by binding with Cl^- binding site of the symporter. They also inhibit Ca^{++} and Mg^{++} reabsorption in the thick ascending limb by abolishing the transepithelial potential difference that is dominant driving force for reabsorption of these cations. They produce following effects:

Renal Effects

- **Effects on serum electrolytes and urinary excretion:** They produce profound increase in the urinary excretion of Na^+ (up to 25% of the filtered load of Na^+) and Cl^- and moderate increase in the urinary excretion of K^+ and H^+ (titrable acid). They also cause marked increase in the urinary excretion of Ca^{++} and Mg^{++}. Frusemide and mefruside have weak carbonic anhydrase inhibiting activity (at site I) and increase the urinary excretion of bicarbonate and phosphate. On acute administration high ceiling diuretics increase the excretion of uric acid and on chronic administration decrease the excretion of uric acid (by increasing reabsorption). By blocking active Na^+ and Cl^- reabsorption in the thick ascending limb they interfere with a critical step in the mechanism that produces a hypertonic medullary interestitium (hypertonic fluid draws more water from ECF). Therefore, they block kidney's ability to concentrate urine during hydropenia. They also markedly impair the kidney's ability to excrete a dilute urine during water diuresis.
- **Effects on renal haemodynamics:** They increase renal blood flow (RBF) and GFR. They block TGF (tuboglomerular feedback).

Other Effects

- **Effects on blood vessels and BP:** They can cause peripheral vasodilatation and lower arterial BP. They cause rapid venous pooling of blood and reduce cardiac preload and afterload. By decreasing left ventricular filling pressure (by venodilatation of capacitance vessels) and pulmonary congestion, they produce benefits in patients of pulmonary oedema even before diuresis ensures.

- **Metabolic effects:** They can cause hyperglycaemia, hyperuricaemia, uraemia, hypocalcaemia and hypomagnesaemia. They may inhibit Na^+/K^+-ATPase, mitochondrial respiration, microsomal Ca^{++} pump, adenylcyclase, phosphodiesterase and PG-dehydrogenase.

Pharmacokinetics

They are well-absorbed orally. Frusemide is given IV for immediate action. They are extensively bound to plasma proteins. They are secreted in the proximal renal tubule by organic acid transport system and thereby gain access to their binding sites on the Na^+-K^+-$2Cl^-$ symporter in the luminal membrane of the medullary thick ascending limb of loop of Henle. Frusemide is excreted within 6 hours of oral administration largely unchanged by both glomerular filtration and tubular secretion. On its IV administration, diuresis begins within 2 minutes and lasts for 2 to 3 hours. It is best administered in a single daily dose.

Clinical Uses

These are as follows:

- **As diuretics:** They are used in the treatment of oedema associated with sodium retention as in cardiac oedema (CCF), hepatic oedema (cirrhosis of liver) and renal oedema (nephrotic syndrome and chronic renal failure) when refractory to other groups of diuretics.
- **As antihypertensives:** They may be used in mild and moderate hypertension but not preferred for long-term therapy because of high dose requirement, short duration of action and high diuretic activity. They are reserved for patients in whom other antihypertensives do not produce satisfactory response.
- **In the treatment of acute pulmonary oedema:** IV frusemide is used. It produces rapid relief of symptoms of pulmonary oedema by increasing venous pooling in capacitance vessels and decreasing left ventricular filling pressure (preload to heart). It is effective in this condition even before the onset of diuresis. Other drugs that may be used in this condition are morphine, aminophylline and nitroglycerine given IV.
- **In the treatment of chronic CCF:** Frusemide is used when diminution of extracellular fluid volume is desirable to minimize venous and pulmonary congestion.
- **To induce forced alkaline diuresis:** Frusemide with sodium bicarbonate is infused IV in patients with anuria due to barbiturate or salicylate poisoning, in order to facilitate more rapid excretion of the offending drug in urine.
- **To treat hypercalcaemia:** Frusemide with normal saline is infused IV in the emergency management of hypercalcaemia in order to increase calcium excretion in urine.
- **To treat life-threatening hyponatraemia:** Frusemide with hypertonic saline is infused IV to correct hyponatraemia.

Preparations and Dosage

- Frusemide (Lasix) tablet (40 mg)—40 to 100 mg daily.
- Frusemide (Lasix) injection (20 mg/2 mL)— 40 to 200 mg IV or IM.
- Bumetanide (Burinex) tablet (1 mg)—1 to 2 mg daily.
- Mefruside (Baycaron) tablet (12.5 mg)— 12.5 to 50 mg daily.
- Ethacrynic acid (Edecrin) tablet (50 mg)— 50 to 150 mg daily
- Sodium ethacrynate (Edecrin) injection (50 mg/2 mL)—0.5 to 1 mg/kg IV.

Adverse Reactions

These are powerful diuretics and can precipitate serious electrolyte and water disturbances due to excessive loss of Na^+, K^+, Cl^- and H_2O. There may be weakness, fatigue, dizziness, muscle cramps, hypotension, acute urinary retention (due to reduced GFR), circulatory collapse, thromboembolic episodes and hepatic encephalopathy/coma (in presence of severe hepatic disease). Increased excretion of K^+ and H^+ causes hypokalaemia and hypochloremic alkalosis. Increased Mg^{++} and Ca^{++} excretion may cause hypomagnesaemia and hypocalcaemia. They can cause ototoxicity, which is manifested as tinnitus, hearing impairment, deafness, vertigo and a sense of fullness in the ear. Ethacrynic acid produces more ototoxicity than frusemide and others. They can cause hyperglycaemia (may precipitate diabetes mellitus) and hyperuricaemia (may precipitate gout). They can increase plasma levels of LDL cholesterol and triglycerides but decrease plasma level of HDL cholesterol. Other adverse effects include skin rashes, nausea, vomiting, diarrhoea, photosensitivity, paraesthesia and rarely acute pancreatitis and bone marrow depression (causing neutropaenia and thrombocytopaenia).

Contraindications

- In individuals hypersensitive to sulphonamides
- During pregnancy
- Severe Na^+ and fluid volume depletion
- Along with lithium and cephalosporins (increase their toxicity)
- Severe hepatic disease

Inhibitors of Renal Epithelial Na+ Channels (K+ Sparing Diuretics)

These are organic bases, e.g. triamterene and amiloride. They are transported (secreted) by the organic base secretory mechanism in the proximal convoluted tubule. Their action is direct and not dependent on the mineralocorticoid aldosterone.

Pharmacological Actions

Mechanism of action: They are Na^+ channel blockers. They act in the late part of distal convoluted tubule and collecting duct, which have in their luminal membranes. Na^+ channels for the entry of Na^+ into the epithelial cells down the electrochemical gradient created by the Na^+ pump in the basolateral membrane. They block the Na^+ channels in the luminal membrane of the epithelial cells and prevent reabsorption of Na^+ in this part of nephron. This results in mild increase in the excretion rates of Na^+ and Cl^- (about 2% of the filtered load). Blocking of Na^+ channels hyperpolarizes the luminal membrane reducing the luminal negative transepithelial voltage. Since the luminal negative potential difference normally opposes cation reabsorption and facilitates cation secretion, so decrease of luminal negative voltage decreases the excretion rates of K^+, H^+, Ca^{++} and Mg^{++}. They produce following effects:

Renal Effects

They increase urinary excretion of Na^+, Cl^-, HCO_3^- and H_2O and decrease excretion of K^+, H^+, Ca^{++} and Mg^{++}. They also increase excretion of uric acid. They have little or no effect on renal haemodynamics and do not alter TGF (tuboglomerular feedback).

Other Effects

They do not produce hyperglycaemia. They have no antihypertensive effect, but when combined with a thiazide or loop diuretic they increase the diuretic and antihypertensive effects of latter drugs.

Pharmacokinetics

They are well-absorbed orally. They are little metabolized in the liver and excreted in urine almost unchanged. They have plasma t½ of 6 to 10 hours.

Clinical Uses

They are seldom used alone in the treatment of oedema or hypertension as they produce mild natriuresis. They are mainly used in combination with a thiazide or loop diuretic to increase diuretic and antihypertensive effects. Moreover, by decreasing potassium loss in urine by other diuretics, they normalize the plasma K^+ level. They are used particularly in the long-term management of persistent oedema due to nephrotic syndrome and cirrhosis of liver.

Preparations and Dosage

- Triamterene (50 mg) with benzthiazide (25 mg) tablet (Ditide)—one to two tablets daily.
- Amiloride (5 mg) with hydrochlorothiazide (50 mg) tablet (Biduret)—one to two tablets daily.

Adverse Reactions

They can cause hyperkalaemia, nausea, vomiting, diarrhoea, headache, leg cramps, dizziness, uraemia and skin rash. They should not be used in hyperkalaemia due to any cause.

Antagonists of Mineralocorticoid Receptors (Aldosterone Antagonists)

Spironolactone is an steroid with structural similarity to the mineralocorticoid aldosterone. It is the commonly used aldosterone antagonist. It is also a K^+ sparing diuretic.

Pharmacological Actions

Mechanism of action: Aldosterone causes retention of salt (NaCl) and H_2O and increases the excretion of K^+ and H^+ by binding to specific mineralocorticoid receptors (MRs) in the epithelial cells of the late part of distal convoluted tubule and collecting duct. Aldosterone antagonist, spironolactone competitively inhibits the binding of aldosterone to the mineralocorticoid receptors and prevents the actions of aldosterone. Aldosterone increases the Na^+ conductance of the luminal membrane and sodium pump activity of the basolateral membrane of the epithelial cells. As a result transepithelial NaCl transport is increased and the luminal negative transepithelial voltage is increased leading to increased driving force for secretion of K^+ and H^+ into the tubular lumen. Spironolactone prevents these actions of aldosterone.
It produces following effects:

- **Renal effects:** These are similar to triamterene and amiloride.
- **Other effects:** It has mild antihypertensive effect. It does not produce hyperglycaemia.

It has antiandrogenic activity at the receptor level. It may increase blood urea nitrogen and serum uric acid levels.

Pharmacokinetics

It is well-absorbed orally. It is metabolized in the liver and excreted slowly in urine. It has a cumulative effect and full response is observed after a few days of therapy.

Clinical Uses

It is used in the treatment of oedema and hypertension either alone or in combination with a thiazide or loop diuretic. It is particularly useful in the treatment of primary hyperaldosteronism (as in adrenal adenomas and bilateral adrenal hyperplasia) and in refractory oedema associated with secondary hyperaldosteronism (as in CCF, cirrhosis of liver, nephrotic syndrome and severe ascites). It is the diuretic of choice in oedema due to cirrhosis of liver, as hyperaldosteronism is present since early stage of this condition. It is also used in female hirsutism (for antiandrogenic activity).

Preparations and Dosage

- Spironolactone (Aldactone) tablet (25 mg)—25 to 200 mg daily.
- Spironolactone (25 mg) with hydroflumethiazide (25 mg) tablet (Aldactide)—2 to 4 tablets daily.
- Spironolactone (50 mg) with frusemide (20 mg) tablet (Lasilactone)—1 to 4 tablets daily.

Adverse Reactions

It can cause hyperkalaemia (by potassium retention) metabolic acidosis (in cirrhotic patients), drowsiness, lethargy, confusion, headache, gynecomastia, impotence, decreased libido and menstrual irregularities. It may induce diarrhoea, gastritis, gastric bleeding and peptic ulcer. Aspirin interacts with it and decreases its action. It should not be used in hyperkalaemia due to any cause. Potassium canrenoate (Spiroctan-M) is an aldosterone antagonist. It has similar actions and uses of spironolactone but it can be given parenterally. It is a metabolite of spironolactone. It is available as injection (20 mg/mL in 10 mL ampoule) and administered IV slowly up to 400 mg/day in divided doses.

Inhibitors of Carbonic Anhydrase (CA)

These are sulphonamide derivatives. They are weak (low efficacy) diuretics, e.g. acetazolamide.

Pharmacological Actions

Mechanism of action: They act by inhibiting the enzyme carbonic anhydrase, present in the proximal convoluted tubule of renal cortex and also in gastric mucosa, pancreas, eye and CNS. It catalyzes the reaction:

$$CO_2 + H_2O \xrightarrow{\text{CA}} H_2CO_3 \rightleftharpoons H^+ + H_2CO_3^-$$

Actual reaction is:

i. $H_2O \rightleftharpoons OH^- + H^+$

ii. $OH^- + CO_2 \rightleftharpoons H_2CO_3^-$

iii. $HCO + H^+ \rightleftharpoons H_2CO_3$

Due to inhibition of the enzyme carbonic anhydrase, H^+ is not available for H^+/Na^+ exchange mechanism, leading to excretion of Na^+ accompanied by H_2O. Due to lack of H^+, bicarbonate (HCO_3^-) is excreted in urine in large amount and so plasma Cl^- is increased leading to metabolic acidosis. As the reabsorption of Na^+, K^+ and $H_2CO_3^-$ is reduced, so they are excreted in urine producing alkaline urine. They also increase phosphate excretion (mechanism unknown), but have no effect on the excretion of Ca^{++} and Mg^{++}. Their effect is self-limiting as they cause metabolic acidosis, which produces loss of diuretic activity.

They produce following effects:

• **Renal effects:** They cause urinary excretion of Na^+, K^+, $H_2CO_3^-$ and PO_4^- ions. By increasing delivery of solutes to macula densa, they trigger TGF (tuboglomerular feedback), which increases afferent arteriolar resistance and decreases renal blood flow and GFR.

• **Other effects:** They reduce intraocular tension by inhibiting the enzyme, carbonic anhydrase. Carbonic anhydrase present in various intraocular structures is important in the formation of aqueous humour, which has a high bicarbonate content. Inhibition of carbonic anhydrase decreases formation of aqueous humour leading to fall of intraocular pressure. They also decrease CSF formation.

Pharmacokinetics

They are well-absorbed orally. They are little metabolized in the liver and excreted almost completely in urine within 24 hours.

Clinical Uses

They have limited uses:

• In the treatment of glaucoma (open angle or secondary) to reduce intraocular pressure.

• For the prevention and treatment of acute mountain sickness. This condition is caused by rapid ascent in mountain to heights of 8000 feet or more, where the partial pressure of atmospheric oxygen is much less than that at sea level. As a result, marked decrease in arterial oxygen saturation (hypoxaemia) occurs leading to tissue hypoxia and pulmonary arterial hypertension. Its manifestations are impairment of memory and judgement, headache, anorexia, malaise and insomnia. There may be cerebral oedema, pulmonary oedema and retinal haemorrhages. Coma and death may occur in some patients. The best approach in prevention and treatment of this condition is gradual ascent in mountain. If it is not possible for some reasons then acetazolamide is given in the dosage of 250 mg thrice daily on the day before, during and for 5 days after the ascent. It probably acts by causing mild metabolic acidosis, which increases respiratory drive and prevents hypoxaemia. It ameliorates symptoms of mountain sickness but cannot reduce the risk of cerebral oedema, pulmonary oedema or retinal haemorrhages. Dexamethasone is highly effective in the treatment of cerebral oedema. It is given in the dosage of 4 mg 6 hourly, begun on the day of ascent and continued for 3 days at high altitude and then tapered for 5 days. Other measures include adequate rest and hydration, mild analgesics and avoidance of alcohol.

- In the treatment of resistant epilepsy (grand mal) as an adjuvant to other drugs (probably act by producing metabolic acidosis).

- In the treatment of familial periodic paralysis of limbs (mechanism unknown).

- To correct metabolic alkalosis caused by some diuretics, e.g. thiazide diuretics, high ceiling diuretics and mercurial diuretics.

Preparations and Dosage

- Acetazolamide (Diamox) tablet (250 mg)—250 to 500 mg once or twice daily.

- Dichlorphenamide (Daranide) tablet (50 mg)—50 to 100 mg once or twice daily.

Adverse Reactions

They can cause metabolic acidosis and hypokalaemia. Sometimes they produce excessive potassium loss without causing significant sodium loss. Metabolic acidosis is dangerous in presence of kidney damage. In high dosage they can cause drowsiness and paraesthesia. Like sulphonamides, they can cause skin rashes, blood dyscrasias, crystalluria and kidney damage. Salicylates increase their toxicity by displacing them from plasma protein binding sites and inhibiting their renal tubular secretion.

Contraindications

- Cirrhosis of liver (can produce hepatic encephalopathy by diversion of ammonia of renal origin from urine into the systemic circulation).

- Severe chronic obstructive pulmonary disease (COPD).

- Patients with hypochloraemic acidosis.

Osmotic Diuretics

These are solutes which have the following properties:

- They are freely filtered at the glomerulus.
- They are poorly reabsorbed by the renal tubules.
- They are not metabolized in the body.
- They are relatively inert pharmacologically.
- They are administered in large doses to increase the osmolality of plasma and tubular fluid.

Mechanism of Action

They act in the proximal convoluted tubule and the loop of Henle and increase delivery of Na^+ and H_2O from them. By extracting water from the intracellular compartments they expand extracellular fluid volume, decrease blood viscosity and inhibit renin release. These effects increase renal blood flow (RBF). The increased renal medullary blood flow removes NaCl and urea from the renal medulla and reduces medullary toxicity, which causes a decrease in the reabsorption of H_2O from the distal tubular lumen. This inturn limits the concentration of NaCl in the tubular fluid entering the proximal tubular lumens and decreases the passive reabsorption of NaCl in the proximal renal tubule. In general osmotic diuretics increase the urinary excretion of nearly all electrolytes including Na^+, K^+, Ca^{++}, Mg^{++}, Cl^-, $H_2CO_3^-$ and PO_4^-.

DISCUSSION OF COMMONLY USED DRUGS

Mannitol

It is a sugar (polyhydroxyaliphatic alcohol with 4-hydroxy groups). It is administered IV in large dosage. It is not metabolized in the body and rapidly filtered by the glomeruli. It is nonabsorbable and so exerts high osmotic activity, which interferes with the reabsorption of Na^+ and H_2O in the tubules causing osmotic diuresis. It is not a suitable diuretic in cases of cardiac oedema with sodium retention, because it increases extracellular fluid volume, which increases further the load on the already decompensated heart.

Clinical uses

It is used in:

- **Barbiturate poisoning:** It increases the urinary excretion of barbiturate when administered by IV infusion. The infusion is continued as long as the urine output remains good. Water and electrolytes are given concurrently to replace those lost in urine. Up to 200 g of mannitol can used by IV infusion.

- **Acute renal failure (due to a rapid decrease in GFR):** It is useful in threatened acute oliguric renal failure from prerenal cases, e.g. severe gastroenteritis, severe burns and severe traumatic injuries which result in hypovolemia and hypotension. In such cases, after initial correction of hypovolemia by adequate amount of fluid 100 mL of mannitol (25% soln) is infused rapidly in 10 to 15 minutes. If the urine flow rate increases, then further mannitol is given to maintain the high urine flow rate. If no diuresis occurs after the initial mannitol infusion then established acute renal failure is diagnosed and no more mannitol is given. Mannitol is also useful in acute renal failure due to renal causes, e.g. acute tubular necrosis produced by nephrotoxins (aminoglycosides, cisplatin, amphotericin-B, radiocontrast media, cyclosporins, sepsis) or by haemoglobinuria and myoglobinuria produced by haemolytic transfusion reactions.

- **Cerebral edema:** It is used by IV infusion in cerebral edema to reduce raised intracranial tension by IV infusion.

- **Glaucoma:** It is used by IV infusion to reduce high intraocular pressure in acute congestive glaucoma by extracting water out of the eye.

Preparation and Dosage

Mannitol injection (10, 20, 25% solution in 50 mL ampoule)—100 to 500 mL by IV infusion.

Adverse Reactions

It can cause headache, nausea, chills, polydipsia, confusion and pain in chest. It may precipitate pulmonary oedema in patients with CCF by increasing blood volume (hypervolemia). It can also cause hyponatraemia by excessive sodium loss in urine. It can produce rebound oedema.

Contraindications

Dehydration, CCF and acute cerebral haemorrhage.

Glycerol Glycerin

It is a sugar (polyhydroxyaliphatic alcohol with 3-hydroxy groups). It is administered orally or IV. It has mechanism of action and clinical uses like mannitol. It has certain advantages over mannitol. It can be administered in presence of dehydration and CCF. It does not produce rebound oedema. It can be used in acute cerebral haemorrhage.

Preparations and Dosage

- Glycerol solution (50 to 75%) for oral use—30 mL 4 times daily. Palatability is increased by chilling the solution or adding lemon juice.

- Glycerol (10%) in 500 mL of normal saline or 5% dextrose solution for injection—500 to 1000 mL daily by IV infusion for 5 days.

Adverse Reactions

It can cause hyperglycaemia on being metabolized. High concentration (30%) of glycerol by IV infusion can cause haemolysis of blood cells (RBCs).

Miscellaneous Diuretics

Ammonium chloride

It is an acidifying salt diuretic. It is administered orally. It is broken down into NH_4^+ and Cl^- ions in the intestine, which are absorbed from the intestine. In the liver, NH_4^+ is converted to urea, leaving excess Cl^- in plasma. Cl^- reacts with $NaHCO_3$ in plasma forming NaCl and CO_2. This lowers alkali reserve and produces acidosis. The excess of NaCl is excreted by the kidney with corresponding loss of H_2O in urine producing diuresis. The diuretic action of ammonium chloride is self-limiting as kidney compensates for the acidosis by producing NH_3 and by secreting more H^+ ions for exchanging with Na^+ ions in the tubular fluid. H^+ combines with Cl^- and saves Na^+ (base saving mechanism).

Clinical Uses

It is now obsolete as a diuretic due to weak action. It is used as a reflex expectorant and an urinary acidifier to promote excretion of basic drugs like chloroquine, amphetamine, pethidine, etc. in their poisoning.

Preparation and Dosage

Ammonium chloride syrup—1 g in 30 mL twice or thrice daily.

Adverse Reactions

It can cause nausea (due to bad taste) and vomiting (by gastric irritation). In the presence of renal damage it can cause severe acidosis, as kidney cannot compensate for it. It is contraindicated in severe renal and hepatic diseases.

Theophylline

It is a xanthine alkaloid diuretic. It is the most effective diuretic amongst the xanthene alkaloids (caffeine, theophylline and theobromine). It produces diuresis by increasing GFR and renal blood flow especially in the medulla. The increase in renal blood flow is due to cardiac stimulant action and renal vasodilatation action. It dilates the afferent arterioles and increases the number of functioning glomeruli. It also directly inhibits the reabsorption of Na^+, Cl^- and H_2O in the proximal convoluted tubule and the diluting segment of the loop of Henle. The loss of K^+ is small and there is no change in acid base balance.

Clinical Uses

It is now rarely used as a diuretic due to weak action. It is mainly used as a bronchodilator in bronchial asthma.

Preparations and Dosage

- Theophylline (Theopa) tablet (100, 300 mg)—100 to 300 mg twice daily.
- Theophylline (Anhydrous) (Theolong) capsule (100, 200 mg)—100 to 200 mg twice daily.
- Aminophylline tablet (100, 200 mg)—100 to 200 mg thrice daily. It is a water-soluble salt.
- Aminophylline injection (250 mg/10 mL ampoule)—250 to 500 mg dissolved in 10 to 20 mL of 5% dextrose solution is given by slow IV injection taking 10 to 20 minutes.

Adverse Reactions

It can produce headache, tremors, anxiety, tachycardia, hypertension, cardiac arrhythmias and convulsions in high dosage. Rapid IV injection of aminophylline can cause cardiac stimulation leading to cardiac arrhythmias, cardiac arrest or sudden severe fall of BP (anaphylactoid shock).

Mersalyl

It is an organic mercurial diuretic. It is a potent diuretic. It is ineffective orally. When administered IM, mercury ions combine with –SH group of enzymes (due to high affinity) in renal tubules which depresses tubular reabsorption of Na^+ and Cl^- leading to excretion of Na^+, Cl^- and H_2O in urine. Loss of K^+ and HCO_3^- in urine is less marked causing hypochloraemic alkalosis.

Clinical Uses

It can be used in severe oedema and ascites, due to cirrhosis of liver. It is contraindicated in severe renal diseases.

Adverse Reactions

It can produce gingivitis, stomatitis, renal impairment (nephrotoxicity), loss of memory, delirium and psychosis.

Carbacrylamine Resin

It is a synthetic cation exchange resin. When administered orally, it exchanges its H^+ ions with the Na^+ ions in the intestine. The resultant compound is not absorbed, thereby preventing the absorption of Na^+ from the intestine. K^+ is also exchanged along with Na^+. So there is significant loss of K^+ in faeces along with Na^+.

Clinical Uses

It is used for removal of sodium from the body in the dosage of 40 to 65 g daily.

Adverse Reactions

It can cause nausea, vomiting and diarrhoea. On prolonged use it produces hypokalaemia and metabolic acidosis.

Treatment of Resistant (Refractory) Oedema

Combination of two diuretics acting at different sites is helpful in resistant oedema.

- Frusemide (40 mg) and amiloride (5 mg) tablet (Frumil/Lasiride).

- Frusemide (20 mg) and spironolactone (50 mg) tablet (Lasilactone).

- Frusemide (20 mg) and triamterene (50 mg) tablet (Frusemine).

- Amiloride (5 mg) and hydrochlorothiazide (50 mg) tablet (Biduret). Triamterene (50 mg) and benzthiazide (25 mg) tablet (Dytide). Combination of two diuretics acting on the same site is not helpful in resistant oedema.

36

Antidiuretics and Drugs Altering Urinary pH

ANTIDIURETICS

Antidiuretics are drugs that decrease urine volume by increasing reabsorption of water in the distal renal tubule and collecting duct or decreasing GFR. They are used in the treatment of diabetes insipidus (DI), which is characterized by persistent excretion of excessive quantities of urine of low specific gravity and by constant thirst. Diabetes insipidus can be subdivided into two main types, *viz.* central (pituitary) diabetes insipidus, in which there is deficient production of the antidiuretic hormone (ADH /vasopressin) in the hypothalamus and nephrogenic diabetes insipidus, in which the distal renal tubule and collecting duct are unresponsive to vasopressin. Central DI is due to head injury, hypothalamic or pituitary tumours, cerebral aneurysms or idiopathic (familial) and nephrogenic DI is due to hypokalaemia, hypercalcaemia, postobstructive renal failure or drug induced (lithium, methoxyflurane, dimethylchlortetracycline or heavy metal poisoning).

Drugs used in diabetes insipidus are antidiuretic hormone, benzothiadiazines, chlorpropamide and carbamazepine.

Antidiuretic Hormone (ADH Vasopressin)

It is a polypeptide (nonapeptide) hormone synthesized in the hypothalamus (by the supraoptic and paraventricular nuclei) and travels along the hypothalamohypophyseal tract to the posterior pituitary, where it is stored along with oxytocin. The rate of secretion or release of ADH is mainly determined by the state of hydration. Thus, dehydration stimulates, whereas hydration inhibits the secretion of ADH. An increase or decrease in circulating blood volume also influences the secretion through volume receptors found in the heart, pulmonary veins and hypothalamus. Drugs like morphine, nicotine and barbiturates stimulate the release of ADH, whereas alcohol and phenothiazines depress the release of ADH.

Physiological and Pharmacological Actions

It has prominent actions on kidneys and cardiovascular system. It produces following effects:

- **Renal effects:** It acts on the distal convoluted tubule and collecting duct of the nephron and increases their permeability to water. As a result, a large amount of water is reabsorbed from that site leading to reduction in the total volume of urine. The electrolyte content of urine is not altered.

  Mechanism of action: The cellular action of ADH is mediated by interaction of the hormone with two types of receptor V_1 and V_2. V_1 receptors are present in vascular smooth muscles (especially in the vasa recta and efferent arteriole), renal medullary interstitial cells, epithelial cells of collecting duct, adenohypophysis, hepatocytes, adepocytes and platelets and mediate actions like vasoconstriction, glycogenolysis, platelet aggregation, ACTH release and growth of vascular smooth muscle cells. V_2 receptors are present in distal renal tubule and collecting duct and mediate water influx by increasing water permeability of those sites leading to anti-diuresis.

- **CVS effects:** It causes an initial tachycardia due to coronary insufficiency (by vasoconstriction), which is followed by bradycardia due to direct depressant effect on the myocardium and rise of BP (by direct stimulation of the vascular smooth muscle) in large dosage.
- **Other effects:** It also stimulates the smooth muscle of the GIT promoting peristalsis in large dosage. It has little oxytocic activity.

Pharmacokinetics

It is not effective orally due to peptide nature. It has to be administered parenterally for therapeutic effect. When administered SC or IM it remains in the body only for a few hours and when administered IV it is rapidly destroyed in liver and kidney. It has a plasma t½ of about 20 minutes. Its effects can be prolonged (24 to 48 hours) when it is administered SC or IM as repository form (vasopressin tannate in oil).

Clinical Uses

It is used in:

- **Diabetes insipidus of central origin:** Desmopressin is the preparation of choice in this condition. Nephrogenic diabetes insipidus does not respond to it.
- **Bleeding oesophageal varices in portal hypertension:** It controls bleeding by splanchnic vasoconstriction and thereby reducing the portal blood flow and venous pressure.
- **Haemophilia:** It prevents bleeding in this condition by releasing and increasing plasma level of factor VIII (antihaemophilic factor).

Preparations and Dosage

- Vasopressin (Pitressin) injection (a sterile aqueous solution containing 20 units/ml)—5 to 10 units SC or IM every 4 to 6 hours.
- Vasopressin tannate injection (an oily suspension containing 5 units/ml)—5 units IM once in 24 to 72 hours.
- Desmopressin acetate (Minirin) spray (a synthetic vasopressin analogue, i.e. desamino-D-arginine vasopressin/DDAVP, containing 0.1 mg/ml)—5 to 10 mcg intranasally twice daily. It can also be given by injection (SC or IM).
- Lyprissin or syntopression spray (Lysine-8-vasopressin containing 50 units/ml)—2 to 8 units intranasally 3 to 6 times daily. It can also be given by injection (SC or IM).

Adverse Reactions

It can produce nausea, belching and abdominal cramps and defecation (due to increased peristaltic activity) and hypotension and shock (due to coronary spasm especially in patients with hypertension or a vascular disease in large dosage). Nasal irritation and ulceration may occur following repeated nasal administration.

Contraindications

It should not be used in patients with ischaemic heart disease, hypertension or chronic nephritis.

Benzothiadiazines Thiazides

Hydrochlorothiazide, polythiazide, chlorthalidone, etc. They are effective in controlling nephrogenic diabetes insipidus. They probably act by causing initially a state of electrolyte depletion (negative sodium balance) which increases reabsorption of electrolytes (Na^+ and Cl^-) along with water from the glomerular filtrate in the renal tubules. They also decrease GFR. This leads to decrease in volume of urine (up to 50%) by volume contraction. They may cause hypokalaemia by excretion of K^+ in urine, which can be corrected by giving a potassium sparing diuretic or by potassium supplementation. Their preparations and dosage are discussed along with diuretics.

Chlorpropamide

It is an oral antidiabetic drug, which is also effective in controlling diabetes insipidus of central (pituitary) origin. It probably acts by increasing the sensitivity of renal tubules to lower concentration of ADH. It is given orally in the dosage of 250 to 500 mg daily. Other closely related drugs like tolbutamide and glibenclamide are not effective in this condition.

Carbamazepine

It is an antiepileptic drug, which is also effective in controlling diabetes insipidus of central (pituitary) origin. It probably acts by stimulating ADH release from the posterior pituitary (neurohypophysis). It is administered orally in the dosage of 200 mg twice daily. Alcohol antagonizes its effect by inhibiting release of ADH.

Drugs Altering Urinary pH

Normal urinary pH is between 5 and 8.5. These are of two groups:
1. Urinary alkalinizers
2. Urinary acidifiers.

Urinary Alkalinizers

These are sodium or potassium bicarbonate, sodium or potassium citrate and sodium or potassium acetate. These drugs when administered orally, react with the gastric HCl forming NaCl or KCl and CO_2 + H_2O/citric acid/acetic acid. In the intestine, NaCl or KCl remains unchanged and is unable to neutralize the sodium bicarbonate of the intestinal contents which is, therefore, absorbed into blood forming systemic alkalosis. Citric acid or acetic acid is converted to sodium citrate or sodium acetate by reacting with sodium bicarbonate in the intestine. They are absorbed into blood and citrate or acetate is converted to bicarbonate in the liver forming systemic alkalosis. The glomerular filtrate contains good deal of sodium bicarbonate. Normally,

the body conserves Na^+ from $NaHCO_3$ by exchanging with H^+ secreted by the renal tubular cells forming H_2CO_3 which makes the urine acidic. But in the excess of $NaHCO_3$ in urine the need of Na^+ preservation by the body is reduced and so $NaHCO_3$ is excreted as such in urine making the urine alkaline.

Clinical Uses

Urinary alkalinizers are used for following purposes:
- To prevent crystalluria during sulphonamide therapy.
- To prevent reabsorption of barbiturate (phenobarbitone) or salicylate (aspirin) in the renal tubules during poisoning.
- In the treatment of urinary tract infections caused by *E. coli*, and other pathogenic microorganisms that grow in acid urine.

They also reduce the pain and burning sensation due to cystitis.

Adverse Reactions

They may cause sodium overloading, which should be guarded.

Urinary Acidifiers

These are ammonium chloride, calcium chloride, sodium acid phosphate and arginine monohydrochloride and vitamin C (in high dose).

Ammonium chloride when administered orally is broken down into NH_4^+ and Cl^- in the intestine, which are absorbed into blood. In the liver, NH_4^+ is converted to H^+ and NH_3 which forms, urea. Excess Cl^- in plasma reacts with $NaHCO_3$ in blood forming NaCl and CO_2. This lowers alkali reserve of blood producing systemic acidosis. Excretion of H^+ and Cl^- in urine produces acidification of urine.

Clinical Uses

It is used for following purposes:
- To promote quick elimination of basic drugs like chloroquine, amphetamine and pethidine in poisoning.

- To correct hypochloremic alkalosis produced by organic mercurials, thiazides and high ceiling diuretics.
- As a reflex expectorant.

Adverse Reactions

It can cause nausea and vomiting. Calcium chloride is less preferred than ammonium chloride as it produces metabolic acidosis and cardiac arrhythmias. Sodium acid phosphate is better tolerated than ammonium chloride but the action is weak. It does not produce metabolic acidosis. Amino acid arginine hydrochloride liberates HCl in the stomach and produces metabolic acidosis. It is weaker than ammonium chloride as an urinary acidifier. High dosage of ascorbic acid also produces urinary acidification but the action is weak.

Section IX

UTERINE PHARMACOLOGY

37

Uterine Stimulants (Ecbolics/Oxytocics)

Drugs increasing uterine motility by acting on myometrium are oxytocin, prostaglandins and ergot alkaloids. Drugs like quinine sulphate, ethacridine lactate and sparteine sulphate are now not used due to toxicity.

DISCUSSION OF DRUGS

Oxytocin

It is a polypeptide (octapeptide) hormone synthesized in the hypothalamus (by the supraoptic and paraventricular nuclei) and travels along the hypothalamohypophyseal tract to the posterior pituitary, where it is stored along with ADH. The rate of secretion or release of oxytocin is mainly determined by dilatation of the cervix and uterus and the stimulus of suckling of the breast by the infant.

Physiological and Pharmacological Actions

It has prominent actions on uterine muscles (myometrium) and myoepithelium of the breast. It produces following effects:

- **Effects on uterus:** It stimulates both the frequency and force of contractile activity in uterine smooth muscles. The nature of contractions of the uterus is dose dependent. Following administration of low dosage (few units) by slow IV infusion, it produces regular coordinated contractions of the upper uterine segment (fundus and body) with relaxation in between con-

secutive lower uterine segments (cervix). By increasing the dose, the frequency and amplitude of contractions are increased but the relaxation period is decreased. In high dosage, it can cause sustained contraction of the upper segment of the uterus. By producing rhythmic contractions of the upper uterine segment and relaxation of the lower uterine segment it helps in labour and delivery.

- **Mechanism of action:** It acts on specific receptors in the myometrium which develop in gravid uterus. Oestrogen increases but progesterone decreases the sensitivity of these receptors to oxytocin. The response of gravid uterus to oxytocin is low during first and second trimesters of pregnancy and progressively increases during third trimester of pregnancy (due to decrease in circulating progesterone level). The response is maximum at the later phase of pregnancy producing labour and delivery.

- **Effects on mammary gland:** The alveolar ramifications of mammary gland are surrounded by a network of modified smooth muscle cells called myoepithelium. Oxytocin causes contraction of these cells and forces milk from the alveolar channels into the large sinuses, where it is easily available to the suckling infant. This function is called milk ejection (let down). Myoepithelium is highly sensitive to oxytocin. Catecholamines inhibit milk ejection. The milk ejection reflex is initiated by the stimulus of sucking by the infant, which causes release of oxytocin. It is not dependent on autonomic innervation.

- **CVS effects:** It causes a marked by transient relaxation of vascular smooth muscle in large dosage. This decreases BP (both systolic and diastolic) and produces flushing, reflex tachycardia and an increase in limb blood flow.
- **Other effects:** It can produce antidiuretic effect in large dosage, probably by constriction of renal cortical vessels and decrease in renal blood flow and GFR. It can suppress the action of ACTH.

Pharmacokinetics

It is not effective orally due to peptide nature. It has to be administered parenterally for therapeutic effect. It is usually administered by IV infusion. It can be administered by nasal spray. It is rapidly inactivated by the enzyme oxytocinase present in the plasma, uterine tissue and placenta in pregnant women. It has a plasma t½ of about 15 minutes. It is removed from circulation by the kidneys and the liver.

Clinical Uses

These are obstetric uses and use during lactation.

Obstetric Uses

- **For induction of labour:** It is the drug of choice for induction of labour. Indications are those situations (e.g. diabetes mellitus, isoimmunization, hypertensive states, intrauterine growth restriction and placental insufficiency), in which the continuation of pregnancy is considered to be of greater risk to the mother or the foetus than the risk of delivery or pharmacological induction. Contraindications are cephalopelvic disproportion, abnormal foetal position, foetal distress, placental abnormalities and previous uterine surgery.
- **For augmentation of labour if labour is progressing normally:** It may be used for maternal benefit.

- **In third stage of labour and puerperium:** It may be used to aid in maintaining uterine tone (in uterine inertia) after delivery. If it is not effective, ergometrine may be used.
- **In postpartum haemorrhage (PPH):** It may be used to control PPH by contraction of uterus, but ergometrine is better in this respect.

Used During Lactation

It is used to promote milk ejection (lactation), if it is inefficient in mother.

Preparations and Dosage

- Oxytocin (Pitocin, Syntocinon) injection (10 units/ml) (1 unit = 2 µg of pure oxytocin)—10 units is mixed with 500 ml of 5% dextrose solution and administered by slow IV infusion at the rate of 1 milliunit per minute and gradually increasing to 4 milliunits per minute for at least 1 hour (to produce uterine contractions).
- Oxytocin (Syntocinon) nasal spray (40 units/ml)—used 2–5 minutes before breastfed.

Adverse Reactions

It can cause hypotension, forcible uterine contractions leading to maternal and foetal soft tissue injury, rupture of uterus, foetal asphyxia and death, if used in large dosage. It may occasionally cause water retention (due to ADH like activity) leading to water intoxication (manifested as nausea, vomiting, anorexia, weight gain and lethargy).

Prostaglandins

These are lipid derived autacoids—synthesized from the polyunsaturated fatty acid, arachidonic acid present in the cell membrane. Their basic structure is prostanoic acid which is a 20C fatty acid with 2 double bonds and a cyclopentane ring. They are derivatives of prostanoic acid. They are discussed in detail in autacoid pharmacology. In the female reproductive system, they are found in the ovary, myometrium and menstrual fluid. Their physiological significance, however, is not well-understood. Majority of prostaglandins in varying doses inhibit the spontaneous motor activity of the uterus but PGE_2 and $PGF_{2\alpha}$ in low doses stimulate both the tone and amplitude of uterine contractions. Their concentrations rise in amniotic fluid, umbilical cord blood and maternal blood at term and during labour. They act as myometrial smooth muscle stimulants causing contraction of uterus and as cervical primers causing cervical ripening (softening and dilatation of cervix).

Pharmacological Actions

Their actions on gravid uterus are similar to that of oxytocin, i.e. they produce regular coordinated contractions of the upper uterine segment with relaxation in between consecutive contractions and relaxation of lower uterine segment. Unlike oxytocin, they are effective throughout the period of gestation (pregnancy). They can induce abortion in the first and second trimesters of pregnancy.

Clinical Uses

- They are used for therapeutic abortion/medical termination of pregnancy (MTP) especially for mid-term abortion. Abortion during the first trimester of pregnancy is commonly done by means of suction curettage. A progesterone antagonist, mifepristone (a synthetic 19-nonsteroid) can be used to inhibit the effect of progesterone on the uterus, which serves as a potent abortifacient during this period. When administered to women during first trimester of pregnancy in combination with a prostaglandin or methotrexate, it induces abortion in more than 95% of cases. In the second trimester of pregnancy several methods for abortion are available. Intra-amniotic injection of a hypertonic (20%) solution of NaCl (100 to 200 ml) has been used but numerous failures occur and serious adverse effects (like hypernatraemia and hypofibrinogenaemia) may occur in patients. Vaginal suppositories of PGE_2 (Dinoprostone/Primiprost—0.5 mg/suppository) inserted at intervals of 3 to 5 minutes can be used effectively. Intramuscular or intra-amniotic injection of 15-methyl $PGF_{2\alpha}$ haemabate (Carboprost trimethomine, Prostodin) (5 mg/ml and repeated after 6 hours if necessary) is also effective. Nausea, vomiting and diarrhoea are frequent side effects of these prostaglandins even after vaginal use. These effects can be prevented by intravaginal administration of misoprostol in the dosage of 0.2 mg every 12 hours.

- They can be used to induce labour in patients not responding to oxytocin.
- They may used to evacuate the uterus in incomplete abortion or hydatidiform mole.

Ergot Alkaloids

Ergot is the product of a fungus—*Claviceps purpurea*, which grows mainly on rye and occasionally on other grains. Ergot spores are carried by insects or wind and deposited on the ovaries of young rye where they germinate and their hyphal filaments penetrate deep into the ovary of the rye. This ultimately results in destruction of the entire grain substance and formation of a hardened, black purple body called sclerotium. This sclerotium is the commercial source of ergot alkaloids.

Classification of Ergot Alkaloids

These are of three groups:

1. Amino acid alkaloids, e.g. ergotamine, ergosine and ergotoxine.
2. Amine alkaloids, e.g. ergometrine (ergonovine) and methylergometrine.
3. Semisynthetic dihydrogenated amino acid alkaloids, e.g. dihydroergotamine (DHE) and hydergine (a mixture of dihydroergocornine, dihydroergocristine and dihydroergokryptine). Besides the alkaloids, ergot also contains histamine, tyramine, acetylcholine, ergosterol, fungisterol, fixed oil and inorganic salts. So ergot is a treasure house of many pharmacological constituents.

Pharmacological Actions

They produce following effects:

- **Effects on uterus:** All the natural ergot alkaloids have the ability to cause contraction of the uterine smooth muscle. The response depends upon the alkaloid used, the dose used, the degree of uterine maturity and the stage of gestation. Ergometrine and its derivative methyl ergometrine produce an immediate and powerful response. Amino acid alkaloids and their dihydrogenated derivatives produce delayed and less powerful response. In small dosage, they increase the force and frequency of contractions of the whole uterus with normal relaxation in between consecutive contractions. As the dose is increased, contractions become more powerful and prolonged and the resting muscle tone is markedly increased. In large dosage a sustained tonic contraction of the uterus results. The uterine blood vessels tend to get squeezed due to muscle contraction. They are effective during any phase of estrous cycle or gestation. Even an immature uterus is stimulated by them but the uterus at full-term and immediately after delivery is highly sensitive to them.

- **Mechanism of action:** They have a direct stimulant action on the uterine smooth muscle. They act as partial agonists of α-adrenoreceptors and 5-HT receptors of uterine smooth muscles (myometrium).
- **Effects on blood vessels:** Amino acid alkaloids have poor α-adrenergic blocking and moderate vasoconstrictor actions and may produce hypertension in high dosage. Dihydrogenated amino acid alkaloids have powerful α-adrenergic blocking and poor vasoconstrictor action is minimum. They can produce fall of BP. Ergometrine has no α-adrenergic blocking action and produces minimum vasoconstriction.

Pharmacokinetics

They are effective orally and parenterally. They are rapidly and almost completely absorbed from GIT. They are metabolized in the liver and excreted in urine. They have plasm t½ of 1 to 2 hours. Their effects last for 2 to 4 hours.

Clinical Uses

- They are used primarily to control postpartum haemorrhage (PPH).
- They are used after caesarean section or forceps delivery to prevent uterine atony.

Table 37.1: Comparison of uterine stimulants

	Oxytocin	Prostaglandin	Ergometrine
1. Chemical nature	Physiological substance, octapeptide.	Physiological substance, fatty acid derivative.	Natural substance, ergot alkaloid.
2. Nature of uterine contraction	Increases frequency of uterine contraction (contraction followed by relaxation).	Increases frequency of uterine contractions (contraction followed by relaxation).	Increases tone of uterus (tonic contraction of whole uterus in large dosage).
3. Sensitivity of uterus	Sensitivity increases with duration of pregnancy. Most sensitive at term. Immature uterus resistant.	Contracts uterus in all stages of pregnancy and also nonpregnant and immature uterus.	Sensitivity increases at term. Nonpregnant and immature uterus also contracts.
4. Duration of action	Short	Medium	Long
5. Uses	Induction of labour. Postpartum uterine atony.	Induction of abortion and labour.	To control postpartum haemorrhage and uterine atony.
6. Route of administration	IV, oral or nasal.	Intravaginally, intra-amniotically, IV or oral.	IM, IV or oral.

- They are used to hasten involution of uterus in the puerperium, especially in multipara, where the uterus is flabby.

Preparations and Dosage

- Ergometrine maleate injection (0.5 mg/ml), tablet (0.5 mg)—0.5 to 1 mg IM or IV, 0.5 to 1 mg orally twice daily.
- Methylergometrine maleate (Methergin) injection (0.2 mg/ml), tablet (0.125 mg)— 0.2 to 0.4 mg IM or IV, 0.25 to 0.5 mg orally twice daily.

Adverse Reactions

They can produce nausea, vomiting, headache, hypertension, blurring of vision and decrease in milk secretion (due to decrease prolactin activity). They should be cautiously used in patients of angina pectoris or peripheral vascular disease and in presence of sepsis (can cause dry gangrene). They are contraindicated during pregnancy and for induction of labour as they may lead to foetal compression, asphyxia and death. Comparison of uterine stimulants is shown in **Table 37.1.**

38

Uterine Relaxants (Tocolytic Agents)

INTRODUCTION

Drugs that inhibit uterine motility by acting on myometrium are magnesium sulphate, β_2-adrenergic receptor agonists, calcium channel blockers, PG-synthetase inhibitors and oxytocin antagonists. Drugs like ethylalcohol, morphine and pethidine are now not used due to toxicity. These are used:

- To delay or prevent premature (preterm) labour in selected individuals.

- To slow or arrest delivery for brief period in order to undertake other therapeutic measures.

Premature births account for a large fraction of perinatal morbidity and mortality. About 50% of patients of premature labour with regular uterine contractions respond to bed rest and hydration. If this fails, a tocolytic agent may be used. It is done in those pregnancies where the gestational age is between 20 and 36 weeks. In it, therapeutic success occurs if the cervical dilatation is less than 4 cm. It should not be attempted—

- If the membrane is ruptured, as there is risk of infection.

- In eclampsia or severe preeclampsia.

- In chorioamnionitis.

- In premature detachment of placenta

- In foetal distress.

DISCUSSION OF TOCOLYTIC AGENTS

Magnesium Sulphate

It is used during pregnancy to control eclamptic seizures. It is also used as a highly effective inhibitor of uterine activity in premature labour. It is an alternative drug, when β_2-adrenergic receptor agonists are contraindicated. It is administered IV in a loading dose of 4 g over a period of 20 minutes, followed by IV infusion at the rate of 1 to 2 g per hour for a total period of 24 hours.

Adverse Reactions

It can produce progressive inhibition of cardiac conduction and neuromuscular transmission leading to cardiac arrest and respiratory depression.

β_2-adrenergic Receptor Agonists

For example, salbutamol, terbutaline, ritodrine and isoxsuprine. They are preferred drugs for the treatment of premature labour. They cause uterine relaxation and produce postponement of delivery for one to few weeks in about 70% of cases.

Preparations and Dosage

- Salbutamol (Asthalin) injection (500 mg/mL)—it is given by IV infusion at the rate of 1 µg/min for first five minutes and then the dose is doubled every five minutes till uterine contractions reduce.

- Terbutaline (Bricaryl) tablet (2.5 mg)—it is given orally in a dose of 2.5 to 5 mg every 6 hourly.
- Terbutaline injection (1 mg/mL)—it is given by IV infusion at the rate of 10 to 80 μg/min for a period of 1 to 4 hours,
- Ritodrine hydrochloride (Yutopar) injection (0.3 mg/mL)—it is given by IV infusion at the rate of 0.1 mg/min and gradually the dose is increased to 0.35 mg/mL till labour is controlled.
- Isoxsuprine hydrochloride (Duvadilan) injection (10 mg/mL)—it is given by IV infusion at the rate of 0.2 to 0.5 mg/min and adjusted according to result and effect on BP and heart rate. It can be injected IM in a dose of 10 mg every 1 to 2 hours.

Adverse Reactions

They can produce many cardiovascular and metabolic side effects such as fall of BP, reflex tachycardia, pulmonary oedema, hyperglycaemia and hypokalaemia. They also produce tremor, nausea and vomiting.

Calcium Channel Blockers

Nifedipine is the most commonly used calcium channel blocker for the treatment of premature labour, if used in the early stages. It is given in a loading dose of 10 mg sublingually initially and repeated every 20 minutes for 2 to 3 doses. Maintenance therapy continues with 10 to 20 mg orally every 4 to 6 hours. Amlodipine can be used orally as uterine relaxant like nifedipine.

Adverse Reactions

Discussed with calcium channel blockers in CVS Pharmacology.

PG-Synthetase Inhibitors

Indomethacin is the most commonly used PG-synthetase inhibitor for treatment of premature labour. It is given in a loading dose of 50 mg rectally as suppository initially and then 25 mg rectally 6 hourly for 2 to 3 days.

Adverse Reactions

It can produce headache, giddiness, mental confusion, blurring of vision, mental depression, sodium retention, skin rashes and blood dyscrasias.

Oxytocin Antagonists

Atosiban and related peptides have been found to inhibit preterm contractions of uterus by blocking the action of oxytocin at cellular level. They are in clinical trials.

Progestational Agents

Progesterone is a physiological uterine relaxant. It is used for prophylaxis of preterm labour. It is administered IM from 14 to 36th week of pregnany to prevent threatened or habitual abortion due to progesterone deficiency. It also reduces uterine sensitivity to oxytocin. It is, however, ineffective to produce significant uterine relaxation at full-term, even on intra-amniotic administration.

Part 2

Section I

CNS PHARMACOLOGY

39

General Considerations

INTRODUCTION

Drugs acting on central nervous system influence the lives of everyone every day. They are very useful therapeutic agents because they can produce specific physiological and psychological effects. They can selectively relieve pain, reduce fever, induce sleep or arousal, suppress disordered movements, reduce appetite or relieve vomiting. They can be used to treat anxiety, mania, depression or schizophrenia without altering consciousness. Modern surgery is not possible without the help of general anaesthetics, which are central nervous system acting drugs. The central nervous system consists of brain and spinal cord. It is an assembly of interrelated neuronal systems that regulate their own and each other's activity in a dynamic complex fashion. Anatomically, it is divided into several parts, which perform different functions (as shown in **Table 39.1**).

Limbic system is made up of hippocampal formation, amygdaloid complex, septum, olfactory nuclei, basal ganglia (corpus striatum and substantia nigra) and some nuclei of diencephalon (thalamus and hypothalamus). Brain stem is made up of pons and medulla oblongata and contains reticular activating system (RAS), which is also present in midbrain (mesencephalon).

Classification of Central Nervous System Acting Drugs

These are given as follows:
- **Central nervous system depressants:** They cause inhibition of cells of central nervous system. They are given as follows:
  - **Nonselective (general) central nervous system depressants**—e.g. sedative hypnotics, alcohols and general anaesthetics.
  - **Selective (local) central nervous system depressants**—e.g. antiepileptics, antiparkinsonian drugs, opioid analgesics, nonopioid analgesics, neuroleptics, anxiolytics, antimanics, etc.
- **Central nervous system stimulants:** They cause excitation of cells of CNS. They are as follows:
  - **Nonselective (general) central nervous system stimulants**—e.g. CNS stimulants and convulsants.
  - **Selective (local) central nervous system stimulants**—e.g. psychostimulants, analeptics, cerebral activators, psychodysleptics (hallucinogens).

Modes of Action of Central Nervous System Acting Drugs

They can affect the central nervous systems by following ways:
- They may act directly on the neurons and modify neuronal functions. The sites of

Table 39.1: Parts of central nervous systems and their functions

Parts of CNS	Functions attributed
Cerebral cortex	Control of higher functions like memory, judgement, intelligence, consciousness, voluntary movements, fine pain, tactile discrimination, special senses like vision, smell, hearing and coordination and inhibitory influence on lower centres.
Limbic system	Primary area of control of autonomic functions, emotion and behaviour.
Basal ganglia	Extrapyramidal control of skeletal muscle tone and coordination of posture. Lesions produce tremors, rigidity and loss of emotional expression.
Thalamus	Relay centre for sensory pathways to cortex. Conscious appreciation of pain, temperature and crude touch sensations. Exerts regulatory control over visceral functions.
Hypothalamus	Control of autonomic nervous system and adenohypophysis, regulation of body temperature, control of appetite and satiety, drinking and sexual behaviour. Lesions cause diabetes insipidus, narcolepsy, autonomic imbalance and sham rage.
Cerebellum	Control of vestibular function, balance and posture.
Reticular formation	Control of BP, respiration, vomiting, skeletal muscle tone and posture, sleep wakefulness cycle, crude pain and stress reflex.
Spinal cord	Control of reflex movements, skeletal muscle tone and upper and lower motor neurons through presynaptic and postsynaptic inhibitions.

action are synapses, receptors and ion channels (Na^+, K^+, Ca^{++}, Cl^-, etc.).

- They may act reflexly by sending afferent impulses to the central nervous system *via* the chemoreceptors, baroreceptors and peripheral nerves and thereby producing psychic, somatic or visceral responses.

- They may affect the nutrition and oxygen supply of the neurons by altering blood supply or affecting metabolism (e.g. by causing hypoglycaemia or ammonia intoxication).

Types or Action of Drugs on Central Nervous System

Drugs may either depress or stimulate central nervous system.

- **Nonselective CNS depression** is due to depression of excitable tissue at all levels of central nervous system leading to decrease in the amount of transmitter released by the nerve impulses as well as general depression of postsynaptic responsiveness and ion movement.

Nonselective CNS stimulation is produced by blockade of inhibition or by direct neuronal excitation, which may involve increased neurotransmitter release, more prolonged transmitter action, labelization of the postsynaptic membrane or decreased synaptic recovery time.

- **Selective CNS depression or stimulation** is caused by local depression or stimulation of the CNS. In some instances, a drug may produce both depression and stimulation simultaneously at different systems. Although selectivity of action may be remarkable, a drug usually affects several CNS functions to varying degrees.

Some Important Aspects of CNS Acting Drugs

- To reach the CNS, a drug must have high degree of lipid solubility (high oil/water partition coefficient) or a specialized transport mechanism. Ionized drugs as a rule cannot penetrate into CNS. For this reason the existence of a blood–brain barrier (BBB) has been postulated. It is a structure of the glial cell lining of the brain capillaries. Lipid-soluble and unionized drugs can easily cross the BBB, while lipid-insoluble and ionized drugs (polar compounds) and macromolecules cannot cross BBB. In the presence of meningeal inflammation (meningitis), a considerable amount of the ionized drugs can cross BBB, e.g. penicillins, streptomycin, etc.

- Drugs may modify the synthesis, storage, release or metabolism of inhibitory or excitatory neurotransmitter, e.g. MAO inhibitors (nialamide, isocarboxazide, etc.) act as antidepressants by inhibiting the destruction of noradrenaline by the enzyme MAO (monoamine oxidase).
- Drugs may act by modifying ionic fluxes across the cell membrane, e.g. phenytoin sodium inhibits influx of Na^+ ions during depolarization producing membrane stabilizing action.
- Drugs may modify the energy supply of CNS, e.g. barbiturates cause local inhibition of synthesis of high energy phosphate bonds (ATP).
- Drugs may specifically act as antagonists of other drugs at receptor sites, e.g. naloxone or naltrexone antagonizes the effects of opioids (morphine, pethidine, etc.).
- Drugs of different groups can be combined to produce better therapeutic effects, e.g. combination of levodopa and anticholinergic drug in Parkinson's disease. However, some combinations of drugs may be detrimental due to potentially dangerous additive or antagonistic effects, e.g. combination of benzodiazepines and alcohol, MAO inhibitors with tricyclic antidepressants.
- Drugs may affect different levels (grades) of CNS depression or stimulation by gradual increase of dose.

Chemical Messengers in CNS

The CNS processes information with the help of some chemical messengers, *viz.* neurotransmitters, neuromodulators, neuromediators and neurotropic factors, which act *via* specific mechanism to mediate neurotransmission.

- **Neurotransmitters:** A neurotransmitter is a substance contained in a neuron and secreted by that neuron to transmit information to its postsynaptic target. The action of the transmitter may be excitatory or inhibitory on the postsynaptic receptors (by depolarization or hyperpolarization of the cell membrane). Central neurotransmitters are acetylcholine, noradrenaline, adrenaline, dopamine, 5-HT, histamine, GABA, glycine, glutamate, aspartate, substance P, opioid peptides (endorphins, enkephalins and dynorphins) and neuropeptides (neuropeptide-Y, vasoactive intestinal peptide, gastrin and cholecystokinin). Their distribution in CNS and functions are shown in **Table 39.2**. Their common properties (characteristics) are discussed in ANS Pharmacology.
- **Neuromodulators:** A neuromodulator is a substance that can influence neuronal activity in a manner different from that of neurotransmitter. It originates from cellular and nonsynaptic sites but influences the excitability of the nerve cells, e.g. CO_2 and NH_3 (arising from neurons and glial cells), circulating steroid hormones, locally released adenosine and other purines, postaglandins and other eicosanoids.
- **Neuromediators:** A neuromediator is a substance that participates in the elicitation of the postsynaptic response to a transmitter, e.g. cAMP, cGMP, NO, IP_3 and DAG.

Levels of CNS depression are:

Sedation $\longrightarrow$ Hypnosis (sleep) $\longrightarrow$ Unconsciousness $\longrightarrow$ Coma $\longrightarrow$ Surgical anaesthesia

$\longrightarrow$ Fatal depression of respiration and cardiovascular system.

Levels of CNS stimulation are:

Excitement $\longrightarrow$ Restlessness $\longrightarrow$ Convulsions/Manic episodes (Psychosis)

- **Neurotropic factors:** A neurotropic factor is a substance produced in the CNS by neurons, astreocytes or glial cells. These are peptides, which produce different functions, e.g. neurotropins (nerve growth factors), neuropoietic factors (cholinergic differentiation factor and myeloid leukaemia inhibiting factor), epidermal growth factor, fibroblast growth factor, insulin-like growth factor and platelet-derived growth factor.

Table 39.2: Distribution and functions of central neurotransmitters

Neurotransmitter	Distribution	Functions	Receptors involved
Acetylcholine	Widely distributed in CNS. Predominantly present in cerebral cortex, RAS, cerebellum and spinal cord.	Both excitatory and inhibitory	M_1, N_N M_2
Noradrenaline Adrenaline	Widely distributed in CNS. Predominantly present in hypothalamus, limbic system and reticular formation of brain stem.	Both excitatory and inhibitory	α_1 α_2, β
Dopamine	Widely distributed in CNS. Predominantly present in basal ganglia. Also present in hypothalamus, adenohypophysis and frontal cortex.	Both excitatory and inhibitory	D_1 D_2
5-HT	Widely distributed in CNS. Predominantly present in hypothalamus, limbic system and reticular formation of brain stem. Also present in cerebral cortex and hippocampal areas.	Both excitatory and inhibitory	$5\text{-}HT_1$ $5\text{-}HT_2$
Histamine	Like 5-HT	Both excitatory and inhibitory	H_1, H_3 H_2
GABA	Widely distributed in CNS	Inhibitory	Specific (GABA)
Glycine	Present in spinal cord and brain stem	Inhibitory	Specific
Glutamate	Widely distributed in CNS	Excitatory	Specific (NMDA)
Aspartate	Widely distributed in CNS	Excitatory	Specific (NMDA)
Substance P	Present in spinal cord, hypothalamus, thalamus and basal ganglia.	Excitatory	Specific
Opioid peptides (enkephalins, endorphins and dynorphins)	Present in spinal cord, limbic system, corpus striatum, thalamus and hypothalamus	Both inhibitory and excitatory	μ, κ, δ
Neuropeptides (somatostatin, cholecystokinin, gastrin, secretin, vasoactive intestinal peptide (VIP), leptin, Pyy, etc.	Present in cerebral cortex, hippocampus, limbic system and hypothalamus	Excitatory	Specific

GABA (Gamma-aminobutyric acid). NMDA (N-methyl-D-aspartate).

40

Sedatives and Hypnotics

INTRODUCTION

Sedatives are drugs that reduce motor activity and excitement and produce calmness and drowsiness without producing sleep. These are used for the treatment of anxiety. Hypnotics are drugs that produce sleep (induction and maintenance) which resembles natural arousable sleep. These are used for the treatment of insomnia (sleeplessness).

Physiology of Sleep

The duration and pattern of sleep vary considerably among individuals. Age has an important effect on the quantity and depth of sleep. It decreases in elderly persons. Adequate sleep is necessary for giving rest to the body. Sleep is divided into three phases based on electroencephalographic (EEC) and electrooculographic (EOG) studies.

- **Awake period (Stage 0):** It is the period from lying down to falling asleep. It constitutes 1 to 2% of sleep time. EEC shows α-activity when eyes are closed and β-activity when eyes are open. Eye movements are irregular or slowly roving.
- **Nonroving eye movements (NREM) sleep:** It has four stages:

  Stage 1: Dozing (3–6%)—in it, α activity is interspersed with θ waves.

  Stage 2: Unequivocal sleep (40–50%)—in it, θ waves are present with intersparsed spindles.

Stage 3: Deep sleep transition (5–8%)—in it, θ and δ waves are present. Spindle activities are present.

Stage 4: Cerebral sleep (10–20%)—in it, δ activity predominates.

In these stages, heart rate, BP and respiration are steady and muscles are relaxed.

- **Roving eye movements (REM) sleep (paradoxical sleep):** In it, waves of all frequencies are present. There are irregular and darting eye movements. Dreams and nightmares occur. Heart rate and BP fluctuate. Respiration is irregular. Muscles are fully relaxed and occasionally irregular body movements occur. It constitutes 20–30% of sleep time.

Normally, stages 0 to 4 and REM sleep occur in succession over a period of 80 to 100 minutes. Then stages 1–4 of REM sleep occur repeatedly in cyclical manner. Hypnotics can effect one or more stages of sleep.

Classification of Sedative-hypnotics

These are mainly of two groups:

- **Benzodiazepines,** e.g. diazepam, nitrazepam, lorazepam, alprazolam, etc.
- **Nonbenzodiazepines:** These are given as follows:
  - Barbiturates, e.g. phenobarbitone, pentobarbitone, secobarbitone, etc.
  - Newer drugs, e.g. buspirone, melatonin, zolpidem, zopiclone.

– Miscellaneous drugs, e.g. chloralhydrate, triclophos, paraldehyde, methaqualone, ethanol, ethchlorvynol, glutethimide, methyprylone, potassium bromide, meprobamate, scopolamine and antihistamines (promethazine and diphenhydramine).

DISCUSSION OF INDIVIDUAL GROUPS OF DRUGS

Benzodiazepines (BDZs)

These are benzodiazepine derivatives. Benzodiazepine contains two benzene rings and a diazepine ring **(Fig. 40.1)**.

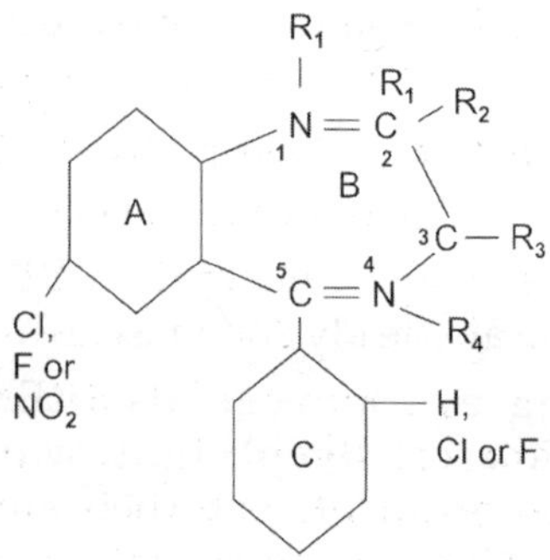

R_1, R_2, R_3 and R_4 are different radicals attached to diazepine ring

Fig. 40.1: Basic structure of benzodiazepines

Classification

These can be classified into two ways:

1. **According to duration of action:** These are of three groups:

   a. Long-acting (8 to 24 hours), e.g. chlordiazepoxide, diazepam, flurazepam, clonazepam, prazepam, clorazepate and clobazam.

   b. Intermediate-acting (4 to 8 hours), e.g. nitrazepam, lorazepam, oxazepam, temazepam and medazepam.

   c. Short-acting (1 to 4 hours), e.g. alprazolam, triazolam, estazolam and midazolam.

2. **According to primary therapeutic use:** These are of four groups:

a. As a sedative (antianxiety drugs), e.g. diazepam, chlordiazepoxide, oxazepam, prazepam and demoxepam.

b. As an hypnotic, e.g. lorazepam, nitrazepam, flurazepam, alprazolam, estazolam and triazolam.

c. As an anticonvulsant (antiepileptic), e.g. diazepam, clonazepam, clorazepate and lorazepam.

d. As an anaesthetic, e.g. midazolam and diazepam.

Pharmacokinetics

Most benzodiazepines are absorbed completely from GIT after oral administration. They differ in their rate of absorption, bioavailability and plasma protein binding. Due to lipid solubility, they rapidly enter the brain by crossing BBB. From the brain they re-enter the blood and equilibrium is produced. Then they are distributed to muscles and adipose tissue. They are metabolized in the liver and excreted through kidneys. Long-acting benzodiazepines produce long-acting metabolite 'nordiazepam', which is converted to oxazepam by a very slow metabolic process and undergoes glucuronide conjugation for excretion in urine. Intermediate- and short-acting benzodiazepines undergo direct glucuronide conjugation and excreted in urine.

Pharmacological Actions

Mechanism of action: Benzodiazepines act by potentiating the inhibitory action of GABA (an inhibitory neurotransmitter). They bind with the specific benzodiazepine receptor in the central nervous system, which modulates GABA receptor and facilitates the GABA-ergic transmission. Benzodiazepine receptor is an integral part of $GABA_A$ receptor–Cl^- ion channel complex. Binding of benzodiazepine with the receptor causes opening of Cl^- ion channel with influx of Cl^- ion leading to hyperpolarization of the neuronal membrane, which makes the neuron hypoexcitable. As a result, depolarization and action potential cannot occur and so neuronal transmission in brain and spinal cord decreases.

Benzodiazepines produce following effects:

- **CNS effects:** Unlike barbiturates, they are not general CNS depressants. They produce sedative-hypnotic, anticonvulsant, muscle relaxant and anaesthetic effects.

  - **Sedative-hypnotic effects:** In smaller doses they cause sedation and relief of anxiety. In larger doses they cause sleep (hypnosis). They shorten the time spent in stage 4 of NREM sleep and REM sleep but increase the total sleep time. Sleep produced by them is more refreshing and with less hangover symptoms such as drowsiness, dysphoria and mental or motor depression on the next day than barbiturates. They act as sedative-hypnotic by facilitating GABA-ergic transmission in the midbrain reticular formation (which maintains sleep-wakefulness cycle) and the limbic system (which controls thought and mental functions).

  - **Anticonvulsant effects:** Some benzodiazepines, e.g. diazepam, clonazepam and clorazepate produce anticonvulsant (antiepileptic) effect by raising the seizure threshold in the cortex, thalamus and limbic system by potentiating GABA action and thus preventing the spread of seizure in the brain. They are used in drug induced convulsions (produced by CNS stimulants) and in convulsions due to epilepsy, eclampsia and tetanus.

  - **Muscle relaxant effects:** They produce relaxation of skeletal muscle by facilitating GABA-ergic transmission in the brain stem and spinal cord. They are used in acute spasm of skeletal muscles due to trauma or inflammation and in skeletal muscle rigidity (spasticity) due to upper motor neuron (pyramidal tract) lesion.

  - **Anaesthetic effects:** Some benzodiazepines, e.g. midazolam and diazepam are used for preanaesthetic medication

(given IM) and for induction of general anaesthesia (given IV). They act by facilitating GABA-ergic transmission in reticular formation and limbic system.

- **Miscellaneous effects:** Their effects on respiration and cardiovascular system are of minor importance (mild). In high doses they can cause respiratory depression, bradycardia and fall of BP. They can reduce nocturnal gastric HCl secretion in peptic ulcer patients. They can produce relief of gastrointestinal disorders like irritable bowel syndrome and spastic colitis, where anxiety is the major etiological factor.

Clinical Uses

They are used in:

- Anxiety states and neuroses: Long-acting benzodiazepines are used.
- Insomnia: Intermediate- and short-acting benzodiazepines are used.
- Convulsions and epileptic seizures: Diazepam, lorazepam, clonazepam and clorazepate are used IV. Diazepam is the drug of choice in status epilepticus.
- Skeletal muscle rigidity: Diazepam or chlorodiazepoxide is used.
- Anaesthesia: Midazolam or diazepam (IV) is used as preanaesthetic medication and for induction of general anaesthesia.
- Delirium tremens during withdrawal of alcohol in chronic alcoholics. Diazepam or chlordiazepoxide is used.
- Mental depression: Alprazolam or triazolam is used as antidepressant.

Some Preparations and Dosage

- Diazepam (Valium, Calmpose) tablet (5 mg)—5 to 15 mg daily. Diazepam (Valiun, Calmpose) injection (5 mg/ml)—10 to 20 mg IM or IV.
- Chlordiazepoxide (Librium) tablet (10 mg)—10 to 30 mg daily.
- Nitrazepam (Hynotex, Nitravate) tablet (5 mg)—5 to 10 mg daily.
- Lorazepam (Larpose, Ativan) tablet (1, 2 mg)— 1 to 2 mg daily.

- Alprazolam (Alzolam, Alprax) tablet (0.25, 0.5 mg)—0.25 to 1 mg daily.
- Triazolam (Halcion) tablet (0.125, 0.25 mg)—0.125 to 0.5 mg daily.
- Oxazepam (Serepax) tablet (15, 30 mg)— 15 to 60 mg daily.
- Clonazepam (Lonazep) tablet (0.5 mg)— 0.5 to 1 mg daily.
- Clorazepate (Traxene) tablet (15 mg)—15 to 30 mg daily.
- Midazolam (Hypnovel) injection (5 mg/2 ml ampoule)—2.5 to 5 mg IM or IV.

Adverse Reactions

They are well-tolerated drugs. They may cause sedation, drowsiness, lethargy and ataxia (immobility) as side effects. They also cause dose dependent impairment of visual-motor incoordination and behavioural changes. They may aggravate schizophrenia. Rarely, they may cause allergic reactions, photosensitization, headache, vertigo, impaired sexual function and menstrual irregularities. With prolonged use they can produce tolerance and dependence. Patients develop tolerance to sedative (but not anxiolytic) action and physical dependence. Withdrawal symptoms include anxiety, sweating, insomnia, agitation, depression and even convulsions. Treatment is similar to barbiturate dependence (discussed later on). They are often misused as drugs of abuse. When administered to the mother before delivery they can produce flappy baby syndrome characterized by reluctance to feed, hypotonia, hypothermia and apnoea in the newborn baby. Acute toxicity (poisoning) due to overdose may occur with benzodiazepines. It is treated by administration of specific antidote (competitive antagonist), flumazenil (Anexate), which is an imidazodiazepine. It binds competitively with benzodiazepine receptors and blocks many of the pharmacological actions of benzodiazepines. It rapidly reverses the central effects of benzodiazepines. It is available as injection (1 mg/ml) and given IV initially in the dose of 0.2 mg over 15 seconds and then repeated in the dose of 0.1 mg every minute to a total dose not more than 1 mg. It can also be given by IV infusion with normal saline. It can cause withdrawal syndrome in patients dependent on benzodiazepines. Other supportive measures as required are also taken in the poisoning case.

Drug Interactions

- Alcohol, barbiturates and antidepressants increase benzodiazepine induced central nervous system depression.
- Oral contraceptives, cimetidine and isoniazid reduce benzodiazepine metabolism and elimination by inhibiting hepatic microsomal enzymes.

Advantages of Benzodiazepines over Barbiturates and other Sedative-hypnotics

- They have wide margin of safety (high therapeutic index).
- They do not depress respiration and cardiovascular functions in therapeutic doses.
- They cause less hangover and rebound REM sleep.
- They do not induce hepatic microsomal enzymes to increase metabolism of other drugs.
- They have low addiction (abuse) liability.

Barbiturates

These are barbituric acid derivatives. Barbituric acid is a condensation product of urea with malonic acid (as shown in **Fig. 40.2**). It consists of a six-membered ring structure.

Barbituric acid was synthesized by Von Bayer on St. Barbara's day in 1864 and so such name was given.

Barbituric acid has no sedative-hypnotic activity but barbiturates produced from it are sedative-hypnotics.

Classification of Barbiturates

These are of four groups according to durations of action:

1. Long-acting (8 to 24 hours), e.g. phenobarbitone, mephobarbitone and barbitone.

2. Intermediate-acting (4 to 8 hours), e.g. amylobarbitone (amobarbitone), allobarbitone and butobarbitone.

3. Short-acting (1 to 4 hours), e.g. pentobarbitone, secobarbitone (quinalbarbitone) and hexobarbitone.

4. Ultrashort-acting (5 to 15 minutes), e.g. thiopentone, kemithal and methohexitone (given IV). These are thiobarbiturates.

Pharmacokinetics

They are well-absorbed from GIT after oral administration. Their sodium salts are more rapidly absorbed from GIT but due to their high alkalinity, they may cause epigastric distress. After absorption they are distributed in all body tissues and fluids. (They readily cross the BBB and the placental barrier.) They are secreted in milk, which can affect breast-fed babies (cause respiratory depression). Distribution of barbiturates in the body depends on lipid solubility, degree of protein binding and extent of ionization. Ultrashort-acting barbiturates are highly lipid-soluble and so enter brain very rapidly, while long-acting barbiturates are poorly lipid-soluble and so enter brain very slowly. Their plasma protein binding also varies, e.g. phenobarbitone (20%), pentobarbitone (35%) and thiopentone (75%). They exist in plasma as both ionized and unionized forms. The ionized form cannot cross biological membranes and cannot be reabsorbed by the renal tubules and so

excreted in urine. The action of barbiturates is terminated by redistribution, metabolism and excretion. After IV injection of thiopentone, it rapidly enters brain due to high lipid solubility and produces unconsciousness within a few minutes, but the consciousness is regained in 15 to 20 minutes due to re-entry into blood and redistribution in tissues like muscles and adipose tissue, which are also highly vascular. This occurs with different barbiturates at different rates. Barbiturates are metabolized in the liver by oxidation and dealkylation with the help of hepatic microsomal enzymes. The inactive metabolites are conjugated with glucuronic acid and are excreted in urine. A small portion of barbiturates is excreted unchanged in urine.

Pharmacological Actions

Mechanism of action: They probably act like benzodiazepines by potentiating the action of GABA (an inhibitory neurotransmitter). They facilitate GABA-ergic transmission in the CNS by binding with $GABA_A$ receptor–Cl^- ion channel complex at a different (allosteric) site than benzodiazepines. This causes opening of Cl^- ion channels and influx of Cl^- ions leading to hyperpolarization of the neuronal membrane. As a result, the neuron becomes hypoexcitable and so depolarization and action potential cannot occur and neuronal transmission decreases. They depress polysynaptic responses and delay synaptic recovery.

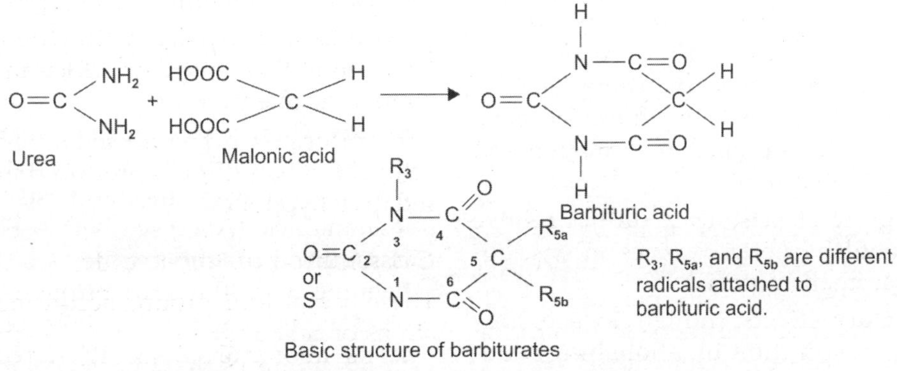

Basic structure of barbiturates

Fig. 40.2. Structures of barbituric acid and barbiturates

They produce following effects:

- **Central nervous system effects:** They are general CNS depressants. They produce dose dependent depth of CNS depression from sedation to coma. At lower dosage, they produce sedation and at higher dosage produce sleep. At still higher dosage they produce general anaesthesia and coma. They produce following CNS effects:

  - **Sedative-hypnotic effects:** Long-acting barbiturates are used as sedatives and anxiolytics, while intermediate- and short-acting barbiturates are used as hypnotics. For induction of sleep, short-acting barbiturates and for maintenance of sleep, long-acting barbiturates are preferred. They act by facilitating GABA-ergic transmission in the midbrain reticular formation. They produce hangover and rebound REM.

  - **Anticonvulsant effects:** In high doses, they can control convulsions due to drugs (CNS stimulants) and diseases (epilepsy, eclampsia and tetanus). Phenobarbitone has a selective anticonvulsant action and used for prevention of grand mal seizures. They act by facilitating GABA-ergic transmission in the limbic system and thus raising the threshold of seizure, which limits the spread of seizure in the brain. For control of status epilepticus, phenobarbitone sodium (IV) can be used, but diazepam (IV) is more preferred.

  - **Anaesthetic effects:** Ultrashort-acting barbiturates are used for induction of anaesthesia before administration of general anaesthetics. They are also used for operation of short duration. They act by facilitating GABA-ergic transmission in the midbrain reticular formation and also in limbic system.

  - **Analgesic effects:** They do not relieve pain until the subject becomes unconscious in anaesthetic dosage.

- **Respiratory effects:** In high dosage, they depress respiration by abolishing/neurogenic chemical and hypoxic drives one after another. Normally, the respiratory centre is controlled by a neurogenic drive (originating in the reticular activating system (RAS)), a chemical drive (which depends on the concentration of blood CO_2 and pH of arterial blood) and a hypoxic drive (which is mediated through chemo-receptors in carotid sinus and aortic body). In chronic obstructive pulmonary diseases (COPDs) like emphysema and bronchial asthma, even a hypnotic dose of a barbiturate can produce dyspnoea by decreasing the ventilatory volume.

- **Cardiovascular effects:** In hypnotic dosage, they can cause slight fall of BP and decrease in heart rate. In very high (toxic) doses they cause severe and sustained fall of BP and bradycardia by a direct depressant action of VMC and heart (myocardium), as well as by hypoxia and blockade of sympathetic ganglia.

- **Skeletal muscle effects:** In hypnotic doses, they have little effect but in anaesthetic doses, they reduce muscle contraction by depressing excitability of the neuromuscular junction.

- **Smooth muscle effects:** Even in hypnotic dosage they slightly reduce tone and motility of GIT. Their actions on bronchial, urinary bladder, ureteric and uterine muscles are not significant.

- **Hepatic effects:** They are potent hepatic microsomal enzyme inducers and increase metabolism of many drugs including oral contraceptives, glucocorticoids, oral anti-coagulants, thyroxine, phenytoin, phenylbutazone, vitamins (D and K), theophylline, chloramphenicol and griseofulvin and reduce their therapeutic effects. They increase the synthesis of porphyrin in the liver by increasing the synthesis of amino levulinic acid (ALA) synthetase. Porphyrin is required for the synthesis of haem of haemoglobin. Phenobarbitone is used in neonatal nonhaemolytic jaundice (kernicterus neonatorus), as it increases the synthesis of glucuronyl transferase in the liver to produce glucuronic acid, which conjugates bilirubin.

- **Renal effects:** In hypnotic dosage, they do not affect urine output, but in anaesthetic dosage, they decrease urine output by decreasing renal blood flow, GFR and also by stimulation of ADH secretion.

Clinical Uses

They have now limited uses due to availability of benzodiazepines. They are used in:

- **Convulsion:** Phenobarbitone is used as an antiepileptic drug to prevent grand mal seizures. Phenobarbitone sodium (IV) can be used in drug or disease induced convulsions.
- **Neonatal nonhaemolytic jaundice (kernicterus neonatorum):** Phenobarbitone is used to produce rapid excretion of bilirubin in urine by forming bilirubin glucuronide.
- **Insomnia:** Secobarbitone or pentobarbitone is occasionally used as hypnotic.
- **For anaesthesia:** Thiopentone sodium (IV) is commonly used for induction of anaesthesia before administration of general anaesthetics. For preanaesthetic medication diazepam is preferred than phenobarbitone; or secobarbitone.

Contraindications

These are given as follows:

- Chronic obstructive pulmonary diseases (COPDs)
- Patients with intermittent porphyria produce acute exacerbation.
- Severe hepatic or renal diseases.

Some Preparations and Dosage

- Phenobarbitone (Gardenal) tablet (30, 60 mg)—30 to 60 mg daily, phenobarbitone sodium (Gardenal) injection (100 mg/ml)—100 to 200 mg IM or IV.
- Secobarbitone (Seconal) capsule (50, 100 mg)—50 to 100 mg daily.
- Pentobarbitone (Nembutol) capsule (50, 100 mg)—50 to 100 mg daily.

- Thiopentone sodium (Pentothal) injection (0.25, 0.5 g/vial)—It is used freshly and prepared as 2.5% solution in distilled water and given in a dose of 0.5 to 1 g by slow IV injection.

Adverse Reactions

They produce following adverse effects:

- **Side effects:** Hangover in the next day, mental confusion, amnesia and impairment of motor functions commonly occur. Road accident may occur during motor driving.
- **Intolerance:** Abnormal reactions like excitement, headache, nausea, vomiting, diarrhoea, lassitude and paroxysmal pain resembling neuralgia, myalgia or arthralgia may occur.
- **Allergic reactions:** Urticaria and other skin rashes, angioneurotic oedema, agranulocytosis and thrombocytopenic purpura may occur.
- **Depression of foetal respiration:** It may occur if they are administered in woman during labour.
- **Megaloblastic anaemia:** It may occur on prolonged use of phenobarbitone in grand mal. It responds to folic acid.
- **Acute attack of intermittent porphyria:** It occurs after administration of barbiturates in some persons.
- **Drug automatism:** If a barbiturate is used as a hypnotic, especially in an elderly person, he or she may repeatedly take the drug due to confusion and amnesia producing poisoning effects. The phenomenon is called drug automatism.
- **Tolerance:** It develops on repeated administration of barbiturates. It can be pharmacokinetic tolerance (due to increased metabolism of barbiturates by induction of hepatic microsomal enzyme system) and tissue tolerance (due to adaptation of nervous tissue to barbiturates).
- **Drug dependence:** It develops on repeated administration of barbiturates. It is both psychological and physical and seen in

chronic barbiturate intoxication in an addict. It is manifested as thick slurred speech, ataxia (inability to move), hypotonia of muscles, decreased superficial and deep reflexes, nystagmus and difficulty in accomodation of eye. The nutrition is usually unimpaired.

If barbiturate treatment is stopped in an addict, then withdrawal symptoms (abstinence syndrome) appear within 2 to 3 days. It is manifested as anxiety, restlessness, tremors, craving for the drug, hypotension, nausea, vomiting, abdominal colics, prostration, visual hallucination, disorientation, delirium, convulsions and cardiovascular collapse. It is treated symptomatically. If desired replacement therapy can be done by administration of a less toxic sedative-hypnotic like diazepam (100 mg daily), chlordiazepoxide (20 mg daily) or chloralhydrate (1 g daily) in divided doses.

- **Acute toxicity (poisoning):** It is due to ingestion of an overdose either accidently or with suicidal intention. The lethal dose of a barbiturate is about 10 times of a hypnotic dose. The clinical picture is characterized by depression of central nervous system, particularly the respiration and a peripheral circulatory collapse. The patient is flabby and comatose and shows weak and rapid pulse, cold and clammy skin and slow or rapid and shallow respiration. Cheyne-Stokes breathing may occur. The pupils may be initially constricted and reacting to light but subsequently develop paralytic dilatation and not reacting to light. Death may occur due to respiratory or renal failure.
- **Treatment:** It is an emergency situation and requires prompt treatment. There is no specific antidote (competitive antagonist) of barbiturates and so supportive and symptomatic treatment is done. The patient should be hospitalized immediately and put in intensive care unit (ICU). Gastric lavage is done with plain water to remove the poison, if administered orally. Maintenance of respiration is done by oxygen administration (inhalation) and in severe case by endotracheal intubation and artificial ventilation. Maintenance of circulation is done by administration of adequate fluids by IV infusion to maintain electrolyte balance and BP. Forced alkaline diuresis is done for rapid excretion of barbiturates in alkaline urine by administration of a diuretic (frusemide—20 mg IV or mannitol—100 ml of 25% solution) with 50 ml of 2.5% sodium bicarbonate solution and 1 litre of 5% dextrose saline solution by IV infusion. It is more helpful in long-acting barbiturates, which are eliminated primarily by renal excretion. In severe renal failure, peritoneal dialysis, haemodialysis or haemoperfusion may be done for elimination of barbiturate. Proper nursing care and maintenance of nutrition must be done. Prophylactic antibiotics are given to prevent respiratory and urinary tract infections.

Analeptics like bemegride or nikethamide should not be given as they can produce convulsions in comatose stage leading to death of the patient.

OTHER SEDATIVE-HYPNOTICS

Chloralhydrate

It is a general CNS depressant like barbiturates. It has sedative (in small dose) and hypnotic (in large dose) actions. It is a prodrug and is converted to an active metabolite, trichloroethanol in the liver. It produces sleep within one hour which lasts for 5 to 6 hours. It does not significantly depress respiration and BP in hypnotic dose. It is a safe hypnotic for all ages in insomnia. It is especially preferred in elderly persons and children. It is administered as a mixture or syrup in a dose of 0.5 to 1 g at bed time. It is metabolized in the liver and is excreted in urine as urochloralic acid (a conjugate of trichloroethanol with glucuronic acid). It can produce nausea and vomiting due to gastric irritation and bad taste. It produces hangover in the next day. Rarely it produces drug dependence and allergic reactions. It is contraindicated in peptic ulcer and severe hepatic or renal disease.

Triclofos (Trichloroethyl phosphate/trichloryl)

It is a stable ester of trichloroethanol. It is available as tablet (0.5 g) and syrup (0.5 g/5 ml) and given in a dose of 0.5 to 1 g at bed time for hypnotic action in insomnia. It produces less gastric irritation than chloralhydrate.

Paraldehyde

It is a polymer of acetaldehyde (containing three molecules of acetaldehyde). It is a general CNS depressant like barbiturates. It has sedative (in small dose), hypnotic and anticonvulsant (in large dose) actions. It produces sleep within 30 minutes, which lasts for 6 to 8 hours. It does not significantly depress respiration and BP in hypnotic dosage. It is metabolized in the liver and excreted in urine and through lungs. It is administered rectally (as it produces gastric irritation) or by IM injection. The dose is 15 to 30 ml rectally or 5 to 10 ml by deep IM injection. It can be used as a hypnotic in insomnia and as an anticonvulsant in convulsions due to epilepsy (grand mal), eclampsia or tetanus. It can cause tissue necrosis, abscess formation and even nerve damage when injected into the muscle. It is contraindicated in peptic ulcer and in severe hepatic, renal or pulmonary disease.

Methaqualone

It is a synthetic drug. It has sedative (in small dose), hypnotic and anticonvulsant (in large dose) actions. It produces vivid dreams. A fixed dose combination of methaqualone (250 mg) and diphenhydramine (25 mg) is available in the name of Mandrex, which is a potent hypnotic. It can produce drug dependence (addiction) on repeated use and so it is now less used.

Antihistaminics

These are synthetic drugs. Promethazine (25 mg at bed time) and diphenhydramine (50 mg at bed time) are potent hypnotics and preferred in children. They are discussed in respective chapter.

Newer sedative-hypnotics such as buspirone (a partial agonist of $5HT_{1A}$ receptor), zolpidem (binds with benzodiazepine receptor) and melatonin (synthesized in pineal gland from 5-HT) act by potentiating GABA effect. They are available for clinical use. These drugs are discussed with anxiolytic drugs.

Older sedative-hypnotics like ethinamate, etomidate, glutethimide, methyprylon, ethchlorvynol, meprobamate and potassium bromide are now rarely used in therapy. Scopolamine is used in motion sickness for sedative action.

Aliphatic Alcohols

INTRODUCTION

Aliphatic alcohols are hydroxy (OH) derivatives of the aliphatic hydrocarbons (ethane, methane, propane, etc.). They are of three groups:

1. Monohydroxy alcohols, e.g. ethyl alcohol, methyl alcohol and propyl alcohol.
2. Dihydroxy alcohols, e.g. ethylene glycol and propylene glycol (glycol means sweet taste).
3. Polyhydroxy alcohols, e.g. glycerol (glycerin), mannitol and sorbitol.

Only ethyl alcohol is commonly consumed by men. Methyl alcohol is of toxicological importance and so not used in men.

Ethyl alcohol (C_2H_5OH): It is also called ethanol. It is a colourless, volatile and inflammable liquid with a characteristic (sweet) smell and taste. It is generally obtained from sugar by fermentation with the help of zymase present in yeast and separated by simple distillation. It is a constituent of various beverages (drinks) such as wine, beer, whisky, brandy, rum, gin, port, sherry, champagne and vodka. Their alcohol content varies from 4 to 55% by volume.

Pharmacokinetics

It is absorbed very rapidly from upper GIT. The absorption is delayed by the presence of food in the stomach (especially milk). It is highly lipid-soluble and diffusible. It passes rapidly through various body membranes and gets distributed throughout the body tissues and fluids. It diffuses back to blood when its blood concentration falls. In the lung it passes from blood to breath, which smells of alcohol. It is metabolized in the liver to the extent of about 95% by two nonmicrosomal enzymes as follows:

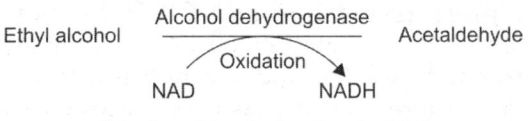

(Nicotinamide adenine dinucleotide)

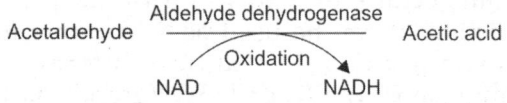

Acetic acid is converted to acetyl coenzyme A (by combining with coenzyme A) and finally oxidized to CO_2 and H_2O in the liver and tissues by entering Krebs cycle.

Acetic acid + Coenzyme A → Acetyl CoA
→ CO_2 + H_2O + Energy (ATP).

Elimination of alcohol from the body: When the blood concentration is more than 50 mg/100 ml it follows zero order kinetics, i.e. a fixed amount of alcohol is eliminated per unit time (say 15 ml per hour).

A small amount of alcohol is excreted unchanged through lungs (3%) and kidneys (2%).

Pharmacological Actions

Mode of action: It probably acts like barbiturates by potentiating the action of GABA and thus facilitating the inhibitory GABA-ergic transmission in the central nervous system. It also inhibits Ca^{++} influx through calcium channels in the cell membrane and antagonizes the action of glutamate in the CNS. It produces following effects:

- **CNS effects:** It is a general CNS depressant. It produces descending and irregular depression of CNS. It first depresses the inhibitory system of CNS, which includes midbrain RAS and certain subcortical centres. This leads to release of cerebral cortex and other areas of the brain from the integrating control or inhibition by the inhibitory system of brain. Thus there occurs apparent/pseudoexcitement and euphoria (feeling of well-being). As the concentration of alcohol in blood rises following changes in CNS gradually occurs (as shown in **Table 41.1**).

Table 41.1: Behavioural changes with rise of blood concentrations of alcohol

Blood concentration (mg/100 ml)	Behavioural changes
Less than 50 mg%	Not significant
50 to 100 mg%	Feeling of exaltation, talkativeness, hilarity, vivid personality.
100 to 200 mg%	Emotionally unstable, frequent mood swings, violent behaviour, loud speech, motor incoordination, nystagmus.
200 to 300 mg%	Loss of self-control, staggering gait, loss of memory, slurring of speech, impairment of vision and other sensory functions.
400 to 500 mg%	Stupor, dead drunk
More than 500 mg%	General anaesthesia, coma
300 to 400 mg%	Respiratory depression and failure, death.

At blood concentration of alcohol above 100 mg%, there are uncoordinated movements and decreased superficial and deep reflexes. Smooth operation of motor processes becomes disturbed and performance of skilled tasks like typing and motor car driving are impaired. There may be road accident by motor car driving due to faulty judgement. The finer grades of discrimination, memory, concentration and insight are gradually dulled and finally lost. Alcohol is not a dependable hypnotic as it produces poor quality of sleep and early morning awakening. It cannot be used as a general anaesthetic due to its narrow margin of safety (low therapeutic index). It can precipitate an attack of fit in epileptic subject.

- **CVS effects:** It causes dilatation of skin vessels by a central action when consumed in moderate amounts. It gives a feeling of warmth, for which people of cold countries have the habit of taking alcoholic beverages at night. It causes fall of BP when consumed in large amount. This is due to depression of myocardiac and vasomotor centre (VMC). Chronic consumption of alcohol in moderate amounts produces cardiomyopathy, which is manifested as cardiomegaly, cardiac failure and cardiac arrhythmias. It is suspected to increase the risk of hypertension.

- **GIT effects:** It increases gastric acid secretion when administered in dilute solution (10 to 20%). It is due to both direct (*via* gastrin) and reflex (*via* taste buds) actions. It has an irritant action on the gastric mucous membrane. It should not be used as an appetizer in peptic ulcer, as it causes gastric irritation and even haemorrhage. Administered in high concentrations, it produces acute gastritis giving rise to nausea, vomiting and epigastric pain. Its chronic administration produces chronic gastritis and achlorhydria due to atrophy of gastric mucosa.

- **Hepatic effects:** In the liver it produces impaired gluconeogenesis, diminished fatty acid oxidation, reduced synthesis of albumin and transferrin and increased synthesis of VLDL with consequent hyper-triglyceridemia. Acute consumption of alcohol inhibits the hepatic microsomal enzyme systems, whereas chronic consumption of alcohol induces (stimulates) them leading to increased rate of metabolism of many drugs and of alcohol itself. It can produce hepatomegaly, fatty degeneration of liver, cirrhosis of liver, hepatitis or hepatoma on chronic use.

- **Renal effects:** It causes diuresis (increases the output of urine) due to decreased tubular reabsorption of water by inhibition of ADH secretion. It also increases the excretion of magnesium and calcium and decreases that of potassium in urine.

- **Metabolic effects:** It produces hypoglycaemia by inhibiting hepatic gluconeo-genesis and depleting hepatic glycogen. It diminishes fatty acid oxidation. It increases synthesis of VLDL and produces hyper-triglyceridaemia. It decreases synthesis of albumin and transferrin.

- **Miscellaneous effects:** It has an erroneous reputation as a sexual stimulant (aphro-disiac). It increases the sex desire but decreases the sex power/performance. It can cause impotence, sterility and gynaeco-mastia on chronic administration. It can also produce prostatic congestion causing acute urinary retention. It produces anaemia by causing folate and iron deficiency. It causes fetal alcohol syndrome in neonates if consumed by mother during pregnancy. These babies are born with birth defects like low birth weight, microcephaly, flat face, mental retardation and congenital heart diseases. Even moderate alcohol consumption during pregnancy increases the risk of abortion.

Food value of alcohol: Alcohol is an energy producing substance. It supplies 7 calories/g, when compared with fat (9 calories/g), carbohydrate (4 calories/g) and protein (4 calories/g). It cannot be considered as a complete food, because the calories available from its hourly oxidation are inadequate even for maintenance of basal metabolism.

Moreover, it cannot be stored in the body and it produces dietary deficiencies, physical dependence and many adverse effects.

Clinical Uses

It has following external and internal uses:

External Uses

- It is used as an antiseptic. Rectified spirit (containing 90% alcohol) or absolute alcohol (98%) is used before injection or minor surgical procedure for sterilization of skin. It acts as a bactericide by precipitation of bacterial protein.
- It is used as a hardening agent in bedsores (to harden the skin).
- It is used as a cleansing agent to wash out phenol from the skin in accidental phenol burn.

Internal Uses

- It is used in methyl alcohol poisoning. Dilute ethyl alcohol (10 to 20% solution) is administered orally by gastric tube or by IV infusion in a dosage of 200 to 400 ml in methyl alcohol poisoning and acts by competing for the same metabolic pathway (competitive antagonist). After entering the liver it utilizes the enzyme, alcohol dehydrogenase for its metabolism, because it has greater affinity for this enzyme than methyl alcohol. It thus blocks metabolism of methyl alcohol to form formaldehyde and formic acid, which are toxic substances. It can be life-saving in methyl alcohol poisoning. If for some reasons, acidosis cannot be prevented by rapid IV administration of alkali solution (sodium bicarbonate). 4-methyl pyrazole, an alcohol dehydrogense inhibitor can also be used in methyl alcohol poisoning.

- It is used as an appetizer (appetite stimulant) in 10% solution (30 to 50 ml) before meals in weak patients and old persons.

- It is used to destroy a nerve by local injection (5 to 10 ml of 70% solution) around the nerve in trigeminal neuralgia to relieve intractable pain.

• It is used as a solvent in elixirs (syrups), tinctures, spirits and extracts.

Adverse Reactions

These are acute alcoholism and chronic alcoholism.

Acute Alcoholism

It is due to ingestion of over dose of concentrated alcohol. It is characterized by severe CNS depression manifestated as stupor, coma, cold skin, noisy respiration, slow and weak pulse, hypotension, hypoglycaemia, ketoacidosis, dilated pupils, hypotonia of muscles, convulsions and cardiovascular collapse.

Treatment

It is an emergency situation. The patient should be hospitalized and put in intensive care unit (ICU). Symptomatic and supportive treatment is done. Gastric lavage with sodium bicarbonate solution (5%) by gastric tube is done to wash out alcohol from the stomach. Maintenance of respiration is done by administration of oxygen or by artificial ventilation (in severe case). Maintenance of circulation is done by administration of IV fluids (normal saline, 5% dextrose saline, etc.) and vasopressor drugs (if required).

To treat hypoglycaemia, 50% glucose solution (50 to 100 ml) along with thiamine (100 mg) is administered IV. To treat ketoacidosis, 2.5% sodium bicarbonate solution (100 to 200 ml) is administered by IV drip. To treat convulsions, diazepam (10 mg) is administered IV. Maintenance of nutrition and electrolyte balance is done and proper nursing care should be given.

In very severe case peritoneal dialysis or haemodialysis is done to remove alcohol from blood.

Chronic Alcoholism

It is due to repeated consumption of alcohol leading to addiction (drug dependence). In addicts, the normal feeling of well-being depends on a continuous availability of alcohol molecules in the body tissues and fluids. There is intense craving for alcohol and the desire of alcohol consumption becomes the only interest in addicts. Sudden withdrawal of alcohol in them may lead to withdrawal syndrome which is manifested as restlessness, anxiety, irritability, nausea, vomiting, hyperexcitability, insomnia, disordered perception and convulsions and later on tremors, hallucinations, disorientation and ANS overactivity (delirium tremens). Moreover, they also suffer from anaemia, hyperlipidaemia, hepatic cirrhosis and neuropsychiatric disorders like Korsakoff's psychosis, Wernicke's encephalopathy, polyneuritis, hallucinosis and suicidal tendencies.

Treatment

It consists of drug therapy and psychotherapy.

• **Drug therapy:** Drugs used for aversion therapy are disulphiram and citrated calcium cyanamide. It should be done in a hospital with proper precautions.

Disulphiram (antabuse)

It is a thiuram compound (tetraethyl thiuram disulphide). It is available as tablet (250 mg). It is administered in following dosage for aversion therapy, first day: 1 g, second day: 0.75 g, third day: 0.5 g, and fourth and subsequent days: 0.25 g for 2–3 months and sometimes up to one year. It is used in those addicts, who are cooperative and willing to give up drinking of alcohol.

Mechanism of action

It is an aldehyde dehydrogenase inhibitor. It blocks conversion of acetaldehyde to acetic acid in the body. Thus, when alcohol is ingested after taking disulphiram, the concentration of acetaldehyde in blood rises producing many unpleasant and severe symptoms called aldehyde syndrome (antabuse reaction). These include flushing, sweating, headache, palpitation, nausea, vomiting, uneasiness, dizziness, severe fall of BP and even cardiovascular collapse. The addict thus realizes that while on this drug, he cannot tolerate even a small dose of alcohol and so he refuses to take alcohol. Severe fall of BP is due to inhibition of the enzyme, dopamine β-oxidase, decreasing synthesis of noradrenaline from dopamine.

Adverse reactions

It can cause drowsiness, nausea, headache, muscle cramps, fatigue and metallic taste in mouth. It is contraindicated in uncontrolled diabetes mellitus, hepatic and circulatory diseases.

Citrated calcium cyanamide (CCC) has similar properties of disulphiram but has a shorter duration of action.

Other aldehyde dehydrogenase inhibitors like metronidazole, chlorpropamide, tolbutamide, phenylbutazone, griseofulvin nitrofurantoin and a few cephalosporins (cefamandole, cefoperazone and moxalactum) should not be used in chronic alcoholics as they produce aldehyde syndrome (antabuse reaction) like disulphiram.

- **Psychotherapy:** It often gives good result when done by a sympathetic doctor. Complete cooperation of the patient is necessary. He should be explained by the doctor that indulgence even in small quantity of alcohol again would lead to a relapse of the condition and so it should be avoided. Drug therapy and psychotherapy can be supported by institutional therapy (in a rehabilitation centre), where the patient can see for himself the ex-alcoholics who have given up drinking of alcohol and are living a happy life. This will help to boost the patient's moral. A religious and spiritual approach in them is also helpful.

Methyl alcohol (CH₃OH)

It is also called methanol. It is not used therapeutically. It has some pharmacological effects like ethyl alcohol but it is a poison. In the liver, it is oxidized to formaldehyde by alcohol dehydrogenase and then to formic acid by aldehyde dehydrogenase. Formic acid can produce toxicities like folate depletion, metabolic acidosis and damage of retinal cells causing blindness. It is of toxicological importance. Methylated spirits containing 5% methyl alcohol and 95% ethyl alcohol is used in varnishing paint of wooden furnitures mixing with salac.

42

General Anaesthetics

INTRODUCTION

General anaesthetics (GAs) are drugs that produce general anaesthesia. The cardinal features of general anaesthesia are reversible loss of all sensations, unconsciousness, relaxation of skeletal muscles and abolition of all reflexes.

In the modern practice of balanced anaesthesia, these modalities are obtained by using combination of drugs, each drug for a specific purpose. With the help of general anaesthesia painful surgical procedures can be carried out painlessly. But these general anaesthetics have narrow margin of safety (low therapeutic index). Even slight overdose of them may produce death of the subject. Hence, they should be administered by trained anaesthesiologists.

History

The first inhalation anaesthetic nitrous oxide is discovered by Pristley in 1776 and used by Horace Wells in 1844 for painless dental extraction. Ether was introduced by Morton in 1846, chloroform by Simpson in 1847 and halothane by Johnstone in 1956. The intravenous general anaesthetic thiopentone sodium is introduced by Lundy in 1935. Gradually other general anaesthetics were introduced in anaesthetic practice.

Classification of General Anaesthetics

These are of following two groups:

1. Inhalation general anaesthetics

- Volatile liquids, e.g. ether, halothane, enflurane, isoflurane, desflurane and sevoflurane. Chloroform, ethylchloride, trichloroethylene and methoxyflurane are now obsolete due to toxicity (cardiotoxicity, hepatotoxicity, neurotoxicity and nephrotoxicity).
- Gases, e.g. nitrous oxide cyclopropane is now obsolete due to toxicities like cardiotoxicity, respiratory depression, shock and capillary oozing.

2. Intravenous general anaesthetics

- Inducing agents, e.g. thiopentone sodium, methohexitone sodium and thiamylal sodium. These are ultrashort-acting barbiturates.
- Slowly acting drugs, e.g. midazolam, diazepam, ketamine, fentanyl/alfentanyl and droperidol combination, althesin and alphadione (steroid anaesthetics), etomidate and propofol.

Site and Mechanism of Action of General Anaesthetics

They act by producing nonselective, irregular and descending depression of central nervous system. The sensory cortex is most sensitive and medullary centres are least sensitive to their action. Motor cortex, midbrain RAS, brain stem and spinal cord are moderately sensitive to their action. They inhibit neuronal cell activity and synaptic transmission in the

CNS but their molecular mechanism of action is not clear. Several theories have been postulated to explain the mechanism of action of which three theories are popular:

- **Lipid theory (proposed by Mayer and Overtone in 1901):** According to this theory, general anaesthetics which are more lipid-soluble than water (high lipid/water partition coefficient) can easily enter the CNS through the neuronal membrane from extracellular fluid (blood) and produce rapid general anaesthesia.

- **Protein theory (proposed by Eyring and Woodbury in 1973):** According to this theory, general anaesthetics which bind with hydrophobic sites of protein molecules of the neuronal membrane of CNS can alter protein structure of the neuronal membrane leading to decreased neuronal cell activity producing general anaesthesia.

- **Hydrate theory (proposed by Pauling and Miller in 1961):** According to this theory, general anaesthetics that freeze water molecules to form anaesthetic gas hydrate crystals (clathrates) on the surface of neuronal cell membrane of CNS can alter (decrease) neuronal cell activity (excitability) by blocking Na^+ channels in the cell membrane. As Na^+ channels cannot open for influx of Na^+ ions during depolarization of AP, so neuronal transmission cannot occur by nerve impulse and this produces general anaesthesia. These agents may also release endogenous opiate-like substances (opioids) which produce analgesia.

Administration of Inhalation Anaesthetics

Following devices are used:
- **Anaesthetic machines:** With these devices, the anaesthesiologist is able to deliver measured quantities of anaesthetic gases and oxygen through accurate flowmeters and with the use of special vapourizers, it is possible to add the vapour of volatile anaesthetic liquid to the gas stream. The mixture of oxygen and anaesthetic agent is then delivered to a breathing circuit for administration by inhalation.

- **Vapourizers:** Liquid anaesthetic agents are vapourized into a stream of oxygen and nitrous oxide by a vapourizer that delivers a precise concentration of a particular anaesthetic agent. The vapourizer is constructed in such a way that anaesthetic concentration is accurately maintained over a range of gas flows and ambient temperatures.

- **Breathing circuits:** The gases and vapours are delivered into a system of wide bore tubes with valves, a distensible bag that provides a reservoir for the gases and a method for elimination of expired CO_2. Gases are administered to the patient by means of a face mask or endotracheal tube. There are two types of gas delivery systems, *viz.* low flow system and high flow system.

Stages of General Anaesthesia

Guedel in 1920 using ether as general anaesthetic described four stages of general anaesthesia which are:

Stage I   : Stage of analgesia (loss of pain sensation).

Stage II : Stage of delirium (excitement).

Stage III : Stage of surgical anaesthesia.

Stage IV : Stage of medullary depression (respiratory paralysis).

Stage III is again divided into four planes depending on the depth of anaesthesia.

Plane I: The pupils are normal in size and the eyeballs are roving. The respiration is full, regular, deep and of thoracoabdominal character. The BP and pulse rate are normal. The skeletal muscles are incompletely relaxed. The eyelid reflex, swallowing, retching and vomiting are gradually lost. The conjunctival reflex is lost but corneal reflex is present.

Plane II: The pupils begin to dilate and the eyeballs are fixed. The respiration is regular but the amplitude is diminished. The skeletal muscles are adequately relaxed. The corneal reflex, pharyngeal reflex and laryngeal reflex are gradually lost. Endotracheal intubation can be performed.

Plane III: The pupils are moderately dilated and the eyeballs are fixed. The respiration is more abdominal character than thoracic. The skeletal muscles are completely relaxed. The BP begins to fall. The intercostal muscles are gradually paralysed and the costal margins retract with the descent of the diaphragm.

Plane IV: The pupils are widely dilated and the eyeballs are fixed. The respiration is abdominal in character and thoracic respiration ceases. There is complete paralysis of intercostal muscles. The skeletal muscles are flaccid and the BP is low.

The secretions are progressively reduced from plane I onwards and are completely abolished in plane IV.

Arrival of stage IV is signalled by severe fall of BP and stoppage of spontaneous respiration due to depression of vasomotor and respiratory centres of the medulla. If no measure is taken, coma and death may occur. Discontinuation of anaesthesia, positive pressure ventilation and IV fluids are life-saving measures. In the modern anaesthetic practice, balanced anaesthetic is done by combination of different anaesthetic agents and so these stages of anaesthesia are never discerned separately. Every effort is made to achieve smooth induction, avoiding the stage of delirium (excitement) with the help of the intravenous agent, thiopentone sodium.

Practical Approach in Evaluating the Depth of Anaesthesia

The following approach is useful for any general anaesthetic. If the eyelids blink when the eyelashes are touched, if the patient is swallowing and if respiration is irregular in rate and depth, then surgical anaesthesia is not produced. The beginning of surgical anaesthesia is indicated by loss of eyelid reflex and the development of rhythmic respiration. Light anaesthesia is suggested by increase in respiratory rate and rise of arterial BP by making a skin incision or there may be gagging, coughing, vomiting or laryngospasm. Deep anaesthesia is suggested by depression of respiration, severe hypotension and cardiac

asystole. Associated blood loss and hypoxia can aggravate the situation. This must be avoided.

Pharmacokinetics of Inhalation Anaesthetics

This can be divided into three stages:
1. Induction of anaesthesia
2. Maintenance of anaesthesia
3. Recovery from anaesthesia.

Induction of anaesthesia is the period (time) between the onset of anaesthetic administration and the development of effective surgical anaesthesia. It is dependent upon how fast the effective anaesthetic concentration reach the brain. Recovery from anaesthesia is the period between cessation of anaesthetic administration and gaining of consciousness of the patient. It is dependent upon how fast the anaesthetic agent is eliminated from the body.

Maintenance of anaesthesia is the period between the induction of anaesthesia and the recovery from anaesthesia.

Inhalation anaesthetics have the advantage that the required depth of anaesthesia can be maintained by suitably altering their concentration in the body.

Factors determining the depth of anaesthesia and potency of an anaesthetic agent (gas or vapour).

- **Partial pressure of the anaesthetic agent:** The higher the alveolar concentration of the anaesthetic agent, the greater is its partial pressure within the alveoli and more is its diffusion from the alveoli to blood and then to brain (Alveoli $\rightleftharpoons$ Blood $\rightleftharpoons$ Brain) and so greater is the depth of anaesthesia. It is a measure of depth of anaesthesia.

- **Minimum alveolar concentration (MAC) of the anaesthetic agent:** It is that concentration of an inhaled anaesthetic in lung alveoli in 1 atmospheric pressure (760 mmHg), which produces immobility in 50% of human subjects by a painful stimulus (i.e. no response is obtained by incision of the skin). It is expressed as percentage of alveolar air. The higher the MAC value, the lower the potency of the anaesthetic agent.

MAC Values of Some Anaesthetic Agents

Ether (1.9%), halothane (0.75%), enflurane (1.68%), isoflurane (1.20%), sevoflurane (2.0%), desflurane (6.0%), nitrous oxide (10.5%) and cyclopropane (9.2%).

- **Lipid solubility of the anaesthetic agent:** Higher the lipid solubility of an anaesthetic agent than water solubility, the greater is the ease of penetration of the anaesthetic into the central nervous system through neuronal membrane to produce anaesthesia. It is measured by oil/water partition coefficient. It is an index of potency of an anaesthetic agent.

- **Blood solubility of the anaesthetic agent:** An anaesthetic agent which has low blood solubility (e.g. nitrous oxide), its partial pressure in blood will rise quickly as the blood becomes quickly saturated with it. As a result, the anaesthetic will rapidly enter the central nervous system neurons from blood and produces rapid anaesthesia. On the other hand, an anaesthetic agent which has high blood solubility (e.g. ether) will take longer time to produce anaesthesia. It is measured by blood/gas partition coefficient. It gives an idea about the speed of onset of anaesthesia.

Elimination of Anaesthetic Agents

Major portion of inhalation anaesthetics is eliminated through lungs by exhalation during recovery from anaesthesia. Some anaesthetics are metabolized in the liver to some extent, e.g. ether (10%), halothane (20%), enflurane (5%) and isoflurane (2%) and are excreted through kidneys (in urine), skin (in sweat) and intestinal mucous membranes (in faeces). Presence of hepatic or renal insufficiency may delay recovery from anaesthesia.

Drugs used in General Anaesthesia

These are of three groups:

1. Drugs used before surgery/anaesthesia: These are preanaesthetic medication and drugs for basal anaesthesia.
2. Drugs used during surgery: These are general anaesthetics and skeletal muscle relaxants.
3. Drugs used after surgery/during recovery from anaesthesia: These are analgesics, sedative-hypnotics, antibiotics, etc.

Preanaesthetic Medication (Premedication)

These are drugs administered in the ward (at night and morning) before bringing the patient to operation theatre for anaesthesia. Aim of premedication is to make anaesthesia safe and acceptable (agreeable) to the patient. Objects of premedication are:

- To allay anxiety and apprehension of the patient.
- To relieve pain (preoperative and operative).
- To obtain an additive/synergistic action, so that induction of anaesthesia becomes smooth, pleasant and rapid and the dose of anaesthetic required can be reduced.
- To counteract the adverse effects of some anaesthetics like ether (excessive salivary and bronchial secretions, bradycardia and vomiting).
- To reduce reflex excitability like laryngospasm and bronchospasm by excessive salivary and bronchial secretions.

Drugs used for Premedication

These are of following groups:

- **Opioid (narcotic) analgesics:** Morphine (8 to 12 mg IM), pethidine (50 to 100 mg IM) and fentanyl (0.05 to 0.1 mg IM) are commonly used. They produce analgesic and sedative actions and reduce the dose of general anaesthetic required. Their disadvantages are:
  - Depression of RC causing decreased respiration (by all).

– Depression of VMC causing fall of BP (by all).

– Interference with the pupillary reactions (signs) of the general anaesthetic (morphine produces miosis and pethidine produces mydriasis).

– Vomiting and antidiuretic effect (by morphine).

– Tachycardia (by pethidine due to vagolytic action).

– Precipitation of acute attack of bronchial asthma due to histamine release (by morphine and pethidine).

– Delay of recovery from anaesthesia as their actions last for 6 to 8 hours.

- **Sedative-hypnotics and antianxiety drugs:** Benzodiazepines are preferred than barbiturates for their wide margin of safety, less respiratory depressant effect and good muscle relaxant activity of the benzodiazepines like diazepam (5 to 10 mg IM or orally), midazolam (0.07 mg/kg IM), lorazepam (1 to 2 mg orally) and alprazolam (0.25 to 0.5 mg orally) are commonly used. Drugs like phenothiazines (chlorpromazine, etc.), butyrophenones (haloperidol, etc.) and antihistaminics (hydroxyzine, etc.) are now rarely used as they cause respiratory depression and hypotension by potentiating the effects of opioid analgesics.

- **Anticholinergic drugs:** Muscarinic antagonists like atropine (0.4 to 0.6 mg IM), scopolamine (0.4 to 0.6 mg IM) and glycopyrrolate (0.1 to 0.3 mg IM) are commonly used to block vagal stimulant actions of general anaesthetics like excessive salivary and bronchial secretions, vomiting, bradycardia, hypotension and reflex excitability. Glycopyrrolate is now preferred than atropine (CNS stimulant) and scopolamine (CNS depressant) as it has little CNS action and it does not cause tachycardia.

- **Antiemetics:** Prokinetic drugs like metoclopramide (10 mg IM or orally), domperidone (10 mg orally) are preferred than antihistaminics like promethazine and cyclizine in stopping emetic episodes in operative and postoperative periods as they do not produce hypotension.

- **Drugs that reduce the acidity and volume of gastric contents:** Antacids like sodium bicarbonate (1 to 2 g orally) and sodium citrate (1 to 2 g orally) and H_2-blockers like ranitidine (150 to 300 mg orally) and famotidine (20 to 40 mg orally) are commonly used to reduce gastric acidity and gastric acid secretion and to prevent gastric regurgitation leading to aspiration pneumonia.

- **Miscellaneous drugs:** Antibiotics, chemotherapeutic agents, antihypertensives, antidiabetics, antithyroids or thyroids, bronchodilators, glucocorticoids, antiepileptic drugs, antiparkinsonian drugs, etc. are used if required by the patients.

Basal Anaesthetics

These are drugs used to produce basal anaesthesia, which is a state of light anaesthesia, on which surgical anaesthesia is built up by a general anaesthetic. These are administered in the ward one hour before surgery. They produce amnesia (loss of memory) and sedation (reduce excitability of the patient). They also reduce the dose of general anaesthetic required.

Preparations and Dosage

- Paraldehyde 10 to 15 ml rectally mixed with normal saline (120 ml).
- Tribromoethanol (Bromethol) 5 to 8 ml rectally mixed with normal saline (120 ml).
- Diazepam (5 to 10 mg) and ketamine (2 to 4 mg) IM or IV. It is now preferred than other two drugs due to less adverse effects.

DISCUSSION OF COMMONLY USED INHALATION OF GENERAL ANAESTHETICS

Ether (Diethyl Ether/C_2H_5—O—C_2H_5)

It is a volatile general anaesthetic. It is a colourless liquid with pungent smell. Its vapour is inflammable and explosive. It is a potent anaesthetic. A concentration of 10 to 15%

of ether with oxygen is required for induction of anaesthesia and a concentration of 4 to 5% of it with oxygen is required for maintenance of anaesthesia. It has some advantages and disadvantages given as follows:.

Advantages

- It is a potent anaesthetic (MAC value is 1.9%).
- It produces good analgesia and adequate skeletal muscle relaxation.
- It can be administered by open drop method and without requiring a special form of anaesthetic apparatus. It allows the use of air as a source of oxygen, because it produces anaesthesia at a low concentration.
- It has high margin of safety. It does not produce cardiac arrhythmias as it does not sensitize heart to catecholamines. It maintains BP and respiration to normal levels during anaesthesia due to reflex stimulation and producing high sympathetic tone. It does not produce hepatotoxicity.
- It is cheap (economical).

Disadvantages

- It produces slow and unpleasant induction of anaesthesia with marked excitement, struggling and breath holding.
- It increases salivary and bronchial secretions and produces coughing, laryngeal spasm and bronchospasm (due to irritant nature of vapour). Nausea and vomiting may occur with it.
- It can cause lung complications like bronchitis and bronchopneumonia due to aspiration of secretions into lungs.
- It can produce explosion hazard due to use of electrocautery.
- It produces slow recovery from anaesthesia.

Halothane (Fluothane)

$$F-C(F)(F)-C(Br)(Cl)(H)$$

It is a halogenated (fluorinated) volatile general anaesthetic. It is a colourless liquid with a characteristic sweet fruity smell. Its vapour is nonirritant, noninflammable and nonexplosive. It is a potent general anaesthetic. A concentration of 2 to 3% of halothane with oxygen is required for induction of anaesthesia and a concentration of 1 to 2% of it with oxygen is required for maintenance of anaesthesia. It has some following advantages and disadvantages:

Advantages

- It is a potent anaesthetic (MAC value is 0.75%).
- It produces rapid and pleasant induction of anaesthesia and rapid recovery from anaesthesia.
- It does not increase salivary and bronchial secretions and does not produce coughing, laryngeal spasm and bronchospasm.
- It produces bronchodilatation by direct relaxation of bronchial smooth muscle and can be used in bronchial asthma.
- It is noninflammable and nonexplosive and so electrocautery can be used during its administration.

Disadvantages

- It cannot be administered by open drop method and requires a special form of anaesthetic apparatus for administration.
- It has poor analgesic and skeletal muscle relaxant activities.
- It can produce cardiac arrhythmias as it sensitizes the heart (myocardium) to the action of catecholamines.
- It can produce cardiovascular depression leading to hypotension.
- It can depress respiration in high concentration (4%).
- It should not be used during labour and caesarean section (CS) because by relaxing the uterine muscle it prolongs labour and increases PPH. It also depresses foetal respiration.
- It can produce malignant hyperthermia (discussed with succinylcholine) and hepatotoxicity.
- It is costly (expensive).

Enflurane and Isoflurane

These are halogenated volatile general anaesthetics. They are very costly and are rarely used. Isoflurane is an isomer of enflurane. They are very stable chemically. They are noninflammable and nonexplosive. They are potent general anaesthetics (isoflurane is 1½ times more potent than enflurane). Their pharmacological properties are similar to halothane. They have poor analgesic activities like halothane but they produce better skeletal muscle relaxation than halothane.

Enflurane can produce hypotension (by cardiovascular depression) and cardiac arrhythmias (by sensitizing the myocardium to the actions of catecholamines) like halothane. Isoflurane does not sensitize the myocardium to the actions of catecholamines and does not produce cardiac arrhythmias. It cannot be used for induction of anaesthesia due to pungent smell. Enflurane and isoflurane rarely produce hepatotoxicity. Enflurane can cause convulsions and so contraindicated in patients of epilepsy, while isoflurane does not produce convulsions and is preferred for neurosurgery.

Nitrous Oxide (N₂O/Laughing Gas)

It is a colourless and odourless gas heavier than air. It is a nonirritant, noninflammable and nonexplosive gas. It is supplied in steel cylinder at under pressure (650 to 800 lb per square inch). It has low potency as a general anaesthetic. A concentration of 70 to 80% of nitrous oxide with oxygen (20 to 30%) is required for induction of anaesthesia. A further increase in the concentration of nitrous oxide produces hypoxia leading to respiratory depression. It cannot be used alone for maintenance of general anaesthesia. It is mainly used as a supplement to other potent inhalation anaesthetics, which can be used in small doses leading to shorter recovery time and less complications. It is used as nitrous oxide + ether/halothane + oxygen mixture. If administered along with air, it produces a stage of excitement (delirium) and also produces amnesia. Hence, it is called laughing gas. It has some following advantages and disadvantages:

Advantages

- It is nonirritant, noninflammable and non-explosive.
- It produces rapid induction of anaesthesia and rapid recovery from anaesthesia.
- It has powerful analgesic action.
- It can produce second gas effect during induction of anaesthesia (discussed later on).
- It is the safest of the anaesthetic agent, having little or no adverse effects on heart, circulation, respiration, liver and kidney.
- It does not produce postanaesthetic nausea and vomiting.
- It is cheap (economical).

Disadvantages

- It is a low potency (weak) anaesthetic (MAC value is 10%).
- It has no skeletal muscle relaxant activity and so a neuromuscular blocker is required during its administration.
- It may produce severe excitement (delirium) during induction of anaesthesia.
- It can produce diffusional hypoxia during recovery from anaesthesia (discussed later on).
- It requires a special form of anaesthetic cavity apparatus for administration.
- It cannot be administered in presence of any closed gas filled in the body, which tends to expand during its administration. It is therefore, contraindicated in patients with collection of air in the pleural, pericardial or peritoneal cavity, intestinal obstruction, obstruction of middle ear, chronic obstructive pulmonary disease or emphysema.

Second Gas Effect, O₂ Concentration Effect and Diffusional Hypoxia

The uptake and distribution of nitrous oxide in the body are influenced by its physical properties. A normal adult breathing 70% N₂O will achieve 90% equilibration in about 15 minutes. During this time, approximately 10 litres of N_2O will have been absorbed from the alveolar gas into the body. This volume change is more than 10 times that which occurs during the inhalation of 1% halothane. This large uptake of N_2O gas produces second gas effect and O_2 concentration effect during induction of anaesthesia, because it increases the rapidity of uptake of a potent inhalation anaesthetic and also increases the alveolar concentration of O_2. Thus, it minimizes hypoxia.

The reverse process occurs when the administration of N_2O is discontinued. Then N_2O rapidly diffuses from the blood into the alveoli and dilutes the alveolar air leading to decrease in volume of O_2 in the alveolar air and resulting in decrease in alveolar tension and hence arterial tension of oxygen. This is termed diffusional hypoxia. It is produced mainly when N_2O is used alone as the sole anaesthetic agent. It can cause postoperative hypoxaemia, particularly when there is also respiratory depression following prolonged hyperventillation. It has a limited time span and so its adverse effects can be avoided by administration of 100% of oxygen during the early recovery period.

Properties of an Ideal General Anaesthetic

- **For patient:** It should be pleasant to inhale without producing any irritation. The induction of anaesthesia produced by it should be rapid and pleasant and the recovery from anaesthesia should be smooth and rapid. It should not produce any adverse effect/toxicity.

- **For surgeon:** It should produce good analgesia and adequate skeletal muscle relaxation. It should not be irritant, inflammable or explosive. It should produce minimum capillary bleeding.

- **For anaesthetist:** It should be stable at room temperature. It should be easily controllable and has a wide margin of safety. It should not require special anaesthetic apparatus for administration. It

should not interact with material used for anaesthesia, e.g. metal and rubber tubes. It should not produce respiratory or cardiovascular depression and should be rapidly eliminated from the body.

- **For manufacturer:** Its cost of manufacture should be cheap. It should be stored at room temperature for a long period.

Of all the general anaesthetics, isoflurane is considered to be a 'near ideal' general anaesthetic.

Intravenous General Anaesthetics

They are mainly used for induction of anaesthesia, dissociative anaesthesia or neuroleptanaesthesia. They serve to reduce the dose of inhalation anaesthetic for maintenance of anaesthesia. They also promote hypnosis, analgesia, skeletal muscle relaxation and control of visceral reflex responses of general anaesthetics.

DISCUSSION OF COMMONLY USED INTRAVENOUS GENERAL ANAESTHETICS

Thiopentone Sodium

It is an ultrashort-acting barbiturate. It is highly soluble in water and yields a very alkaline solution, which must be prepared freshly before injection. It is injected IV slowly. It produces unconsciousness in the patient in 15 to 20 seconds. Its undissociated form has high lipid solubility and enters brain almost instantaneously. Unconsciousness in the patient lasts for 10 to 15 minutes due to redistribution of the drug from the brain to other like adipose and muscle tissues. It produces rapid and pleasant induction of anaesthesia, which is maintained by a potent inhalation anaesthetic (ether/halothane). When used alone, it can be used for short surgical procedure. It is also used as an anticonvulsant in the emergency treatment of convulsions.

Preparation and Dosage

Thiopentone sodium (Pentothal, Intrakel) injection (0.5 g powder per vial).

It is dissolved in 20 ml of purified water or solvent supplied to make 2.5% solution and administered IV slowly in the dose of 3 to 5 mg/kg body weight.

Advantages

- It produces rapid and pleasant induction and rapid recovery from anaesthesia.
- It does not produce postanaesthetic excitement, nausea and vomiting.
- It does not produce irritation of mucous membranes.
- It does not sensitize the myocardium to the actions of catecholamines.
- It does not produce hepatic toxicity.

Disadvantages

- It cannot be used for maintenance of anaesthesia.
- It has weak analgesic and muscular relaxation actions.
- It can produce coughing, hiccough, laryngospasm and bronchospasm, as the pharyngeal and laryngeal reflexes are not abolished.
- It can depress respiratory centre (RC) in high dosage leading to apnoea and respiratory failure.
- It can depress vasomotor centre (VMC) in high dosage leading to severe fall of BP (hypotension).
- It may depress myocardium in high dosage leading to cardiac arrhythmias.
- It may produce acute intermittent porphyria.

Midazolam (Hypnovel, Mezolam)

It is a short-acting benzodiazepine. It is used for induction of anaesthesia and for sedation during endoscopic procedures. It is also used IM for premedication. It is available as injection (5 mg/mol). The IV dose is 2.5 to 7.5 mg and IM dose is 5 mg. It is better than diazepam, because it is water-soluble and less irritant to the veins. It has also been used as an anticonvulsant by subcutaneous infusion with a syringe pump.

Ketamine

It is a short-acting general anaesthetic which is chemically and pharmacologically related to phencyclidine (a hallucinogen). It produces dissociative anaesthesia, which is characterized by complete analgesia, amnesia, light sleep and peculiar feelings of dissociation of one's own body with the surrounding. There is no loss of consciousness and the patient remains in a trance like state. It produces anaesthesia within one minute, which lasts for about 15 minutes but analgesia lasts for about 40 minutes and amnesia lasts for 1–2 hours. It probably acts on the cerebral cortex, particularly the limbic system and not the reticular activating system (RAS). It interferes with the action of glutamic acid (an excitatory neurotransmitter in the brain) by acting on NMDA (N-methyl-D-aspartate) receptors. It is used for short operations on the head and neck in patients with severe haemorrhage, burn dressings, dental extraction, angiocardiography, cardiac catheterization and trauma surgery. It is preferred in children and asthmatic patients. It is suitable for single-handed surgery.

Preparation and Dosage

Ketamine hydrochloride (Ketalar) injection (0.5 g/10 ml ampoule). It can be administered IV or IM. IV dose is 1 to 2 mg/kg body weight and IM dose is 5 to 10 mg/kg body weight.

Advantages

- It is a safe anaesthetic (greater margin of safety).
- It does not produce respiratory depression and CVS depression.
- It can be used for induction of anaesthesia, which is maintained by a potent inhalation anaesthetic.
- It is suitable for single-handed surgery.
- It is suitable for paediatric surgery.

Disadvantages

- It may cause delirium, hallucinations and unpleasant dreams during induction and recovery from anaesthesia. Diazepam must be used before its administration to reduce these effects.

- It produces poor muscular relaxation.
- It increases salivation.
- It sometimes causes nystagmus, involuntary movements and hyponeas.
- It cannot be used in patients with past history of mental illness as it produces delirium and hallucinations.
- It cannot be used in intraocular or intracranial surgery as it increases intraocular or intracranial pressure.
- It cannot be used alone in major surgery.

Fentanyl and Droperidol Combination (Innovar)

Fentanyl is a synthetic opioid analgesic and droperiodol is in butyrophenone neuroleptic. In combination, they produce a state called neuroleptanalgesia. Further combination with N₂O and O₂ produces neuroleptanaesthesia. In neuroleptanalgesia, there is strong analgesia and neuroleptic syndrome (discussed with chlorpromazine), but the patient remains conscious and cooperative. It is used for short painful surgical procedures like tooth extraction, proctoscopy, orthopaedic manipulations and burn dressings.

Preparation and Dosage

Fentanyl (50 mg/ml) and droperidol (2.5 mg/ml) injection—1 to 2 ml IV slowly (as respiratory depression may occur).

Adverse Reactions

Common side effects are vomiting, confusion, mental depression, hypotension and bradycardia. Extrapyramidal symptoms may rarely occur. Alfentanil and droperidol combination (Rapifen) is now popular, because it produces less adverse effects than fentanyl–droperidol combination.

Skeletal Muscle Relaxants (Neuromuscular Blockers)

These are important adjuvants in modern anaesthetic practice. Their use during anaesthesia would provide relaxation of skeletal muscles without the need to deepen the anaesthetic level. They are discussed in ANS pharmacology.

43

Local Anaesthetics

INTRODUCTION

Local anaesthetics are drugs that produce reversible loss of function or sensation by preventing or diminishing the conduction of nerve impulses to the site of their application or injection. They decrease permeability of the nerve cell membrane and produce membrane stabilizing effect. When applied locally to nerve tissue in appropriate concentration, they reversibly block the action potential (AP) responsible for nerve conduction. They act on any part of nervous system and on every type of nerve fibre. Thus local anaesthetic in contact with a nerve trunk can cause both sensory and motor paralyses in the area innervated. Their action is reversible in therapeutic concentrations and their use is followed by complete recovery in nerve function with no evidence of damage to nerve fibres or cells.

History

The first local anaesthetic, cocaine is isolated from the leaves of the coca plant. (*Erythroxylon coca*) by Albert Niemann in 1860. Carl Koller introduced cocaine into clinical practice as a topical anaesthetic for ophthalmological surgery in 1884. Shortly thereafter, Halstead popularized its use in infiltration and conduction block anaesthesia. The first synthetic injectable local anaesthetic procaine is introduced into clinical practice by Einhorn and his colleagues in 1905. Lidocaine was introduced by Lofgren in 1948. Gradually other synthetic local anaesthetics are introduced in clinical practice.

Classification

They can be classified in two ways:

1. **Chemical classification (according to chemical structure):** These are of two groups:

   a. Esters, e.g. cocaine (natural drug) and synthetic drugs like procaine, chlorprocaine, tetracaine (amethocaine), benzocaine, orthocaine and proparacaine.

   b. Amides, e.g. lidocaine, bupivacaine, mepivacaine, ropivacaine, etidocaine, prilocaine and dibucaine (cinchocaine). These are synthetic drugs.

2. **According to duration of action:** These are of three groups:

   a. Short-acting (½ to 1 hour), e.g. procaine and chlorprocaine.

   b. Moderately long-acting (1 to 2 hours), e.g. cocaine, lidocaine and prilocaine.

   c. Long-acting (2 to 6 hours), e.g. bupivacaine, mepivacaine, tetracaine, dibucaine, ropivacaine, editocaine, benzocaine, orthocaine and oxethazine.

Other drugs possessing local anaesthetic activity are propranolol, bucricaine, phenol, cloveoil, quinine and some antihistaminics.

Chemistry

Cocaine is an ester of benzoic acid, procaine is an ester of paraminobenzoic acid (PABA) and lidocaine is an amide. The structural formula of a local anaesthetic contains a lipophilic (hydrophobic) group and a hydrophilic group, which are separated by an intermediate ester or amide linkage (as shown in **Fig. 43.1**).

Ester type versus amide type local anaesthetics:

- Ester type local anaesthetics are readily hydrolyzed by plasma and liver cholinesterases at the ester linkage (bond) and have shorter duration of action. Amide type local anaesthetics are metabolized by the liver microsomal amide hydrolyzes and have longer duration of action.
- Allergic reactions are common with ester type local anaesthetics due to presence of PABA portion in the structure. Amide type local anaesthetics can produce CNS and cardiac depression.

Pharmacological Actions

Mechanism of action: Local anaesthetics prevent the generation and the conduction of the nerve impulse. Their primary site of action is the cell membrane. They block conduction of nerve impulse by decreasing or preventing the large transient increase in the permeability of the excitable membrane to Na^+ that normally is produced by a slight depolarization of the membrane. This action of local anaesthetics is due to their direct interaction with the specific binding sites (receptors) within the voltage-gated Na^+ channels. As the anaesthetic action progressively develops in a nerve, the threshold for electrical excitability gradually increases, the rate of rise of the action potential decreases and impulse conduction slows. These decrease the propagation of nerve action potential and so nerve conduction fails to produce local anaesthesia.

Differential Sensitivity of Nerve Fibres to Local Anaesthetics

Small nerve fibres are more sensitive to the action of local anaesthetics than the large nerve fibres. The smallest mammalian nerve fibres are nonmyelinated and are blocked more readily than the larger myelinated fibres. In general, autonomic fibres, small non-myelinated C fibres (mediating pain sensation) and small myelinated Aδ fibres (mediating pain and temperature sensations) are blocked before larger myelinated Aγ, Aβ and Aα fibres (carrying postural, touch, pressure and motor information). Smaller nerve fibres are blocked first because they have greater surface area per unit volume for the action of a local anaesthetic than the larger nerve fibres.

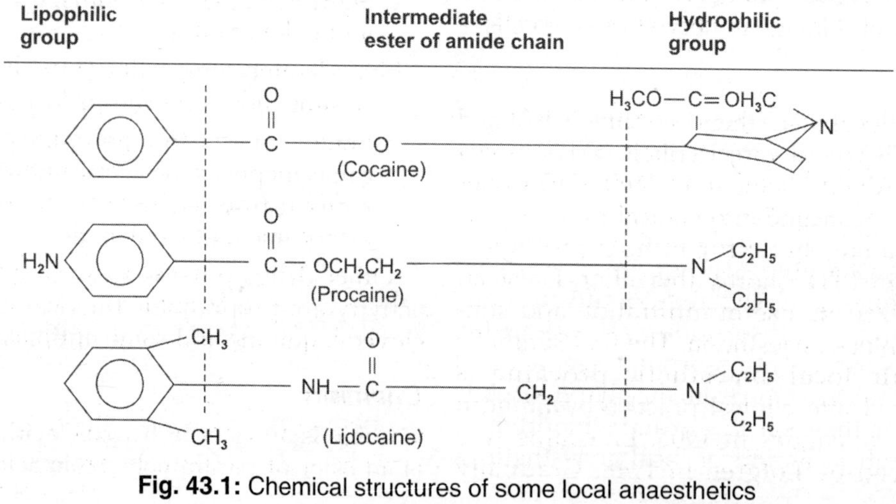

Fig. 43.1: Chemical structures of some local anaesthetics

Effect of pH on Local Anaesthetic Activity

Local anaesthetics are weak bases and are usually water-insoluble. Their hydrochloride salts are acidic, water-soluble and stable. In the tissues where the pH is alkaline (pH 7.4), the free base of the local anaesthetic is released by hydrolysis, which produces local anaesthetic action.

Prolongation of Duration of Action of Local Anaesthetics by Vasoconstrictors

When used by infiltration, the absorption of local anaesthetics can be retarded by using a vasoconstrictor agent like adrenaline or phenylephrine along with the drug. This prolongs the duration of action and reduces the systemic toxicity of the drug.

Other Actions of Local Anaesthetics

Cocaine is a central nervous system stimulant and can produce restlessness, tremors and convulsions. Lidocaine is a CNS depressant and can produce drowsiness and mental clouding. Procaine is a vasodilator by sympatholytic action and can produce hypotension. Cocaine has sympathomimetic action by inhibiting uptake of noradrenaline by the adrenergic nerve endings and can produce hypertension, tachycardia and even cardiac arrhythmias. Lidocaine and bupivacaine in therapeutic doses produce antiarrhythmic action, while in toxic doses they can produce cardiac arrhythmias and even cardiac arrest. Prilocaine can produce methaemoglobinaemia by causing accumulation of its metabolite 'O-toluidine' in blood. Tetracaine and amethocaine can produce vasodilation and hypotension like procaine. Dibucaine (cinchocaine) can produce cinchonism.

Pharmacokinetics

Local anaesthetics are not absorbed from unbroken skin. Applied to the mucous membrane, the absorption varies with the mucous surface. The absorption is more rapid from the trachea than from the pharynx, while it is poor through the urinary bladder. A considerable amount of local anaesthetic is absorbed from a raw granulating surface. Metabolism of local anaesthetic has been discussed previously. They are excreted in urine as metabolites.

Clinical Uses of Local Anaesthetics

They are used for following purposes:

- **Topical (surface) anaesthesia:** The local anaesthetic solution is applied to the mucous membrane or abraded skin to block the sensory nerve endings. It is applied as solution, ointment, cream or powder to the site at which anaesthesia is required. Commonly used local anaesthetics for this purpose are lidocaine (2 to 4%), tetracaine (1 to 2%), dibucaine (1 to 2%), benzocaine (1 to 4%) and oxethazine (1 to 5%).

- **Infiltration anaesthesia:** The local anaesthetic solution (2 to 5 ml) is injected subcutaneously at the site of operation or at one or more places around the area to be anaesthetized to block sensory nerve endings. It has rapid onset of action than topical anaesthesia. It is used for minor operations like incision, excision, hydrocele operation and herniorrhaphy. Commonly used local anaesthetics for this purpose are lidocaine (0.5 to 2%), bupivacaine (0.25 to 0.5%), procaine (0.25 to 0.5%) and tetracaine (0.5 to 1%).

- **Field block anaesthesia:** The local anaesthetic is injected subcutaneously in a manner that all nerves coming to a particular field is blocked. It is used in operation of scalp, anterior abdominal wall and the lower extremity. Its advantage over infiltration anaesthesia is that it requires lesser amount of drug to produce greater area of anaesthesia. Local anaesthetics used are same as infiltration anaesthesia.

- **Nerve block anaesthesia:** The local anaesthetic is injected very close to the nerve or plexus, e.g. intercostal nerve, ulnar nerve, sciatic nerve, trigeminal nerve, lingual nerve, ophthalmic nerve and branchial plexus. It is used in tooth extraction and operations on eye, tongue, limbs, thoracic wall and abdominal wall. By it, a large area can be anaesthetized with less amount of drug. Local anaesthetics used are same as infiltration anaesthesia.

- **Spinal anaesthesia:** The local anaesthetic solution is injected in the subarachnoid space between L_2 and L_3 or L_3 and L_4, i.e. below the lower end of the spinal cord to block the nerve roots in the cauda equina. It is used to anaesthetize lower abdomen and hind limbs in obstetrics, prostatectomy, fracture setting and operation of lower limbs. It is safer than general anaesthesia as it produces good analgesia and skeletal muscle relaxation without loss of consciousness. It has less cardiac, pulmonary and renal complications. It can be used in diabetics. Commonly used drugs for this purpose are lignocaine (2 to 5%), bupivacaine (0.5 to 1%), tetracaine (1 to 2%) and procaine (5 to 10%). The level of anaesthesia depends on the volume and specific gravity of the anaesthetic solution and the posture of the patient. The anaesthetic solution becomes heavy, i.e. hyperbaric (high specific gravity) when mixed with 10% glucose solution or light, i.e. hypobaric (low specific gravity) when mixed with normal saline as the vehicle. The position of the patient is also important in limiting the block to the desired level.

Disadvantages (complications): It can cause spinal shock by producing severe hypotension. It can cause respiratory paralysis, headache (by seepage of CSF), septic meningitis (by introduction of bacteria) or cauda equina syndrome (due to damage of nerves supplying urinary bladder and intestine causing urinary retention and intestinal atony).

- **Epidural anaesthesia:** The local anaesthetia is injected into the spinal extradural space through which spinal nerve roots travel. It is safer than spinal anaesthesia and so preferred. Drugs used are same as spinal anaesthesia.

- **Intravenous regional anaesthesia (intravascular infiltration anaesthesia):** The local anaesthetic is injected into a vein which is occluded by a tourniquet) so as to anaesthetize the area distal to it (in the periphery). It is now rarely used due to toxicity like tissue necrosis.

Properties of an Ideal Local Anaesthetic

- It should be nonirritant to the tissue.
- It should not produce damage of nerve tissue.
- It should be free from systemic toxicity.
- It should have quick onset and sufficient duration of action.
- It should be effective by all routes (topical as well as by injection).
- It should be potent.
- It should be stable at room temperature of all the local anaesthetics, lidocaine is a near ideal local anaesthetic.

DISCUSSION OF SOME LOCAL ANAESTHETICS

Cocaine

It is a natural local anaesthetic. It is an alkaloid obtained from the leaves of the coca plant, *'Erythroxylon coca'*, that grows in South America. It is the methylbenzoyl ester of ecgonine, which is chemically related to atropine. It was previously used for ocular anaesthesia, but now not used in eye, as it produces constriction of conjunctival vessels, mydriasis, dimness of vision and sloughing of cornea by irritation. It is a surface anaesthetic. It is used illegally by some persons for psychotropic (psychic stimulant) effects. It is absorbed from the mucous membrane and abraded skin. It is metabolized (hydrolyzed) by plasma and liver cholinesterases and excreted in urine as metabolites. Beside the local anaesthetic action, it exerts an stimulant action on the CNS. It acts on cerebral cortex and autonomic centres in the brain. It potentiates the actions of adrenaline and noradrenaline. It produces euphoria by acting on dopaminergic neuronal system (stimulating dopaminergic neurotransmission by blocking the presynaptic reuptake of dopamine). The euphoric effect of cocaine, consumed by smoking, lasts for about 30 minutes and that following intranasal administration lasts for about two hours. It abolishes the sense of fatigue and hunger. It is a drug of addiction or abuse. It produces strong psychic dependence but little tolerance and physical dependence. Cocaine addicts show paranoid and homicidal tendencies.

It also activates the sympathetic nervous system by blocking the presynaptic reuptake of noradrenaline and thus producing an excess of neurotransmitter at the postsynaptic receptor sites. This causes vasoconstriction, rise in BP, tachycardia and even cardiac arrhythmias and convulsions. It can also cause mydriasis, hyperglycaemia and hyperthermia.

Adverse Reactions

- Applied locally it is a protoplasmic poison. It produces poisonous effects on tissue cells and leucocytes.
- It can produce allergic reactions, cardiac arrhythmias, myocardial infarction, convulsions, respiratory failure and even sudden death after acute systemic administration by any route.
- Its chronic use may produce anorexia, emaciation, restlessness, insomnia, sexual dysfunction, sexual disinterest, tremors, disturbances of sensation and emotion, hallucinations and insanity. Diazepam (IV) is used to control convulsions produced by cocaine.

Procaine/Novocaine

It is a synthetic local anaesthetic. It is the diethyl aminoethyl ester of para-aminobenzoic acid. It is nonirritant and as effective as cocaine as a local anaesthetic. It is poorly absorbed from the mucous membrane and abraded skin and so it has no topical use. It is used as injection for infiltration, spinal and epidural anaesthesia. It has vasodilator property. It is rapidly metabolized (hydrolyzed) by plasma and liver cholinesterases and is excreted in the urine conjugated with glucuronic acid and glycine. It releases PABA on hydrolysis, which can antagonize the antibacterial action of sulphonamides. It is combined with benzyl-penicillin to prolong the duration of action of penicillin by delaying the absorption due to vasodilator action. It produces mild CNS stimulant action. It does not produce euphoria and drug dependence (addiction).

Adverse Reactions

It can produce allergic reactions including anaphylactic shock. So before its injection skin test for hypersensitivity reactions must be done.

Chlorprocaine is more potent and less toxic than procaine.

Lidocaine/Lignocaine/Xylocaine

It is a synthetic local anaesthetic. It is an amide. Chemically, it is an acetanilide derivative. It is the most commonly used (popular) local anaesthetic. It is stable and can be stored at room temperature for a long time and can be autoclaved repeatedly. It has rapid onset of action and sufficient duration of action (1 to 2 hours). It has high degree of tissue penetration. It can be used by all routes (topical as well as by injection). It does not produce allergic reactions and can be safely used in patients allergic to procaine or other ester type local anaesthetics. It is metabolized in the liver by microsomal amide hydrolyzes and is excreted in urine mainly as metabolites. Addition of a vasoconstrictor like adrenaline or phenyl-ephrine prolongs its duration of action (2 to 3 hours) by delaying its absorption.

It is an all-purpose LA used for topical anaesthesia, infiltration anaesthesia, field block anaesthesia, nerve block anaesthesia, spinal anaesthesia and epidural anaesthesia. It is also used for dental analgesia and in cardiac arrhythmias.

Adverse Reactions

It can produce drowsiness and mental clouding by CNS depressant action. In toxic dose, it can produce ventricular arrhythmias and even cardiac arrest. With procainamide it produces ventricular fibrillation by synergism.

Bupivacaine (Marcaine)

It is a synthetic local anaesthetic. It is an amide. Its chemical structure is similar to lidocaine, except the amine containing group is replaced by butylpiperidine group. It is about 4 times as potent as lignocaine and has more prolonged duration of action (up to 8 hours). It provides more sensory than motor block, which has made it a popular drug for producing prolonged anaesthesia during labour or the postoperative period. It is not used for topical anaesthesia but used as injection for other types of anaesthesia.

Adverse Reactions

It has adverse effects like lidocaine. It is more cardiotoxic than lidocaine and can produce severe ventricular arrhythmias and myocardial depression in toxic dose.

Mepivacaine has N-methyl substituent in the place of the butyl group of bupivacaine. It is less potent than bupivacaine.

Tetracaine/Amethocaine (Pontocaine)

It is a synthetic local anaesthetic. It is an ester. It is a long-acting and potent local anaesthetic. It is effective both topically and parenterally (by injection). It should not be used on inflamed, injured or very vascular surfaces, as death may occur due to rapid absorption. It is less suitable than lidocaine for operation of shorter duration as it has longer duration of action following spinal injection.

Dibucaine/Cinchocaine (Nupercaine)

It is a synthetic local anaesthetic. It is a quinoline derivative. It is a long-acting and potent local anaesthetic but it is very toxic. It can produce cinchonism like quinine. It can be used topically in the form of ointment. It should not be used parenterally (by injection).

Bucricaine (Centbucridine/Centoblock)

It is a synthetic local anaesthetic. It is not an ester or amide. It is an acridine derivative. It has longer duration of action (6 to 8 hours) than lidocaine. It has some intrinsic vasopressor activities and so does not require the addition of a vasopressor agent for infiltration anaesthesia. It has uses like lidocaine. It can be used in patients allergic to lidocaine. It has less CNS and cardiac toxicity than lidocaine. It is available as solution for injection in 5 mg/mL of 30 mL ampule.

Oxethazine (Mucaine)

It is a synthetic local anaesthetic. It is not an ester or amide. It is used as local anaesthetic of gastric mucosa to relieve pain of peptic ulcer and gastritis. It is available as mucaine gel along with aluminium hydroxide and magnesium hydroxide.

44

Antiepileptic Drugs

INTRODUCTION

Epilepsy is a collective term for a group of chronic paroxysmal seizure disorders characterized by sudden and transient episodes of loss of consciousness (seizure), with or without a characteristic body movements (convulsions) and sometimes with autonomic hyperactivity. During seizure there is abnormal discharge of brain neurons. Seizures may be partial (focal/local seizures recorded in EEC as sharp and spiky waves) or generalized seizures (convulsive or non-convulsive).

Common Types of Epilepsy

- **Grand mal (major epilepsy/generalized tonic-clonic seizures):** It is characterized by sudden loss of consciousness without any warning (aura), tonic spasm of all body muscles, clonic jerking movements, prolonged sleep and depression of all CNS functions. The initial tonic extensor spasm is followed by repeated clonic jerking movements, which last for a few minutes. The attack may be accompanied by tongue biting, frothing at the mouth and urinary incontinence.

- **Petit mal (minor epilepsy/absence seizure):** It is characterized by sudden brief loss of consciousness (5 to 15 seconds) and minimum motor manifestations. There is no convulsive movement or loss of postural control. The patient appears to go blank for about one minute, which may be accompanied by fluttering of eyelids or small chewing movement of the mouth. It is common in children.

- **Psychomotor epilepsy (temporal lobe epilepsy):** It is characterized by attacks of bizarre and confused behaviour (1 to 2 minutes) and emotional changes with or without loss of consciousness.

- **Cortical focal epilepsy (myoclonic seizure/ Jacksonian epilepsy):** It is characterized by localized sensory disturbances and convulsive movements confined to a group of muscles without loss of consciousness.

- **Status epilepticus:** It is characterized by rapid repetitive grand mal seizures without intermission (recovery of consciousness). It is an emergency condition, as it can be fatal due to repetitive convulsions (producing brain damage), hyperpyrexia, lactic acidosis and respiratory failure. It must be treated promptly, preferably in a hospital (in ICU).

Etiology of Epilepsy

Most of the cases are primary (idiopathic). Some cases are secondary to trauma/surgery on head, intracranial tumour, tuberculoma, cerebral ischaemia and cysticercosis of brain. Treatment of epilepsy is symptomatic and same whether primary or secondary. Some drugs are effective in grand mal, while other drugs are effective in petit mal. So correct diagnosis is essential for proper treatment.

Secondary epilepsy should be treated by appropriate measure if possible.

Classification of Antiepileptic Drugs

These can be classified into two ways:

1. **Chemical classification** (according to chemical structure). These are as follows:
   - Hydantoin derivatives, e.g. diphenyl hydantoin (phenytoin), mephenytoin (mesantoin) and ethotoin.
   - Barbiturates, e.g. phenobarbitone, mephobarbitone and primidone (a deoxybarbiturate).
   - Iminostilbines, e.g. carbamazepine and oxcarbazepine.
   - Succinimides, e.g. ethosuximide, methsuximide and phensuximide.
   - Propylacetic acid derivatives, e.g. sodium valproate.
   - Benzodiazepines, e.g. diazepam, donazepam, clorazepate and clobazam.
   - Newer drugs, e.g. gabapentin, lamotrigine, vegabatrin, felbamate and topiramide
   - Miscellaneous drugs, e.g. trimethadione (troxidone), phenacemide, acetazolamide, progabide, sulthiam and bromides.

2. **Therapeutic classification** (according to clinical use). These are as follows:
   - Drugs used in grand mal, e.g. phenytoin, carbamazepine, sodium valproate, phenobarbitone and primidone.
   - Drugs used in petit mal, e.g. ethosuximide, sodium valproate, clonazepam, clorazepate, lamotrigine and troxidone.
   - Drugs used in psychomotor epilepsy, e.g. carbamazepine, sodium valproate, phenytoin, primidone and vigabatrin.
   - Drugs used in cortical focal epilepsy, e.g. carbamazepine, sodium valproate, phenytoin, phenobarbitone and primidone.
   - Drugs used in simple or complex partial seizures, e.g. sodium valproate, carbamazepine, phenytoin, phenobarbitone, primidone, gabapentin, lamotrigine and vigabatrin.

   - Drugs used in status epilepticus, e.g. diazepam, phenytoin sodium, phenobarbitone sodium and lorazepam given IV slowly. In resistant case, general anaesthesia with ether may control seizures by muscle relaxant activity.

General Considerations of Antiepileptic Therapy

The objective (aim) of the therapy of epilepsy is to keep the patient seizure-free as far as possible without drug induced impairment of functions. This is done by:

- **Appropriate selection of drugs:** Some drugs are of value only in certain types of seizures and may worsen other types of seizures, e.g. phenytoin worsens petit mal and ethosuximide aggravates grand mal. So selection of drugs should be based on clinical as well as EEG-findings of the type of seizures.

- **Individualization of therapy:** Each patient requires adjustment of dosage of the most effective drug that provides minimum adverse effects. One should always start with low dose and then gradually increased until seizures are controlled and continued for at least 2 years maintenance dose.

- **Consideration of pharmacokinetic factors:** This is required for prolonged treatment to prevent seizures or emergency treatment to control seizures.

- **Use of serum/plasma level data of the drug:** To prevent seizures an effective serum/plasma concentration of the drug should be maintained. The dose interval of the drug is determined by the plasma half-life (t½) of the drug. Most drugs can be given twice daily. Drugs which have long plasma t½, e.g. barbiturates and sometimes phenytoin are given once daily.

- **Long-term monitoring** of drug action and follow-up of the drug treatment must be done. Sudden withdrawal of the drug should not be done as it aggravates the condition.

- **Combination of antiepileptic drugs:** Usually the treatment is started with a single drug. A second drug is added if seizures are not controlled by the first drug. Use of more than two drugs should be avoided as drug interactions may occur due to enzyme induction by some drugs (phenytoin, phenobarbitone and carbamazepine).
- **Cautious use of drugs** in pregnancy, hepatic or renal disease must be done.

DISCUSSION OF SOME ANTIEPILEPTIC DRUGS

Phenytoin Sodium

It is a hydantoin derivative. Its chemical structure is shown in **Fig. 44.1.** It is highly lipid-soluble and poorly water-soluble. It can easily cross the BBB.

Pharmacokinetics

It is a weak acid and is slowly and incompletely absorbed from gastrointestinal tract. It is precipitated at the IM injection site and its absorption from that site is unpredictable. It is widely distributed in the body tissues. It is highly plasma protein bound (about 90%). It is metabolized in the liver by hydroxylation and glucuronide conjugation. At plasma concentration below 10 µg/mL, its elimination follows first order kinetic and plasma $t\frac{1}{2}$ ranges between 6 to 24 hours. At higher concentrations (above 10 µg/mL) its elimination follows zero order kinetics and plasma $t\frac{1}{2}$ ranges between 20 to 60 hours. It is excreted in urine mainly as inactive metabolites and slightly (5%) as free form.

Pharmacological Actions

Mechanism of action: It exerts antiepileptic action without causing general depression of the CNS. It may produce slight sedation in therapeutic dose, but this does not increase with increase of dose. In toxic dosage it may produce excitatory signs and at lethal level a type of decerebrate rigidity.

It selectively inhibits the sustained high frequency repetitive firing of the cortical neurons (which cause the seizures) and limits the spread of impulse from an active focus to adjacent normal brain tissue. This effect is mediated by a slowing of the rate of recovery of voltage activated Na^+ channels from inactivation. It targets those Na^+ channels which are repetitively opening and closing. It prevents the opening of these Na^+ channels. This effect is produced at therapeutic concentrations of phenytoin in CSF. As it inhibits the opening of Na^+ channels in the cell membrane (neuronal/myocardial), so it is said to have a membrane stabilizing action on the excitable cell membrane. In higher dosage, it also inhibits the pumping of K^+ (from ICF) leading to longer refractory period. By decreasing the neuronal Na^+ concentration, it leads to a reduction in the post-tetanic potential (PTP) and an increase in the neuronal K^+ concentration. PTP is an enhancement of synaptic transmission following repeated tetanic, high frequency stimulation of the presynaptic fibres. Enhancement of synaptic transmission due to PTP leading to spread of seizures occurs in grand mal. It blocks this process and stops the spread of seizure discharge. At concentrations 5 to 10 folds higher than the therapeutic concentration several effects are produced such as reduction of spontaneous activity and enhancement to responses to GABA and 5-HT, phenytoin produces following effects:

- **CNS effects:** It exerts a selective antiepileptic action without causing central nervous system depression. It is effective in grand mal and other varieties of seizures but ineffective in petit mal, which may worsen by phenytoin. In higher dosage it produces CNS stimulation (excitement).
- **CVS effects:** It is an antiarrhythmic drug. It is discussed with antiarrhythmic drugs in CVS pharmacology.
- **Miscellaneous effects:** It is effective in certain types of neuralgia including trigeminal neuralgia, glossopharyngeal neuralgia and diabetic neuropathy. It has been found to be useful in chorea (nonrhythmical involuntary jerking movements

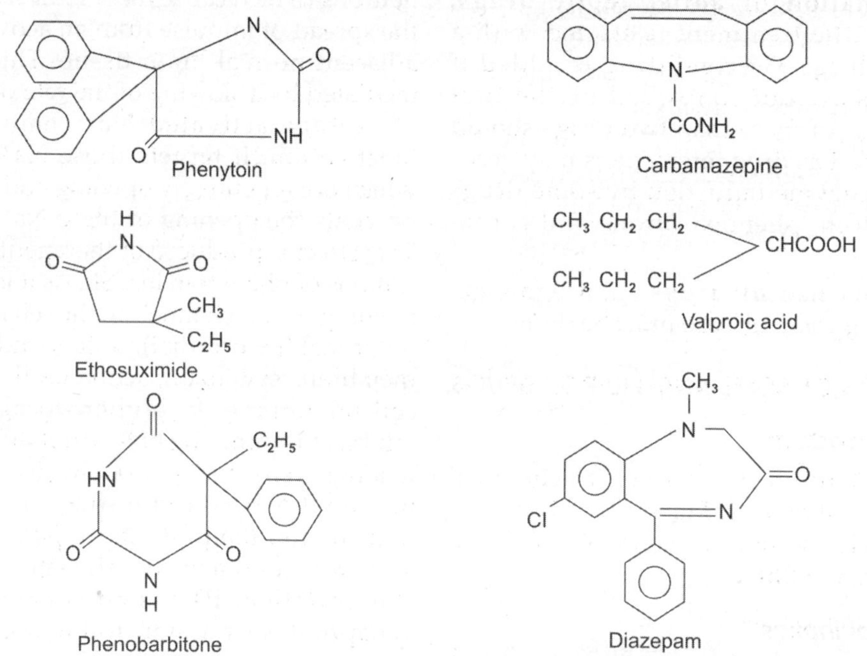

Fig. 44.1: Chemical structures of some antiepileptic drugs

affecting different areas of the body in an irregular unpredictable fashion). These effects are probably due to stabilization of the neuronal membrane.

Clinical Uses

It is used in following cases:

- **Epilepsy:** It is an widely used antiepileptic drug effective against grand mal and other types of epilepsy except petit mal. It aggravates petit mal seizures.
- **Cardiac arrhythmias:** It is used in cardiac arrhythmias especially in digitalis induced cardiac arrhythmias.
- **Neuralgias:** It is used in trigeminal neuralgia, glossopharyngeal neuralgia and diabetic neuropathy to relieve pain.
- **Chorea:** It is used in Sydenham's chorea (rheumatic chorea), Huntington's chorea and senile chorea to control involuntary movements. Dopamine blockers like tetrabenazine, haloperiod and pimozide are also used in this condition.

Preparations and Dosage

- Phenytoin sodium (Ditantin/Eptoin tablet) capsule (100 mg)—100 to 200 mg once or twice daily.
- Phenytoin sodium paediatric suspension (100 mg/5 ml)—10 mg/kg body weight/ day.
- Phenytoin sodium injection (50 mg/ml)—100 to 200 mg IV slowly.

Adverse Reactions (Toxicity)

The toxic effects of phenytoin depend upon the route of administration, the duration of exposure and the dosage. When it is given IV at an excessive rate in the emergency treatment of status epilepticus, it can produce cardiac arrhythmias with or without hypotension and/or CNS depression. These complications can be minimized by administration of phenytoin at a rate less than 50 mg/ minute.

- **Adverse effects at therapeutic dose level (on chronic use)**

– CNS effects like behavioural changes and increased frequency of seizures.

– GIT effects like nausea, vomiting, epigastric pain and anorexia.

– Miscellaneous effects like gingival hyperplasia, osteomalacia, hyperglycaemia, megaloblastic anaemia and hirsutism (in young females). Gingival hyperplasia is due to increased collagen proliferation. It can be minimized by maintaining oral hygiene. Hyperglycaemia is due to inhibition of insulin release from β cells of pancreas. Osteomalacia is due to desensitization of the target tissues to vitamin D and interference with calcium metabolism. Megaloblastic anaemia is due to altered folate absorption and metabolism. It responds to folic acid. Hirsutism is due to endocrine disturbance in young females. All these effects can be prevented by proper adjustment of dosage.

• **Adverse effects at toxic dose level** (due to overdose) is cerebellovestibular syndrome (characterized by vertigo, diplopia, nystagmus and choreoathetoid movements of limbs). It can also produce foetal hydantoin syndrome.

• **Teratogenic effect if used during pregnancy:** It is characterized by hypoplastic phalanges, cleft palate, harelip and microcephaly in the foetus.

• **Hypersensitive (allergic)** reactions (usually involving skin, bone marrow and liver). These are skin rashes (morbilliform), leucopenia, agranulocytosis, thrombocytopaenia, lymphadenopathy and rarely Stevens-Johnson syndrome, SLE and liver damage.

Drug Interactions

• Phenytoin is a hepatic microsomal enzyme inducer and can increase the metabolism of corticosteroids and oral contraceptives decreasing their therapeutic effects.

• Phenobarbitone and carbamazepine increase the metabolism of phenytoin by induction of hepatic microsomal enzyme system, whereas ethanol decreases the metabolism of phenytoin by inhibition of hepatic microsomal enzyme system.

• Sodium valproate and phenylbutazone decrease both the rate of metabolism and plasma protein binding of phenytoin.

• Sulphisoxazole, salicylates and tolbutamide increase the concentration of free phenytoin in plasma by competing for the binding sites on plasma proteins.

• Chloramphenicol, dicoumerol, disulphiram, isoniazid, cimetidine and some sulphonamides increase the concentration of phenytoin in plasma by decreasing the rate of metabolism of phenytoin by inhibiting hepatic microsomal enzyme system.

Mephenytoin (Mesantoin) and ethotoin are less potent and more toxic than phenytoin and so rarely used in epilepsy.

Phenobarbitone

It is a long-acting barbiturate. It is effective in grand mal, partial seizures (both simple and complex), status epilepticus and febrile convulsions in children. It is not effective in petit mal, rather it aggravates petit mal seizures.

Mechanism of Action

It produces antiepileptic action by raising the seizure threshold in the cerebral cortex and decreasing the spread of seizure discharges to the other parts of brain. It inhibits seizures by potentiation of synaptic inhibition through an action on the $GABA_A$ receptor. At levels exceeding therapeutic concentrations, it also limits sustained repetitive firing of action potential (as in status epilepticus). Its main advantages for use are:

• It is well-tolerated by most patients.

• It has long plasma half-life and so a single dose a day therapy is possible, thereby ensuring better patient compliance.

• It is cheap.

• It has low toxicity.

It is administered in grand mal and other types of epilepsy as phenobarbitone tablet (30, 60 mg) in the dosage of 30 to 60 mg once daily.

It is used in status epilepticus as injection (phenobarbitone sodium—200 mg/ml) in the dosage of 200 to 400 mg IV slowly. It is also available as paediatric suspension (20 mg/5 ml) and used in the dosage of 5 to 10 mg/kg/day.

It is a hepatic microsomal enzyme inducer and increases metabolism of it as well as of many lipid-soluble drugs. Mephobarbitone is methyl phenobarbitone. It is incompletely absorbed from GIT. It is less potent (about ½) than phenobarbitone and so less used in epilepsy.

Primidone

Primidone is a deoxybarbiturate. Its active metabolite is phenobarbitone. It is less potent than phenobarbitone and so less used in epilepsy. It is useful in cases of essential tremors resistant to propranolol or when propranolol is contraindicated.

Carbamazepine

It is an iminostilbine derivative with structural resemblance to the tricyclic antidepressant, imipramine. Its chemical structure is shown in **Fig. 44.1**.

Pharmacokinetics

It is slowly but almost completely absorbed from GIT. It is metabolized in the liver (98%). Children metabolize the drug faster than the adults. Its plasma half-life is initially high (24 to 36 hours) which later on falls to 12 hours on chronic administration because of auto-induction. It is a hepatic microsomal enzyme inducer, by which it accelerates its own metabolism (auto induction) as well as of many lipid-soluble drugs. It is excreted in urine mostly as inactive metabolites.

Pharmacological Actions

It is effective in grand mal and other types of epilepsy except petit mal.

Mechanism of Action

Like phenytoin it inhibits the sustained repetitive firing of the cortical neurons from inactivation. This effect is its active metabolite 10, 11-epoxide produces this effect mediated by slowing of the rate of recovery of voltage activated Na^+ channels from inactivation.

It is also useful to relieve pain in trigeminal neuralgia, glossopharyngeal neuralgia and diabetic neuropathy like phenytoin. It is a specific drug for these neuralgias.

Clinical Uses

- It is used in grand mal, psychomotor epilepsy, cortical focal epilepsy and partial seizures. It is ineffective in petit mal.
- It is used in trigeminal neuralgia, glosso-pharyngeal neuralgia and diabetic neuropathy to relieve pain.
- It is used in diabetes insipidus of pituitary origin as an alternative to ADH and in manic depressive psychosis (MDP) as an alternative to lithium carbonate.

Preparations and Dosage

- Carbamazepine (Tegretol/Mezetol) tablet (100, 200 mg)—100 mg twice daily and gradually increased to a maximum of 1200 mg per day.
- Carbamazine paediatric syrup (100 mg/5 ml)—10 mg/kg/day.

Adverse Reactions

On chronic use it can produce GIT side effects (anorexia, nausea and vomiting), CNS side effects (sedation, mental confusion, vertigo and ataxia), visual disturbances (diplopia and blurring of vision), allergic reactions (skin rashes, eosinophilia, lymphadenopathy, dermatitis, hepatitis and nephritis) and blood dyscrasias (megaloblastic anaemia, agranulocytosis, thrombocytopaenia and even aplastic anaemia). It has been reported to produce obstructive jaundice, peripheral neuritis and teratogenic effect (in foetus). Its long-term use may cause mental and physical sluggishness due to loss of physical and mental drive. During its use haematological, hepatic and renal functions should be regularly checked up.

Drug Interactions

- Phenobarbitone, phenytoin and sodium valproate increase the metabolism of carbamazepine by hepatic microsomal enzyme induction. Again carbamazepine may increase the metabolism of these drugs by hepatic microsomal enzyme induction.

- Erythromycin, isoniazid, verapamil and d-propoxyphene inhibit the metabolism of carbamazepine by hepatic microsomal enzyme inhibition.

Oxcarbazepine is closely related to carbamazepine. It is claimed to be less toxic than carbamazepine.

Ethosuximide

It is a succinimide derivative. Its chemical structure is shown in **Fig. 44.1**. It is effective in petit mal.

Pharmacokinetics

It is completely absorbed from the GIT. It is present in the plasma mostly in free form. It is metabolized in the liver and excreted in urine mostly as inactive metabolites (glucuronides) and partly (20%) as free form. It has a plasma half-life of 45 to 60 hours.

Pharmacological Actions

It is effective only in petit mal, where it is more effective than trimethadione (troxidone).

Mechanism of Action

It acts by inhibiting T-type of Ca^{2+} currents (low threshold) in thalamic neurons. The thalamus plays an important role in the generation of 3 Hz spike wave rhythms of petit mal.

Clinical Uses

It is used only in petit mal. It has a lower risk of serious adverse reactions than trimethadione. Concurrent administration of phenytoin or phenobarbitone may be required to control associated or unmasked grand mal.

Preparations and Dosage

- Ethosuximide (Zarantin) capsule (250 mg)—250 mg daily and gradually increased (at weekly intervals) to a maximum of 1000 mg per day until control is achieved.
- Ethosuximide syrup (250 mg/5 ml)—same dose.

Adverse Reactions

On chronic use it can cause GIT side effects (anorexia, nausea and vomiting), central nervous system side effects (drowsiness, dizziness, headache and extrapyramidal symptoms), allergic reactions (skin rashes and dermatitis) and blood dyscrasias (agranulocytosis, thrombocytopaenia, rarely aplastic anaemia).

It has been reported to produce systemic lupus erythematosus and psychiatric disturbances. It can aggravate or unmask grand mal.

Methsuximide and phensuximide are less potent than ethosuximide and so less used in epilepsy.

Sodium Valproate

It is a derivative of propyl acetic acid. Its chemical structure is sodium dipropyl acetate. The structure of valproic acid (a liquid fatty acid) is shown in **Fig. 44.1**.

Pharmacokinetics

It is rapidly and almost completely absorbed from GIT. It is highly (about 95%) plasma protein bound. It is metabolized in the liver and is excreted in urine as inactive metabolites (90%) and free form (10%).

Pharmacological Actions

It is a broad spectrum antiepileptic drug effective against all types of epilepsy. It is the drug of choice in petit mal epilepsy.

Mechanism of Action

It produces effects on brain neurons similar to those of both phenytoin and ethosuximide. In therapeutic concentrations, it inhibits sustained repetitive firing of action potential induced by depolarization of neurons. In slightly higher concentrations it inhibits I-type of calcium currents in thalmic neurons like ethosuximide. It also stimulates the activity of the GABA synthetic enzyme. Glutamic acid decarboxylase and inhibit GABA degradative enzymes, GABA transaminase and succinic semialdehyde dehydrogenase leading to increase in concentration of GABA in brain.

Clinical Uses

It is a valuable drug in petit mal. It is also effective in a wide variety of partial and generalized seizures. In patient having both grand mal and petit mal, it is an ideal drug.

Preparations and Dosage

- Sodium valproate (Epilex, Epilin) tablet (100, 200 mg)—initially 300 mg twice daily and then gradually increased (at weekly intervals) to a maximum of 1 to 2 g per day until control is achieved.
- Sodium valproate syrup (200 mg/5 ml)—initially 20 mg/kg body weight/day and then gradually increased until control is achieved.

Adverse Reactions

On chronic use it can cause GIT side effects (nausea, vomiting and increased appetite causing weight gain), CNS side effects (sedation, drowsiness and ataxia), alopecia (loss of hair), hepatic damage, pancreatitis, skin rashes, thrombocytopaenia and coagulation defect (by reducing prothrombin, fibrinogen and platelet levels leading to prolongation of bleeding time). Liver function tests should be done before starting sodium valproate. It is a teratogenic drug and can produce spina bifida in foetus if used during pregnancy.

Drug Interactions

- It increases the plasma concentration of phenobarbitone by inhibiting its metabolism.
- It increases the plasma concentrations of phenytoin by displacing it from plasma protein binding sites.

Benzodiazepines (Diazepam, Lorazepam, Clonazepam and Clorazepate)

Diazepam, lorazepam and clonazepam are used in status epilepticus. Clonazepam and clorazepate are used in petit mal.

They act by enhancing GABA induced increase in the conductance of Cl^-. At therapeutic concentrations they increase the inhibitory effects produced by GABA within the CNS and enhance GABA induced changes in membrane potential.

Preparations and Dosage

- Diazepam (Valium) injection (5 mg/mL in 2 mL ampoule)—10 mg IV slowly (over 5 minutes) in adults (5 mg in children over 7 years of age and 2.5 mg for children below 7 years of age).

  It may be repeated twice more at 15 minutes intervals. Rapid IV injection may cause cardiac arrest, severe hypotension and respiratory depression.
- Clonazepam (Lonazep) injection (1 mg/ mL in 2 mL ampoule)—2 mg IV slowly (over 5 minutes) in adults (lower doses in children like diazepam).
- Clonazepam tablet (0.5, 2 mg)—0.5 mg twice daily and gradually increased to maximum of 4 to 8 mg per day. Similar doses are used in younger children for treatment of petit mal. Benzodiazepines are not good for long-term treatment of epilepsy because tolerance can develop and dose related adverse reactions like drowsiness and ataxia can occur. These are discussed in detail in sedative-hypnotics.

NEWER ANTIEPILEPTIC DRUGS

Gabapentin (Neurontin)

It is an amino acid chemically related to GABA. It does not interact with GABA receptors but promote the release of GABA by an unknown mechanism. It is used in partial seizures and generalized toniclonic seizures in the dose of 900 to 1800 mg per day in 3 divided doses. Used alone it is not much effective but when used in combination with other antiepileptic drugs it is very useful especially in resistant cases of epilepsy. It can cause drowsiness, dizziness, ataxia and fatigue as side effects.

Lamotrigine (Lamitor)

It is a phenyltriazine compound with antiepileptic action. It blocks the influx of Na^+ ions and thus inhibits the release of excitatory amino acid glutamate in brain. Reduction of release of glutamate produces stabilizing effect on neuronal membranes. It has uses like gabapentin. It is used in the dose of 50 mg twice daily initially and then the dose is gradually increased to a maximum of 200 mg per day. It can cause drowsiness, ataxia, nausea, headache and diplopia as side effects.

Vigabatrin (Sabril)

It is a GABA analogue with GABA-like structure. It inhibits GABA transaminase and so increases the concentration of GABA in the CNS.

It has uses like gabapentine. It is used in the dose of 500 mg twice daily. It can cause drowsiness, weight gain, mental confusion and even psychiatric symptoms.

Felbamate

It increases GABA activity and decreases NMDA activity. It has uses like gabapentine. It is claimed to be less toxic than gabapentine.

Miscellaneous antiepileptic drugs: These are trimethadione (troxidone), phenacemide, acetazolamide, progabide, sulthiam and bromides. These are now rarely used in epilepsy due to toxicity and availability of better drugs.

Treatment of Status Epilepticus

Diazepam is the drug of choice. It is administered IV slowly in the dose mentioned before. It is a short-acting drug and so a long-acting drug like phenytoin sodium or phenobarbitone sodium (100 to 200 mg IV slowly) must be administered after its administration and repeated as necessary. Alternate drugs to diazepam are clonazepam and lorazepam given IV slowly. If seizures are not controlled by these drugs, then general anaesthesia with ether (has neuromuscular blocking effect) is used to control seizures. Paraldehyde injection (5 to 10 ml deep IM) may be used if ether anaesthesia is not possible. Supportive treatment includes oxygen inhalation and administration of IV fluids to maintain water and electrolyte balance and acid–base balance.

45

Antiparkinsonian Drugs

INTRODUCTION

Parkinson's disease (parkinsonism/paralysis agitans) is an extrapyramidal motor disorder characterized by tremor, skeletal muscle rigidity, bradykinesia (hypokinesia) or akinesia (loss of movement), mask-like face, festinant gait (posture), excessive salivation and sweating, aphonia (loss of voice), mental depression and dementia (loss of memory). It was first described by a British physician named **James Parkinson** in 1817 and so the disease is called Parkinson's disease. It is due to imbalance between dopaminergic system (inhibitory) and cholinergic system (excitatory) in the basal ganglia of brain (corpus striatum, subthalamic nucleus and substantia nigra). Corpus striatum consists of caudate nucleus, globus pallidus and putamen. Progressive degeneration of the dopaminergic neurons in the substantia nigra and nigrostriatal tract leads to the deficiency of dopamine in the corpus striatum. As a result, there is increased cholinergic transmission (by Ach) in the basal ganglia. Decreased dopaminergic activity leading to increased cholinergic activity in the corpus striatum is responsible for parkinsonism.

Causes of Parkinsonism

Majority (90%) of the cases are idiopathic (unknown). A few cases are due to viral infection (postencephalitic), vascular disease (arteriosclerotic), brain tumour or trauma, drugs (e.g. chlorpromazine and other phenothiazines, haloperidol, triperidol, reserpine, methyldopa and metoclopramide) and toxic chemicals (e.g. carbon monoxide, manganese or copper poisoning and methylphenyl tetrahydropyridine/MPTP).

In drug induced parkinsonism, the dopamine receptors in the corpus striatum are blocked and so dopaminergic drugs are ineffective in the treatment. Anticholinergic drugs are used for the treatment.

Classification of Antiparkinsonian Drugs

These are of two groups:

1. **Drugs that act through dopaminergic system (by increasing dopaminergic activity)**—These are as follows:

   - Dopamine precursor, e.g. levodopa (l-Dopa).

   - Drugs that inhibit dopamine metabolism, e.g. selegiline.

   - Drugs that release dopamine, e.g. amantadine.

   - Dopamine agonists (dopamine receptor stimulants). These are as follows:

     – Ergolines, e.g. bromocriptine, lisuride and pergolide.

     – Aporphines, e.g. apomorphine and peribedil.

2. **Drugs that act through cholinergic system (by decreasing cholinergic activity)**—These are as follows:

- Central anticholinergics, e.g. trihexy-phenidyl (Benzhexol), benzotropine, biperiden and procyclidine.
- Antihistaminics with anticholinergic properties, e.g. diphenhydramine, orphenadrine, promethazine, etc.

DISCUSSION OF INDIVIDUAL DRUGS

Levodopa

It is the main drug used in the treatment of parkinsonism. It is an amino acid precursor of dopamine. It is a prodrug which is converted to dopamine (the active drug) in the body by the help of the enzyme dopa decarboxylase. Dopamine cannot cross BBB and so not used in parkinsonism. Levodopa can cross BBB and is converted to dopamine in the brain to produce actions.

Pharmacokinetics

It is rapidly absorbed from GIT and peak plasma level is reached in ½ to 2 hours. Its plasma half-life is 2 to 3 hours. More than 95% of orally administered levodopa is rapidly decarboxylated peripherally in the lumen of GIT, liver and other tissues and very little amount of levodopa enters the brain. Hence, large dosage of levodopa is required to raise the dopamine concentration of brain. The blood concentration of levodopa can be increased by inhibiting peripheral decarboxylation of levodopa by the enzyme, dopa decarboxylase (present in the intestine, liver and other tissues) by using a peripheral decarboxylase (DC) inhibitor like carbidopa or benserazide. As these DC-inhibitors do not easily penetrate the BBB, so conversion of levodopa to dopamine in the brain is not prevented. Pyridoxine accelerates the peripheral decarboxylation of levodopa, as the decarboxylase enzyme is pyridoxine dependent. So pyridoxine should not be administered during levodopa therapy. High protein content of a meal interferes with the absorption of levodopa, so levodopa is best taken ½ hour before or 1 hour after a meal. The drug is metabolized in the liver and other tissues and is excreted in urine partly unchanged and partly as dopamine and its principal metabolite, homovalinic acid (HVA). Some amount of the drug is converted to noradrenaline and is excreted in urine as vanillylmandelic acid (VMA).

Pharmacological Actions

Mechanism of action: It acts by supplying dopamine in the brain, which acts on dopamine receptors of dopaminergic system. It produces following effects:

- **CNS effects:** It produces improvement in muscle tone and movement in patients with parkinsonism but not in normal individuals. It can be called universal antiparkinsonian drug, because it improves all the manifestations of parkinsonism. Bradykinesia or akinesia is first improved, followed by rigidity and tremor. Gradually other manifestations such as sialorrhoea, seborrhoea, aphonia and depressed mood are improved. The patients become more alert and intersted on themselves and to the surroundings. Feelings of apathy are replaced by increased vigour and sense of well-being. In general, about 30% of patients show impressive improvement, whereas another 30% of patients show worthwhile improvement. Younger patients with milder symptoms derive greater benefit than elderly, debilated patients, who cannot tolerate full dosage due to adverse effects. Drug induced parkinsonism does not respond to levodopa as dopamine receptors are blocked by the drug. It also produces a nonspecific awakening effect in hepatic encephalopathy (coma).
- **CVS effects:** It can cause some CVS effects on being converted to dopamine in the periphery. Dopamine acts on CVS by stimulating:
  - β_1-adrenergic receptors in the heart producing cardiac acceleration, i.e. increase the force of cardiac contraction and heart rate.
  - α_1 receptor in blood vessels producing vasoconstriction and rise in BP (in large dosage of levodopa).

– specific dopaminergic receptors causing renal and mesenteric vasodilatation leading to fall in BP (in small dosage of levodopa).

- **Endocrine effects:** It inhibits prolactin secretion from the anterior pituitary leading to fall in prolactin level of blood. It increases growth hormone level in blood in normal persons but not in patients with parkinsonism. This is probably due to altered mechanism in regulating growth hormone secretion in patients with parkinsonism.

Clinical Uses

It is used in the treatment of:

- **Parkinsonism except drug induced parkinsonism:** It is the drug of choice in parkinsonism. It improves all the manifestations of parkinsonism. It is combined with a peripheral decarboxylase inhibitor (carbidopa or benzserazide) in order to achieve a good therapeutic level in brain. It is ineffective in drug induced parkinsonism as dopamine receptors are blocked by the drug.
- **Hepatic encephalopathy (coma):** It produces a nonspecific awakening effect in these patients.
- **Hyperprolactinaemia:** It inhibits lactation by decreasing prolactin secretion from the anterior pituitary.

Preparations and Dosage

- Levodopa (Levopa) tablet (0.5 g): The initial dose is 125 mg twice daily. The total daily dose is gradually increased once in a week till satisfactory control is achieved or adverse reactions appear. Maximum dose is 4 to 6 g per day in 3 or 4 divided doses.
- Levodopa (100 or 250 mg) with carbidopa (10 or 25 mg) tablet (Syndopa/Sinemet/Levopa-C).
- Levodopa (100 or 200 mg) with benzserazide (25 or 50 mg) tablet (Benspar/Madopar). Their dose is expressed as levodopa. Initial dose is 100 to 125 mg 3 to 4 times a day and

the maintenance dose is 750 to 1500 mg per day in 3 or 4 divided doses.

Advantages of adding DC-inhibitor (DCI) with levodopa

- The dose of levodopa can be reduced by as much as 25%.
- Adverse effects of levodopa like nausea, vomiting and cardiac side effects can be prevented.
- The control of symptoms is smoother.
- The number of daily doses can be reduced without loss of control.
- Degree of improvement is higher than levodopa alone.

Contraindications

- Psychiatric disorders
- Ischaemic heart disease (angina pectoris or history of myocardial infarction)
- Narrow angle glaucoma
- Peptic ulcer
- Pregnancy
- Lactation.

Adverse Reactions

Side effects of levodopa are frequent and often troublesome. Most of the side effects are dose dependent and limit the dose that can be administered. Common side effects are:

- GIT side effects like nausea, vomiting and anorexia. They are of central origin (action on CTZ) and are minimized by taking levodopa with food (which reduces its absorption) and gradually increasing the dose of levodopa.
- CVS side effects like postural hypotension with syncope, palpitation, sinus tachycardia, increased A-V conduction, exacerbation of angina (especially in patients with pre-existing heart disease) and ventricular arrhythmias. These can be counteracted by a DC-inhibitor and a β-blocker such as propranolol.
- CNS side effects like abnormal involuntary movements (mainly choreiform) involving

head, neck and extremities (dyskinesias and dystonias) on prolonged therapy (within one year). These are not prevented by DC-inhibitor but abolished by pyridoxine, which, however, reduces the clinical efficacy of levodopa.

- Behavioural side effects like mental depression with suicidal tendency, agitation, restlessness, confusion, hypomania, auditory or visual hallucinations and delusions. It exacerbates latent or active psychotic states (both organic and functional). Sudden withdrawal of levodopa after prolonged treatment can produce neuroleptic malignant syndrome.

- Miscellaneous adverse effects: It can produce transient rise of blood urea nitrogen (BUN) and SCOT and decrease in serum cholesterol level and carbohydrate tolerance during prolonged treatment.

Besides these adverse effects, it can produce tolerance and two phenomena on prolonged use:

- Tolerance, i.e. gradual loss of efficacy of levodopa may occur especially to vomiting and postural hypotension due to down-regulation (hyposensitivity) of postsynaptic dopamine receptors.

- Wearing off phenomenon (end of dose) effect: In it, the duration of effect by a dose of levodopa is decreased and so the frequency of drug administration is to be increased. It may be due to pharmacokinetic tolerance.

- On/off phenomenon effect: It is characterized by sudden loss of clinical efficacy (off phenomenon) of levodopa with reappearance of symptoms, which last for several hours and is followed by 'on phenomenon', i.e. disappearance of symptoms or recovery of clinical efficacy of levodopa. The cause of this phenomenon is not clear but it correlates with the fluctuations of blood levels of levodopa.

A drug holiday (stopping of the drug) of 3 days to 3 weeks may help in relieving some of the neurological and behavioural adverse effects of levodopa but it does not relieve on/off phenomenon. The patient must be under close medical supervision during the break of treatment. Up to two-thirds of patients show improved responsiveness to levodopa when the drug is reinstituted because they can be managed on lower dosage than before and adverse mental effects and dyskinesias are less troublesome. But drug holiday carries the risk of aspiration pneumonia, pulmonary embolism and venous thrombosis due to immobility of the patient in severe parkinsonism.

Drug Interactions

- Pyridoxine decreases clinical effects of levodopa by increasing peripheral decarboxylation.

- Selegiline (a MAO-B inhibitor) prolongs the effects of levodopa.

- MAO inhibitors potentiate the effects of levodopa by preventing the metabolism of dopamine. They can precipitate severe hypertension when used with levodopa.

- Neuroleptics (chlorpromazine, haloperidol, reserpine, etc.) decrease the effects of levodopa by blocking dopamine receptors.

- Methyldopa intensifies the adverse effects of levodopa.

- Anticholinergic drugs increase the stay of levodopa in the stomach and increase its degradation. They should be taken at least 2 hours before levodopa.

- Sympathomimetic drugs increase the cardiovascular toxicity of levodopa.

Selegiline

It is a selective MAO-B inhibitor used in parkinsonism. Two isoenzymes of MAO, *viz.* MAO-A and MAO-B oxidize monoamines (adrenaline, noradrenaline and dopamine). Both are present in the periphery and inhibit monoamines of intestinal origin. The isoenzyme MAO-B is the main form in the CNS and degrades mainly dopamine. It is inhibited by selegiline. At low or moderate dosage (10 mg/day) selegiline selectively inhibits MAO-B leading to irreversible inhibition of the enzyme. Unlike nonspecific MAO-inhibitors, it does not inhibit peripheral metabolism of catecholamines. Thus it can be taken safely with levodopa. Given alone, it has no effect in parkinsonism in dosage up to 15 mg/day. Given with levodopa or levodopa plus carbidopa, it increases the duration of action of levodopa and is beneficial in overcoming early morning stiffness and immobility and decreasing on/off phenomenon. It is very effective in patients having wearing off effect.

Preparation and Dose

Selegiline (Deprenyl) tablet (5 mg)—5 mg twice daily along with levodopa or levodopa plus carbidopa.

Adverse Reactions

It can produce postural hypotension, syncope, nausea, vomiting, mental confusion, hallucination, dyskinesia (abnormal movements) and psychotic episodes. It is contraindicated in patients with convulsive disorder.

Amantadine

It is an antiviral drug used for the prophylaxis and treatment of influenza-A disease. It has moderate antiparkinsonian action. It probably acts by releasing dopamine from dopaminergic nerve endings and preventing neuronal uptake of dopamine. It has also anticholinergic properties, which also contribute to its antiparkinsonian action. It is used in the initial treatment of mild parkinsonism. It may also be useful as adjunct in patients on levodopa with dose related fluctuations.

Preparation and Dosage

Amantadine (Amantrel) tablet (100 mg)—100 mg twice daily.

Adverse Reactions

It is well-tolerated. It may produce dizziness, lethargy, insomnia, nausea and vomiting, which are mild and reversible.

Bromocriptine

It is a synthetic ergot derivative. It has specific dopamine D_3-receptors agonist action. It can easily cross BBB. Unlike levodopa, it does not have to be converted to an active metabolite. It is useful in the treatment of late parkinsonism but it is slower acting than levodopa. It is also used in galactorrhoea and hepatic encephatopathy.

Preparation and Dosage

Bromocriptine mesylate (Proctinal/Perodel) tablet (2.5 mg)—2.5 mg twice daily and gradually increased to a maintenance dose of 20 to 30 mg per day. This dose is almost ten times that required to suppress galactorrhoea (due to hyperprolactinaemia).

Adverse Reactions

It can cause nausea and vomiting by its dopaminergic action on the medullary CTZ. This is treated by domperidone but not by metoclopramide, which may worsen parkinsonism.

Lisuride and pergolide dopamine (D_1) agonists with pharmacological properties and uses like bromocriptine. They are more potent and longer-acting than bromocriptine. They can be used in patients who have developed tolerance to bromocriptine.

Apomorphine and peribidil act on both D_1 and D_2 receptors and so less preferred in parkinsonism.

Anticholinergic Drugs (Muscarinic Receptor Antagonists)

They were widely used for the treatment of parkinsonism before the discovery of levodopa. They act by blocking muscarinic receptors in the basal ganglia (especially in corpus striatum). They are the only drugs which the patients can afford for prolonged periods.

Preparations and Dosage

- Trihexyphenidyl (Benzhexol) hydrochloride (Pacitane) tablet (2 mg)—2 to 4 mg thrice daily.
- Biperiden hydrochloride (Dyskinon) tablet (2 mg)—Same as above.

- Benzotropine mesylate (Cogentin) tablet (1 mg)—1 to 2 mg twice daily.
- Diphenhydramine hydrochloride (Benadryl) tablet (25 mg)—25 to 50 mg thrice daily.
- Orphenadrine hydrochloride (Orphipal) tablet (50 mg)—50 to 100 mg thrice daily.

Adverse Reactions

They can produce sedation, mental confusion (especially in elderly persons), constipation, blurring of vision (due to mydriasis and cycloplegia), narrow angle glaucoma and urinary retention.

46

Opioid Analgesics and Antagonists

INTRODUCTION

Analgesics are drugs that relieve pain without causing loss of consciousness. They act on CNS or peripheral pain mechanism. Pain is an unpleasant sensation felt only by the subject. It is a symptom of many diseases and demands immediate relief by drugs to give comfort to the subject.

Pathophysiology of Pain

Pain receptors are distributed throughout the body. Noxious stimuli stimulate pain receptors and other nociceptive receptors of sensory nerve endings. In most cases this stimulation is mediated by pain producing substances like histamine, 5-HT, bradykinin, kallidin and acetylcholine. These are released in tissues during inflammation, tissue injury, ischaemia and by thermal or mechanical stimuli. Of these chemical substances, bradykinin is most potent and acts partly by releasing prostaglandins which sensitize the pain receptors in the sensory nerve endings to the action of pain producing substances.

Sensations from pain receptors are transmitted through sensory afferent nerve fibres of pain (A-δ and C) to the dorsal horn of spinal cord *via* the dorsal nerve root ganglia and terminate in the substantia gelatinosa (SG) of the spinal cord situated at the tip of the dorsal horn. The first neuron ends here and the second neuron arises, which then crosses the opposite side and travels in the spinothalamic

tract (STT) (as shown in **Fig. 46.1).** The nerve fibres of STT terminate in the intermediate relaying centres in the midbrain stem (called spinoreticular thalamic tract) and also in thalamus (called direct spinothalamic tract). Spinoreticular thalamic tract carries affective (autonomic) component of pain and direct spinothalamic tract carries nociceptive component of pain. Pain sensations (signals) received in the thalamus, midbrain stem (periaqueductal gray matter) and magnus raphe nucleus are processed and transmitted to the sensory cortex, where pain is finally perceived. A descending pain inhibiting pathway from thalamus and midbrain ends in substantia gelatinosa of dorsal horn of spinal cord.

Gate Control Mechanism of Pain Sensation Transmission

Gate Control Theory was proposed by Melzack and Wall in 1965. According to this theory, the substantia gelatinosa at the tip of the dorsal horn of spinal cord is considered as the gate. It is subjected to modulating influence by some neurotransmitters (substance P and endogenous opioids). The primary afferents of both the pain and touch sensations enter the dorsal horn of spinal cord. Pain fibres terminate at the substantia gelatinosa (SG), whereas crude touch fibres do not terminate directly at the SG but turn upward to form the dorsal lemniscal fibres (Tract of Goll and Burdach) and while turning upward, they give collaterals which terminate

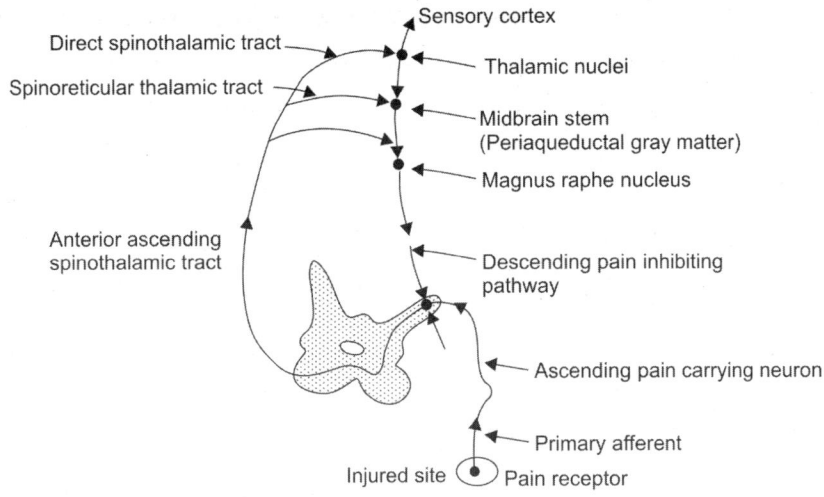

Fig. 46.1: Pain pathway

at the SG. When pain sensation alone is passing through the gate (SG), there is no problem in transmission of pain though the STT, but when crude touch sensation is passing along with pain sensation through the gate (SG), then the transmission of pain to the anterior ascending spinothalamic tracts (STT) is obstructed due to presynaptic inhibition by the released endogenous opioids (inhibitory) and decreased release of substance P (excitatory) from the descending pain inhibiting neurons.

Classification of Analgesics

These are of two groups:
1. Opioid analgesics (narcotic analgesics), e.g. morphine, codeine, pethidine, methadone, pentazocine, etc. They are used mainly in visceral pain, i.e. pain arising from viscera. They are addicting drugs.
2. Nonopioid analgesics (nonnarcotic analgesics/analgesic antipyretics/nonsteroidal anti-inflammatory drugs), e.g. aspirin, paracetamol, ibuprofen, diclofenac, piroxicam, etc. They are used in somatic pain, i.e. pain arising from skin, muscles, joints, ligaments and bones. They are nonaddicting drugs.

Opioid Analgesics

These are drugs or neurotransmitters that produce effects by acting on opioid receptors.

These are of following two groups:
1. Exogenous opioids, e.g. opium alkaloids (opiates) like morphine and codeine; semisynthetic and synthetic morphine substitutes like diacetylmorphine (heroin), ethylmorphine (dionine), pethidine, pentazocine, methadone and buprenorphine.
2. Endogenous opioids, e.g. enkephalins (methionine-enkephalin and leucine-enkephalin), endorphins (α-endorphin and β-endorphin), and dynorphins (α-dynorphin and β-dynorphin). These are peptides present in brain and spinal cord and also in peripheral tissues at the sites of opioid receptors and behave like morphine. They are synthesized locally from precursor molecules like proenkephalin-A, proenkephalin-B and prodynorphin and metabolized by peptidases like enkephalinase-A and enkephalinase-B. They act as physiological agonists at opioid receptors and modulate pain sensation.

Opioid Receptors

These are receptors (peptides), with which morphine and other opioids (exogenous and endogenous) combine to produce actions. They are widely distributed in the CNS (brain and spinal cord) and peripheral tissues (intestine, pancreas, adrenal cortex and medulla). Their main sites in CNS are substantia gelatinosa (SG), periaqueductal gray matter (PAG), amygdaloid nucleus, thalamus, hypothalamus, area prostrema, locus caeruleus, magnus raphe nucleus and trigeminal nucleus. There are five types of opioid receptors, *viz.* mu (μ), kappa (κ), delta (δ), sigma (σ) and epsilon (ϵ). Of these receptors, μ, κ and δ receptors have physiological role in man but σ and ϵ receptors have no physiological role. μ, κ and δ receptors have different subtypes, *viz.* μ_1, μ_2, κ_1, κ_2, κ_3, δ_1 and δ_2. Of the exogenous opioids, morphine and codeine have high affinity for κ receptors; pethidine and pentazocine have high affinity for κ receptors; nalorphine and nalbuphine have high affinity for κ receptors.

Of the endogenous opioids, endorphins have high affinity for μ receptors; dynorphins have high affinity for κ receptors and enkephalins have high affinity for δ receptors (as shown in **Table 46.1**).

Molecular mechanism of action of opioids: At molecular level, they decrease the generation of phospholipase-C mediated IP_3/DAG and also cAMP leading to inhibition of Ca^{++} influx through calcium channels in the neuronal membrane. This decreases neuronal activity.

Table 46.1: Physiological functions/pharmacological actions of opioid receptors by combining with agonists

Receptors	Functions/Actions
Mu (μ)	Supraspinal analgesia (μ_1), spinal analgesia (μ_2), sedation (μ_1 and μ_2), respiratory depression (μ_2), miosis (μ_2), constipation (μ_2), euphoria and physical dependence (μ_1).
Kappa (κ)	Supraspinal analgesia (κ_3), spinal analgesia (κ_1), sedation (κ_1 and κ_3), respiratory depression (κ_3), miosis (κ_1), constipation (κ_1 and κ_3), dysphoria and physical dependence (κ_1 and κ_3).
Delta (δ)	Supraspinal analgesia (δ_1), spinal analgesia (δ_2).

Classification of Exogenous Opioids

These are of three groups:

1. Natural opium alkaloids (opiates), e.g. morphine and codeine.

2. Semisynthetic opiates, e.g. diacetylmorphine (heroin), ethylmorphine (dionine), hydromorphone, oxymorphone, hydrocodone and oxycodone.

3. Synthetic opioids, e.g. pethidine (meperidine), fentanyl, pentazocine, cyclazocine, nalbuphine, buprenorphine, methadone, dextropropoxyphene, levallorphan, tramadol, etc.

Opium is the sun-dried juice of poppy capsule (*Papaver somniferum*) obtained by incising the unripe seed capsule. On exposure to sunlight, the milky exudate becomes dark brown resinous material which is then powdered. It contains alkaloids (about 20), gum, resin and volatile oils.

Alkaloids of opium (about 20% of opium powder) are of two groups:

1. Phenanthrene alkaloids, e.g. morphine (10%), codeine (0.5%) and thebaine (0.2%).

2. Benzyl isoquinoline alkaloids, e.g. papaverine (1%), noscapine (6%), and narcine (0.2%).

Of these alkaloids, only morphine and codeine are analgesics, thebaine is spinal stimulant, papaverine is smooth muscle relaxant and noscapine is antitussive and smooth muscle relaxant and narcine is not used.

Examples of some opioid agonists/antagonists:

1. Pure opioid agonists, e.g. morphine, codeine, pethidine, fentanyl, etc.

2. Pure opioid antagonists, e.g. naloxone, naltrexone.

3. Mixed opioid agonist-antagonists, e.g. Pentazocine, buprenorphine, nalbuphine.

4. Partial opioid agonists, e.g. nalorphine cyclazocine, propiram, profadol.

DISCUSSION OF SOME OPIOID ANALGESICS

Morphine

It is the principal alkaloid of opium. It is a phenanthrene derivative. Its chemical structure is shown in **Fig. 46.2**. It was isolated from opium by Serturner in 1806 and he named it morphine after the name of the Greek God of dream—**Morpheus**. It is discussed as a prototype drug of opioids.

Pharmacokinetics

It is slowly and incompletely absorbed from GIT after oral administration. It has bioavailability of about 20 to 40% due to extensive first pass metabolism in the liver and gut wall. Hence it is administered parenterally (SC or IM), when it produces a demonstrable analgesic effect within 15 to 20 minutes. The peak effect occurs in 60 to 90 minutes and the effect persists for 4 to 6 hours. Given IV, it produces an immediate effect. It circulates in the plasma partly bound with plasma proteins (35 to 50%) and partly in free form. It is widely distributed in the body. Its concentrations in liver, spleen and kidneys are higher than that in plasma. It crosses the BBB inefficiently due to low lipid solubility. It can cross the placental barrier readily and is also secreted in milk. It is metabolized in the liver by N-dealkylation and oxidation followed by glucuronide or sulphate conjugation. It is excreted in urine as active and inactive metabolites and slightly as free form. Morphine-6-glucuronide is more potent than morphine. It is also excreted in bile and undergoes enterohepatic circulation. Its plasma t½ is about 2 hours. It is noncumulative and completely excreted in 24 hours. It is also excreted in sweat in small amount.

Pharmacological Actions

Mechanism of action: It produces its main actions by binding with opioid receptors (μ, κ and δ) in the brain and spinal cord. μ receptor is mainly responsible for analgesic action. It suppresses mainly the affective (psychological or central) component of pain and has a minor effect on the nociceptive (peripheral) com-

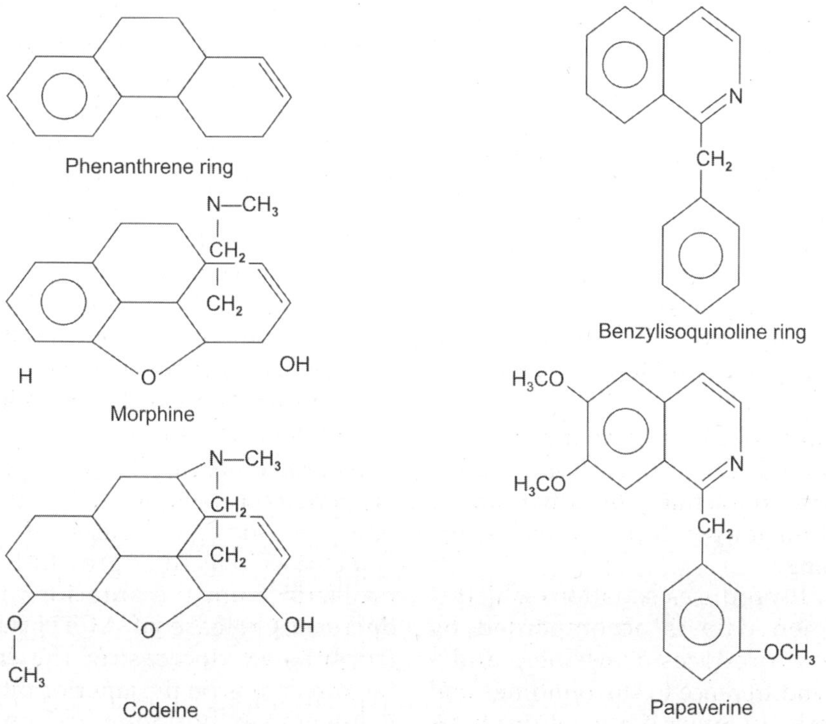

Fig. 46.2: Basic rings and chemical structures of some opiates

ponent of pain. It inhibits the release of substance P (an excitatory neurotransmitter) from the descending pain inhibiting neurons into the substantia gelatinosa (SG) of the dorsal horn of spinal cord and thus prevents the carriage of pain sensation from primary afferent neurons to the neurons of anterior ascending spinothalamic tract (STT). It also inhibits the action of already released substance P. In addition, it decreases the activity of noradrenergic, dopaminergic and GABA-ergic systems and increases the activity of cholinergic, histaminergic and serotonergic (5-HT) systems. Morphine produces following effects:

CNS effects—It has site specific CNS depressant and stimulant effects. CNS depressant effects are:

- **Analgesia:** It is a potent analgesic. It relieves both acute and chronic pains. It relieves visceral pain better than somatic pain. In larger dosage it relieves all types of severe pain (both visceral and somatic pains). It relieves pain by following mechanisms:
  - It suppresses pain perception at the supraspinal sites (sensory cortex, thalamus and midbrain stem) by raising the threshold of pain perception acting on opioid receptors. It also inhibits the cells of substantia gelatinosa of spinal cord by inhibiting release of substance P from the descending pain inhibiting neurons (presynaptic site).
  - It suppresses associated emotional reactions to pain such as apprehension, fear and autonomic effects by an inhibitory action on the limbic system and sensory cortex.
  - It produces euphoria (feeling of well-being and relief of anxiety) which makes the patient to tolerate pain better and so pain is no longer felt unpleasant or distressing.
- **Sedation:** It produces sedation, which is useful when pain is accompanied by insomnia. It produces drowsiness and a feeling of indifference to surroundings and to own body. In larger dosage it produces sleep and coma.

- **Depression of respiration:** It depresses the brain stem respiratory centre (RC) directly in a dose dependent manner and decreases respiratory rate and tidal volume. It also decreases the sensitivity of the medullary respiratory centre to increased plasma CO_2 concentration. In larger dosage it produces respiratory failure by depressing neurogenic drive, hypercapnic drive and hypoxic drive to the respiratory centre in succession.
- **Depression (suppression) of cough:** It depresses the cough reflex probably by a direct depressant action on the medullary cough centre.
- **Depression of vomiting centre (VC)** and **Vasomotor centre (VMC)** in medulla and temperature regulating centre in hypothalamus in large dosage.

CNS stimulant effects are:
- Stimulation of vagal centre in medulla producing bradycardia.
- Stimulation of CTZ in the area prostema of medulla (at the floor of 4th ventricle) producing nausea and vomiting.
- Stimulation of oculomotor centre (Edinger-Westphal nucleus) of oculomotor nerve in the midbrain (at the floor of cerebral aqueduct) producing miosis.
  Pinpoint pupils are characteristic of acute morphine poisoning. Applied by drops in the eye, it does not produce miosis and so it is a central action.
- Stimulation of certain spinal centres: It increases the reflex excitability of the spinal cord and produces muscular rigidity and even convulsions in occasional individuals.

Neuroendocrine effects: It increases release (secretion) of ADH from the posterior pituitary producing a decrease in urine output. It increases release of growth hormone and prolactin from the anterior pituitary but decreases release of ACTH and gonadotrophins by decreasing the influence of hypothalamus on the anterior pituitary. Thus it lowers sex hormone and corticosteroid levels.

CVS effects: It has little or no direct effect on the heart. It may produce bradycardia by vagal stimulation or reflex tachycardia due to fall of BP (hypotension). It produces cerebral vasodilatation and increasses intracranial (CSF) pressure by retaining CO_2. It produces peripheral vasodilatation, which is partly due to histamine release and inhibition of sympathetic tone of blood vessel. In large dosage it also depresses VMC leading to severe fall of BP. By inhibiting sinoaortic baroreceptor reflex, it can produce postural hypotension on standing from recumbent position.

GIT effects: It increases the tone of GIT and decreases secretions and peristaltic movements of GIT. On chronic use, it produces constipation by following mechanisms:

- It decreases gastric motility and increases tone of pyloric antrum, thus decreasing gastric emptying.
- It increases the tone of the smooth muscles of the small and large intestine and decreases propulsive peristaltic movements (motility).
- It causes spasm of ileocaecal and anal sphincters.
- It decreases all GIT secretions.
- It inhibits defaecation reflex making the subject inattentive to defaecation.

All these effects result in greater transit time (for the content) in the GIT, more complete absorption of water causing drying of faecal mass and inability to defaecate producing constipation.

Effects on other smooth muscles

- **On biliary tract:** It causes spasm of biliary sphincter (sphincter of Oddi) leading to increase in intrabiliary pressure (about ten folds) and may cause biliary colic. This action can be partly antagonized by atropine but completely antagonized by opioid antagonist (naloxone) or direct smooth muscle relaxant (glyceryltrinitrate).
- **On respiratory tract:** It causes bronchospasm by a direct stimulant action on the bronchial muscle and also by causing release of histamine from the bronchial mucosa, especially in asthmatic patients.
- **On urinary tract:** It causes spasm of the ureter and the sphincter of urinary bladder. It may produce retention of urine, especially in enlarged prostate patients.
- **On uterus:** It may cause contraction of uterus and prolongs the labour. It can cause respiratory depression in foetus by crossing placental barrier.
- **On tail of mice:** It produces erection and stiffening of the tail of mice due to contraction of the smooth muscles at the base of the tail (Straub tail reaction). It can be used as a diagnostic test of a morphine poisoning case in the tail of a mice.

Clinical Uses

These are given as follows:

- **For relief of pain:** Morpine is one of the most powerful analgesics. It is used to relieve severe pain such as acute myocardial infarction (AMI), fractures of long bones, severe burns, pulmonary embolism, acute pericarditis, pleurisy with effusion, spontaneous pneumothorax and terminal stage of cancer. For relief of sudden excruciating pain, it is usually administered IV, when it produces prompt relief of pain and thus minimizes shock. It is the drug of first choice in acute myocardial infarction. It is highly effective in this condition due to following reasons:

  - It is a potent analgesic and relieves severe pain.
  - It is sedative and anxiolytic and suppresses anxiety, apprehension and fear of the patient.
  - It reduces both preload (by causing venodilatation) and afterload (by causing arteriolar dilatation) to the heart. So it decreases myocardial oxygen demand and cardiac work.
  - It minimizes shock due to severe pain.
  - It reduces reflex sympathetic stimulation.

For the same reasons it can be used in internal bleeding like haematemesis and threatened abortion.

It can be used for relief of pain in renal and biliary colic. But for this purpose, it must be combined with atropine, which produces smooth muscle relaxation and thus helps to relieve spasm. It has been used for the prevention and treatment of labour pain and for the treatment of cancer pain by epidural or intrathecal route. Such analgesia is essentially segmental in distribution and there is no interference with motor function or autonomic activity.

- **In acute left ventricular failure (LVF):** In it, there is congestion of blood in the pulmonary circuit, which precipitates pulmonary oedema leading to severe dyspnoea and even death. It is an emergency situation and requires prompt treatment. Morphine is valuable in this condition due to following reasons:

  - It has analgesic, sedative and anxiolytic effects, which decrease effort of breathing, apprehension, fear and anxiety of the patient.

  - It has venodilator and vasodilator properties, which help in reducing pulmonary congestion and peripheral resistance. It decreases both preload and afterload to the heart. Due to peripheral vasodilatation, it produces shunting of the blood from the pulmonary arteries to the dilated peripheral blood vessels and this reduces pulmonary artery blood flow, pulmonary artery pressure and central venous pressure. Thus it decreases the cardiac work provided oxygenation is maintained.

  - It decreases the sensitivity of the respiratory centre to excessive stimuli coming from congested lung tissue and thus relieves air hunger (dyspnoea).

- **As preanaesthetic medication:** It is used before operation to produce analgesia, sedation and anxiolytic effect. It also reduces the dose of general anaesthetic required.

- **Miscellaneous uses:** It can be used to suppress severe cough but codeine is preferred. It can be used to produce constipation in severe diarrhoea as tincture of opium (1–2 ml) but diphenoxylate or loperamide is preferred. It has been used IV along with other drugs to produce general anaesthesia, especially in subjects who are considered as bad anaesthetic risks.

Preparations and Dosage

- Morphine hydrochloride/sulphate injection (10 mg/mL/ampoule)—10 to 20 mg SC or IM, 2.5 to 5 mg IV slowly.
- Controlled release morphine/sulphate tablet (10, 30 and 60 mg)—10 to 60 mg once or twice daily (for prolonged action).

Contraindications of Morphine

These are given as follows:

- **Head injuries:** Diagnostic features of head injuries are mydriasis, vomiting and respiratory depression. Morphine produces miosis, vomiting and respiratatory depression and also increases intracranial (CSF) pressure by cerebral vasodilation (retaining CO_2) and may aggravate the condition. By producing miosis and mental clouding it may interfere with the diagnosis and assessment of head injuries.

- **Bronchial asthma:** Morphine can precipitate an acute attack of bronchial asthma by causing bronchospasm due to a direct stimulant action on the bronchial smooth muscles as well as by cerebral vasodilation releasing histamine from the bronchial mucosa. It also causes depression of respiration by acting directly on the RC and also by abolishing the sensitivity of the RC to increase plasma CO_2 concentration (PCO_2).

- **Chronic obstructive pulmonary diseases (COPDs)** like emphysema, pulmonary fibrosis and cor pulmonale: In these persons, there is respiratory insufficiency and diminished respiratory reserve. They are on the verge of hypoxia, which they avert by increasing respiratory rate. Morphine by decreasing ciliary activity, depressing cough reflex and respiration and increasing tone of bronchial muscles may aggravate these conditions and can precipitate respiratory failure.

- **Undiagnosed abdominal pain:** Morphine relieves pain without modifying the underlying pathological process. It interferes with the diagnosis of the condition by masking pain and creating a false sense of security. It may aggravate biliary colic, pancreatitis and diverticulitis. Acute appendicitis (inflamed appendix) may rupture after its use.

- **Extremes of age:** Old people and infants are more prone to develop respiratory depression with morphine.

- **Hypovolemic shock:** Morphine produces further fall of BP in hypovolemic shock leading to serious state.

- **Hypothyroidism (myxoedema):** These patients have lower basal metabolic rate (BMR) and decreased rate of metabolism of drugs. They are more sensitive to morphine and frank coma may be precipitated by even conventional therapeutic dosage of morphine.

- **Labour:** Morphine can produce respiratory depression of foetus or neonate by crossing placental barrier.

- **Enlarged prostate:** Morphine can produce urinary retention by causing spasm of trigonal sphincter of urinary bladder.

- **Persons with unstable personality:** They are liable to continue the use of morphine and become addicted to it.

Adverse Reactions

These are given as follows:

- **Side effects:** It can produce drowsiness, mental clouding, euphoria or dysphoria, constipation, dryness of mouth, headache, nausea, vomiting, dizziness, vertigo, fatigue, paraesthesia and increased biliary pressure.

- **Intolerance:** It may occasionally produce tremors and delirium. It can produce allergic skin reactions like rashes, pruritus and contact dermatitis by releasing histamine. Anaphylactoid reaction with fall of BP rarely occurs.

- **Respiratory depression:** It may occur even with therapeutic dose.

- **Hypotension:** It occasionally produces hypotension as a result of peripheral vasodilatation. Patients with reduced blood volume are more susceptible to the hypotensive effect of morphine.

- **Urinary retention:** It may produce urinary retention in old people with enlarged prostate due to spasm of trigonal sphincter.

- **On the foetus:** It may produce respiratory depression in foetus or neonate leading to asphyxia neonatorum.

- **Tolerance:** Repeated administration of morphine leads to the development of tolerance. It occurs with respiratory depressant, analgesic, sedative and euphoriant effects of morphine but the pupils and the GIT do not show tolerance. Thus, a morphine addict has pinpoint pupils and habitual constipation.

- **Drug dependence:** Morphine is a drug of addiction due to its euphoriant effect. It produces psychological and physical dependence. Morphine addicts are usually malnourished and debilitated. They do not suffer from motor incoordination and are capable of performing complex motor and intellectual tasks, but they become a great social problem. Withdrawal of morphine in an addict produces severe abstinence syndrome characterized by drug seeking behaviour (intense craving for the drug), lethargy, weakness, yawning, lacrimation, sweating, rhinorrhoea, tremors, anorexia, restlessness, anxiety, insomnia, fever, rise of BP, tachycardia, mydriasis, intestinal cramps and back and leg pains. The mechanism of morphine withdrawal syndrome is not known but the involvement of the neurotransmitters, noradrenaline and dopamine are suspected. The treatment of morphine dependence is similar to that of alcohol or barbiturate dependence. The result of treatment may be unsatisfactory due to severity of withdrawal syndrome and the high relapse rate. Gradual withdrawal of morphine with substitution of another opioid analgesic methadone decreases the severity of withdrawal syndrome. Methadone is preferred for replacement therapy in morphine dependence because it can be administered orally and has a longer duration of action than morphine. One milligram of methadone will substitute 4 mg of morphine. When the patient is stabilized on methadone, then its dose is gradually reduced by 10% daily and the drug is completely stopped after 10 days. To prevent relapse in addicts, naltrexone tablet (50 mg) in the dose of 100 to 200 mg daily may be used. Acute morphine withdrawal symptoms and signs can be controlled to some extent by drugs like clonidine, propranolol and chlorpromazine, which counteract the noradrenergic and dopaminergic overactivities of morphine.

- **Acute morphine poisoning:** It may occur from clinical overdose, accidental overdose in an addict or from suicidal or homicidal intention. Administration of 60 mg of morphine in an adult subject can produce serious toxicity, but rarely fatal. The fatal (lethal) dose of morphine in an adult subject is about 250 mg. In morphine addicts, the toxic and fatal doses are much higher than the normal subjects. Clinical manifestations of morphine poisoning are respiratory depression (producing slow, shallow and irregular respiration), cyanosis, fall of body temperature, pinpoint pupils, decreased urinary output, fall of BP, slow, weak and irregular pulse, flaccidity of skeletal muscles, circulatory collapse (shock) and coma. Convulsions may occur in children. Death is usually due to respiratory failure or as a result of shock, pulmonary oedema and secondary infection.

Treatment

It consists of:
- Gastric lavage by potassium permanganate solution (1 in 4000) to oxidize morphine to oxymorphone (less toxic) and to remove unabsorbed and secreted morphine from the stomach.
- Administration of antidote (specific opioid antagonist), naloxone in the dosage of 0.4 to 0.8 mg IV (as bolus) and repeated every 5 minutes till respiration becomes normal or a total dose of 10 mg is given. If it is not available, the partial opioid agonist, nalorphine in the dosage of 3 to 10 mg IV (as bolus) may be used and repeated every 30 minutes to a total dose of 40 mg.
- Supportive measures like oxygen inhalation or positive pressure respiration and administration of IV fluids and vasoconstrictors to maintain normal respiration and BP. Proper nursing care should be given. Opioid antagonists should be used carefully in treating acute morphine poisoning in addicts as they may produce severe withdrawal syndrome. The duration of action of opioid antagonists is shorter than the morphine and so the patient has to be carefully monitored to prevent the development of coma.

Drug Interactions

- Metabolism of morphine is inhibited by cimetidine.
- Antihypertensive drugs potentiate the hypotensive effect of morphine.
- Phenothiazines, MAO inhibitors and tricyclic antidepressants potentiate the sedative and respiratory depressant effects of morphine.

Codeine

It is a naturally occurring alkaloid of opium belonging to phenanthrene group. Chemically it is methyl morphine. It is now prepared synthetically by substituting a methyl group in morphine. Its structure is shown in **Fig. 46.2.** It has less affinity for opioid receptors than morphine. It is less potent than morphine as analgesic (only 1/10th activity) and antitussive (only 1/3rd activity). It does not produce significant respiratory depression. It has low addiction liability. It is much better absorbed than morphine when given orally and its bioavailability on oral administration is about 50%. It is mainly used as an antitussive to relieve irritating cough. It is combined with salicylates to enhance the analgesic effect. Unlike morphine, it does not relieve acute (severe) pain. It is available as codeine phosphate syrup (15 mg/5 mL), tablet (30 mg) and injection (15 mg/mL). It is used in the dosage of 30 to 60 mg orally 3 to 4 times daily. Its main disadvantage is constipation. It may produce excitement and convulsions in toxic dosage. Dihydrocodeine and oxycodone are derivatives of codeine. These are used orally for similar purposes as codeine.

Heroin/Diamorphine

It is a semisynthetic derivative of morphine. Chemically, it is diacetylmorphine. It is converted to morphine in the body. It is more potent (three times) analgesic than morphine. It can easily cross the BBB due to more lipid solubility than morphine. It has greater euphoric effect than morphine and so has a higher addiction liability. It is rarely used therapeutically due to high addiction liability. It is extensively used as brown sugar (a drug of abuse). Newborn children of heroin addict mothers develop a severe withdrawal syndrome within few hours after birth. Treatment of heroin addiction is similar to that of morphine addiction. One mg of methadone can substitute for 2 mg of heroin.

Dihydroxymorphine (Dilandid), oxymorphone (Numorphan) and methyl dihydromorphinone (Metopan) and other semisynthetic derivatives of morphine are used orally as analgesics in the dosage of 1.5 mg, 1.5 mg and 3.5 mg respectively. They produce less adverse reactions than morphine.

Synthetic Opioid Analgesics

Pethidine/Meperidine

It is a synthetic opioid. Chemically it is a phenyl piperidine derivative (not related to morphine), but it has analgesic activity by binding with opioid receptors. It is less potent analgesic (1/10th activity) than morphine. Its onset of action is more rapid but duration of action is shorter than morphine. It is less sedative, less constipating and much less cough suppressant than morphine. In equianalgesic dosage, it produces same degree of euphoria, emesis and respiratory depression as morphine. It has atropine like spasmolytic, mydriatic and antisecretory effects. It produces tachycardia by vagolytic action. It produces corneal anaesthesia and inhibits corneal reflex. It can produce hypotension and shock by peripheral vasodilatation. It increases intracranial (CSF) pressure by producing cerebral vasodilatation (retaining CO_2). It also rises intrabiliary pressure by producing spasm of sphincter of Oddi but it is less than morphine.

Pharmacokinetics

It is absorbed from all routes. It has a bioavailability of about 50% after oral administration. It is metabolized in the liver by hydrolysis (forming major metabolite, meperidinic acid) and demethylation (forming minor metabolite, norpethidine). These are then conjugated with glucuronic acid and excreted in urine. Only a small amount of the drug is excreted unchanged in urine. It crosses the placental barrier and is also secreted in milk.

Clinical Uses

It is used for analgesia and preanaesthetic medication. As an analgesic it is used in acute myocardial infarction, burns, biliary, intestinal or renalcolic and for diagnostic procedures like gastroscopy, cystoscopy and pyelography. It is also used for obstetrical analgesia (especially in dilatation and curettage) and epidural and intrathecal analgesia. Its use as preanaesthetic medication is discussed in general anaesthesia.

Preparations and Dosage

- Pethidine hydrochloride tablet (50 mg)—25 to 100 mg orally and repeated if necessary after 4 hours.
- Pethidine hydrochloride injection (50 mg/ml in 2 ml ampoule)—50 to 100 mg SC or IM, 25 to 50 mg IV and repeated if necessary after 4 hours.

Adverse Reactions

It has less adverse effects than morphine. Its common side effects are euphoria or dysphoria, dizziness, sweating, mydriasis, dryness of mouth, vomiting, weakness and palpitation. It produces local irritation at injection site. It can produce bronchospasm and drying of bronchial secretion. It may produce depression of foetal respiration when administered to pregnant woman during labour. Tolerance to analgesic and emetic effects develops on prolonged use of pethidine. Addiction to pethidine commonly occurs in medical persons. Pethidine addicts show dilated pupils, tremors, mental confusion, muscular twitchings and occasionally convulsions. Withdrawal of pethidine in an addict produces abstinence syndrome, which is less severe than morphine. There is little nausea, vomiting or diarrhoea but the patient may show more excitement than during morphine withdrawal. Treatment of pethidine addiction is similar to that of morphine addiction. One mg of methadone can substitute for 20 mg of pethidine. Acute poisoning due to overdosage of pethidine is manifested as respiratory depression, tremors, mydriasis, hyperreflexia, delirium, convulsions and coma. Naloxone or nalorphine can antagonize the respiratory depression and coma but cannot modify the excitant effect (due to nor-pethidine) of pethidine. Acute pethidine poisoning is treated in the similar way as acute morphine poisoning.

Fentanyl, alfentanil and sufentanil are pethidine congeners. They are more potent analgesics than morphine and pethidine. They are used with the neurolepticdroperidol to produce neuroleptanalgesia (discussed in General Anaesthesia).

Methadone

It is a synthetic opioid. Chemically it is dimethylamine diphenyl heptanone (not related to morphine). It is a µ-receptor agonist. It has analgesic activity equivalent to morphine. Its advantages over morphine are orally effective and longer duration of action (12 to 24 hours). It is well-absorbed from GIT and has bioavailability of about 80%. It is metabolized in the liver and excreted in urine as metabolites and free form (10%). It has similar pharmacological actions as morphine. It is mainly used as a substitute of morphine, heroin and pethidine during withdrawal to prevent relapse of acute withdrawal syndrome in the addicts. It can also be used as an analgesic to relieve mild to moderate visceral pain. It is available as methadone hydrochloride (Physeptone) capsule (10 mg) and used in the dosage of 10 to 20 mg twice daily. It has less adverse effects and lower addiction liability than morphine.

Dextropropoxyphene is a methadone congener. It is well-absorbed orally. It is used as an analgesic to relieve mild to moderate visceral pain. It is combined with paracetamol and dicyclomine (Spasmoproxyron) to relieve spasmodic pain like renal, biliary or intestinal colic and dysmenorrhoea. It is available as capsule (65 mg of dextropropoxyphene with 400 mg of paracetamol and 10 mg of dicyclomine) and administered 2 to 3 times daily. It has less adverse effects and lower addiction liability than methadone.

Pentazocine

It is a synthetic drug (a benzomorphan derivative). It is not related to morphine but has analgesic activity. It is a mixed opioid agonist-antagonist. It differs from morphine in following aspects:

- It does not produce euphoria rather causes dysphoria.
- It has lower addiction liability.
- It has less (about ½) analgesic activity.
- It has less spasmodic and constipating actions.
- It produces less sedation and respiratory depression.
- It produces tachycardia and rise of systemic and pulmonary BP by sympathomimetic action and thus increase cardiac workload. It is not recommended in myocardial infarction.
- It has shorter duration of action (2 to 3 hours).

Pharmacokinetics

It is well-absorbed high orally but has only 20% bioavailability due to first pass metabolism in liver. It can be administered rectally and parenterally. It is metabolized in the liver and excreted in urine as glucuronides and partly as free form (10%).

Clinical Uses

It is used as analgesic like morphine except myocardial infarction. It is not effective in acute LVF. It is preferred for obstetric analgesia because it cannot cross placental barrier easily.

Preparations and Dosage

- Pentazocine (Fortwin) tablet (25 mg)—25 to 100 mg every 3 to 4 hours.
- Pentazocine lactate injection (30 mg/ml)—30 to 60 mg SC, IM or IV every 3 to 4 hours.

Adverse Reactions

It can cause dysphoria, vomiting, sweating, dizziness, hallucinations, unpleasant dreams, palpitation, hypertension, respiratory depression and precipitation of acute withdrawal syndrome in an opioid addict. It has low incidence of tolerance and physical dependence. Cyclazocine and phenazocine are less potent than pentazocine and so rarely used. Levorphanol and butorphanol are morphinan congeners with properties similar to those of pentazocine. They are more potent analgesics than morphine and pentazocine. They have high addiction liability and so less used.

Buprenorphine (Tidigesic/Buprine)

It is a semisynthetic derivative of thebaine (an opium alkaloid with convulsant activity). It is a mixed opioid agonist-antagonist. It acts as a partial μ agonist but it has antagonist action on κ receptors. It is 25 to 30 times more potent than morphine as an analgesic and has longer duration of action than morphine. It has similar cardiovascular actions like morphine and can be used in myocardial infarction as an analgesic. It can be administered orally, sublingually and IM. After sublingual admini-stration it has a bioavailability of about 50%. It is highly plasma protein bound. It is metabolized in the liver and excreted in urine and faeces as metabolites and partly as unchanged form. It is used as an analgesic like morphine. It is available as buprenorphine (Tidigeric) tablet (0.2 mg) and injection (0.3 mg/mL). Its dose is 0.2 to 0.4 mg sublingually and 0.3 to 0.6 mg IM or slow IV every 4 to 6 hours.

It can cause respiratory depression like morphine. This action is not readily reversed by naloxone. Doxapram, a respiratory stimu-lant may be useful to reverse respiratory dep-ression. Its other adverse effects include drowsiness, nausea, vomiting, constipation, miosis, bradycardia and hypotension. It has less addiction liability (abuse potential) than morphine.

Tramadol

It is a synthetic opioid (a codeine analogue). It is mainly a μ-receptor agonist. It has excellent analgesic activity but little respiratory depression or GIT effects. It is well-absorbed from GIT and has bioa-vailability of 68%. It is metabolized in the liver and excreted in urine. Its analgesic action lasts for about 6 hours. It is used in the treatment of moderate to severe visceral pain, where it is as effective as morphine or pethidine. In the treatment of chronic pain it is less effective. It is as effective as pethidine in the treatment of labour pain and causes less respiratory depression of foetus. It is also used in postoperative pain. It is available as tablet (50 mg) and injection (50 mg/ml) and admini-stered in the dosage of 50 mg orally thrice daily and 50 to 100 mg IM or IV. It can cause nausea, vomiting, dizziness, dry mouth, sed-ations and headache. It can produce tolerance and physical dependence like codeine.

Opioid Antagonists

These are drugs that antagonize the effects of morphine and other opioid analgesics by blocking opioid receptors (competitive antagonism). Some of them also exert other actions not related to opioid receptors. They are classified into two groups:

- Pure (specific) opioid antagonists, e.g. naloxone and naltrexone.
- Partial opioid agonists with antagonist activity, e.g. nalorphine, cyclazocine, levallorphan, propiram and profadol.

DISCUSSION OF SOME DRUGS

Naloxone (Narcan/Narcotan)

It is a pure competitive antagonist of morphine and other opioid analgesics. It is a synthetic drug. Chemically it is N-allyl analogue of oxymorphone. It has affinity for all types of opioid receptors but the highest affinity for μ receptors. It antagonizes the actions of morphine and other opioid analgesics by binding with opioid receptors. In the absence of morphine or other opioid analgesics, it has no effect of its own. It does not produce respiratory depression, euphoria or analgesia when used alone. Given orally, it is only 1/50th as potent as when given parenterally due to first pass metabolism in the liver. After IV administration its duration of action is 3 to 4 hours.

It is used in the treatment of morphine or other opioid poisoning and to reverse neonatal asphyxia due to respiratory depression produced by administration of morphine in pregnant woman during labour.

Preparation and Dosage

Naloxone injection (0.4 mg/ml)—0.4 to 0.8 mg given as IV bolus and repeated every 5 minutes till respiration becomes normal or a total dose of 10 mg is administered. It does not produce tolerance and physical dependence on prolonged administration. No abstinence syndrome develops on withdrawal of this drug.

Naltrexone

It is a synthetic drug. Chemically, it is related to naloxone. It is a pure opioid antagonist and has actions like naloxone. Its advantage over naloxone are orally effective and long-acting. It is used for maintenance therapy in opioid addicts during withdrawal of the drug to prevent relapse. It is not used in opioid poisoning. It is available as naltrexone (Nalorex) tablet (50 mg) and administered in the dosage of 100 to 200 mg daily. It can produce GIT side effects, nervousness, insomnia and muscle pain. It does not produce tolerance and physical dependence. No abstinence syndrome develops on withdrawal of this drug.

Nalorphine

It is a synthetic drug. Chemically, it is N-allyl normorphine. It is a partial opioid agonist. In the absence of morphine or other opioid analgesic, it produces some effects of its own such as analgesia, sedation, respiratory depression, miosis and euphoria. It precipitates withdrawal syndrome in opioid addicts (used for diagnosis of opioid addiction). It is used in the treatment of acute morphine or other opioid posioning if naloxone is not available. It is available as nalorphine (Lethidrone) injection (10 mg/mL) and administered as IV bolus in the dose of 5 to 10 mg and repeated every 30 minutes till respiration becomes normal or a total dose of 40 mg is given. It can produce drowsiness, dysphoria (anxiety, confusion and visual hallucinations), nausea, vomiting, sweating, miosis and respiratory depression. It does not produce tolerance and physical dependence.

47

Nonsteroidal Antiinflammatory Drugs (NSAIDs)

INTRODUCTION

Nonsteroidal antiinflammatory drugs (NSAIDs) relieve somatic pain and inflammation. They also lower body temperature and so they are called analgesic antipyretics. They differ from narcotic (opioid) analgesics in the following aspects:

- They have no central depressant (sedative) action.
- They relieve pain without binding with opioid receptors but by inhibiting prostaglandins synthesis.
- They are less potent analgesic and effective in mild and moderate pain.
- They possess antiinflammatory and antipyretic activities.
- They are nonaddicting (as they do not produce euphoria).

Classification

They are of two groups:

A. Nonselective COX inhibitors/Conventional NSAIDs

- Salicylates and their congeners, e.g. acetyl salicylic acid (Aspirin), sodium salicylate, methyl salicylate, salicylamide, diflunisal and benorylate.
- Para-aminophenol derivatives, e.g. paracetamol (Acetamenophen), acetanilide and phenacetin are now obsolete.
- Pyrazolone derivatives, e.g. phenylbutazone, oxyphenbutazone and metamizol.

- Indole derivatives, e.g. indomethacin and sulindac.
- Phenyl acetic acid derivatives, e.g. diclofenac, fenclofenac and aceclofenac.
- Pyrrole acetic acid derivatives, e.g. ketorolac, etodolac and tolmetin.
- Propionic acid derivatives, e.g. ibuprofen, fenoprofen, naproxen, ketoprofen and flurbiprofen.
- Fenamic acid derivatives (fenamates), e.g. mefenamic acid, meclofenamic acid and flufenamic acid.
- Enolic acid derivatives (oxicams), e.g. piroxicam, tenoxicam and meloxicam.

B. Preferential COX-2 inhibitors:

For example, nimesulide and nabumetone.

C. Selective COX-2 inhibitors

For example, celecoxib and rofecoxib.

General Pharmacokinetic Properties

- They are weakly acidic drugs with ionizing constants between 3 and 5.
- They have varying degrees of lipid solubility and are well-absorbed from GIT.
- They are highly plasma protein bound and have small volume of distribution in the body.
- They produce gastric irritation in varying degrees.
- They are metabolized in liver and excreted in urine by glomerular filtration and tubular secretion in the kidney.

DISCUSSION OF INDIVIDUAL GROUP OF DRUGS

Salicylates and Related Drugs

Salicylates are esters of salicylic acid (ortho-hydroxybenzoic acid). Chemical structures of salicylic acid and its derivatives are shown in **Fig. 47.1.**

The word salicylate is derived from Salicaceae, which is the botanical name of the willow plant *(Salix alba)*. The extract of willow bark contains a glycoside called salicin, which on hydrolysis yields salicylic acid and glucose. Salicylates are prepared from salicylic acid by structural modification.

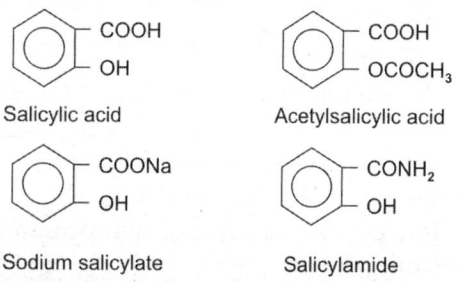

Fig. 47.1: Chemical structures of salicylic acid and its derivatives

Acetyl Salicylic Acid (Aspirin)

It is the most widely used salicylate and is discussed as a prototype drug. It is rapidly converted to salicylic acid in the body, which is responsible for most of the actions.

Pharmacokinetics

It is rapidly absorbed from the stomach and upper part of small intestine in an acidic medium. It is highly plasma protein bound (78%). It is distributed to most of the body tissues and fluids. It crosses blood–brain barrier slowly but placental barrier rapidly. It is metabolized in the gut wall, liver, plasma and other tissues by deacetylation to salicylic acid. Salicylic acid conjugates with glycine forming salicyluric acid and with glucuronic acid forming salicylic acid glucuronide in the liver. These are excreted in urine by glomerular filtration and tubular secretion in the kidney. It has a plasma half-life of 3 to 4 hours. Alkalinization of urine promotes renal excretion of salicylic acid due to ionization in alkaline urine.

Pharmacological Actions

Mechanism of action: This will be discussed with individual effects. It produces following effects:

• **CNS effects**

These are discussed as follows:

– **Analgesic action (analgesia):** It relieves mild to moderate pain of somatic origin arising from integumental structures such as muscles and joints. It also relieves headache, toothache, neuralgia and dysmenorrhoea. It acts by inhibiting the synthesis of prostaglandins in the central (especially thalamus) and peripheral sites. Centrally it acts by raising the threshold of pain perception in the thalamus and thus blocking the transmission of pain sensation from the thalamus to the sensory cortex. Peripherally it acts by preventing the sensitization of the peripheral pain receptors in the sensory nerve endings to the action of pain producing (algogenic) substances like bradykinin, substance P, 5-HT and histamine, which are released by mechanical stimulation (by trauma) or chemical stimulation (by mediators). Unlike opioids, it does not have any cortical action on psychic (mental) processing or on the reaction component of pain and has no sedative, hypnotic or euphoric action in the therapeutic dosage. It does not produce tolerance and addiction. In toxic dosage it produces CNS stimulation followed by CNS depression.

– **Antipyretic action:** It decreases raised body temperature in fever but does not lower normal body temperature. In fever, the hypothalamic thermostat (temperature regulating centre) is set at a higher point. It causes resetting of the thermostat to normal temperature set point and thus brings down the raised body temperature. It also produces peripheral vasodilatation leading to sweating and heat loss. It does not decrease heat production. Its antipyretic action is due to inhibition of synthesis of prostaglandins in the hypothalamus and peripheral sites. It also blocks the pyretic action of pyrogens (proteins) released from leucocytes, which increase prostaglandins synthesis in the hypothalamus leading to rise of body temperature.

– **Respiratory action:** It increases the rate and depth of respiration by both direct and indirect stimulation of the respiratory centre. In therapeutic dosage, it increases the consumption of oxygen primarily by the skeletal muscles resulting in increased production of CO_2 by the skeletal muscles. High concentration of CO_2 in plasma stimulates the respiratory centre through chemoreceptors (indirect action). In high dosage, it causes stimulation of respiratory centre (direct action) leading to hyperventilation. As a result, plasma CO_2 is washed out producing respiratory alkaloids. This is compensated by renal excretion of alkaline urine containing bicarbonate of sodium and potassium and also water. In toxic dosage it can cause hypokalaemia, dehydration and respiratory acidosis (due to retention of CO_2 as a result of depression of RC).

• **Antiinflammatory effects:** It is a potent antiinflammatory drug. It produces antiinflammatory effect in high dosage. It suppresses the signs of inflammation like pain, tenderness, swelling, vasodilatation and leucocyte infiltration but does not affect (arrest) the progression of the underlying disease (rheumatic fever, rheumatoid arthritis or osteoarthritis). It acts by following mechanisms:

– It inhibits the synthesis of prostaglandins (important mediators of inflammation) by inhibiting the enzyme cyclooxygenase (COX), i.e. PG-synthetase.

– It reduces the capillary permeability and thus minimizes the exudation of fluid and development of inflammatory oedema.

– It stabilizes the lysosomal membranes of leucocytes (polymorphonuclear neutrophils) and macrophages and thus prevents the release of lysosomal enzymes, which cause damage of articular cartilage and other tissues producing inflammation.

– It antagonizes the inflammatory action of bradykinins.

– It has antioxidant action. It prevents the generation of free reactive oxygen radicals by the inflammatory cells (neutrophils and macrophages) during inflammation.

• **Immunosuppressive effects:** It suppresses a variety of antigen-antibody reactions including systemic anaphylaxis and serum sickness. It inhibits antibody formation and prevents antigen-antibody reaction and release of histamine from tissue mast cells. It may reduce the cell mediated immunity but this action is controversial in relieving inflammation.

• **Haematological effects:** It does not affect the normal leucocyte count but it reduces leucocytosis and high ESR in inflammatory diseases. In small dosage (50 to 100 mg/day) it has antiplatelet action. It inhibits platelet aggregation by inhibiting the synthesis of thromboxane A_2 (TxA_2) by the platelets, which causes platelet aggregation by releasing ADP from platelets. In the same dose it does not inhibit the synthesis of PGI_2 (prostacyclin) by the vascular endothelium, which inhibits platelet aggregation. This prevents thrombus formation and intravascular clotting. In large dosage (> 5 g/day) it prolongs the clotting time and plasma prothrombin time leading to bleeding tendency. It decreases the synthesis of prothrombin and other vitamin K-dependent clotting factors (VII, IX and X) by the liver by antagonizing the action of vitamin K. Thus, it produces bleeding by preventing coagulation of blood. This can be prevented by prophylactic vitamin K therapy, which prevents hypoprothrombinaemia produced by aspirin.

- **GIT effects:** It can cause epigastric distress, nausea and vomiting due to irritation of gastric mucosal cells. It also produces vomiting by stimulation of CTZ in large dosage. It remains unionized and diffusible in the acid gastric juice, but on entering the mucosal cells, it ionizes and becomes indiffusible. This ion trapping in the mucosal cells increases gastric toxicity Moreover, aspirin particle coming in contact with the mucosal cells promotes local back diffusion of salicylic acid leading to necrosis of mucosal cells and capillaries. This produces gastric ulceration, erosive gastritis, congestion and haemorrhages (haematemesis and melena). It also reduces the cytoprotective action of PGE_2 and PGI_2 on gastric mucosal cells and decreases secretion of mucus and bicarbonate by the gastric mucosal cells. On prolonged use it can cause hypochromic anaemia due to chronic blood loss.

- **Metabolic effects:** It produces certain metabolic effects in large dosage. It increases cellular metabolism especially in skeletal muscles due to uncoupling of oxidative phosphorylation leading to increased heat production. It increases utilization of glucose in peripheral tissues. Blood sugar level may decrease especially in diabetics and liver glycogen is depleted. However, in toxic dosage it produces hyperglycaemia and glycosuria by central sympathetic stimulation and release of adrenaline and corticosteroids from the adrenal gland. Its chronic use in large dosage produces negative nitrogen balance due to increased conversion of protein to carbohydrate (neoglucogenesis) and increased nitrogen excretion in urine by protein breakdown. It also decreases lipogenesis by increasing oxidation of fatty acids in the muscles and liver. It decreases plasma fatty acids, phospholipids and cholesterol levels. It increases oxidation of ketones. In toxic dosage, it can produce metabolic acidosis by accumulation of lactic acid and pyruvic acid (due to inhibition of the enzymes of Krebs cycle) and acetoacetic acid and β-hydroxybutyric acid (due to increased lipid metabolism).

- **Endocrine effects:** In large dosage, it stimulates the hypothalamic sympathetic centre leading to increased release of adrenaline and corticosteroids from the adrenal gland. It also displaces thyroid hormones from plasma protein binding sites (especially thyroxine binding to plasma albumin) by competitive displacement and increases their metabolism.

- **Cardiovascular effects:** In therapeutic dosage, it has no direct effect on CVS. In large dosage, it increases cardiac output to meet increased peripheral oxygen demand and causes direct vasodilatation. In toxic dosage, it depresses vasomotor centre and causes a fall in BP. In patients with low cardiac reserve, it can precipitate CCF by increasing cardiac work and retention of Na^+ and H_2O.

- **Effects on urate excretion:** It produces dose related effect (biphasic action) on renal urate excretion. In small dosage (< 2g/day) it inhibits urate excretion by inhibiting uric acid secretion by the distal renal tubule and increases plasma urate level (hyperuricaemia) by urate retention. In large dosage (> 5 g/day), it inhibits the reabsorption of urate by the proximal renal tubule and produces increased excretion of uric acid in urine (uricosuria). It is not suitable for use in gout as it produces hyperuricaemia in low dose and many adverse reactions in high dose.

- **Hepatic and renal effects:** It increases secretion of bile (choleretic action) by stimulating the liver parenchymal cells. In large dose, especially in children, it causes abnormal liver function tests and even acute hepatic necrosis. It produces transient increase in the urine cell count with traces of albumin and tubular casts in urine. It can produce analgesic nephropathy (renal tubular damage or necrosis) on prolonged use.

Clinical Uses

These are given as follows:

- **For analgesia:** It is used to relieve mild to moderate pain of somatic origin such as headache, backache, myalgia, arthralgia, neuralgia, toothache and dysmenorrhoea. (primary dysmenorrhoea is thought to be due to increased prostaglandin activity in the uterus).

- **As antipyretic:** It is used to decrease temperature in fever of any origin. Dose used is same as for analgesia.

- **As antirheumatic:** It is used as an antiinflammatory drug in rheumatic fever, rheumatoid arthritis, osteoarthritis and fibromyositis. It suppresses the inflammatory reaction but cannot arrest the inflammatory process and so it cannot prevent the progress of the underlying disease.

- **As antiplatelet (cardioprotective and cerebroprotective):** It is used in small dose for prophylaxis (primary or secondary prevention) of myocardial infarction. It is also used for prophylaxis of cerebral strokes and in the treatment of transient cerebral ischaemia.

- **Miscellaneous uses**
  - It is used in the treatment of migraine.
  - It is used in cholera or radiation induced diarrhoea, where it decreases excessive gut secretions by prostaglandins.
  - It is used for closure of patent ductus arteriosus.
  - It is used to delay onset of labour (where prostaglandins are involved for initiation of labour).
  - It is used as a preventive of colorectal cancer (by inhibiting COX-2)
  - Salicylic acid is used locally as an antifungal drug. It has fungistatic, keratolytic and mild antiseptic actions.

- Methyl salicylate (oil of wintergreen) is used as analgesic liniment in arthritis and fibromyositis.

Preparations and Dosage

- Aspirin (Dispirin) tablet (300, 500 mg): As an analgesic and antipyretic—300 to 600 mg thrice daily. In rheumatic fever—900 to 1200 mg 4 to 6 hourly daily. In rheumatoid arthritis, osteoarthritis or fibromyositis—600 to 900 mg 3 to 4 times daily.
- Low dose aspirin (ASA/Loprin) tablet (50, 75 mg)—50 to 100 mg once daily.
- Aspirin with lysine (450 mg) and glycine (50 mg) injection (in vial) is available (Biospirin) for IV infusion in postoperative pain.

Adverse Reactions

These are given as follows:

- **GIT side effects:** It can produce epigastric distress, heart burn, nausea, vomiting, abdominal pain, peptic ulceration and erosion of gastroduodenal mucosa leading to haemorrhage (haematemesis and melena). Occult blood loss in stool is common and may produce hypochromic anaemia. Rarely a single large dose of aspirin may produce severe gastroduodenal haemorrhage, which may be an idiosyncratic reaction. These effects of aspirin can be reduced by taking the drug after meal and administering antacids, which delay gastric absorption of aspirin by making it ionized. Enteric coated tablet of aspirin is also available, which is absorbed from small intestine and thus preventing gastric irritation.

- **Hypersensitivity (allergic) reactions:** It may produce skin rashes, eruptions, urticaria, rhinorrhoea, angioneurotic oedema, bronchial asthma and anaphylactoid shock in susceptible persons with allergic disorders.

- **Salicylism:** In high dosage or on chronic use it may produce a clinical syndrome called salicylism, which is characterized by tinnitus, vertigo, dizziness, impairment of hearing, blurring of vision, excitement, mental confusion, hyperventilation, nausea, vomiting and diarrhoea. It is reversed on stopping the drug.

- **Reye's syndrome:** It can produce this condition in infants and children suffering or recovering from febrile viral infections like influenza and chickenpox. It is characterized by hepatic damage and encephalopathy.

- **Acute poisoning (toxicity):** It is due to overdose of aspirin especially in children and is manifested as vomiting, diarrhoea, dehydration, electrolyte imbalance, acidotic breathing, hyperpyrexia, bleeding from various sites, restlessness, excitement, delirium, hallucinations, hyperexcitability, convulsions and coma. Death may occur due to respiratory failure or cardiovascular collapse.

Treatment

- Gastric lavage with plain water to remove the unabsorbed drug from the stomach.
- External cooling by application of cold water or ice to reduce high temperature.
- Administration of IV fluids, sodium bicarbonate and potassium chloride to maintain fluid and electrolyte balance.
- Administration of vitamin K (10 mg IV) and in severe cases blood transfusion is done to stop bleeding (haemorrhage).
- In serious cases, peritoneal dialysis, haemodialysis or exchange transfusion may be done.

Contraindications

These are given as follows:

- Hypersensitive patients
- Peptic ulcer
- Ulcerative colitis
- Bleeding diseases like haemophilia and purpura
- Metabolic diseases like gout and diabetes mellitus—it produces severe hypoglycaemia.

- In infants and children suffering from viral diseases—it produces Reye's syndrome.
- During labour—it prolongs labour, produces low birth weight babies and increases postpartum haemorrhage.

Drug Interactions

- It displaces warfarin sodium from plasma protein binding sites leading to increased concentration of free warfarin sodium in blood producing bleeding tendency.
- It displaces chlorpropamide from plasma protein binding sites leading to increased concentration of free chlorpropamide in blood producing severe hypoglycaemia.
- It displaces methotrexate from plasma protein binding sites leading to increased concentration of free methotrexate in blood leading to methotrexate toxicity.
- Prednisolone when used with it causes induction of hepatic microsomal enzyme leading to increased metabolism of aspirin, decreasing its therapeutic effect.

Other Salicylates and Salicylate Congeners

Sodium salicylate has similar actions, uses and adverse reactions like aspirin. It is used as mixture in the dosage of 1 to 2 g thrice daily. Methyl salicylate (oil of wintergreen) is used as liniment in rheumatic pain of joints and muscles.

Salicylamide, a salicylate congener is hydrolyzed to salicylic acid in the body. It is available as tablet (0.5 g) and used in the dose of 1 to 2 g thrice daily for the treatment of rheumatic fever and rheumatoid arthritis. It is claimed to be less toxic than salicylates.

Diflunisal (Dolobid), a nonacetylated difluorinated salicylate, has greater potency, better tolerance and longer duration of action than aspirin. It is available as tablet (250 mg) and used in the dose of 250 to 500 mg twice daily as an analgesic and antiinflammatory drug.

Benorylate is an ester of aspirin and paracetamol. It is available as tablet.

Para-aminophenol Derivatives

Paracetamol/Acetaminophen

It is the most widely used analgesic-anti-pyretic. Chemically it is n-acetyl-p-amino-phenol. It is the diethylated active metabolite of phenacetin. Its chemical structure is shown in **Fig. 47.2.**

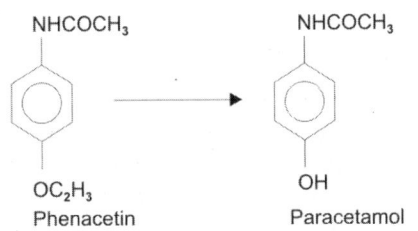

Fig. 47.2: Chemical structures of phenacetin and paracetamol

Pharmacokinetics

It is rapidly absorbed from GIT. Its peak plasma concentration is reached within ½ to 1 hour. It is bound to plasma protein to the extent of about 40%. It is uniformly distributed in the body. It is metabolized in the liver and the metabolites are excreted in urine as conjugation products of glucuronic acid and sulphuric acid. The ability of infant liver for glucuronidation of paracetamol is poor and this may produce increased toxicity of the drug in infants. It has a plasma t½ of 2 to 3 hours and its effects last for 4 to 6 hours.

Pharmacological Actions

It has analgesic and antipyretic actions like aspirin. It has poor antiinflammatory action in comparison to aspirin because it has weak inhibitory activity on prostaglandin synthe-tase (cyclooxygenase) at peripheral sites (sites of inflammation). However, it has equal inhibitory activity of aspirin on this enzyme in the brain and spinal cord. Unlike aspirin, it does not produce acidbase imbalance, electrolyte disturbances, respiratory stimu-lation, GIT irritation, antiplatelet action, hypoprothrombinemic action and uricosuric action.

Clinical Uses

It is a popular analgesic antipyretic drug due to low toxicity than aspirin. It is used in fever, headache, backache, toothache, myalgia, arthralgia and neuralgia.

Preparations and Dosage

- Paracetamol (Calpol/Crocin) tablet (500 mg)—250 to 500 mg 3 to 4 times daily (maximum dose 2.5 g).
- Paracetamol syrup (125 mg/5 mL)—65 to 125 mg 3 to 4 times daily for children.

Adverse Reactions

It is a safe and well-tolerated drug in thera-peutic dosage. It can rarely produce skin rashes, fever, neutropaenia, thrombocytopaenia, haemolytic anaemia and methaemoglo-binaemia. Acute paracetamol poisoning due to overdosage may occur in infants producing extensive liver damage and may cause death due to liver failure. This liver toxicity is due to the toxic metabolite n-acetyl-p-benzo-quinoneimine (n-hydroxy-n-acetyl-p-hydroxy-aniline) produced as a result of inability of glucuronidation of paracetamol in the liver. It causes depletion of glutathione stores in the liver cells producing liver damage. It is treated by administration of sulphhydryl compounds like n-acetylcysteine, l-methionine and cyste-amine. n-acetylcysteine is commonly used. It is administered orally or IV as 5% solution in the dosage of 140 mg/kg initially, followed by 70 mg/kg every 4 hours for three days.

Acetanilide and phenacetin are no longer used in therapeutics due to toxicity. They produce methaemoglobinaemia, cyanosis, haemolytic anaemia (in individuals with glucose-6-phosphate dehydrogenase defi-ciency) and analgesic nephropathy (renal tubular damage or necrosis).

Pyrazolone Derivatives

Phenylbutazone

It is a potent antiinflammatory drug. It has much less analgesic-antipyretic activity and more antiinflammatory activity than aspirin.

It has uricosuric effect like aspirin. It is a potent prostaglandin synthesis inhibitor like aspirin. It is well-absorbed from GIT. It is extensively plasma protein bound (about 98%). It is metabolized in the liver by hydroxylation and glucuronidation. Its active metabolite is oxyphenbutazone. It is excreted in urine mainly as metabolites. Its plasma t½ is long (about 60 hours). It is used in rheumatoid arthritis, ankylosing spondylitis, osteoarthritis and acute gouty arthritis. It should not be used for more than two weeks due to its toxic potential. It is available as phenylbutazone (Zolandin) tablet (100 mg) and injection (200 mg/ml) and administered in the dosage of 100 to 200 mg orally twice daily after meal. It is a more toxic drug than aspirin. It can produce GIT side effects and allergic reactions like aspirin. It also produces oedema and hypertension (by sodium and water retention), hypothyroidism (by reducing iodine uptake by the thyroid gland), hepatitis (by liver cell damage), nephritis (by tubular cell damage, i.e. analgesic nephropathy) and blood dyscrasias (by bone marrow depression). It can produce agranulocytosis, thrombocytopaenia, megaloblastic anaemia and aplastic anaemia. It is contraindicated in peptic ulcer, hypertension, blood dyscrasias, allergic patients and liver, kidney or thyroid disease.

Oxyphenbutazone

It is the active metabolite of phenylbutazone. It has pharmacological actions, pharmacokinetics and adverse reactions like phenylbutazone but it causes less gastric irritation than phenylbutazone. It is used mainly in musculoskeletal pains like myalgia, arthralgia, headache and backache and to prevent swelling and inflammation after blunt injuries, fractures, etc. It is available as oxyphenbutazone (Reducin) tablet (100 mg) and used in the dosage of 100 to 200 mg twice daily after meal. It is also available as 10% eye ointment.

Metamizol

It is a potent and promptly acting analgesic-antipyretic drug. It has poor antiinflammatory and no uricosuric effects. It causes less gastric irritation than phenylbutazone. It has uses and adverse reactions like oxyphenbutazone. It is available as metamizol (Analgin) tablet (500 mg) and injection (500 mg/mL) and administered in the dosage of 500 to 1000 mg orally twice daily after meal. Its advantage over aspirin is that it can be administered IM in emergency.

Indole Derivatives

Indomethacin

It is a potent antiinflammatory drug. It has more analgesic, antipyretic and antiinflammatory actions than phenylbutazone. It has uricosuric effect like phenylbutazone. In patients with rheumatoid arthritis with swollen joints, it produces a quick reduction of the joint swellings. It is a potent prostaglandin synthesis inhibitor. It is also effective in osteoarthritis and ankylosing spondilytis to relieve pain. It is very useful in the treatment of acute attacks of gout, where it relieves pain within 2 hours of the first dose. It is rapidly absorbed from GIT. It is highly plasma protein bound (about 90%). It is metabolized in the liver and is excreted in urine mainly as glucuronide. It has a plasma t½ of 4 to 6 hours. It has uses like phenylbutazone. It is available as indomethacin (Idicin) capsule (25, 50 mg) and administered in the dosage of 25 to 50 mg twice daily after meal. It is also available as suppository (50 mg). It can produce GIT side effects and allergic reactions like aspirin. It produces CNS side effects like headache, giddiness, mental confusion, blurring of vision, depression, and psychotic disturbances. It can cause reduction in renal clearance of lithium and thus a rise in serum lithium level occurs in patients on lithium therapy. It may cause retention of sodium and water leading to oedema.

Sulindac

It is a fluorinated derivative of indomethacin. It has longer duration of action and less adverse reactions than indomethacin. Its antiinflammatory action is weaker than indomethacin. It has uses like indomethacin. It is available as sulindac (Clinoril) tablet (150 mg) and administered in the dosage of 150 to 300 mg twice daily after meal.

Phenyl Acetic Acid Derivatives

Diclofenac

It is a potent antiinflammatory drug. It has more analgesic, antipyretic and antiinflammatory actions than indomethacin. It is a potent prostaglandin synthesis inhibitor (inhibits cyclooxygenase). It may inhibit lipooxygenase (inhibiting synthesis of leukotrienes). It has no uricosuric effect and is not used in gout. It is rapidly absorbed from GIT but 50% of it undergoes first pass metabolism in liver and so only 50% reaches the systemic circulation. It is highly plasma protein bound (about 90%). It is metabolized in the liver and is excreted in urine mainly as glucuronide. It accumulates in the synovial fluid, which probably is responsible for its longer duration of action than its plasma t½ suggests.

It is used in rheumatoid arthritis, severe osteoarthritis, ankylosing spondylitis, bursitis and posttraumatic or postoperative inflammatory conditions. It is available as diclofenac (Voveran) as tablet (50 mg) and injection (25 mg/ml). It is administered orally in the dosage of 50 to 100 mg twice daily after meal. It is given by deep IM injection in the dosage of 75 mg once or twice daily. It is also available as 0.1% eye drops (used to prevent postoperative inflammation in cataract surgery) and as gel for topical use. It has less adverse reactions than indomethacin and phenylbutazone and so better tolerated by the patients. Fenclofenac and aleclofenac have similar properties of diclofenac but less potent.

Pyrrole Acetic Acid Derivatives

Ketorolac

It is a potent analgesic with moderate antiinflammatory activity. It has equal efficacy as morphine in relieving posttraumatic or postoperative pain. It inhibits platelet function like other NSAIDs. It has no uricosuric effect. It is well-absorbed after oral and IM administration. It is metabolized in the liver by glucuronidation and about 50% is excreted unchanged in urine. It has a plasma t½ of about 7 hours. It is used to relieve posttraumatic or postoperative pain and acute musculoskeletal pain and inflammation. It is available as ketorolac (Ketorol) tablet (10 mg) and injection (10 mg/mL). It is administered in the dosage of 20 to 30 mg orally or IM once or twice daily. It has less adverse reactions than diclofenac.

Etodolac and tolmetin have similar properties of ketorolac but less potent.

Propionic Acid Derivatives

Ibuprofen

It is a potent analgesic, antipyretic and antiinflammatory drug. It has poor uricosuric effect. It is a potent prostaglandin synthesis inhibitor like aspirin. It has antiplatelet action. It is well-absorbed from GIT. It is highly plasma protein bound (about 95%) and like aspirin can displace phenytoin, warfarin and chlorpropamide from plasma protein binding sites. It is metabolized in the liver and is excreted in urine mainly as glucuronide. It has a plasma t½ of about 8 hours. It is used in fever, musculoskeletal pain, rheumatoid arthritis, osteoarthritis, ankylosing spondilytis and acute gouty arthritis. It can also be used in posttraumatic or postoperative pain and inflammation. It is available as ibuprofen (Brufen) tablet (200, 400 mg) and administered in the dosage of 200 to 400 mg twice or thrice daily. It is better tolerated orally and has less adverse reactions than diclofenac and indomethacin.

Fenoprofen, naproxen, ketoprofen and flurbiprofen have similar properties of ibuprofen but more potent and expensive. They are also longer-acting than ibuprofen. Flurbiprofen is also available as eye drops.

Fenamic Acid Derivatives (Fenamates)

Mefenamic Acid

It is a less potent (weaker) analgesic, antipyretic and antiinflammatory drug than aspirin. It has no uricosuric effect. It is well absorbed from GIT. It is metabolized in the liver and excreted in urine mainly as glucuronide. It is used in chronic and dull aching musculoskeletal pain and in some cases of rheumatoid arthritis and osteoarthritis. It is available as mefenamic acid (Ponstan) capsule (250, 500 mg) and administered in the dosage of 250 to 500 mg twice daily. It has less adverse reactions than diclofenac and indomethacin.

Meclofenamic acid and flufenamic acid have similar properties of mefenamic acid but less potent and so less used.

Enolic Acid Derivatives (Oxicams)

Piroxicam

It is a potent analgesic, antipyretic and antiinflammatory drug like aspirin. It has uricosuric effect. It is a longer-acting drug and effective in a single daily dose. Its analgesic action is greater than aspirin. It is a potent prostaglandin synthesis inhibitor. It is well-absorbed orally. It is partly metabolized in the liver and slowly excreted in urine. It has long plasma t½ (about 40 hours). It has uses like phenylbutazone. It is available as piroxicam (Dolonex) tablet (20 mg) and administered in the dosage of 20 to 40 mg once daily. It is also available as gel for topical use. It is better tolerated and has less adverse reactions than phenylbutazone and indomethacin.

Tenoxicam and meloxicam have similar properties of piroxicam but more potent and expensive. They are administered in the dosage of 7.5 to 15 mg once daily.

COX–2 Inhibitors

Nimesulide

It is a potent analgesic, antipyretic and antiinflammatory drug like aspirin. It differs from aspirin in its mechanism of action. It is a preferential COX-2 inhibitor. It also inhibits lipo-oxygenase pathway thus decreasing the synthesis of leukotrienes. During inflammation, WBCs (neutrophils) are activated and release various cytokines, which in turn increase synthesis of prostaglandins. Nimesulide inhibits the release of cytokines from the WBCs by stabilizing the cytokine membrane. It is well-absorbed orally, metabolized in the liver and excreted in urine. It has uses like ibuprofen and piroxicam. It is available as nimesulide (Nise) tablet (100 mg) and administered in the dosage of 100 to 200 mg twice daily. It is also available as gel (5%) for topical use. It is well-tolerated and has highest gastric safety. It is much less toxic than phenylbutazone and indomethacin. Nabumetone has similar properties as nimesulide but more expensive.

Celecoxib

It is a diaryl substituted pyrazole. It is a potent analgesic, antipyretic and antiinflammatory drug like aspirin. It is a selective COX-2 inhibitor. It differs from aspirin in some aspects. It does not produce gastric ulceration and intolerance. It does not inhibit platelet function. It is well-absorbed orally, metabolized in the liver and excreted in urine. It is used in rheumoid arthritis and osteoarthritis. It is available as celecoxib (Zycel) capsule (200 mg) and administered in the dosage of 200–400 mg once or twice daily. It is well-tolerated.

Refecoxib has similar proterties as celecoxib and so now obsolete.

48

Drug Therapy of Rheumatoid Arthritis and Gout

RHEUMATOID ARTHRITIS

It is a chronic inflammatory, destructive and deforming polyarthritis associated with systemic disturbance, a variety of extra-articular lesions and the presence of ciculating antiglobulin antibodies (rheumatoid factors). The pattern of joint involvement is usually symmetrical and peripheral. Its course is typically prolonged with exacerbations and remissions. It is thought to be an autoimmune disease, involving both cellular and humoral components of the immune system. The initial stimulus may be injury or microbial toxins leading to joint damage because of in-appropriate immune and inflammatory responses. Toxic oxygen radicals elaborated by neutrophils and macrophages damage immunoglobulins (IgG, IgM and IgA), which then function as autoantigens. These autoantigens stimulate the formation of antiglobulin antibodies (rheumatoid factors), which activate neutrophils and macrophages to initiate a self-sustaining cycle. These activated cells release interleukin-1 (IL-1), which has wide range of actions including increase in the synthesis of prostaglandins (especially PGE_2) by the inflamed synovial lining cells, fibroblast stimulation leading to collagen synthesis, increased wasting of muscles, bone resorption and destruction of cartilage and induction of immune response mainly be facilitating B and T lymphocytes responses to antigen. Thus, IL-1 is an impor-

tant factor in the initiation and perpetuation of the chronic inflammatory condition, rheumatoid arthritis.

Drugs used in the treatment of rheumatoid arthritis are given below.

Classification

These are of four groups:

1. Antiinflammatory analgesic drugs (NS-AIDs), e.g. aspirin, ibuprofen, diclofenac, piroxicam, nimesulide, celecoxib, refecoxib, indomethacin and phenylbutazone. These are drugs of 1st choice (1st line drugs).
2. Antiinflammatory drugs without direct analgesic action, e.g. glucocorticoids like hydrocortisone, cortisone and predni-solone. These are adjuvant drugs when combined with NSAIDs.
3. Remission inducing drugs with unknown action (disease modifying antirheumatic drugs, DMARDs), e.g. gold salts, peni-cillamine, chloroquine, hydroxychloro-quine, and sulphasalazine. These are 2nd line drugs.
4. Immunosuppressive drugs, e.g. metho-trexate, cyclophosphamide, azathioprine and cyclosporine. These are 3rd line drugs.

DISCUSSION OF INDIVIDUAL GROUP OF DRUGS

Antiinflammatory Analgesics (NSAIDs)

These drugs are discussed in detail in the previous chapter. They relieve pain, decrease the swelling and improve the joint movements. This facilitates the practising of exercises designed from rheumatoid arthritis to promote the maintenance of function and the prevention of deformity. Any of the drugs may be choosen and used for at least 2 to 3 weeks in optimal dosage before switching on to an alternate drug. Combination of these drugs should be avoided, as unacceptable synergistic toxicity may occur. The duration of treatment depends upon the course of the disease and patient response. In mild cases, intermittent therapy is adequate. For acute condition (with flare up of symptoms) short-term therapy may be adequate. For chronic condition (with pain, stiffness and functional disability of joints) prolonged treatment will be required. If the disease does not respond to NSAID therapy and symptoms remain severe, then a glucocorticoid or a disease modifying drug can be combined with NSAID.

Glucocorticoids

Their use in rheumatoid arthritis is usually restricted to patients not responding to NSAIDs or DMARDs. They act as adjuvants with these drugs. They are also used during acute exacerbation of symptoms, as they can slow down the rapid progress of the disease. Although they give dramatic relief of the condition, but they do not alter the natural course of the disease and do not correct pre-existing deformities. The relief lasts as long as the drug is used. During prolonged therapy adverse reactions can be minimized by using small daily dosage (e.g. prednisolone 5 to 10 mg). Intra-articular glucocorticoid therapy (e.g. cortisone or hydrocortisone acetate 25 to 50 mg) in a joint cavity is advocated when there is involvement of 1 or 2 major joints and pain, swelling and immobility of joints are very marked. Injections into a particular joint should not exceed 2 to 3 per year.

Disease Modifying Antirheumatic Drugs (DMARDs)

These drugs are used when NSAID therapy is not able to provide relief to the patient or arrest the course of the disease even after six months of use. These are slow-acting antirheumatic drugs (SAARDs).

- **Gold salts:** Commonly used gold salts in rheumatoid arthritis are sodium aurothiomalate (Myocrisin), and aurothioglucose.

  Sodium aurothiomalate injection (25 mg/ml) is given in the dose of 25 to 50 mg IM weekly for 6 months. Aurantofin capsule (3 mg) is given orally in the dosage of 3 mg twice daily for 6 months. It is better tolerated than injectable gold salt. Their effect develops slowly taking 3 to 4 months for optimum therapeutic response as indicated by reduction in joint pain and swelling and arrest of bone and joint damage. Their mechanism of action in rheumatoid arthritis is not clear. They have anti-inflammatory and immunosuppressive actions. They suppress cell mediated immune reactions leading to reduction in circulating rheumatoid factors and inhibition of synthesis and release of IL-1 from macrophages and neutrophils. They are cumulative drugs. They produce dermatitis, mucosal ulceration, bone marrow depression (producing agranulocytosis and thrombocytopaenia), liver and kidney damage, peripheral neuropathy and encephalopathy. Dimercaprol is used as antidote in gold toxicity. Gold salts should not be used with penicillamine (chelation and antagonism occur) and chloroquine (increases exfoliative dermatitis).

- **d-penicillamine:** It is a sulphur-containing amino acid used as a chelating agent. It chelates a number of heavy metals including copper and gold. It is useful in rheumatoid arthritis. It probably acts by inhibiting the synthesis and release of IL-1 from macrophages and neutrophils. It is administered orally as d-penicillamine (Artamin) capsule (250 mg) in the dosage of 250 mg once daily initially and then gradually increasing every 4 to 8 weeks by 250 mg up to 1 to 1.5 g daily. Treatment is continued for six months and then the dose is gradually decreased. Its common adverse effects are anorexia, nausea, vomiting, impaired taste and buccal ulceration. It can produce serious adverse effects like agranulocytosis, thrombocytopaenia, myositis, skin rashes, SLE and kidney damage.

- **Chloroquine:** It is an antimalarial drug effective in rheumatoid arthritis. It has antiinflammatory and immunosuppressive actions. Its antiinflammatory effect is due to inhibition of phospholipase-A and decrease of arachidonic acid level. Its immunosuppressive effect is due to decrease in synthesis and release of IL-1 from macrophages and neutrophils. It also stabilizes lysosomes and inhibits breakdown of collagen. It is administered as tablet (250 mg) in the dosage of 250 mg daily for one year with gradual withdrawal of the drug thereafter. A drug holiday for three months after six months of therapy allows prolonged treatment. Its common side effects are headache, nausea, vomiting, anorexia, abdominal pain, skin rashes and pruritus. Its serious adverse effects are myopathy, hypotension, deafness and ocular complications like blurring of vision, diplopia, loss of accommodation of vision, lenticular opacity, subcapsular posterior cataract and retinopathy. It should not be used in patients with psoriasis and porphyria and along with gold and phenylbutazone. Hydroxychloroquine is better than chloroquine due to less adverse effects.

- **Sulphasalazine (Salazopyrin):** It is a combination of sulphapyridine with a salicylate. It is used in the treatment of ulcerative colitis. It has been found to be useful and much safer than gold salts in the treatment of rheumatoid arthritis. Its mode of action is not clear, though its active metabolite-5-aminosalicylic acid is known to be a neutrophil derived toxic oxygen metabolite. It is administered as tablet (500 mg) in the dosage of 1g 3 to 4 times daily. It is poorly absorbed and its systemic toxic effects are uncommon even after prolonged use.

IMMUNOSUPPRESSIVE DRUGS (IMMUNOSUPPRESSANTS)

These are anticancer drugs with immunosuppressant action. They are sometimes used in rheumatoid arthritis to produce remission of the disease. These are toxic drugs and so they are reserved for patients with rapidly progressing rheumatoid arthritis not responding to other drugs. Methotrexate (Amethopterin) given intermittently has been found to be effective and less toxic than other drugs. It is administered as tablet (250 mg) in the dosage of 500 to 750 mg once in a week. Clinical response is usually seen in 4 to 8 weeks. If no response is seen after 8 weeks of therapy, the dose may be increased by 2.5 mg every other week to a maximum of 15 mg once weekly and maintained until improvement occurs. After improvement sets in, it is given at lowest effective dose indefinitely, as relapse occurs following discontinuation of therapy. It should not be used during pregnancy (as it is teratogenic) and in liver and kidney diseases. Its long-term use may produce cirrhosis of liver.

GOUT

It is a metabolic disease due to an error in purine metabolism leading to overproduction or decreased renal excretion of urate and hyperuricaemia (high plasma level of uric acid) (shown in **Table 48.1**). It is manifested clinically by arthritis, tenosynovitis, bursitis or cellulitis due to deposition of monosodium urate crystals in the soft tissues like synovial membrane, cartilage, bursa and tendon sheath (in acute gout) and later on development of tophi in the cartilage of ear, nose, bursa and tendon sheath; urolithiasis (urate stone in kidney) and nephropathy (in chronic gout). The metacarpophalangeal joint of a great toe is the site of first attack of acute gouty arthritis in 70% of patients. The ankle, knee, small joints of feet and hands, wrist and elbow follow decreasing order of frequency. The affected joint is hot, red and swollen with shiny

Table 48.1: Causes of hyperuricaemia and gout

Increased production of urate	Decreased renal excretion of urate
Genetic causes	**Genetic causes**
• Deficiency of the enzyme, hypoxanthine-guaninephosphoribosyl transferase (HGPRT). • Overactivity of the enzyme, phosphoribosyl pyrophosphate (PRPP) synthetase. • Deficiency of the enzyme, glucose-6-phosphatase idiopathic.	Decreased fractional renal excretion of urate inspite of overall normal renal function (commonest cause). Type I glycogen storage disease.
Acquired causes	**Acquired causes**
• High purine intake • High fructose intake • Excessive alcohol consumption • Myeloproliferative disorders (e.g. polycythaemia vera). • Lymphoproliferative disorders (e.g. chronic lymphatic leukaemia) • Psoriasis (severe, exfoliative).	• Renal failure • Drugs (some diuretics, pyrazinamide, ethambutol, niacin, cytotoxic drugs, aspirin in small doses). Lead poisoning. • Myxoedema • Hyperparathyroidism • Hypertension • Lactic acidosis (by drugs like alcohol and biguanides and in starvation, severe vomiting and toxaemia of pregnancy).

overlying skin and dilated veins and extremely painful and tender. The inflammatory response is due to local generation of inflammatory mediators like leukotrienes (LTs) and prostaglandiens (PCs) and migration of neutrophil cells (granulocytes) to the inflammed area to engulf urate crystals by phagocytosis and to liberate toxic free oxygen radicals, which in turn cause lysis of the cells with release of proteolytic enzymes that sustain the inflammation.

Drugs Used in Gout

Classification

These are of two groups:

1. **Drugs used in acute gouty arthritis (for short-term therapy):** These are colchicine, NSAIDs (piroxicam, indomethacin, ibuprofen, phenyl butazone, oxphenbutazone, etc.) and glucocorticoids (prednisolone, β-methasone, hydrocortisone, etc.).

2. **Drugs used in chronic gout (for long-term therapy):** These are as follows:
   – Uric acid synthesis inhibitors, e.g. allopurinol.
   – Uricosuric drugs, e.g. probenecid, sulphinpyrazone, benzbromarone, azapropazone and aspirin (in high dosage).

DISCUSSION OF INDIVIDUAL GROUP OF DRUGS

Colchicine

It is an alkaloid obtained from the bulb of autumn crocus (*Colchicum autumnale*). Demecolchine is a semisynthetic product.

Pharmacokinetics

It is rapidly absorbed from GIT. It is partly metabolized in the liver. It undergoes enterohepatic circulation. It is excreted in urine and faeces as metabolites and unchanged form.

Pharmacological Actions

It has selective antiinflammatory action in acute gouty arthritis. It is not an analgesic but it produces dramatic relief of pain in acute attack of gout but not in other types of pain.

Mechanism of Action

It causes inhibition of migration of granulocytes into the inflammed area. It does not prevent the phagocytosis of urate crystals by the granulocytes but prevents the production and release of the glycoprotein by the granulocytes after phagocytosis of urate crystals. The intra-articular release of glycoprotein and other substances (proinflammatory enzymes) by the granulocytes is responsible for acute inflammation. It prevents this inflammatory process.

Other Effects

It is an antimitotic agent (arrests cell division in animal and plant cells). It arrests mitosis at metaphase. It binds microtubular protein tubulin and interfers with the function of mitotic spindles. Cells with highest rate of division are affected earlier. It also inhibits the release of histamine from mast cells and the secretion of insulin from β-cells of islets of Langerhans. It depresses body temperature.

Clinical Uses

It is used in the treatment and prevention of acute attacks of gouty arthritis.

Preparations and Dosage

- Colchicine (Goutnil) tablet (0.5 mg): For treatment in acute gout—initially 1 mg, then 0.5 mg every two hours until pain is relieved or diarrhoea starts (maximum total dose 10 mg)
- For prevention—0.5 mg once or twice daily.

Adverse Reactions

Its common side effects are nausea, vomiting, abdominal pain and diarrhoea, which may be severe. Prolonged therapy (chronic use) may cause anaemia, alopecia, leucopenia, agranulocytosis, myopathy, peripheral neuropathy, renal damage, haemorrhagic gastroenteritis and rarely azoospermia and chromosomal abnormalities. Cimetidine and erythromycin reduce the metabolism of colchicine and thus increase its toxicity.

NONSTEROIDAL ANTIINFLAMMATORY AGENTS

These drugs are used to relieve pain and inflammation in acute gouty arthritis. They have mild uricosuric action in high doses. Piroxicam (20 mg orally twice daily) or indomethacin (50 mg orally thrice daily) is highly effective, but the incidence of intolerance is high. Other drugs can be used but have high toxicity.

Glucocorticoids

These drugs can be used in very severe cases of acute gout, which are refractory (not responding) to colchicine and nonsteroidal antiinflammatory agents (NSAIDs). They should not be used routinely as their action is not specific and the relapse rate is high following their withdrawal. Prednisolone is commonly used. It is given in the dose of 30 to 40 mg orally in divided doses on the first day and then the dose is progressively reduced by 5 to 10 mg everyday. If it is withdrawn suddenly acute attack of gout may be precipitated. When a large joint like knee joint is affected, aspiration of fluid and intra-articular injection of cortisone or hydrocortisone acetate (25 to 50 mg) can produce dramatic relief.

Uric Acid Synthesis Inhibitors
Allopurinol

It is an analogue of hypoxanthine. It is useful for long-term treatment of chronic gout.

Pharmacokinetics

It is well-absorbed from GIT. A small portion of it binds with plasma proteins. It is metabolized in the liver by the enzyme—xanthine oxidase to alloxanthine. Both allopurinol and alloxanthine inhibit xanthine oxidase and excreted in urine. Allopurinol has a short plasma t½ (2 hours), while alloxanthine has a long plama t½ (about 20 hours).

Pharmacological Actions

It lowers blood urate level by increasing excretion of oxypurines, hypoxanthine and xanthine in urine.

Mechanism of Action

It is an uric acid synthesis inhibitor. During purine metabolism, the purine nucleotides are degraded to hypoxanthine and xanthine by the action of the enzyme, xanthine oxidase. These oxypurines are finally oxidized to uric acid by the action of xanthine oxidase (as shown in **Fig. 48.1**). Allopurinol and its metabolite alloxanthine are potent inhibitors of xanthine oxidase and thus interfere with the oxidation of hypoxanthine and xanthine to uric acid. This results in decrease of relatively insoluble urates in tissues with concomitant increase in soluble hypoxanthine and xanthine in tissues and blood which are then excreted by the kidney.

It also inhibits denovosynthesis of purine. It has an inhibitory action on hepatic microsomal enzyme system and thus potentiates the action of warfarin by inhibiting its metabolism. It prolongs the duration of action of probenecid when used concurrently. It also prolongs the duration of action of 6-mercaptopurine, which is metabolized by xanthine oxidase.

Clinical Uses

It is used in the treatment of chronic gout and in the prevention of acute attacks of gout. It is particularly useful in patients with gouty tophi or uric acid renal calculi (urolithiasis).

Preparation and Dosage

Allopurinol (Zyloric) tablet (100 mg)—100 mg daily initially in a single daily dose and then gradually increased in 2 to 3 weeks to 300 to 500 mg daily.

Adverse Reactions

It has low incidence of adverse reactions. It can occasionally cause GIT side effects (nausea, vomiting and diarrhoea), allergic reactions (skin rashes and urticaria), bone marrow depression (leucopenia and agranulocytosis), hepatic and renal damage. There is increased risk of acute attack of gout during initial treatment in chronic gout by mobilizing uric acid from tophi, bones, muscles and joints and producing hyperuricaemia. This can be prevented by concurrent use of colchicine in the initial treatment of chronic gout.

Uricosuric Drugs

Probenecid

It is a derivative of benzoic acid. It was introduced originally to reduce the renal excretion of penicillin. It is completely absorbed from GIT. It is highly (about 90%) plasma protein bound. It is metabolized in the liver and excreted in urine mainly as glucuronide. It is an effective uricosuric drug. In large therapeutic dosage, it inhibits (blocks) renal tubular reabsorption of filtered urate (by active transport) and increases excretion of urate in urine. However, in small dosage, it decreases renal excretion of uric acid, penicillins, cephalosporins, dapsone, indomethacin and sulphonylureas by inhibiting (blocking) distal tubular secretion of these substances.

Clinical Uses

- It is used as an uricosuric agent in chronic gout and hyperuricaemia.

- It is used to prolong the duration of actions of penicillins and cephalosporins by decreasing their renal secretions.

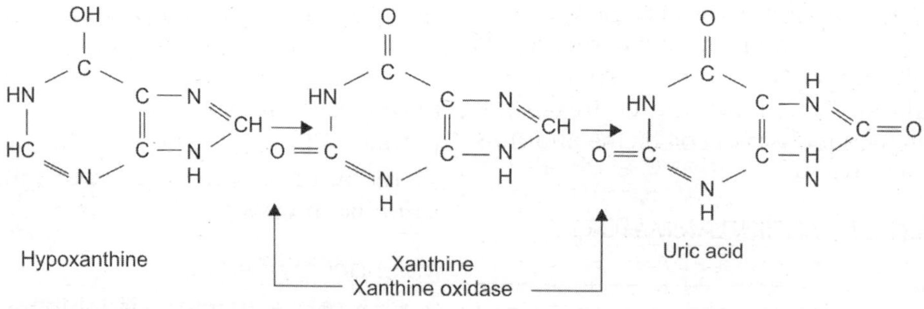

Fig. 48.1: Synthesis of uric acid

Preparation and Dosage

Probenecid (Benemid) tablet (500 mg)—500 mg once daily and then gradually increased to three times daily.

Adverse Reactions

It is relatively nontoxic and well-tolerated. It can occasionally produce GIT upsets (anorexia and dyspepsia), allergic reactions (skin rashes and urticaria) and deposition of urate crystals in the renal tubules or pelvis. It may precipitate haemolytic anaemia in patients with G-6-phosphate dehydrogenase deficiency in RBCs. It can precipitate acute attack of gout by massive mobilization of urate crystals from tophi and other places causing hyperuricaemia. This can be prevented by concurrent use of colchicine like allopurinol. Aspirin blunts the uricosuric effect of probenecid.

Hence, probenecid should not be used in combination with salicylates, as the efficacy of such combination is much less than that of probenecid.

Sulphinpyrazone

It is a congener of phenylbutazone but it has no anti-inflammatory and analgesic actions. Its mechanism of uricosuric action is like that of probenecid, i.e. inhibition of renal tubular reabsorption of filtered urate. It is more potent uricosuric drug than probenecid on weight basis. It is available as sulphinpyrazone (Artiran) capsule (100 mg) and administered in the dosage of 100 mg twice or thrice daily. It is now rarely used in chronic gout due to its serious toxicities like blood dyscrasis (by bone marrow depression) and hypersensitivity reactions. It can also aggravate an existing peptic ulcer.

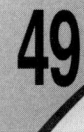

49

Psychopharmacology: Antipsychotic Drugs

INTRODUCTION

Mental disorders (psychiatric illness/behavioural disorders) are common diseases (incidence about 5%).

They are broadly divided into two groups: Psychoses and Neuroses.

Psychoses are serious mental disorders and are divided into two groups:
1. Organic/toxic mental disorders such as delirium (acute state) and dementia (chronic state).
2. Functional mental disorders such as schizophrenia personality (paranoid) disorder, alcoholic psychosis (during withdrawal), psychoses due to old age or brain tumour, and affective disorders like mental depression and mania. Neuroses are less serious mental disorders and are anxiety disorders such as generalized anxiety disorder, phobic disorder, panic disorder and obsessive-compulsive disorder.

Biochemical Basis of Mental Disorders

The neurochemical etiology of mental disorders is still controversial. They are thought to be due to alterations of the central neurotransmitter activity in the mesolimbic system of brain, e.g. schizophrenia is due to increased dopaminergic activity, mental depression is due to decreased mono-aminergic activity and anxiety is due to decreased GABA-ergic activity.

Psychotropic/Psychoactive Drugs

These are drugs capable of modifying mental activity in psychiatric illness/behavioural disorders. These are of five groups:

1. Antipsychotic drugs (neuroleptics), e.g. chlorpromazine, haloperidol, clozapine, molindone, sulpiride, etc.
2. Antianxiety drugs (anxiolytics), e.g. diazepam, alprazolam, meprobamate, buspirone, zolpidem, etc.
3. Antidepressants (mood elevators), e.g. imipramine, amitriptyline, trazadone, fluoxetine, nialamide, tranylcypromine, etc.
4. Antimanic drugs (mood stabilizers), e.g. lithium carbonate, sodium valproate, carbamazepine, etc.
5. Psychostimulants, e.g. amphetamines, methyl phenidate, etc.

Antipsychotic Drugs (Neuroleptics/Major Tranquilizers)

These are drugs used in the treatment of schizophrenia and other types of psychosis.

Schizophrenia is a disorder of thought process and the patient fails to comprehend the reality. It is manifested as split mind, hallucination (auditory or visual), delusion (firmed false belief), incoherent talking and thinking, aggressive mood, excitement and loss of interest to anybody in the society.

Classification of Antipsychotic Drugs

These are of two groups:

1. Typical (classical) neuroleptics (block both dopaminergic D_1 and D_2 receptors):

These are as follows:

- Phenothiazines, e.g. chlorpromazine, triflupromazine, trifluperazine, prochlorperazine, perphenazine, fluphenazine, thioridazine and mesoridazine.
- Butyrophenones, e.g. haloperidol, droperidol and trifluperidol.
- Thioxanthenes, e.g. chlorprothixene, thiothixene and flupenthixol.
- Indoles, e.g. reserpine.

2. Atypical neuroleptics (block only D_2 receptor selectively):

These are as follows:

- Dibenzazopines, e.g. clozapine, loxapine, quetiapine and olanzapine.
- Dihydroindolones, e.g. molindone.
- Piperidines, e.g. pimozide, resperidone and fluspirilene.
- Benzamides, e.g. sulpiride and remoxipride.

DISCUSSION OF SOME NEUROLEPTICS

Chlorpromazine

It is discussed as prototype drug of neuroleptics. It was named largactil by Madam Courvoisier in 1953 for its large number of actions.

Chemically it is a phenothiazine derivative. Phenothiazine has a three ring structure, in which two benzene rings are joined by S and N atoms.

R_1 and R_2 are radicals

Pharmacokinetics

After oral administration it is irregularly and incompletely absorbed from GIT due to high first pass metabolism in the gut wall and liver. It is well-absorbed when administered IM. It is highly plasma protein bound (about 80%). It is lipophilic and can easily cross BBB and PB. Its concentration in brain is higher than that in plasma. It is metabolized in the liver by hydroxylation followed by glucuronidation, sulphoxidation or demethylation. Its inactive metabolites are slowly excreted in urine. It has a plasma t½ of about 30 hours and so it is administered once daily. On chronic use it accumulates in body tissues producing cumulative toxicity.

Pharmacological Actions

Mechanism of action: It acts by blocking both dopaminergic D_1 and D_2 receptors in the mesolimbic system and other parts of brain. It produces following effects:

- **CNS effects:** These are as follows:

  - **Behavioural effects**

    - **In human beings:** In a psychotic patient it produces neuroleptic syndrome, characterized by emotional quietening, psychomotor slowing, indifference to surroundings and diminution of initiative and anxiety without affecting wakefulness. The patient becomes calm and drowsy, sits in silence and shows indifference to the events around him (responding minimally to external stimuli). Spontaneous motor activities (movements) are reduced but avoidance reaction to punishment (e.g. withdrawal of limb after pin prick) persists. There is little ataxia and incoordination (unlike sedative hypnotics). Gradually all the symptoms of psychosis, i.e. hallucinations, delusions, agitation, aggressive behaviour, thought disorder, anxiety, tension and disturbed sleep are ameliorated and the patient becomes more communicative and responsive.

    - **In a normal person,** it produces drowsiness, lethargy, apathy and discomfortness (unpleasantness).

- **In experimental animals (rats, mice and monkeys):** It has ability to tame animals, e.g. Rhesus monkeys which are intractable, become easy to handle after its administration. At low dosage, it reduces aggressive behaviour and spontaneous locomotor activity and at higher dosage, it produces catalepsy, which is an abnormal motor state, in which the animal is positioned in an unusual posture. It also selectively blocks conditioned avoidance (trained) response without blocking unconditioned avoidance (escape/untrained) response. For this test rats are trained to respond to a light (from a bulb) or a sound (from a bell) (conditioned stimulus), which proceeds a punishing foot shock from an electrified grid floor (unconditioned stimulus). Once trained the rat will avoid the unconditioned stimulus (foot shock) by escaping to a safe place (unshocked) in the cage after climbing a pole from the floor of the cage.

At low dosage, chlorpromazine interferes with the ability of the rat to avoid the shock (conditioned response), but not with the ability to escape the shock once it is applied (unconditioned response). On the other hand, sedative hypnotics block both conditioned avoidance response and unconditioned escape response due to greater decrease in motor performance than chlorpromazine.

- Other CNS effects
  - **Sedative effects:** It initially produces sedation causing drowsiness and lethargy, but these gradually disappear due to development of tolerance.
  - **Antiemetic effects:** It prevents nausea and vomiting by blocking the dopaminergic D_2 receptor in CTZ in subneuroleptic dosage.
  - **Hypothermic effects:** It produces lowering of body temperature by interfering with the normal regulation of body temperature by disrupting thermostat mechanism in the hypothalamus.
  - **Muscle relaxant effects:** It causes relaxation of skeletal muscles in some types of spastic disorders, probably by blocking gamma motor neuron discharge (motor activity). It can produce catatonia in some schizophrenic patients, which is similar to cataleptic immobility observed in animals. It can produce extrapyramidal effects like parkinsonism in large dosage by blocking the dopaminergic D_1 receptor in basal ganglia.
  - **Epileptogenic effects:** It can produce epileptic fits (seizures) in untreated epileptic patients by lowering seizure threshold in the motor cortex. The dose of antiepileptic drug is to be increased during its use.
  - **Potentiation of analgesic effects:** It has no analgesic effect but it potentiates narcotic or non-narcotic analgesia.

- **ANS effects:** It produces antiadrenergic and anticholinergic effects. By blocking adrenergic α_1 receptors it produces postural hypotension, nasal stuffiness and failure of ejaculation. By blocking cholinergic-muscarinic (M_1, M_2 and M_3) receptors it produces dryness of mouth, blurring of vision, decreased sweating, urinary retention and constipation.

- **CVS effects:** It has quinidine like cardiac depressant action on the heart and produces bradyarrhythmias. It produces postural hypotension by central and peripheral actions on sympathetic tone (by blocking adrenergic α_1 receptors leading to vasodilatation). This can produce syncope and reflex tachycardia.

- **Renal effects:** It produces mild diuretic effect by either direct inhibition of reabsorption of water and electrolytes in renal tubules or inhibition of ADH secretion/release. It does not change GFR.

- **Endocrine effects:** On chronic use it produces marked changes in the endocrine system. It increases the secretion of prolactin by inhibiting the release of hypothalamic prolactin release inhibitory hormone and produces hyperprolactinaemia. It inhibits the secretion/release of ACTH, growth hormone, gonadotropins, oestrogens, progestogen, insulin and ADH from the respective endocrine glands. It can produce amenorrhoea by blocking ovulation due to decreased gonadotropins secretion.

- **Miscellaneous effects:** It has a procaine like local anaesthetic action, but it is not used as local anaesthetic as it is locally irritant. It has sedative and antipruritic actions by blocking histaminic H_1 and serotonergic 5-HT_1 receptors.

Clinical Uses

These are given as follows:

- **In the treatment of psychoses** such as schizophrenia, paranoid disorder, alcoholic psychosis (during withdrawal of alcohol) and manic depressive psychosis. It relieves symptoms in the psychotic patient within 2 to 3 weeks but cannot cure the disease by removing the cause. Hence, long-term (even lifelong) treatment is required in schizophrenia and paranoid disorder. In acute psychosis, the treatment is started by parenteral (IM) therapy, which is followed by oral medication when symptoms are controlled. In resistant patient, another neuroleptic drug from a different chemical group may be used. It is also effective in behavioural disorders in children.

- **In the treatment of vomiting (as an antiemetic):** It controls nausea and vomiting due to various causes including drug induced vomiting, vomiting due to radiation and uraemia, but it is ineffective in motion sickness (where dopaminergic pathway through the CTZ is not involved). It is effective in morning sickness, but it should not be used in this condition as it effects foetus by crossing PB.

- **In the treatment of intractable hiccups:** It controls this condition when administered parenterally but the mechanism of action is unknown.

- **As preanaesthetic medication:** It is used parenterally to cause sedation, tranquillization and antiemesis and to potentiate the analgesic and muscle relaxant effects of general anaesthetics.

- **For lytic cocktail:** It is used parenterally along with promethazine and pethidine two hours before cardiovascular or neurosurgery to produce bloodless field of operation by hypothermia.

Preparations and Dosage

- Chlorpromazine hydrochloride (Largactil) tablet (25, 100 mg) or syrup (25 mg/mL).
  - As antiemetic—25 to 50 mg orally.
  - As antipsychotic—200 to 800 mg daily in divided doses.
- Chlorpromazine hydrochloride injection (25 mg/mL in 2 mL ampoule).
  - As antiemetic—25 to 50 mg IM.
  - As antipsychotic—100 to 400 mg IM daily.

Adverse Reactions

These are given as follows:

- CNS side effects like sedation, drowsiness, lethargy, mental confusion and extrapyramidal effects (parkinsonism, acute dystonias, akathisia and tardive dyskinesia).

- ANS side effects like dryness of mouth, blurring of vision, urinary retention, postural hypotension, nasal stuffiness and failure of ejaculation.

- CVS side effects like bradycardia, bradyarrhythmias and hypotension.

- Endocrine side effects like amenorrhoea, infertility and galactorrhoea in female and decreased libido and gynaecomastia in male.

- Hypersensitivity (allergic) reactions like skin rashes, urticaria, various types of dermatitis including photosensitivity reaction, blood dyscrasias (agranulocytosis and eosinophilia) and cholestatic (obstructive) jaundice with portal infiltration of bile pigments.

- Miscellaneous adverse effects like blue pigmentation of exposed skin, corneal and lenticular opacities and retinal degeneration can occur on long-term use in high dosage. It can produce a serious condition called neuroleptic malignant syndrome (manifested as catatonia, hyperpyrexia, muscular rigidity, altered consciousness, autonomic instability, i.e. tachycardia and unstable BP and increased sweating) when used in high dose. It is associated with increased serum creatinine kinase activity. In it, myoglobin is found in blood (myoglobinaemia). It occurs within 1 week of treatment and persists for about 4 weeks. It is due to marked decrease of central dopaminergic activity with marked increase of central cholinergic activity. It may be fatal (20% mortality). It is treated by stopping the drug, external cooling by ice or cold water application and administration of dantrolene (a direct muscle relaxant) or bromocriptine (a dopaminergic D_2 agonist). **Tolerance and physical dependence:** Only sedative and hypotensive effects develop tolerance to it after a few weeks of treatment. Antipsychotic and other effects, which are based on dopamine antagonism, do not develop tolerance to it. It does not produce physical dependence.
Acute toxicity (poisoning): It may occur due to overdose. It is manifested as severe hypotension, respiratory depression and coma. Treatment is symptomatic and supportive.

Drug Interactions

- It potentiates the effects of all CNS depressants.
- It blocks the effect of levodopa in parkinsonism by dopamine antagonism.
- It decreases the antihypertensive effects of guanethidine, methyldopa and clonidine by inhibiting their neuronal uptake.

- Phenobarbitone and phenytoin (microsomal enzyme inducers) decrease its effects by increasing metabolism.
- Antacids reduce its absorption from GIT and anticholinergics increase its transit time in GIT leading to its decreased bioavailability.

Trifluperazine (Espazine)

It is a phenothiazine derivative. It has pharmacological properties like chlorpromazine. It is a highly potent antipsychotic drug (dosage 5 to 10 mg/day) but it produces marked extrapyramidal effects.

Fluphenazine (Anatensol)

It is a phenothiazine derivative. It has pharmacological properties like chlorpromazine. It is a highly potent antipsychotic drug (dosage 2 to 4 mg/day) but it produces marked extrapyramidal effects.

Thioridazine (Melleril)

It is a phenothiazine derivative. It has pharmacological properties like chlorpromazine. It is a moderately potent antipsychotic drug (dosage—150 to 600 mg/day) but it produces moderate sedative and hypotensive effects and mild extrapyramidal effects.

Haloperidol (Serenase)

It is a butyrophenone derivative. It has pharmacological properties like chlorpromazine. It is a highly potent antipsychotic drug (dosage—5 to 10 mg/day) but it produces marked extrapyramidal effects and moderate autonomic effects.

Reserpine (Serpasil)

It is a rauwolfia alkaloid and an indole derivative. It has pharmacological properties like chlorpromazine. It differs from chlorpromazine in that it has no antihistaminic, anticholinergic or direct antiadrenergic effects. It acts by depletion of endogenous catecholamines and 5-HT from the brain and peripheral sites. It has antipsychotic and antihypertensive effects. It is a highly potent antipsychotic drug (dosage—1 to 5 mg/day) but it produces many adverse effects including extrapyramidal effects (moderate), epileptic and severe mental depression (precipitating suicidal tendency). Hence, it is now obsolete.

Clozapine (Clozaril)

It is an atypical antipsychotic belonging to dibenzazopines. It has selective effects in the dopaminergic mesolimbic system. It has also antiadrenergic, anti-5-HT and anticholinergic effects. It differs from chlorpromazine in that it produces very little extrapyramidal effects

and does not cause hyperprolactinaemia. It is a moderately potent antipsychotic drug (dosage—50 to 100 mg/day) but it produces agranulocytosis and epileptic fits. Loxapine (Loxapac) and olanzapine (Olzap/Olimez) are similar drugs to clozapine.

Pimozide (Orap)

It is an atypical antipsychotic drug belonging to piperidines. It has selective effects like clozapine. It is a highly potent antipsychotic drug (dosage—1 to 5 mg/day) but it produces marked extrapyramidal effects and cardiotoxicity.

50

Antianxiety Drugs (Anxiolytics)

INTRODUCTION

Antianxiety drugs are used to decrease anxiety and tension. They are also called minor tranquillizers. They can produce mild sedation and hypnosis.

Anxiety is an unpleasant feeling characterized by uneasiness and apprehension. It is due to decreased GABAergic activity in the mesolimbic system of brain. It may be primary (generalized anxiety disorder, phobic disorder, panic disorder and obsessive-compulsive disorder) or secondary (disease induced anxiety, i.e. myocardial infarction, angina pectoris, hypertension, peptic ulcer, ulcerative colitis, cholelithiasis, appendicitis, irritable bowel syndrome or sexual disorder). Treatment of anxiety is instituted only when the cause of anxiety cannot be removed. Earlier barbiturates and allied sedative hypnotics were used to relieve anxiety but they produce marked sedation, respiratory depression and addiction liability. Hence, they are now not used in anxiety. The introduction of benzodiazepines and selective anxiolytics has changed the concept of anxiolytic therapy.

Classification of Anxiolytics

These are of five groups:
1. Benzodiazepines (BDZs), e.g. diazepam, chlordiazepoxide, lorazepam, oxazepam, nitrazepam, alprazolam, triazolam and ketazolam.
2. Azapyrones, e.g. buspirone and ipsapirone.

3. Imidazole pyridines, e.g. zolpidem and zopiclone.
4. 5-HT antagonists, e.g. kitanserin and ondansetron.
5. Miscellaneous drugs, e.g. meprobamate, propranolol, amitriptyline, hydroxyzine and diphenhydramine.

DISCUSSION OF INDIVIDUAL GROUP OF ANXIOLYTICS

Benzodiazepines

At present these are the most commonly used antianxiety drugs. They have similar pharmacological properties but they differ in their pharmacokinetic profiles. They act by potentiating the GABAergic activity by binding with specific BDZ receptors, which are closely associated with $GABA_A$ receptors and Cl^- channels. They increase $GABA_A$ receptor sensitivity and Cl^- conductance (by opening of Cl^- channels) leading to hyperpolarization of the neuronal membrane. They have been discussed in detail in the chapter of sedative-hypnotics.

Commonly used Preparations and Dosage

- Alprazolam (Alprax/Alzolam) tablet (0.25, 0.5 mg)—0.5 to 1 mg daily in divided doses.
- Lorazepam (Larpose; Ativan) tablet (1 mg)—1 to 2 mg daily in divided doses.
- Diazepam (Valium; Calmpose) tablet (5 mg)—10 to 20 mg daily in divided doses.

Azapyrones

These are selective anxiolytic drugs. They do not act directly on GABAergic receptors but act indirectly *via* serotonergic (5HT$_{1A}$) receptors, resulting in an inhibition of the dorsal raphe discharge. They lack the sedative-hypnotic, muscle relaxant and anticonvulsant properties of benzodiazepines. They do not potentiate the effects of CNS depressant drugs. They are particularly useful in anxious elderly patients. Their onset of action is slow and may take one week to develop. They have weaker anxiolytic effect than benzodiazepines. They cause less psychological impairment than benzodiazepines.

Preparation and Dosage

Buspirone (Buspar/Buscalm) tablet (5, 10 mg)—10 to 20 mg daily in divided doses.

Imidazole Pyridines

These are non-benzodiazepine compounds but act by binding with benzodiazepine receptors to potentiate GABA effect. They have also sedative-hypnotic effect.

Preparations and Dosage

- Zolpidem (Nitrest) tablet (5, 10 mg)—5 to 10 mg daily.
- Zopiclone (Zopicon) tablet (7.5 mg)—7.5 mg to 15 mg daily.

5-HT Antagonists

Kitanserin is a 5-HT$_{2A}$ antagonist and ondansetron is a 5-HT$_3$ antagonist with central sedative action. They are discussed with 5-HT antagonists in the section of autacoids.

Miscellaneous Anxiolytics

Meprobamate is an interneuronal blocking agent. It has central sedative and muscle relaxant activities. In the patient with anxiety, it relieves tension, fear and tremulousness and produces a sense of well-being. It is a weaker anxiolytic than benzodiazepines. It can produce tolerance and drug dependence.

Propranolol is a nonselective β-blocker. It acts by decreasing the peripheral autonomic manifestations of anxiety such as tachycardia, hypertension and tremors. Amitriptyline is a tricyclic antidepressant with anxiolytic activity. Hydroxyzine and diphenhydramine are H$_1$ receptor antagonists with sedative and anxiolytic activities. They are discussed in respective chapters.

51

Antidepressant Drugs (Mood Elevators)

INTRODUCTION

Antidepressants are drugs used in the treatment of mental depression, especially endogenous (major/unipolar) depression. Thymoleptics are mood modifiers used in affective disorders like mental depression and mania. These are antidepressants and antimanic drugs.

Mental depression is a state of alteration of mood characterized by melancholy (sadness), hopelessness, worry and anxiety. The patient also suffers from insomnia, anorexia, weight loss, and decreased energy and sexual activity (libido) and shows total disinterest in normal activities and to the surroundings and there is suicidal tendency. It is thought to be due to decreased monoaminergic activity in the mesolimbic system of brain.

Types of Mental Depression

These are of three types:

1. **Endogenous (primary) depression (about 65%):** In it, the cause of depression is unknown.
2. **Exogenous (secondary/reactive) depression (about 25%):** In it, the cause is known. It may be psychoneurotic or drug induced (reserpine, methyldopa, etc.). Both endogenous and exogenous depressions are unipolar depression (only depression is present) and are treated by antidepressant drugs.

3. **Manic depressive psychosis (bipolar depression) (about 10%):** In it, there is episode of depression followed by episode of mania (characterized by agitation, aggressiveness and grandiosity). It is treated by antimanic drugs. Severe depression may require electroconvulsive therapy (ECT), which works quickly by increasing postsynaptic receptor response.

Classification of Antidepressant Drugs

These are divided into two groups:

1. Tricyclic antidepressants (TCADs)

These are given as follows:

- Typical antidepressants (classical antidepressants).
  - Predominantly noradrenaline (NA) reuptake inhibitors (NA selective). These are:
    - Secondary amines, e.g. desipramine, nortriptyline, protriptyline, meprotiline, amoxapine, viloxazine and mianserin.
    - Tertiary amines, e.g. imipramine, trimipramine, clomipramine, amitriptyline, doxepin and dothiepin.
  - Predominantly serotonin (5-HT) reuptake inhibitors (5-HT selective), e.g. fluoxetine, paroxetine, fluvoxamine, venlafaxine and sertraline.

- Atypical antidepressants (chemically unrelated to classical antidepressants), e.g. trazodone, nefazodone, bupropion and normifensine.

  These are both dopamine and noradrenaline reuptake inhibitors.

2. **Monoamine oxidase (MAO) inhibitors**

   These are given as follows:

   - Nonselective MAO inhibitors (inhibit both MAO-A and MAO-B), e.g. phenelzine, tranylcypromine, nialamide, isocarboxazid and iproniazid. These are 1st generation MAO-inhibitors.
   - Selective MAO inhibitors, e.g. clorzyline (inhibits MAO-A) and selegiline (inhibits MAO-B). These are 2nd generation MAO inhibitors.

DISCUSSION OF INDIVIDUAL GROUP OF ANTIDEPRESSANTS

Tricyclic Antidepressants

The term tricyclic is a misnomer because all these compounds are not tricyclic, some are bicyclic, e.g. viloxazine, fluoxetine and paroxetine and some are tetracyclic, e.g. trazodone, nefazodone, amoxapine and meprotiline. The basic structure of these compounds is similar to that of phenothiazine except the sulphur atom is replaced by an ethylene bridge.

R_1, R_2 and R_3 are radicals

Imipramine

It is the parent compound of tricyclic antidepressants. It is a dibenzazepine derivative and a tertiary amine. It is discussed as prototype drug of tricyclic antidepressants.

Pharmacokinetics

It is highly lipid-soluble and so rapidly and almost completely absorbed from GIT. It is highly plasma protein bound (about 80%). It is widely distributed in the body. It is more concentrated in brain and cardiac tissues than in other tissues. It is metabolized in the liver by hydroxylation, demethylation and glucuronidation. It is slowly excreted in urine mainly as in active metabolites and slightly (3%) as free form taking about 2 to 3 weeks. It has a plasma t½ of about 20 hours. Hence, it is administered once daily for maintenance therapy. It has narrow therapeutic window.

Pharmacological Actions

Mechanism of action: It acts by inhibiting neuronal reuptake of biogenic monoamines (NA and 5-HT) at presynaptic nerve endings and thus producing accumulation of these amines at respective postsynaptic receptor sites in the mesolimbic system of brain. It thus corrects the deficiency of monoamines or decreased monoaminergic activity that occurs in mental depression, especially in endogenous depression.

It produces following effects:

1. **CNS effects:** In normal persons it produces drowsiness, light headedness, lethargy and anxiety. In depressed patients it produces elevation of mood and normal sleep to those who suffer from insomnia. These patients become more communicative and show more interest to themselves and to surroundings. In high dosage it can produce epileptic fits in untreated epileptics as it is a proconvulsant. It can also produce ataxia and extrapyramidal effects. In experimental animals (rats, mice and monkeys), it depresses spontaneous motor activity but stimulates a variety of behaviour patterns including potentiation of CNS stimulant effects of amphetamines and methyl phenidate and increase of aggressive behaviour induced by hypothalamic lesion.

2. **ANS effects:** It produces anticholinergic effects like dryness of mouth, blurring of vision, palpitation, constipation and urinary retention by blocking muscarinic receptors. It also produces antiadrenergic effects like postural hypotension, nasal stuffiness (nasal vasodilatation and congestion of nasal mucosa) and failure of

ejaculation by blocking α_1-adrenergic receptors.

3. **CVS effects:** It produces bradycardia (due to inhibition of NA reuptake and blockade of muscarinic receptors) and postural hypotension (partly due to α_1-adrenergic receptor blockade and partly due to bradycardia). In large dosage it produces cardiac depressant effect like quinidine and causes ECG changes like inversion or flattening of T-wave and prolongation of PR interval. In toxic dosage it produces cardiac arrhythmias especially ventricular arrhythmias.

Clinical Uses

It is used in:

- Mental depression especially endogenous depression. It relieves symptoms of depression and restores normal social behaviour in these patients. It takes about 2 to 3 weeks time for suppression of all symptoms of depression and full benefit occurs in 4 to 6 weeks time, after which it is continued at a maintenance dose for several (3 to 6) months to prevent relapse of the condition. ECT may be given in severly depressed patients, especially in the initial stage, when the effect of the drug is developing.

- Severe anxiety disorders like obsessive-compulsive neurosis with depression, phobic and panic anxiety disorders with depression. It can be used in these conditions, but trazodone, fluoxetine and clomipramine are better drugs than it.

- Nocturnal enuresis in children and urinary incontinence in elderly persons. It is given at bedtime and continued for 3 to 6 weeks.

- Psychosomatic disorders like bulimia nervosa, chronic pain disorders (neuralgia due to diabetic, alcoholic or other peripheral neuropathy), fibromyalgia, peptic ulcer, irritable bowel syndrome, chronic fatigue (asthenia), migraine and catalepsy (muscular weakness and hypotonia of muscles).

Preparation and Dosage

Imipramine (Depsonil, Depranil) tablet (25, 75 mg)—50 to 150 mg daily in divided doses.

Adverse Reactions

These are given as follows:

- CNS side effects like sedation, drowsiness, dizziness, confusion, ataxia, nystagmus, tremors and rarely seizures.

- ANS side effects like dryness of mouth, blurring of vision, palpitation, constipation, retention of urine, postural hypotension, nasal stuffiness and impotence.

- CVS side effects like bradycardia, postural hypotension, cardiac depression and cardiac arrhythmias.

- Hypersensitivity reactions like skin rashes, agranulocytosis and jaundice.

- Other adverse effects like increased sweating and weight gain (mechanisms unknown).

  Acute toxicity (poisoning) due to overdose is usually suicidal. It is manifested as severe hypotension, respiratory depression and coma. Treatment is symptomatic and supportive.

Tolerance and Physical Dependence

Tolerance to sedative and hypotensive effects develops after a few weeks of treatment. It does not produce physical dependence.

Drug Interactions

- It potentiates the hypertensive action of directly acting sympathomimetic amines (Adr, NA and phenylephrine) but inhibits the hypertensive action of indirectly acting sympathomimetic amines (amphetamines, tyramine and ephedrine).

- It decreases the antihypertensive action of guanethidine, reserpine and clonidine by preventing their transport into adrenergic neurons.

- It potentiates the action of CNS depressants like alcohol and antihistaminics.

- It produces serious reactions (like atropine poisoning) with MAO inhibitors (hypertensive crisis, hyperpyrexia, hallucinations and convulsions leading to coma).
- Enzyme inducers like phenobarbitone and phenytoin decrease its therapeutic effects by increasing its metabolism.
- Highly plasma protein binding drugs like aspirin and phenylbutazone displace it from plasma protein binding sites leading to toxicity.

Other tricyclic antidepressants have similar pharmacological properties and uses of imipramine but they differ in potency and side effects.

Amitriptyline (Tryptomers Amitryn)

It is moderately potent tricylic antidepressant (dosage—100 to 200 mg/day). It has marked sedative, hypotensive, anticholinergic and cardiac effects and moderate epileptic (seizures producing) and weight gain effects.

Clomipramine (Clofranil, Clomil)

It is a moderately potent tricyclic antidepressant (dosage—100 to 200 mg/day). It has marked anticholinergic and cardiac effects, moderate sedative, epileptic and hypotensive effects and mild weight gain effect.

Trimipramine (Surmontil)

It is a moderately potent tricyclic antidepressant (dosage—100 to 200 mg/day). It has side effects like clomipramine.

Nortriptyline (Sensival, Nortin)

It is a moderately potent tricyclic antidepressant (dosage 75 to 150 mg/day). It has moderate cardiac effects and mild sedative, hypotensive, anticholinergic, epileptic and weight gain effects.

Fluoxetine (Fludac, Prodes)

It is a highly potent bicyclic antidepressant (dosage—20 to 40 mg/day). It has mild sedative and epileptic effects and no hypotensive, cardiac, anticholinergic and weight gain effects.

Trazodone (Trazonil, Trazodep)

It is a moderately potent tetracyclic antidepressant (dosage—150 to 200 mg/day). It has marked sedative effect, moderate hypotensive effect, mild cardiac and weight gain effects and no anticholinergic and epileptic effects.

Monoamine Oxidase (MAO) Inhibitors

These are drugs that prevent the action of MAO, which is involved in the metabolism of monoamine neurotransmitters (NA, Adr, DP and 5-HT) and thus increase the store of these transmitters in the brain. Deficiency of monoamines in the mesolimbic system of brain produces mental depression. MAO inhibitors are as effective as tricyclic antidepressants in treating endogenous depression, but their toxicity and potentially toxic interactions with other drugs and with tyramine containing foods (cheese, chocolates, wine, meat, liver and yeast) led to withdrawal of these drugs from antidepressant therapy. Renewed interest in these drugs began, when MAO was found to exist in two forms (isoenzymes)—MAO-A and MAO-B. MAO-A is present in the mesolimbic system of brain, peripheral adrenergic nerve endings, intestinal mucosa, liver and placenta and MAO-B is present in basal ganglia, liver and platelets. MAO-A preferentially metabolizes, (deaminates) NA and 5-HT and is inhibited by clorgyline. MAO-B preferentially metabolizes phenylethyl amine and is inhibited by deprenyl. Dopamine is deaminated by both types of MAO. Nonselective MAO inhibitors produce irreversible inhibition of both MAO-A and MAO-B. It takes about 2 weeks for the body to replenish MAO levels after discontinuation of MAO inhibitor therapy. Though MAO inhibition occurs rapidly but clinical antidepressant effect occurs only after 2 to 3 weeks (lag period) when about 80% of MAO is inhibited. They are hit and run drugs. Nonselective MAO inhibitors, e.g. phenalzine, tranylcypromine, nialamide, isocarboxazid and iproniazid also inhibit intestinal and hepatic oxidases, which is responsible for many of the interactions of these drugs.

Clinical Uses

They can be used in depressed patients not responding to tricyclic antidepressants. They are particularly useful in panic disorder with depression.

Preparations and Dosage

- Tranylcypromine (Parnate) tablet (10 mg)—10 to 20 mg daily.
- Phenalzine (Nardil) tablet (15 mg)—15 to 30 mg daily.
- Clorgyline tablet (15 mg)—15 to 30 mg daily.

Adverse Reactions

Their common adverse effects are postural hypotension, dizziness, vertigo, insomnia, lethargy, headache, tremors, agitation, mental confusion, constipation and allergic reactions (skin rashes). Isocarboxazid and iproniazid are hepatotoxic drugs and produce cholestatic (obstructive) jaundice.

Drug Interactions

- They potentiate the action of many drugs including alcohol, amphetamines, general anaesthetics, anticholinergics, antihistaminics, barbiturates, morphine and pethidine by blocking their degradation in the liver.
- They produce hypertensive crisis with tricyclic antidepressants and foods containing tyramine by releasing monoamines from adrenergic nerve endings in brain and peripheral sites.

52

Antimanics (Mood Stabilizers) and Hallucinogens

INTRODUCTION

Antimanics are drugs that cause stabilization of mood and used in manic depressive psychosis (MDP), i.e. bipolar depression. Manic depressive psychosis or illness (MDI) is a condition of extreme changes in mood characterized by cyclical mood swings, hyperactivity and uncontrolled thought and speech followed by severe depression. There is high suicidal tendency.

Classification of Antimanics

These are of three groups:

1. Lithium salts, e.g. lithium carbonate and lithium citrate.
2. Antipsychotic drugs, e.g. chlorpromazine, haloperidol and pimozide (used in severely manic patients for initial urgent treatment).
3. Miscellaneous drugs, e.g. carbamazepine, sodium valproate, clonazepam, verapamil and clonidine (used as adjuvant or prophylactic drugs).

DISCUSSION OF INDIVIDUAL GROUP OF DRUGS

Lithium Salts

Lithium is a small inorganic monovalent cation, which has the tendency to replace sodium and potassium ions from the biological fluids. It is the lightest of the alkali metal. It was introduced as a psychotropic drug by Cade in 1949, following the observation that it caused lethargy in guinea pigs. It is available as lithium carbonate and lithium citrate for clinical use. Lithium carbonate is preferred than lithium citrate, as it produces less gastric irritation. It is converted to lithium chloride by gastric hydrochloric acid.

Pharmacokinetics

Lithium salt is completely absorbed from GIT. Its peak plasma concentration is reached in 4 to 6 hours. It does not bind to plasma proteins and has low volume of distribution. It is distributed nonuniformly throughout extracellular and intracellular fluids. It has a plasma $t\frac{1}{2}$ of about 20 hours and its equilibrium is reached after one week of regular intake. It crosses BBB slowly and at steady state its CSF concentration is about half of that of plasma concentration. It crosses PB easily. It is secreted in breast milk. It is not metabolized in the body and is entirely eliminated by the kidney in urine. In renal insufficiency its serum concentration is highly increased. It has a narrow therapeutic window and so its serum concentrations need to be monitered during treatment (it should be in between 0.8 to 1.4 mEq/L).

Pharmacological Actions

Mechanism of action: The exact mechanism of action of lithium is unknown. It may act by following mechanisms:

- It alters the activity of some neurotransmitters in the brain by affecting their synthesis. It decreases the rate of synthesis of NA, DP and Ach in the brain and increases their neuronal uptake. It increases the synthesis of 5-HT and GABA in the brain and increases their brain concentrations.

- It decreases the synthesis of second messengers, IP_3 (inositol triphosphate) and DAG (diacylglycerol) in the brain by inhibiting the phosphatidyl inositol biphosphate (PIP_2) formation in the cell membrane. As PIP_2 is the precursor of the two 2nd messengers (IP_3 and DAG), so deficiency of PIP_2 leads to decreased production of the 2nd messengers and loss of effects of neurotransmitters like NA and Ach.

It produces following effects:

- **CNS effects:** It is neither sedative nor euphoriant but on prolonged use it acts as a mood stabilizer in MDP. It is devoid of neurological or behavioural effects in normal persons. If patients with acute mania, it suppresses the episode and on continued treatment prevents cyclic mood swings. It also normalizes the disturbed sleep pattern in manic patient.

- **Other effects:** It inhibits the action of ADH in distal renal tubules and can produce nephrogenic diabetes insipidus. It has some insulin-like actions on glucose metabolism and it increases body weight. It increases leucocyte count and can be used in drug induced leucopenia or agranulocytosis. It decreases the response of thyroid cell to TSH and can produce hypothyroidism with thyroid enlargement.

Clinical Uses

It is used in:

- **Manic depressive psychosis (MDP):** It is effective in both the short-term treatment and prevention of MDP in about 70 to 80% patients. Since lithium treatment takes 7 to 10 days for full therapeutic effect, so an antipsychotic drug (chlorpromazine or haloperidol) is administered along with lithium in the initial phase to control acute episode of mania. Lithium can prevent recurrences and reduce the severity of manic depression. For prophylactic effect, lithium takes several months of treatment.

- **Endogenous depression:** It can be used if the patient does not respond to conventional antidepressant treatment. It converts the patient to a responder.

- **Behavioural disorder (hyperkinetic syndrome) in children:** It prevents episodic outbursts of anger and violence in these mentally disturbed children.

- **Drug induced leucopenia:** It can be used to increase leucocyte count after cancer chemotherapy.

Preparation and Dosage

Lithium carbonate (Lithoril/Lithosun) tablet/capsule (150/300 mg)—initial dose: 300 to 600 mg twice or thrice daily till control of acute mania and maintenance dose: 150 to 300 mg once daily.

Adverse Reactions

Lithium toxicity is closely related to its serum concentrations. Acute toxicity (poisoning) occurs when the serum concentration of lithium exceeds 2.0 mEq/L.

Mild to moderate adverse effects include diarrhoea, vomiting, abdominal pain, thirst, drowsiness, blurring of vision, muscular weakness, tremors, fatigue, ataxia, slurred speech and impaired cognition. Serious adverse effects include cardiac arrhythmias, conduction defects, cardiac failure, hypotension, cerebelar disturbances, choreoathetoid movements, epileptiform seizures and coma. It can also produce allergic reactions. Its chronic administration may give rise to goitre formation, hypothyroidism, nephrogenic diabetes insipidus (manifested as polyuria and polydipsia) and glycosuria. It can produce teratogenicity (foetal malformation) when administered in pregnant women during 1st trimester. It produces neonatal toxicity (manifested as lethargy, cyanosis, decreased reflexes, tremors and hepatomegaly) when administered in lactating mothers. It should be administered very cautiously in patients with cardiovascular, renal or brain damage.

Treatment of Acute Toxicity of Lithium (Due to Overdose)

- Gastric lavage with plain water and administration of a saline purgative.
- Administration of mannitol (IV) and sodium bicarbonate (IV).
- Supportive and symptomatic measures to maintain BP and respiration and to control cardiac arrhythmias and convulsions by drugs.
- Haemodialysis or peritoneal dialysis to remove lithium from the body in serious cases.

Drug Interactions

- Diuretics (thiazides and loop diuretics) produce retention of lithium by producing sodium depletion. Thiazides also reduce renal clearance of lithium.
- NSAIDs decrease renal clearance and increase serum concentrations of lithium by inhibiting renal PG synthesis. Aspirin and paracetamol have little effects in therapeutic doses.
- Lithium increases toxicity of neuroleptic drugs and carbamazepine.

Other Antimanic Drugs

Antipsychotic Drugs (Neuroleptics)

These are used in severely manic patients for initial urgent treatment in high dosage, e.g. chlorpromazine (100 to 200 mg thrice daily), haloperidol (10 to 20 mg twice daily) and pimozide (10 to 20 mg twice daily). Treatment is to be continued for several weeks after the patient becomes normal and then the dose is gradually reduced. They can produce iatrogenic parkinsonism.

Carbamazepine

It is an antiepileptic drug. It is used either alone or in combination with lithium in MDP, when the patient is not responding to lithium. Its mechanism of action is not clear.

It is known to reduce Na^+ influx into neurons, increase serotonergic and dopaminergic activities and block adenosine receptors. It is used in the dosage of 200 to 400 mg twice daily till the patient becomes normal. It is discussed with antiepileptic drugs.

Sodium Valproate

It is another antiepileptic drug, which has been found useful as a substitute for or as an adjuvant to lithium in the treatment of resistant cases of MDP. It is used in the dosage of 200 to 400 mg twice daily till the patient becomes normal. It is discussed with antiepileptic drugs.

Other drugs like clonazepam (an antiepileptic drug), verapamil (a calcium channel blocker) and clonidine (an α_2-adrenoreceptor agonist) have been found effective in resistant cases of MDP. They are discussed in respective chapters.

Hallucinogens (Psychogenic Drugs/ Psychomimetic Drugs/Psychedelics)

These are drugs that produce psychosis like symptoms including hallucinations and schizoid (schizophrenia like) alterations in mood, behaviour and perception. Toxic psychosis is produced by toxic doses of many drugs, but these are associated with other organic and neurological disturbances like delirium, nystagmus and disturbances of equilibrium, gait and speech. Psychotogenic drugs, however, produce selective psychotic states without producing organic and neurological disturbances.

Classification of Hallucinogens

These are of two groups:

1. Drugs with indole ring, e.g. lysergic diethylamide (LSD), psilocybine, bufetenine and harmine.

2. Drugs without indole ring, e.g. cannabis, mescaline and phencyclidine.

DISCUSSION OF SOME HALLUCINOGENS

Lysergic Acid Diethylamide (LSD)

It is a semisynthetic drug chemically related to the ergot alkaloid 'ergometrine' and possesses oxytocic action. It is a potent hallucinogen. It alters visual perception more than auditory, olfactory, tactile and other sensations. Different colours become more intense and visual illusions occur. It produces marked changes in mood with emotional outbursts. The subject may laugh or cry on slightest provocation. It produces distortion of body images and alterations of perception of size, distance or direction. Sometimes these alterations of perception may be frightening or extremely unpleasant. Many subjects experience a fear of disintegration of the self, the syndrome lasts for about 12 hours after oral administration. In addition to these behavioural effects, it produces prominent central sympathetic stimulation leading to tachycardia, dilatation of pupil, tremors, piloerection and hyperglycaemia. It decreases serotonergic (5-HT) activity in brain and periphery. It produces tolerance and drug dependence (especially psychological). It is not used clinically. It is used as an experimental tool to produce model of psychosis for the evaluation of antipsychotic drugs.

Cannabis/Marijuana

It is a plant product obtained from the hemp plants: *Cannabis indica* and *Cannabis sativa*. It contains many active principles which are psychoactives and called cannabinoids. The most important active principle is A^9 THC (A^9 tetrahydrocannabinol). Other less active principles are *ganja* (from flowering tops), *bhang* (from leaves), *charas* (from resinous exudate of the plant) and *hashis* (from the whole plant). Nabilone is a synthetic derivative of THC. When smoked, THC is rapidly absorbed and effects appear within a few minutes and last for about 2 to 3 hours. Given orally, the onset of action is delayed up to t½ to 1 hour. The behavioural effects of cannabinoids are euphoria, drowsiness, dreamy state and hallucinations. The individual may become garrulous and hilarious, sometimes exhibiting uncontrollable laughter even with minimum stimuli. Time sense is altered. Hearing becomes less discriminating. Vision becomes apparently sharper with many visual distortions. Colours look more brighter and vivid. Cognitive functions are suppressed and mental and motor coordination is reduced. Sleep pattern is altered and vivid dreams occur. Besides these behavioural effects, they produce tachycardia, hypotension, bronchodilatation conjunctival congestion, antiemetic, analgesic, muscle relaxant and anticonvulsant effects. Only naboline is used as an antiemetic and analgesic in cancer patients on cytotoxic drug therapy. Other cannabinoids are not used clinically due to high addiction liability. They produce depersonalization, tolerance and drug dependence (especially psychological). Mild abstinence symptoms like insomnia, nausea, diarrhoea, sweating and tremors are produced on withdrawal of these drugs.

Mescaline

It is obtained from Mexican *Peyote cactus*. It is used as a hallucinogen (low potency) by the natives of Mexico during festivals. It produces visual hallucinations and psychic effects. It is not used clinically.

Phencyclidine

It is related to ketamine. It was introduced to produce dissociative anaesthesia but now not used as it produces hallucinations and drug dependence. It binds with opioid σ receptor.

53

Central Nervous System Stimulants and Cerebroactive Drugs

INTRODUCTION

Central nervous system (CNS) stimulants are drugs whose primary action is to stimulate the CNS. They are not much used because they have nonselective (generalized) action and in higher doses can cause convulsions. Many other drugs can produce CNS stimulation (by secondary action) as side effects or at high doses. Nicotine, lobeline, ammonium carbonate, etc. stimulate CNS reflexly.

Classification of CNS Stimulants

These are of three groups:

1. **Cerebral stimulants (psychostimulants),** e.g. caffeine, cocaine, amphetamines, methyl phenidate, ephedrine, atropine, etc.
2. **Medullary stimulants:** These are as follows:
   - Analeptics, e.g. nikethamide, doxapram, ethylbutamide and propylbutamide.
   - Convulsants, e.g. pentyline tetrazole, picrotoxin and bicuculine.
3. **Spinal stimulants (convulsants),** e.g. strychnine and brucine.

DISCUSSION OF INDIVIDUAL GROUP OF DRUGS

Cerebral Stimulants (Psychostimulants)
Caffeine

It is an alkaloid obtained from coffee seeds and tea leaves. Of the three naturally occurring methylxanthines (caffeine, theophylline and theobromine), only caffeine is used as a psychostimulant. It produces more rapid and clear flow of thought and reduces drowsiness and fatigue. It stimulates heart and dilates coronary and other blood vessels. It increases the strength of skeletal muscle contraction. It relaxes nonvascular smooth muscles. It has a diuretic effect like theophylline. It increases gastric secretion by stimulating secretion of gastrin.

It acts by three cellular mechanisms of action:

1. It releases Ca^{2+} from sarcoplasmic reticulum, especially in skeletal and cardiac muscles.
2. It inhibits the enzyme, phosphodiesterase, which degrades cyclic nucleotides (cAMP and cGMP).
3. It blocks adenosine receptors, especially in smooth muscles.

It is used in combination with aspirin to relieve headache, mental exhaustion and fatigue. It is also used in combination with ergotamine to relieve headache due to migraine.

It is used as caffeine or caffeine citrate in the dosage of 50 to 200 mg orally.

It can produce adverse effects like nausea, vomiting, hyperacidity, nervousness, insomnia, agitation, muscular twitchings, rigidity, tremors, tachycardia, cardiac arrhythmias, pyrexia, delirium and convulsions.

Acute toxicity with caffeine is rare. It produces tolerance and habituation after prolonged use.

Other psychic stimulants are discussed in respective chapters.

Medullary Stimulants

Analeptics

These are drugs that stimulate respiration, when it is failing. They stimulate the RC both directly and reflexly (through stimulation of chemoreceptors in carotid sinus and aortic body). They also rises BP when it is failing. They resuscitate the patient in fainting or coma. They have limited clinical uses in ventilatory failure like hypnotic or narcotic drug poisoning, apnoea of premature infants, suffocation on drowning, respiratory failure after general anaesthesia or due to pulmonary diseases.

Preparations and Dosage

- Doxapram (Dopram) injection (200 mg/mL)— 0.5 to 1.5 mg/kg by IV infusion.
- Ethylbutamide and propylbutamide (Restimulen) injection (125 + 125 mg/1.5 mL)— 125 to 250 mg IM or IV slowly.
- Nikethamide (Coramine) injection (2 mL of 25% solution)—1 to 2 mL IM or IV. They have narrow margin of safety (T_1) and can produce convulsions in higher doses.

Convulsants

They have no clinical use as they have low margin of safety. They are of toxicological importance. Their poisoning is treated by IV diazepam. Their mechanism of convulsant action is important. Pentyline tetrazole (Leptazol) acts by direct depolarization of central neurons and may interfere with GABAergic inhibition. Picrotoxin is a glycoside obtain from fish berry and acts by blocking presynaptic inhibition mediated through GABA. It does not block GABA receptor but acts on a distal site to increase Cl^- conductance and produce hyperpolorization of the neuronal membrane. Bicuculine is a competitive GABA-A receptor antagonist but GABA-B receptor is insensitive to it.

These are used as experimental tools to produce convulsions in mice for evaluating the activity of anticonvulsant drugs.

Spinal Stimulants (Convulsants)

Strychrine and brucine are alkaloids obtained from nux-vomica seeds and by blocking the postsynaptic inhibition produced by the inhibitory transmitter 'glycine' especially in Renshaw cell—motor neuron junction in the spinal cord, through which inhibition of antagonistic muscle is achieved. Due to loss of synaptic inhibition, any nerve impulse becomes generalized resulting in apparent excitation and convulsions. They are not used clinically due to low margin of safety. Their poisoning is treated by IV diazepam.

Cerebroactive Drugs (Nootropic Drugs)

(Greek: 'Noos' means mind). These are drugs that improve memory by activating cerebral functions. They are memory/cognition enhancers. They have positive effects on organically impaired cognition (meaning to know), which includes all aspects of perceiving, thinking, learning and remembering. They are piracetam, pyritinol tetrahydroaminoacridine, pentoxifylline, codergocrine and cyclandelate. They facilitate the aquisition of learning and enhance memory retention. They act either by improving cerebral metabolism and energy utilization or improving cerebral circulation or increasing cerebral cholinergic activity.

Clinical Uses

They are used in following conditions:
- Congnition (memory) deficits associated with presenile dementia (Alzheimer's disease) and senile dementia.
- Learning and attention deficits in children.
- Memory deficits associated with neurological and mental diseases.
- Transient cerebral ischaemic attacks
- Amnesia following cerebral trauma, seizures and alcoholism.

Preparations and Dosage

- Piracetam (Nootropil/Piratam) capsule (400 mg)—400 to 800 mg twice daily.
- Pyritinol (Mentat/Encephabol) tablet (100 mg)—100 to 200 mg twice daily.
- Tetrahydroaminoacridine (Cognex) tablet (40 mg)—40 to 80 mg twice daily.
- Pentoxifyline (Trental) tablet (400 mg)—400 to 800 mg twice daily.
- Codergocrine (Hydergine) tablet (1 mg)—1 mg twice daily.

Adverse Reactions

They can produce nausea, vomiting, diarrhoea, insomnia and skin rashes.

Section II

ENDOCRINE PHARMACOLOGY

54

Hypothalamic and Pituitary Hormones

INTRODUCTION

Hormones are chemical substances of intense biological activity, which are secreted by endocrine (ductless) glands or nonendocrine tissues and transported through circulation to act on the target cells. They regulate body functions and maintain homeostasis. The word hormone is derived from the Greek word 'Hormao' means to impel. A hormone may act on other endocrine glands, e.g. hypothalamic regulatory (releasing or release inhibiting) hormones and tropic hormones of the anterior pituitary gland or may act directly on the tissues, e.g. thyroid hormones, parathyroid hormone, calcitonin, insulin, growth hormone, prolactin and hormones of adrenal glands and gonads (testes and ovaries).

Classification of Hormones

Chemically they are of four groups:
1. Polypeptides, e.g. hypothalamic regulatory hormones, anterior pituitary hormones, posterior pituitary hormones, hormones of islet cells of pancreas and gut hormones.
2. Steroids, e.g. adrenocortical hormones and gonadal hormones.
3. Catecholamines, e.g. adrenal medullary hormones (adrenaline and noradrenaline).
4. Iodothyronines, e.g. thyroid hormones (thyroxine and triiodothyronine).

Storage of Hormones

Generally, a hormone is stored in the same gland, which synthesizes it but hypothalamic regulatory hormones are synthesized in various areas of the hypothalamus and stored in the median eminence of the hypothalamus. Posterior pituitary hormones (vasopressin and oxytocin) are synthesized in the hypothalamus but stored in the neurohypophysis (posterior pituitary).

Regulation and Release of Hormones

A hormone is directly released into venous blood from the endocrine gland or nonendocrine tissue at a slow basal rate, which in the case of many hormones may show a natural diurnal rhythm. Factors which modulate (increase or decrease) the hormone synthesis and release are:

- Hypothalamic regulatory (releasing or release inhibiting) hormones act on the anterior pituitary to modify the synthesis and release of the tropic hormones of the latter.
- Anterior pituitary hormones stimulate synthesis and release of hormones of the target glands (e.g. thyroid, adrenal cortex and gonads). In the absence of these hormones, the target glands undergo atrophy with decrease of functions. Hence these hormones are called tropic hormones. Thus increased plasma concentrations of hormones produced by the target glands act on the hypothalamus to alter the rate of release of regulatory hormones and on the pituitary to reduce the secretion of the respective tropic hormones (TSH, ACTH,

FSH and LH). On the other hand, decrease in the plasma concentration of a hormone of the target gland leads to a greater release of the corresponding tropic hormone. This mechanism of mutual regulation of hormone activity between two glands is called feedback control. It helps to maintain the plasma concentration of the target gland hormones within a balanced narrow range.

- Concentrations of nonhormonal chemical substances in the plasma can influence the rate of release of a hormone, e.g. hyperglycaemia stimulates the release of insulin from the islet cells of the pancreas but decreases the release of growth hormone from the normal anterior pituitary. Hypoglycaemia has the opposite effects. Hypocalcaemia stimulates the release of parathyroid hormone but decreases the release of calcitonin. Hypercalcaemia has the opposite effects. This is another feedback control.

- Psychoneurogenic factors can alter the rate of secretion of a hormone, e.g. anxiety may inhibit gonadotropins secretion and acute stress increases the release of catecholamines from the adrenal medulla and corticosteroids from the adrenal cortex.

Sites and mechanisms of action of hormones: Hormones act on their specific receptors located on or within the target cells by following mechanisms (shown in Table 54.1).

Transport and Metabolism of Hormones

Hormones are carried in the plasma partly in the free form and partly bound to plasma proteins. The free form is the active form and the protein bound form is the inactive form, which has a reservoir function, releasing more free hormone as it is utilized by the body. Metabolic degradation of hormones occur mainly in liver and partly in the target endocrine glands and the tissues on which

Table 54.1: Sites and mechanisms of hormonal action

Sites	Mechanisms of action	Hormones
Cell membrane receptors	Through alteration of intracellular cAMP (second messenger) concentration leading to alteration of protein kinase activity.	Adrenaline, noradrenaline glucagon, TSH, FSH, LH, parathyroid hormone, calcitonin, ACTH, some hypothalamic regulatory hormones.
	Through IP_3/DAG generation, release of intracellular Ca^{2+} and activation of protein kinase-C.	Vasopressin, oxytocin
	Direct effect on membrane transport processes leading to increased rate of glucose entry into the cells of adipose tissue and muscle.	Insulin
Cytoplasmic receptors (cytosol receptors)	Steroid-receptor complex formed in the cytoplasm enters the nucleus and binds with the specific area of a specific DNA to modify gene transcription and forming mRNA for the synthesis of specific enzymes or other proteins to produce biological actions.	Steroid hormones (corticosteroids and sex steroids)
Nuclear receptors	Steroid-receptor complex formed in the nucleus alters DNA-RNA mediated cellular protein (enzyme) synthesis to produce biological actions.	Thyroid hormones

they act. Conjugation with sulphuric acid and glucuronic acid to form sulphates and glucuronides occurs in the liver. Both conjugated hormone and free (original) hormone are excreted in urine through kidneys.

Hypothalamic Regulatory Hormones

These are of two groups:

1. **Releasing hormones (RH) or factors (RF)**

   These are as follows:
   - Thyrotropin (TSH)-releasing hormone (TRH).
   - Corticotropin (ACTH)-releasing hormone (CRH).
   - Growth hormone (GH)-releasing hormone (GHRH).
   - Gonadotropin (Gn)-releasing hormone (GnRH).
   - Prolactin releasing factor (PRF).
   - Melanocyte-stimulating hormone (MSH)-releasing factor (MSH-RF).

2. **Release inhibiting hormones (RIH) or factors (RIF)**

   These are given as follows:
   - Growth hormone (GH)-release inhibiting hormone (GH-RIH)/somatostatin
   - Prolactin release inhibiting factor (PRIF).
   - Melanocyte-stimulating hormone (MSH)-release inhibiting factor (MSH-RIF). Chemical nature of the hormone is known (i.e. polypeptide) but the chemical nature of the factor is unknown.

Anterior Pituitary Hormones

These are of three groups:

1. Somatotropic hormones, *viz.* growth hormone (GH) and prolactin.
2. Glycoprotein hormones, *viz.* thyroid-stimulating hormone (TSH/thyrotrophin), follicle-stimulating hormone (FSH) and luteinizing hormone (LH). FSH and LH are gonadotropins.
3. Pro-opiomelanocortin (POMC) derived hormones, *viz.* adrenocorticotropic hormone (ACTH/corticotropin) and melanocyte-stimulating hormone (MSH).

Growth hormone and prolactin are secreted by acidophil cells and other hormones are secreted by basophil cells of anterior pituitary. Hypothalamic regulatory hormones control the secretion of anterior pituitary hormones. Secretions of some hormones are stimulated while others are inhibited.

Clinical Uses

Growth hormone (synthetic), ACTH (natural and synthetic) and human chorionic gonadotropin are available as injections (IM) and used in deficiency diseases (dwarfism, adrenal-hypocorticism and infertility respectively).

Preparations and Dosage

Growth hormone

- Somatrem (methionyl HGH) is available as:
  - Protropin (5 mg = 13 IU per vial).
  - Somatonorm (2 mg = 5.2 IU per vial).
- Somatropin (nonmethionyl HGH) is available as:
  - Genotropin (12 and 16 IU per vial).
  - Humatrope (4 and 16 IU per vial). The dose is 0.4 to 0.7 IU/kg/week. 1/7th of the calculated dose is injected IM daily.

ACTH (Corticotropin)

- Natural ACTH with gelatin or zinc hydroxide (40 IU of ACTH/mL)—initially 40 IU, IM daily. Initially maintenance dose 20 IU IM twice or thrice a week.
- Synthetic ACTH (Tetracosactrin/Synacthen)—1 mg IM every 48 hours (1 mg = 10 IU of natural ACTH).

Human chorionic gonadotropin/HCG (Pregnyl/Profasi). It is available as powder in a vial containing 5,000 or 10,000 IU and 10 mL of diluent.

The dose is 3,000 to 5,000 IU IM twice in a week.

Human menopausal urinary gonodotropin/hMG (Menotropin/Pergonal) is rarely used.

Posterior Pituitary Hormones

These are vasopression/ADH and oxytocin. These are discussed in respective chapters.

55

Thyroid Hormones and Antithyroid Drugs

THYROID HORMONES

These are three in numbers, *viz.* tetraiodothyronine (thyroxine) and triiodothyronine (liothyronine) secreted by the follicular cells and thyrocalcitonin (calcitonin) secreted by the interfollicular 'C' cells of the thyroid gland. Thyroxine (T_4) and triiodothyronine (T_3) have been discussed in this chapter. Calcitonin has been discussed in the Chapter 56.

Chemistry

Thyroxine (T_4) and triiodothyronine (T_3) are iodine-containing amino acids. They contain two phenyl rings linked with an ether (–O–) bridge. The left hand side and right hand side rings are called the outer and inner rings respectively. In thyroxine there are 4 iodine atoms at 3, 5 (inner ring) and 3', 5' (outer ring) positions and in triiodothyronine there are three iodine atoms at 3, 5 (inner ring) and 3' (outer ring) positions (as shown in **Fig. 55.1**).

Triiodothyronine is biologically very active.

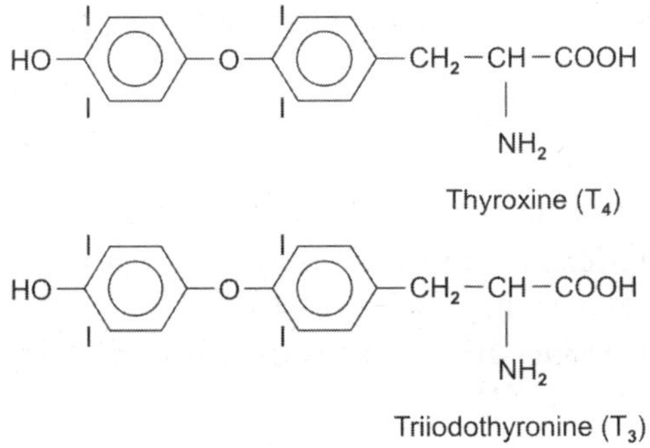

Biosynthesis

Sea fish, eggs and milk are good dietary sources of iodide. Dietary iodide is absorbed from the upper part of GIT and is carried in the plasma as inorganic iodide. Synthesis of thyroid hormones involves following steps:

- **Iodide trapping (uptake):** Thyroid gland traps the plasma iodide circulating through it by an energy dependent active process

Fig. 55.1: Thyroid hormones

(against a concentration gradient of 25 to 100). This uptake is stimulated by TSH and inhibited by the thiocyanate and perchlorate ions. The other organs which compete with thyroid gland are kidneys (excrete iodine in urine) and to some extent the salivary glands, GIT, liver and mammary glands (for excretion).

- **Oxidation of iodide to iodine:** Within the thyroid follicular cells the iodide ion is oxidized to inorganic iodine with the help of the enzyme peroxidase.

- **Organic binding of iodine:** Iodine binds with the amino acid 'tyrosine' in the thyroglobulin (TG) molecule (a large glycoprotein) within the follicular cells to form monoiodotyrosine (MIT) and diiodotyrosine (DIT) successively. These two reactions are very rapid and stimulated by TSH and inhibited by thiouracils.

- **Coupling:** Thyroxine (T_4) is formed by coupling (union) of two molecules of DIT and triiodothyronine (T_3) is formed by coupling of one molecule of MIT with one molecule of DIT. Coupling reactions occur while MIT and DIT are bound by peptide bonds within the thyroglobulin molecule (which contains about 115 tyrosine residues). These are oxidative reactions and require the enzyme *'peroxidase'*. These are stimulated by TSH and inhibited by thiouracils.

Release of Thyroid Hormones

Thyroglobulin which contains the thyroid hormones is secreted by the follicular cells into the follicular lumen, where it is stored. Under the influence of TSH, a proteolytic enzyme (protease) acts on the thyroglobulin molecule to release T_4 and T_3, as well as MIT and DIT. MIT and DIT are deiodinated within the follicular cells and the iodine is reutilized for iodinating thyroglobulin molecule. T_4 and T_3 enter the circulation directly from the follicular cells.

Transport of Thyroid Hormones

One of the thyroid hormones in circulation is thyroxine (T_4), which is largely deiodinated (80%) in peripheral tissues to the active form triiodothyronine (T_3). T_3 is 3 to 5 times more potent than T_4. Both T_4 and T_3 are extensively bound with plasma proteins (globulin and albumin). Salicylates and phenytoin displace thyroid hormones from plasma protein binding sites.

Metabolism of Thyroid Hormones

Thyroid hormones are metabolized in the liver by deiodination, deamination and conjugation. Free form and conjugated metabolites are excreted in bile and urine.

Physiological Functions and Pharmacological Actions of Thyroid Hormones

These are given as follows:

- **Calorigenic action:** Thyroid hormones stimulate oxygen consumption and heat production in all tissues except the brain, gonads, lymph nodes, spleen, thymus and dermis. Total thyroidectomy lowers the BMR by 40%, while in hyperthyroidism, the BMR is markedly raised. In hypothyroid individuals, the calorigenic response of externally administered thyroid hormones is prominent.

- **On growth and development:** Thyroid hormones are essential for intra- as well as extrauterine growth and tissue differentiation. Intrauterine thyroid deficiency leads to cretinism, characterized by physical and mental retardation. Deficiency of thyroid hormones appearing after birth leads to lack of physical, mental and sexual growth. Hence the child is short statured (physical) and idiot (mental) with infantile sex. There is marked delay in the bone maturation (retarded bone age) due to abnormality of calcification in the epiphyseal cartilages. Deficiency of thyroid hormones in adults produces myxoedema.

- **Metabolic actions:** In small doses, thyroid hormones produce anabolic effects by promoting growth and protein synthesis but in large doses, they produce catabolic effects by stimulating carbohydrate, protein and lipid metabolism. They increase the rate of absorption of glucose from the gut. In peripheral tissues, they increase the rates of cellular entry and intracellular utilization of glucose, but in larger doses they produce glycogenolysis in the liver and skeletal muscle. They increase the rate of cholesterol synthesis by the liver. They also increase the rate of biliary excretion, its conversion to bile acids and increase its faecal loss. They affect the water and electrolyte metabolism. Thus, hypothyroid subjects retain water and sodium and cannot excrete an added load of water and sodium. Administration of thyroid hormone in such subjects produce diuresis and natriuresis.

- **CNS effects:** Thyroxine is essential for myelination in CNS. Deficiency of thyroxine during foetal life leads to irreversible CNS damage. In hypothyroidism, various neurological changes like mental retardation and slow tendon reflexes are seen. Various types of psychosis are also seen in hypothyroidism. On the other hand, nervousness, anxiety, mental irritability, tremors and hyperkinaesia are characteristic features of hyperthyroidism.

- **CVS effects:** Thyroxine produces tachycardia, rise of systolic BP, cardiac arrhythmias and excessive sensitivity of the heart to catecholamines (can be inhibited by β-blockers).
- **Reproductive effects:** In hypothyroidism, oligospermia, decreased libido and infertility occur in males and menorrhagia and infertility occur in females. No specific changes are observed in hyperthyroidism.
- **Miscellaneous effects:** In hypothyroidism (myxoedema), there is deposition of a complex mucopolysaccharide material in the connective tissue of the skin, which is responsible for the pallor and roughness of the skin. Anaemia, especially megaloblastic anaemia is seen in hypothyroidism. Constipation occurs in hypothyroidism, while diarrhoea occurs in hyperthyroidism. Various types of myopathies as well as a periodic paralysis are seen in hyperthyroidism.

Clinical Uses

Thyroid hormones are used for following purposes:
- **As substitution therapy:** They are used in cretinism (children) and myxoedema (adults). Once started the treatment must be continued lifelong. Treatment is started with a small dose, which is increased only at fortnightly intervals. The entire daily dose is given once a day. The effect of treatment is monitored clinically and by periodic determination of plasma levels of T_3, T_4 and TSH. The lethargic obese patients need slightly larger doses than the anxious thin patients. The dose must be smaller in the children and older patients than the adults.

- **In nontoxic (simple) goitre**, in which size of the thyroid gland increases but secretion of thyroid hormones is low. In it, plasma TSH level is normal. It is thought to be due to locally released growth factors. It is corrected by administration of thyroid hormones.
- **In myxoedema coma** (characterized by coma, hypothermia, marked bradycardia and hypotension occurring in elderly patients especially during cold season). It is treated by administration of thyroid hormones, glucocorticoids and antimicrobial drugs, preferably in a hospital.

Preparations and Dosage

- Levothyroxine sodium (Eltroxin) tablet (100 µg)—50 to 300 µg daily in single dose.
- Liothyronine sodium (Tetroxin) tablet (20 µg)—20 to 60 µg daily in three divided doses.

Adverse Reactions

These include diarrhoea, weight loss, palpitation, tremors, hyperkinesia, irritability and occasionally anginal pain (similar to the symptoms of thyrotoxicosis). Prolonged administration of thyroid hormones in large doses can cause osteoporosis especially in menopausal women, left ventricular hypertrophy and pseudotumour cerebri.

Antithyroid Drugs

These are drugs used in hyperthyroidism to inhibit the synthesis or release of thyroid hormones. The clinical manifestations of hyperthyroidism are due to an excess of circulating thyroid hormones. There are two major forms of hyperthyroidism, *viz.* diffuse toxic goitre (thyrotoxicosis/Graves' disease) and toxic nodular goitre. Graves' disease is an autoimmune disease in which autoantibodies (IgG) called 'long-acting thyroid stimulators' (LATS) are found in blood. They bind to and stimulate thyroid cells and have TSH-like actions. Exophthalmus producing substance (EPS), which is also an autoantibody is found in blood and produces protrusion of eyeball due to deposition of retro-orbital fat and inflammatory oedema. In toxic nodular goitre, thyroid hormones are secreted independent of TSH actions and occur mostly in elderly persons over nontoxic goitre. In it, ocular changes are generally absent.

Classification of Antithyroid Drugs

These are of four groups:

1. Inhibitors of iodide trapping (ionic inhibitors), e.g. sodium or potassium perchlorate, sodium or potassium thiocyanate.

2. Inhibitors of thyroid hormone synthesis (thioamides/thiouracils). These are thiourea derivatives, e.g. carbimazole, methimazole and propylthiouracil.

3. Inhibitors of thyroid hormone release (iodides), e.g. sodium or potassium iodide and Lugol's iodine solution (5% iodine in 10% potassium iodide).

4. Destroyers of thyroid tissue (radioactive isotopes of iodine), e.g. ^{131}I (commonly used); ^{125}I and ^{123}I (rarely used).

Goitrogens

These are substances that produce goitres by interfering with the synthesis or release of thyroid hormones, e.g. vegetables like cabbage, turnip, mustard, etc. (which contain goitrin) and drugs like sulphonamides, PAS, lithium, amiodarone, aminoglutethimide/resorcinol, phenylbutazone, thiouracils, ionic inhibitors and iodides.

DISCUSSION OF INDIVIDUAL GROUP OF ANTITHYROID DRUGS

Ionic Inhibitors

These drugs act by competitive inhibition of trapping of iodide by the thyroid gland and thus decreasing the formation of thyroid hormones. They are now obsolete drugs due to potential toxicity. The toxicity includes gastric irritation, fever, skin rashes, lymphadenopathy, agranulocytosis, aplastic anaemia, methaemoglobinemia, hepatic and renal damage.

Thioamides

These drugs act by reducing the biosynthesis of thyroid hormones by inhibiting iodination of tyrosine and coupling of iodotyrosines to form T_4 and T_3. In addition, propylthiouracil inhibits the peripheral conversion of T_4 to T_3 and hence the metabolic response to T_4 but not to T_3. Carbimazole is also claimed to produce a remission in Graves' disease by suppressing the autoimmune process in the thyroid gland.

Pharmacokinetics

These drugs are rapidly absorbed (in 20 to 30 minutes) after oral administration. After absorption, they are concentrated in the thyroid gland. The duration of action of a single oral dose is less than 8 hours. So they are administered every 6 to 8 hours. They are partly metabolized in the liver and thyroid gland and excreted in urine as metabolites and unchanged (free) form. Carbimazole is metabolized to the active metabolite methimazole. They are secreted in mother's milk and cross the placental barrier in significant amounts. Hence they should be used cautiously in pregnant women and lactating mothers, as they can cause hypothyroidism in foetus and infants.

Clinical Uses

These are used in following cases:

- Diffuse toxic goitre (thyrotoxicosis/Graves' disease)

- Toxic nodular goitre

- Before thyroidectomy in all cases

- Along with radioactive iodine to decrease symptoms before radiation effects are manifested.

- Thyrotoxic crisis/storm (due to aggravation of thyrotoxic state). Large doses of an antithyroid drug (propylthiouracil or carbimazole) and also hydrocortisone and propranolol are used in this condition.

Preparations and Dosage

- Carbimazole (Neomercazole) tablet (5, 10 mg): Initial dose—30 to 60 mg/day in three divided doses until remission of symptoms occurs. Maintenance dose—5 to 20 mg daily.
- Methimazole (Tapazole) tablet (5, 10 mg): Dosage like carbimazole.
- Propylthiouracil tablet (50 mg): Initial dose—300 to 600 mg daily in three divided doses. Maintenance dose—50 to 200 mg daily.

Adverse Reactions

Milder adverse effects include skin rash, drug fever, pruritus, urticaria, oedema of feet, arthralgia, lymphadenopathy and alopecia. More serious adverse effects are leucopenia, agranulocytosis, thrombocytopaenia and liver damage. Hypothyroidism due to over-treatment is common but reversible on stopping the drug. Carbimazole is more potent and less toxic than propylthiouracil, but propylthiouracil is preferred in lactating mothers because it is less secreted in the milk.

Precautions to be taken during thiouracil treatment:

- Regular examination of blood (TC and DC), preferably at two weeks interval to detect blood dyscrasias.
- Cautious use in pregnant women and lactating mothers to avoid hypothyroidism in foetus and infants.

Iodides

These drugs (in large doses) act by inhibiting the release of the preformed thyroid hormones (probably by preventing proteolysis of the thyroglobulin molecule). They produce the so-called thyroid constipation. They are quickest acting drugs (onset of action within 24 hours). They cause decrease in size and vascularity of the thyroid gland. When given along with a thiouracil drug, they prevent the increase in the size of the gland (goitre), which usually occurs following administration of the drug alone. This is probably due to decreased responsiveness of the iodine-rich thyroid gland to the circulating TSH.

Pharmacokinetics

They are well-absorbed after oral administration and distributed throughout the body. They are selectively trapped by the thyroid gland, uptake being increased in hyperthyroidism and decreased in hypothyroidism. They can cross the placental barrier and may produce cretinism in the foetus. They are excreted in urine by the kidneys.

Clinical Uses

These are used for following purposes:

- Preoperative preparation of a hyperthyroid patient to reduce the size and vascularity of the thyroid gland. They are given for 10 to 14 days preoperatively (before subtotal thyroidectomy) along with a thiouracil drug.
- Rapid control of hyperthyroidism in a patient with thyrotoxic crisis or CCF. They should be given along with a thiouracil drug.
- Blocking the thyroidal uptake before administration of a ^{131}I labelled compound (radioactive iodine uptake test) to diagnose thyroid disorders.

Preparations and Dosage

- Lugol's iodine solution (it is prepared by dissolving 5 g of iodine in 100 mL of 10% potassium iodide solution and it provides 150 mg of iodine per mL)—0.1 to 0.3 mL thrice daily.
- Saturated solution of potassium iodide (It is prepared by dissolving 30 g of potassium iodide in 20 mL of water to give 30 mL of solution and it provides 1 g of potassium iodide per mL)—0.1 to 0.2 mL thrice daily.

Adverse Reactions

They can produce iodism in susceptible individuals which is manifested as soreness of throat, lacrimation, rhinorrhoea, increased salivation, gingivitis, swelling of eyelids and skin rashes. These symptoms disappear on withdrawal of the drug. On prolonged use they can produce goitre and even myxoedema. They cross the placental barrier and may cause goitrous cretinism in the foetus.

Radioactive Iodine (^{131}I)

When it is given orally it is taken up by the thyroid gland by iodide trapping and concentrates within the thyroidal follicles. It acts by ionizing radiation emeting beta (β) and gamma (γ) rays. It has a t½ of 8 days. Beta rays are particles that penetrate and destroy cells of thyroidal follicles up to 5 mm distance producing fibrosis of tissues. Gamma rays are more penetrative and can be detected by Geiger-Müller counter (for external counting) in thyroid function tests.

Clinical Uses

It is used in the treatment of diffuse toxic goitre (thyrotoxicosis/Graves' disease), toxic nodular goitre and thyroid carcinoma and in the diagnosis of thyroid disorders in all patients above 35 years of age.

Preparation and Dosage

Radioactive sodium iodide (Na ^{131}I) capsule or solution.

For treatment—5 to 10 millicurie (mCi) orally in an empty stomach or after light breakfast.

For diagnosis—50 to 100 microcurie (mCi).

Adverse Reactions

It can produce hypothyroidism, thyroid carcinoma and damage to the foetal thyroid (if administered in pregnant woman). Precautions to be taken during radioactive iodine treatment:

- Persons handling radioactive iodine should be alert from radiation hazards.
- Urine and faeces of patients receiving radioiodine should be carefully disposed.
- Pregnant and lactating women and young children should be treated very cautiously.

56

Parathyroid Hormone and Calcitonin

PARATHYROID HORMONE/PTH (PARATHORMONE)

It is a polypeptide hormone (containing 84 amino acids) secreted by the chief cells of the parathyroid glands (4 in numbers). It is the major regulator of calcium homeostasis in the body. Its secretion is regulated by plasma ionic calcium concentrations. Rise in the plasma ionic calcium concentration inhibits its secretion, while a fall in the plasma ionic calcium concentration stimulates its secretion.

Physiological Functions and Pharmacological Actions

It increases plasma ionic calcium concentration by acting on GIT, bones and kidneys.

- *On GIT:* It promotes the active absorption of calcium and phosphorus from GIT with the help of vitamin D.
- *On bones:* It mobilizes calcium and phosphorus from old bones into the extracellular fluid by promoting osteoclastic bone resorption with the help of vitamin D. It does not influence the ionic exchange of calcium occurring between the extracellular fluid and the newly laid down bone mineral.
- *On kidneys:* It decreases the urinary excretion of calcium by increasing its reabsorption from the glomerular filtrate in the distal renal tubules with the help of vitamin D. At the same time, it increases the urinary

excretion of phosphorus by decreasing its reabsorption in the proximal renal tubules with the help of vitamin D. It also converts the vitamin D to its final active form 1,25-dihydroxycholecalciferol (calcitriol) in the kidneys (vitamin D is a prohormone and calcitriol is a hormone).

The effect of PTH on the kidneys is of more rapid onset than that on the bones.

Pharmacokinetics

It is ineffective orally because it is hydrolyzed by proteolytic enzymes of gut. It is administered SC or IM. It is partly metabolized in the liver and partly excreted in urine.

Clinical Uses

It can be used for the treatment of hypoparathyroidism, but vitamin D and calcium salts are preferred. It is used only for the diagnosis of pseudohypoparathyroidism, which does not respond to it due to end organ resistance.

Preparation and Dosage

Parathyroid hormone (Bovine or Porcine) injection (contains not less than 100 MRC units of the calcium raising activity per mL)—40 to 80 units SC or IM daily.

Adverse Reactions

It can cause hypercalcaemia and allergic reactions (urticaria, anaphylaxis, etc.).

CALCITONIN/THYROCALCITONIN

It is a polypeptide hormone (containing 32 amino acids) secreted by the interfollicular 'C' cells of the thyroid gland. Its secretion is regulated by plasma ionic calcium concentrations. Rise in plasma ionic calcium concentration increases its secretion, while a fall in plasma ionic calcium concentration decreases its secretion.

Physiological Functions and Pharmacological Actions

It decreases plasma ionic calcium concentration by acting on bones and kidneys.

- *On bones:* It promotes deposition of calcium in bones by stimulating osteoblastic activity. It inhibits PTH induced osteoclastic activity and bone resorption of calcium and phosphorus. Thus calcium from the circulation is shunted to bones.

- *On kidneys:* It increases the urinary excretion of calcium and phosphorus by inhibiting their renal tubular reabsorption.

The net result of calcitonin action is to reduce plasma calcium and phosphate levels. Its action of lowering plasma calcium level is rapid and of short duration.

Pharmacokinetics

Like PTH.

Clinical Uses

It is used in Paget's disease of bones, osteoporosis and hypercalcaemia associated with hyperparathyroidism, vitamin D intoxication and osteolytic bone metastasis. In Paget's disease of bones it can be combined with oral phosphate administration.

Preparations and Dosage

- Salmon calcitonin (Salcatonin) injection (very expensive): 50 to 100 MRC units SC or IM thrice in a week for 3 to 6 months (in Paget's disease of bones).
- Porcine calcitonin (Calcitare) injection: 50 to 100 MRC units SC or IM for 2 to 3 times in a week for 3 to 6 months.

Adverse Reactions

These include nausea, oedema of hands, flushing and allergic reactions (urticaria, anaphylaxis, etc.).

Sodium etidronate can be used as an alternative to calcitonin in Paget's disease of bones. Its advantages are oral efficacy and lack of antigenicity. It acts by inhibiting bone resorption of calcium and phosphorus. It is administered daily orally for 6 to 12 months.

57

Hormones of Islets of Pancreas

INTRODUCTION

Pancreas contains exocrine part (about 80%) and endocrine part (about 20% containing islets of Langerhans).

Hormones of islets of Langerhans of pancreas are:

- Insulin (secreted by beta cells)
- Glucagon (secreted by alpha cells)
- Somatostatin (secreted by delta cells)
- Pancreatic polypeptide hormone (secreted by F cells).

DISCUSSION OF INDIVIDUAL HORMONES

Insulin

It is a polypeptide hormone (containing 51 amino acids) secreted by the beta cells of islets of Langerhans of pancreas. It has two amino acid chains (A and B) joined together by two disulphide linkages (−S−S−), which are essential for biological activity of insulin. It has a molecular weight of 6,000. It was discovered by Banting and Best in 1922.

Synthesis and Storage

It is synthesized within the β-cells as a single chain polypeptide precursor called prepro-insulin (containing 110 amino acids), which is converted to proinsulin (containing 86 amino acids). Proinsulin is biologically only 1/8th as active as insulin. From proinsulin, a portion called connecting peptide (c peptide) is removed by the proteolytic enzyme and thus insulin (containing 51 amino acids) is formed.

Insulin is packaged within granules and stored in the β-cells, from which it is released at a slow rate by exocytosis in repeated bursts into the circulation. The plasma concentration of insulin shows fluctuations throughout the day and peak plasma concentrations are produced after meals.

Regulation of Secretion of Insulin

Insulin secretion is regulated by many factors including blood glucose concentration, certain hormones and CNS. High blood glucose concentration (hyperglycaemia) stimulates insulin secretion. Rise of blood amino acids and fatty acids concentrations also stimulate insulin secretion. Gut hormones like gastrin, CCK-PZ and secretin, which are secreted after meal stimulate insulin secretion. Glucagon, growth hormone, ACTH, thyroxine, cate-cholamines and glucocorticoids stimulate insulin secretin. These are anti-insulin or diabetogenic hormones. CNS regulates insulin secretion *via* the ANS. α_2-adrenergic stimulation and vagotomy inhibit insulin secretion, whereas β_2-adrenergic stimulation and vagal stimulation increase insulin secretion. Nonspecific β-blockers, (e.g. propranolol) thus causes inhibition of insulin secretion. Drugs like sulphonylureas and xanthines stimulate insulin release, whereas thiazides, frusemide, diazoxide and phenytoin inhibit insulin release.

Pharmacokinetics of Insulin

Insulin is ineffective orally as it is rapidly destroyed by proteolytic enzymes in the gut. It is administered SC or IV. It circulates in the plasma as a free, nonprotein bound form. In the presence of antibodies, it may be strongly bound to them. It disappears rapidly from the plasma with a plasma t½ of 5 to 6 minutes. It is metabolized in the liver, kidneys and skeletal muscles. It is excreted in urine mainly as metabolities and slightly as unchanged form. In chronic renal disease, its metabolism and excretion is reduced.

Physiological Functions and Pharmacological Actions

Insulin regulates metabolism of carbohydrate, fat and protein by acting on the cells of target organs like liver, adipose tissue and skeletal muscle (as shown in **Table 57.1**).

Mechanism of Action

Insulin acts on the cell membrane, where it exerts following actions:

- It stimulates carrier mediated transport of glucose by recruiting glucose transporters (GLUTs) from the cytoplasm to the cell membrane. The rise of intracellular glucose concentration to very high levels can stimulate many of the chemical reactions involved in glucose utilization. It also directly stimulates certain reactions concerned in glucose utilization within the cell. It increases the uptake of amino acids and potassium by the cell, which is not dependent on increased glucose uptake. Liver cells are freely permeable to glucose, which enters them by the glucose transporters. Insulin promotes glucose uptake by the liver cells.

- It binds with the specific receptors (insulin receptors) in the cell membrane of the insulin-sensitive and insulin-insensitive cells. Binding of insulin with the receptors in the insulin sensitive cells activates tyrosine kinase activity, which is present inside the insulin receptors. The activated receptor phosphorylates a protein called insulin receptor substrate-1 (IRS-1), which then catalyzes the phosphorylation of various enzyme proteins in the cells leading to their activation. This action is independent of the carrier mediated transport of glucose and other substrates into the cells. Insulin also decreases the intracellular concentration of cAMP in the hepatocytes (liver cells) and adipocytes (adipose tissue cells).

- It stimulates the synthesis of DNA leading to cell proliferation and differentiation. It is

Table 57.1: Actions of insulin on the target organs

Metabolism	Liver cells	Adipose tissue cells	Skeletal muscle cells
Carbohydrate	Increased glycogen synthesis and storage. Decreased glycogenolysis and gluconeogenesis.	Increased glucose uptake and utilization.	Increased glucose uptake and utilization. Increased glycogen synthesis and deposition.
Fat	Increased lipogenesis Decreased ketogenesis	Decreased lipolysis. Increased lipogenesis (promotes formation of triglycerides).	Decreased lipolysis.
Protein	Increased protein synthesis. Decreased protein breakdown.		Increased protein synthesis by promoting entry of amino acid and potassium into cells. Decreased protein breakdown.

considered as an anabolic and growth promoting hormone.

Effects of Insulin Deficiency

These are given as follows:

- Hyperglycaemia and glycosuria (due to decreased peripheral utilization of glucose, increased glycogenolysis and increased gluconeogenesis; these may be partly due to unopposed actions of the diabetogenic hormones).
- Diabetic ketoacidosis (due to increased breakdown of lipids especially triglycerides leading to increased levels of free fatty acids and ketones like acetoacetic acid and β-hydroxybutyric acid in blood).
- Abnormal blood lipid pattern (hypercholesterolaemia, hypertriglyceridaemia and high LDL level with susceptibility to atherosclerosis).
- Muscle wasting.
- Nephropathy, retinopathy, neuropathy, etc.
- Susceptibility to bacterial infections (acute as well as chronic).

Clinical Uses

Insulin is indicated in:

- Diabetes mellitus (DM): It is a chronic metabolic disease due to deficiency of insulin and characterized by hyperglycaemia, glycosuria, polyurea, polydipsia, hyperlipidaemia, ketonaemia and azoturia and in severe cases ketoacidosis. It is of two types, *viz.* Type I (juvenile onset DM/insulin dependent DM) (IDDM) and type II (maturity onset DM/noninsulin dependent DM) (NIDDM). Insulin is used in:
  - All cases of juvenile onset DM (IDDM).
  - Those cases of maturity onset DM (NIDDM), where oral hypoglycaemic drugs are not effective (primary or secondary failure).
  - All cases of DM with complications such as severe infection, severe trauma, ketosis, intractable pruritus, gangrene of extremities, CCF and progressive retinopathy.

  - Diabetic emergencies like diabetic pre-coma and coma.
  - Diabetes following pancreatectomy.
  - Pregnant diabetics.
  - Diabetics during surgical procedures.
- Hyperosmolar nonketotic diabetic coma in type II diabetics. It is characterized by severe dehydration due to osmotic glucose diuresis, severe hyperglycaemia, hypovolaemia and hyperosmolarity. Insulin with normal saline IV drip is used in this condition.
- Hyperkalaemia: Insulin with glucose (10%) IV drip is used to promote intracellular influx of potassium.
- Schizophrenia: Insulin coma is induced in schizophrenia as a therapeutic measure.
- Diagnostic tests:
  - Insulin tolerance test with determination of plasma growth hormone or ACTH is used to test anterior pituitary function and to diagnose hypopituitarism.
  - Hollander's test, i.e. decreased response of gastric acid secretion by insulin induced hypoglycaemia is used to test the completeness of vagotomy.

Preparations and Dosage of Insulin

A variety of insulin preparations are available for clinical use. They differ in their source and duration of action. Conventional insulin preparations of bovine origin is shown in **Table 57.2**. Plain (regular/soluble) insulin is commonly injected about ½ hour before each major meal. Intermediate- and long-acting insulin preparations are injected once or twice a day, before the breakfast and/or before dinner. The action of short-acting insulins is so short that several injections per day are required to control diabetes adequately. The action of long-acting insulins starts too late to cover the breakfast (first meal of the day) when an injection is taken in the morning. So appropriate mixtures of two insulin preparations are commonly used in clinical practice. Such insulin mixtures have rapid

Table 57.2: Conventional insulin preparations of bovine origin

Preparation	pH and appearance		Activity in hours		
			Onset	Peak	Duration
Short-acting:					
Plain (regular/soluble)	3.2	Clear	½ to 1	2 to 4	6 to 8
Insulin zinc suspension (amorphous/semilente)	7.2	Cloudy	1 to 2	4 to 8	12 to 16
Intermediate-acting:					
Isophane (NPH) insulin	7.2	Cloudy	1 to 2	6 to 10	18 to 24
Insulin zinc suspension (lente)	7.2	Cloudy	1 to 2	6 to 10	18 to 24
Long-acting:					
Protamine zinc insulin (PZI)	7.2	Cloudy	5 to 7	12 to 18	24 to 36
Insulin zinc suspension (crystalline/ultralente)	7.2	Cloudy	4 to 6	10 to 16	24 to 36

onset and act for about 24 hours. They are given before breakfast.

Insulin mixtures commonly used are:

- PZI (protamine zinc insulin) and plain insulin (1 part: 2 or 3 parts): PZI contains free protamine, which combines with added plain insulin.

- NPH (Neutral protamine Hagedron) insulin: It is a modified PZI, which contains just enough protamine to combine with insulin. It behaves like a 1:3 mixture of PZI and plain insulin. It can also be mixed with plain insulin if necessary.

- Lente insulin (insulin zinc) suspension made by mixing amorphous (semilente) and crystalline (ultralente) insulins in the proportion of 3:7.
  Insulin mixtures except lente insulin are unstable and must be prepared immediately before use. Their main advantage is that they can be prepared according to the requirement of an individual patient.

Newer Insulins (Purified Porcine and Human Insulins)

- Porcine (p) insulins (highly purified by gel filtration and crystallization).
  These are:
  – Actrapid/Rapidica (plain insulin)

  – Insulatard (isophane insulin)
  – Lentard/Zinulin (insulin zinc suspension)
  – Mixtard/Rapimix (30% actrapid + 70% insulatard).

- Human (H) insulins (monocomponent by gel filtration and ion exchange chromatography). These are prepared by recombinant DNA technology in bacteria (E. coli). These are:
  – Actrapid-H/Rapidica-H/Huminsulin-R (plain insulin).
  – Insulatard-H/Huminsulin-R (isophane insulin).
  – Monotard-H/Huminsulin-L (insulin zinc suspension).
  – Mixtard-H/Rapimix-H/Huminsulin 30/70 (like that of porcine insulin).
  – Huminsulin-U (ultralente insulin).

Advantages of Purified Preparations of Insulin

- They are purer than the older conventional preparations of insulin, as proinsulin and intermediate breakdown products of proinsulin are removed.
- They are neutral in reaction and do not cause subcutaneous fat atrophy (lipodystropy).

- They are less antigenic (allergenic) than porcine and bovine insulins.
- They are more stable than bovine insulins.

Human insulin is ideal but is expensive at present. It is now used in economically developed countries, replacing bovine and porcine insulins.

Calculation of Dose of Insulin

The dose of insulin is very important. It should be carefully adjusted according to the need of the patient. It is determined by the doctor according to the severity of diabetes mellitus. It can be calculated by testing blood sugar (glucose) levels (fasting and postprandial) or urine sugar concentration. Roughly, 1 unit of insulin is given for 10 mg of blood sugar level (if above 180 mg%) or 1 g of sugar excreted in urine. The dosage of insulin is expressed as international unit (IU). 1 mg of insulin is equal to 22 IU. Thus, limit = 45 µg. Preparations of insulin are available in 40 or 100 units/ml in 10 ml vials and injected by insulin syringe or pen injector.

New Routes of Administration of Insulin

Nowadays insulin can be administered orally by encapsulating or incorporating into lyposomes for its protection from destruction by proteolytic enzymes of gut. Implantable pellets of insulin is also available which releases insulin slowly over days or weeks.

Factors Influencing Insulin Requirements

Insulin requirement is increased by

- Drugs like glucocorticoids, growth hormone, thyroxine, oral contraceptives, thiazides, frusemide, diazoxide, etc. which increase blood sugar level.
- Stress of all types such as physiological stress (by pregnancy, severe infection, severe trauma, surgery and thyrotoxicosis) and psychological stress (by anxiety and depression).
- Obesity increases the dose of insulin.

Insulin requirement is decreased by

- Exercise: It promotes entry of glucose into muscle cells and releases muscle bound insulin.
- Drugs like sulphonamides and anticoagulants which can release insulin and thereby decrease insulin requirement.
- Eating pattern (dieting): Alterations of diet (less carbohydrate and more protein) or a change in eating time decreases insulin requirement.

Adverse Reactions of Insulin

These are given as follows:

- **Hypoglycaemia:** This is due to overdose of insulin and is quite common. It is manifested as sweating, tachycardia, hunger, weakness, headache, blurring of vision, mental confusion, incoherent speech, convulsions and coma. It is treated by administration of sugar/glucose or fruit juice orally if the patient is conscious or IV glucose (50 ml of 50% solution) if the patient is unconscious. Glucagon injection (1 mg IM) can be used for rapid awakening of the patient. If coma persists after correction of hypoglycaemia, mannitol and large dose of hydrocortisone can be administered IV to relieve the cerebral oedema.
- **Allergy:** It may consist of local itching, redness, swelling and pain at the site of injection or generalized urticaria and lymphadenopathy. It may be due to insulin itself or to protamine (protein) in the preparation. Nonprotein insulin such as lente insulin is thus preferred than protamine insulin. Similarly, pork or human insulin is devoid of antigenicity (allergenicity) and so preferred than beef insulin.
- **Lipoatrophy:** It consists of atrophy of the local subcutaneous fat at site of frequent insulin injections leading to irregular depression in the skin and subcutaneous tissue, where from absorption of insulin is erratic. It can be prevented by frequently changing the site of injections.

- **Presbyopia:** When a diabetic is rapidly controlled by insulin, he may develop loss of visual accommodation due to alteration of the physical properties of the lens. It is usually corrected within a few weeks and does not require new glasses.
- **Obesity:** Insulin may increase the body weight (by anabolic action and preventing lipolysis in the already obese diabetic patient), if dietary restriction is not done.

Insulin Resistance

It is a condition where daily requirement of insulin exceeds 200 units in a diabetic patient. It may be acute or chronic due to resistance at prereceptor, receptor or postreceptor sites. Prereceptor resistance is due to development of antibodies (IgG) against exogenous insulin. Receptor resistance is due to decrease in number or sensitivity of insulin receptors (downregulation). Postreceptor resistance is due to increase in activity of tyrosine kinase, which decreases insulin actions. Antigenicity (to develop antibodies) is less common with purified porcine and human insulins than conventional bovine insulins. Acute insulin resistance occurs with infection, severe trauma, surgery, strees or corticosteroid therapy. It is treated by removing the cause and administration of insulin (as much as is required to attain normal blood sugar levels) as well as fluids and electrolytes. Chronic insulin resistance occurs with endocrine disorders like acromegaly, adrenal hypercorticism and pheochromocytoma and development of antibodies in patients receiving insulin. It is treated by removing the cause and administration of human insulin in place of bovine or pig insulin.

MANAGEMENT OF EMERGENCIES IN THE DIABETIC PATIENT

Ketoacidotic Diabetic Coma

Uncontrolled diabetes mellitus can lead to severe catabolism of fatty acids of adipose tissue leading to excessive formation of ketone bodies (acetoacetic acid and β-hydroxybutyric acid) resulting in diabetic ketoacidosis (diabetic or by acute infection) which causes the plasma levels of anti-insulin (diabetogenic) hormones to rise. Failure of glucose entry into peripheral tissue cells leads to hyperglycaemia. Formation of excessive ketone bodies leads to metabolic acidosis. These organic acids are excreted in urine as salt of sodium and potassium and thus deplete the body sodium, potassium and water. Metabolic acidosis causes a shift of phosphorus out of the cells and increases excretion of phosphorus in urine producing severe phosphate depletion. Increased hepatic glycogenolysis results in depletion of liver glycogen. Increased catabolism of muscle protein results in increased urinary excretion of nitrogen. The urine is loaded with sugar and ketone bodies and the breath smells of ketone. The blood sugar level is in the region of 600 to 800 mg/100 mL (dL). Hyperglycaemia and glycosuria promote solute diuresis leading to dehydration and hypovolemia.

Management

This is done by:
- Hospitalizing the patient, as it is a medical emergency.
- **Insulin therapy:** Soluble (plain) insulin is administered IV to lower blood sugar level. Initially a bolus dose of 50 to 100 units is administered IV. This is followed by 5 to 10 units/hour (0.1 to 0.2 unit/kg/hour) by IV infusion. In 4 to 6 hours, the blood sugar level comes to 300 mg/dL. If the blood sugar level does not lower satisfactorily (10%/hour) then the dose of insulin is doubled and continued until the patient becomes conscious. This treatment is followed by conventional SC insulin therapy when the blood sugar level falls below 300 mg/dL.
- **Fluid therapy (saline infusion):** Initially normal (1 N) saline solution is administered by IV infusion at the rate of 1 L/hour and then half normal (½ N) saline is administered by IV infusion at the rate of 1 L/4 hours. A 5% dextrose solution is added to

½ N saline when the glucose level of blood falls to 300 mg/dL, because before the ketoacidosis subsides, the blood sugar level falls to hypoglycaemic level.

- **Potassium therapy (KCl infusion):** During ketoacidosis, the potassium level of blood is normal, but as potassium is excreted in urine, so there occurs movement of intracellular potassium into blood as compensatory mechanism. When ketoacidosis subsides, potassium level of blood decreases due to intracellular withdrawal from blood. This can produce severe hypokalaemia. Hence, a small amount of KCl is added to saline infusion to prevent hypokalaemia. The rate of KCl infusion is 10 to 20 mEq/hour. Continuous monitoring of plasma potassium level and BP must be done during KCl administration.

- **Bicarbonate therapy (NaHCO$_3$ infusion):** When the arterial blood pH is less than 7.0, then sodium bicarbonate (50 to 100 mEq at a time) administered along with saline infusion to correct metabolic acidosis.

- **Phosphate therapy:** Sodium or potassium phosphate is administered IV at the rate of 5 to 10 mmol/hour along with saline infusion to correct hypophosphatemia due to urinary phosphorus loss.

- **Treatment of the precipitating cause:** Presuming presence of infection, proper antibiotics should be administered. Prophylactic administration of antibiotic is, however, not recommended.

- **Proper nursing care:** This is essential in the management of a patient in diabetic coma. Attention should be given to skin, mouth, urinary bladder and position of the patient to avoid complications.

Hyperosmolar Nonketotic Diabetic Coma

This is typically seen in elderly NIDDM diabetics, who are suffering from severe infection, which decreases their water intake. There is severe hyperglycaemia (blood sugar level is more than 1000 mg/dL) and severe water loss through urine leading to hyperosmolar plasma and dehydration (by plasma volume depletion). They do not develop ketoacidosis because they have some endogenous insulin (as they are NIDDM cases), which acts on the liver preventing formation of ketone bodies.

Treatment consists of:
- Heavy fluid therapy (by ½ N saline).
- Insulin therapy (in moderate doses).

Insulin therapy should be stopped if the blood sugar reaches about 250 mg/dL.

Glucagon

It is a polypeptide hormone (containing 29 amino acids) secreted by the alpha cells of islets of Langerhans of pancreas. Its secretion is stimulated by a fall in blood glucose level and rise of plasma amino acid level. It has opposite effects of insulin. It raises blood sugar level by stimulating hepatic glycogenolysis (glycogen is converted into glucose and released into the blood). It also inhibits glycogen synthesis. It stimulates lipolysis in peripheral tissues, which in turn stimulates ketogenesis. Its hyperglycaemic action is seen particularly in the presence of insulin deficiency. It is thought to be involved in insulin secretion by stimulation of β-cells of islets of Langerhans. It has also a significant positive inotropic action on the heart.

Pharmacokinetics

It is ineffective orally, as it is rapidly destroyed by proteolytic enzymes in the gut. After parenteral administration it is rapidly absorbed and produces short-lasting effect. It is metabolized in the liver and kidneys and excreted in urine. It has a short plasma t½.

Clinical Uses

It is used for treating insulin induced hypoglycaemia and in cardiogenic shock. It can be used for the diagnosis of insulinoma for its insulin releasing property and in the diagnosis of pheochromocytoma for its catecholamine releasing property.

Preparation and Dosage

Glucagon hydrochloride (Bovine or Porcine) injection (1 or 10 mg of the dry powder in the ampoule)—0.5 to 1 mg IM or IV.

Adverse Reactions

It has no toxic effect.

Somatostatin (Somatosan)

It is a polypeptide hormone (containing 14 amino acids) secreted by the delta cells of islets of Langerhans of pancreas. It was first isolated from the hypothalamus of pig and shown to inhibit the release of growth hormone from the anterior pituitary. It also inhibits the release of insulin and glucagon from the pancreas and polypeptide hormones (gastrin, secretin, etc.) from the GIT. It is available as injection (3 mg/mL). A synthetic somatostatin analog called octreotide (sandostatin) is used to control severe diarrhoea due to carcinoid tumour and metastatic vasoactive intestinal polypeptide (VIP) tumour (vipoma). It is also used in peptic ulcer, dumping syndrome and oesophageal varicosal bleeding.

58

Oral Hypoglycaemic Drugs Used in DM

ORAL ANTIDIABETIC DRUGS

These drugs reduce hyperglycaemia in type II (maturity onset) diabetes mellitus when administered orally. The first clinically acceptable oral hypoglycaemic drug 'Tolbutamide' was introduced in 1957. Gradually other oral hypoglycaemic drugs were introduced in clinical practice.

Classification of Oral Hypoglycemic Drugs

These are of three groups:

- Sulphonylureas:
  - First generation (older), e.g. tolbutamide, chlorpropamide, acetohexamide and tolazamide.
  - Second generation (newer), e.g. glibenclamide (glyburide), glipizide, gliclazide and glimepiride.
- Biguanides, e.g. metformin and phenformin.
- Meglitinides, e.g. repaglinide and nateglinide.
- Thiazolidinediones, e.g. pioglitazone, rosiglitazone and troglitazone.
- α-glucosidase inhibitors—acarbase and miglitol drugs of sulphonylureas and meglitinides improve insulin availability, whereas biguanides, thiazolidinediones and α-glucosidase inhibitors overcome insulin resistance.

DISCUSSION OF INDIVIDUAL GROUP OF DRUGS

Sulphonylureas

These drugs are chemically related to sulphonamides but have no antibacterial action.

Pharmacological Actions

They lower blood sugar level in nondiabetic as well as in type II (maturity onset) diabetes mellitus, i.e. NIDDM. They are effective only in the presence of a functioning pancreas. They lower postprandial rise of blood sugar and normalize the metabolic status of the diabetic patient. They also lower the elevated plasma free fatty acid levels. They increase the body weight like insulin.

Mechanism of Action

They have pancreatic and extrapancreatic actions:

- **Pancreatic action:** They stimulate the release of insulin from β-cells of islets of Langerhans but do not stimulate synthesis of insulin. They probably act by increasing the sensitivity of β-cells to glucose, so that more insulin is released at every glucose level. They act on specific sulphonylurea receptors on the cell membrane of β-cells. These receptors are linked to the ATP sensitive K^+ channels in the cell membrane of β-cells. Activation of these receptors by sulphonylureas causes closing (blocking) of K$^+$ channels (i.e. decreased repolarization) leading to depolarization of the cell membrane. This produces influx of Ca^{++} resulting in release of insulin from β-cells by exocytosis (degranulation). They also reduce the release of glucagon from the α-cells of pancreas.

- **Extrapancreatic action:** They inhibit gluconeogenesis and glycogenolysis in the liver but the exact mechanism of action is not known. They increase the sensitivity of insulin receptors in the peripheral tissues such as skeletal muscle; so that small amount of insulin can produce greater action.

The basic action of all sulphonylureas is similar. They differ from each other in pharmacokinetics (rate of absorption, metabolic fate and excretion).

Pharmacokinetics

They are rapidly absorbed from the GIT. In the blood they are extensively (> 90%) plasma protein bound. They are metabolized in the liver and excreted in urine as metabolites and unchanged form (20%). Their duration of action and plasma half-life vary. They can cross the placental barrier and may produce neonatal hypoglycaemia.

Clinical Uses

They are used in:

- Maturity onset type of diabetics (in fresh cases of NIDDM).
- Insulin resistant diabetes (in some cases).
- Diabetes insipidus—chlorpropamide is usually used.

Limitations

They are ineffective in IDDM, very long-standing NIDDM, diabetic coma, diabetes due to pancreatectomy or destruction of pancreas by disease, surgical diabetics and in the presence of severe infection.

Preparations and Dosage

- Chlorpropamide (Diabenes, Copamide) tablet (250 mg)—250 to 500 mg once daily.

- Glimepiride (Amaryl, Betaglim) tablet (1 mg)—1 to 2 mg once daily.
- Glibenclamide (Daonil, Euglucon) tablet (5 mg)—5 to 20 mg once daily.
- Glipizide (Glynase, Glyzip) tablet (5 mg)—5 to 20 mg once daily.
- Gliclazide (Glucozid, Glizid) tablet (80 mg)— 80 to 180 mg once daily.

Adverse Reactions

They are well-tolerated drugs and their toxicity is low. They can produce:

- **Hypoglycaemia** which is precipitated by an excessive dose, decreased food intake, vomiting and hepatic or renal disease. Some drugs like oral anticoagulants, sulphaphenazole, salicylates and phenylbutazone can potentiate the hypoglycaemic effect of sulphonylureas by displacing them from plasma protein binding sites. Propranolol and MAO-inhibitors can produce hypoglycaemia unresponsiveness when combined with sulphonylureas or insulin. Alcohol may produce aldehyde reaction with chlorpropamide and severe hypoglycaemia in patients receiving any sulphonylurea.
- **Allergic reactions** like skin rashes and bone marrow depression producing leucopenia, thrombocytopaenia and agranulocytosis.
- **Other reactions:** Cholestatic jaundice (by chlorpropamide) and goitre (by all).

Contraindications

Hypersensitivity, hypoglycaemia, type I diabetes mellitus and diabetic ketoacidosis with or without coma.

Biguanides

Chemically they are made up of two guanidine molecules joined together.

Pharmacological Actions

They lower blood sugar level only in diabetic patients. They potentiate the hypoglycaemic action of insulin and sulphonylureas.

Mechanism of Action

They do not act by releasing insulin from beta cells of islets of Langerhans. They act by stimulating the uptake/utilization of glucose by the peripheral tissues. But the presence of either exogenous or endogenous insulin is necessary for their action. They produce inhibition of aerobic glycolysis, which stimulates anaerobic glycolysis leading to increased glucose uptake by the cells. They inhibit hepatic gluconeogenesis. They also reduce glucose absorption from the intestine. Unlike insulin and sulphonylureas, they decrease body weight and do not cause hypoglycaemia.

Pharmacokinetics

They are rapidly absorbed from the GIT and give adequate plasma levels. Phenformin is 1/3rd metabolized in the liver and 2/3rd is excreted unchanged in urine. Phenformin is largely excreted unchanged in urine. Metformin has longer duration of action (about 12 hours) than phenformin.

Clinical Uses

They are used in maturity onset type of diabetics (NIDDM), who are obese (i.e. have some resistance to insulin action), or where sulphonylureas alone is not effective.

Preparations and Dosage

- Metformin (Glycomet, Glyciphage) tablet (250–500 mg)—250 to 500 mg, 2 to 3 times daily with meals.
- Phenformin (DBI) tablet (25 mg)—50 to 100 mg twice daily with meals. Phenformin (DBITD) capsule (50 mg)—50 to 100 mg once daily.

Adverse Reactions

They can produce metallic taste, anorexia, nausea, vomiting, abdominal discomfort, diarrhoea, lethargy, muscular weakness and weight loss. Rarely they can produce anaphylaxis or generalized urticaria. Phenformin usually produces lactic acidosis (lactacidaemia) and ketonuria and so it is now rarely used. They also cause malabsorption of vitamin B_{12} on prolonged use.

Contraindications

Severe ketoacidosis, diabetic coma, severe hepatic or renal insufficiency, cardiac failure, pregnancy, type I diabetes mellitus and severe thyroid disorder.

α-GLUCOSIDASE INHIBITORS

Meglitinides

These are oral insulin secretagogues. They stimulate insulin secretion by blocking (closing) ATP-sensitive potassium channels in the pancreatic β-cells. This results in depolarization of β-cells and opening of voltage-dependent calcium channels, which increase influx of calcium into the β-cells and causes release of insulin. They are used in maturity onset (type II) diabetes mellitus.

Preparations and Dosage

- Repaglinide (Novonorm) tablet (0.5, 1 mg)—0.5–1 mg twice daily before meals.
- Nateglinide (Natelide) tablet (60, 120 mg)—60 to 120 mg twice daily before meals.

Adverse Reactions

They can produce hypoglycaemia, dizziness, diarrhoea, nausea, vomiting, constipation, skin rashes, visual disturbances, arthropathy, upper respiratory infection, bronchitis and myalgia.

Contraindications

They should not be used in hypersensitivity, type I diabetes mellitus and diabetic ketoacidosis with or without coma.

Thiazolidinediones

These are selective agonists for nuclear peroxisome proliferator-activated receptor gamma (PPAR-γ). They bind to PPAR-γ, which in turn activates insulin responsive genes that regulate carbohydrate and lipid metabolism. They require insulin to be present for their action. They exert their main effects by lowering insulin resistance in the peripheral tissues, but an effect to lower glucose production by the liver is also present. They increase glucose transport in muscle and adipose tissues by increasing the synthesis and translocation of speczific forms of the glucose transporter proteins. They also can activate genes that regulate FFA metabolism in the peripheral tissue. They are used in type II diabetes mellitus.

Preparations and Dosage

- Pioglitazone (Pionorm) tablet (15, 30 mg)— 15 to 30 mg once daily.
- Roziglitazone (Rosinorm) tablet (2, 4 mg)— 2 to 4 mg once daily.

Adverse Reactions

They can produce pharyngitis, sinusitis, headache, myalgia, fatigue, diarrhoea, hypoglycaemia, oedema and iron deficiency anaemia.

Contraindications

They should not be used in hypersensitivity, type I diabetes mellitus and diabetic keto-acidosis with or wihtout coma. Troglitazone is not available in India.

Acarbose

It is obtained by fermentation of *Actinoplanes utahensis*.

It is an inhibitor of intestinal α-glucosidase. It reduces the breakdown and absorption of carbohydrates and thus reduces postprandial rise in blood sugar level. When used as a single drug it does not cause hypoglycaemia but when used with sulphonylureas it potentiates their hypoglycaemic effects in NIDDM.

Preparation and Dose

Acarbose (Glucobay) tablet (50 mg)—50 to 100 mg with each meal.

Adverse Reactions

It can produce flatulence, abdominal discomfort, diarrhoea and even hepatotoxicity.

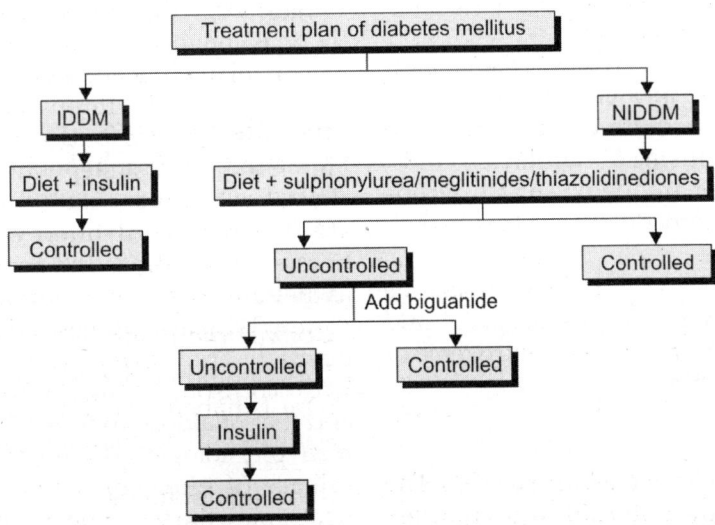

59

Adrenocortical Hormones

CORTICOSTEROIDS

Adrenal cortex is vital for survival and secretes several steroidal hormones called corticosteroids. It has three zones, *viz.*

- Zona glomerulosa (outermost zone) secretes mineralocorticoids.
- Zona fasciculata (intermediate zone) secretes glucocorticoids.
- Zona reticularis (innermost zone adjacent to adrenal medulla) secretes adrenal androgens and oestrogens (sex steroids).

Glucocorticoids, e.g. hydrocortisone (cortisol), cortisone and corticosterone are mainly concerned with carbohydrate and protein metabolism. Mineralocorticoids, e.g. aldosterone and deoxycorticosterone are mainly concerned with electrolyte (Na^+ and K^+) balance.

Sex steroids, e.g. dehydroepiandrosterone (DHEA), androstenedione (androgens) and traces of oestrogens have weak androgenic or oestrogenic activities.

Chemistry

All adrenocortical hormones are steroids. The basic structure of a steroid is a complex cyclopentanophenanthrene (CPP) ring with various functional groups ($-H$, $-CH_3$, $-OH$, $=O$) attached to different carbon atoms. They are 21-carbon compounds. They have similar basic structure with minor differences, which cause striking alteration in their biological activity. They are sparingly soluble in water but soluble in lipids and in various organic solvents. Their conjugates with glucuronic acid and sulphuric acid are soluble in water.

Biosynthesis and Release

Corticosteroids are biosynthesized from cholesterol, the major part of which comes from the exogenous source and a smaller amount is synthesized in the adrenal cortex. Cholesterol, mostly low density lipoprotein (LDL) is converted to corticosteroids with the help of mixed function oxidases (contained in cytochrome P-450) through a series of steps. The biosynthetic pathways is shown in **Fig. 59.1**. The first step is the conversion of cholesterol to pregnenolone (a rate limiting step) and is controlled by ACTH. Corticosteroid synthesis is a continuous process as they are not stored preformed in the adrenal cortex. They are synthesized and released as needed. The normal rate of secretion of hydrocortisone in man is about 20 mg/day and that of aldosterone is 0.125 mg/day. The main physiological stimulus for synthesis and release of glucocorticoids is ACTH (corticotropin), the secretion of which is regulated partly by corticotropin-releasing hormone (CRH) of hypothalamus and partly by the blood levels of glucocorticoids. The synthesis and release of mineralocorticoids is regulated by the renin-angiotensin system. Certain drugs, e.g. mitotane, metyrapone, trilostane,

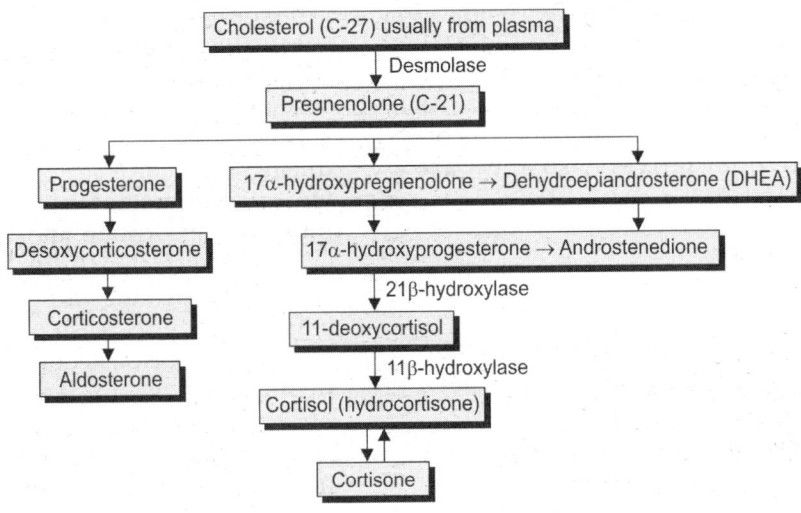

Fig. 59.1: Biosynthetic pathways of corticosteroids

etc. inhibit the biosynthesis of corticosteroids by interfering with chemical reactions. These drugs will be discussed later on as corticosteroid antagonists.

Classification of Corticosteroids

These are given as follows:

1. **According to source**—these are of two groups:
   a. Natural corticosteroids: These are:
      - Glucocorticoids, e.g. hydrocortisone, cortisone and corticosterone.
      - Mineralocorticoids, e.g. aldosterone and desoxycorticosterone (DOCA).
   b. Synthetic corticosteroids: These are:
      - Glucocorticoids, e.g. prednisolone, prednisone, methyl prednisolone, triamcinolone, betamethasone, dexamethasone, paramethasone, beclomethasone and budisonide.
      - Mineralocorticoids, e.g. fludrocortisone and desoxycorticosterone.

2. **According to duration of action**—these are of three groups:
   a. Long acting (biological half-life is 6 to 12 hours), e.g. hydrocortisone, cortisone and fludrocortisone.
   b. Intermediate-acting (biological half-life is 12 to 36 hours), e.g. prednisolone, prednisone, methyl prednisolone and triamcinolone.
   c. Long action (biological half-life is 36 to 72 hours), e.g. betamethasone, dexamethasone, beclomethasone and fluticasone. Natural corticosteroids are obtained from animal source (bovine, porcine). Synthetic corticosteroids are produced by chemical modification of hydrocortisone (obtained from diosgenin of *Dioscorea* plants). They are cheaper substitutes of natural corticosteroids.

Physiological Functions and Pharmacological Actions of Corticosteroids

Mechanism of Action (at cellular/molecular level)

Corticosteroids by crossing the cell membrane bind with specific intracellular (cytosolic) receptors of the target cells. The steroid-receptor complex thus formed enters the nucleus and binds with a specific site of a specific DNA to modify gene transcription and forming mRNA for the synthesis of specific enzymes or other proteins to produce biological actions.

Corticosteroids exert a wide variety of physiological functions and pharmacological actions in the body. They also enable the body to resist various types of noxious stimuli and environmental changes known as stress. As actions of glucocorticoids and mineralocorticoids differ qualitatively, so they are discussed separately.

GLUCOCORTICOIDS

They produce following effects:

1. **Metabolic effects:** They affect the metabolism of carbohydrates, proteins, fats, electrolytes, water and calcium.

   a. **On carbohydrate metabolism:** They increase blood sugar concentration by stimulating hepatic glycogenesis and gluconeogenesis and decreasing peripheral utilization of sugar. Although, increase in hepatic glycogenesis should cause fall in blood sugar concentration, but the increased gluconeogenesis and decreased peripheral utilization of sugar compensate this and the net result is hyperglycaemia. Persons predisposed to diabetes can develop frank diabetes or persons with frank diabetes are worsen by administration of glucocorticoids.

   b. **On protein metabolism:** They increase protein catabolism leading to increased plasma concentrations of amino acids. They inhibit incorporation of amino acids into protein in the peripheral tissues and produce a negative nitrogen balance and wasting of skeletal muscles. Amino acids by deamination are converted to glucose in the liver (gluconeogenesis) and the nitrogen residue is excreted in urine.

   c. **On fat metabolism:** They play a permissive role in the mobilization of fat from the peripheral fat depots by the lypolytic hormones like adrenaline and growth hormone. On prolonged use they cause redistribution of fat in the body, with a loss from the extremities and a deposition in the neck (buffalo hump), supraclavicular area and face (moon face). The mechanism of this action is not known.

   d. **On electrolyte and water metabolism:** They have a milder sodium and water retaining and potassium excreting activity in comparison to mineralocorticoids. In larger doses they can cause sufficient salt and water retention producing oedema.

   e. **On calcium metabolism:** They decrease intestinal absorption and increase renal excretion of calcium by an antivitamin D action and produce a negative calcium balance. They increase osteoclastic activity and decrease osteoblastic activity. On prolonged use in large doses they produce osteoporosis of bones and may lead to fracture of bones. They also interfere with the development of cartilage and inhibit linear growth in children. As a result of the protein catabolic action, they inhibit the formation of new bones.

2. **Antiinflammatory effects:** They suppress the clinical features of inflammation such as local heat, redness, swelling and tenderness, irrespective of the cause of inflammation (injury or insult). At the tissue level they attenuate (relieve) the early phenomena (oedema, fibrin deposition, capillary dilatation, migration of phagocytes (neutrophils and macrophages) into the inflamed area and phagocytosis as well as the late manifestations (capillary proliferation, fibroblast proliferation, collagen deposition and cicatrization of tissue). Fibrous tissue, once formed cannot be dissolved by glucocorticoids.

The probable mechanisms of antiinflammatory action of glucocorticoids are:

- Inhibition of chemotactic factor, involved in migration of inflammatory cells (neutrophils and macrophages) to the area of inflammation.

- Decreased production of prostanoids and leukotrienes (eicosanoids) by inhibiting the enzyme phospholipase-A_2 (through synthesis of lipocortin-1).

- Decreased generation of cytokines (IL-1 to IL-6) in the tissue.

- Decreased generation of induced nitric oxide (NO) in the tissue.
- Decreased histamine release from basophils.

3. **Antiallergic and immunosuppressive effects:** They suppress all types of hypersensitivity (allergic) reactions in larger doses. They also suppress cell mediated immunity (CMI) by causing lysis of thymus derived lymphocytes (T lymphocytes) but they do not suppress the humoral antibody production by B lymphocytes. They decrease the concentration of compliment component in the plasma. They decrease the production of gamma globulin (IgG) by the plasma cells. They interfere with the immune mechanism by influencing the functions of macrophages as follows:

- They inhibit the action of macrophage migration inhibitor factor (MIF) and hence decrease the migration of macrophages from the involved site.
- They inhibit the processing and displaying of antigen by interfering with the action of gamma interferon.
- They inhibit the synthesis and release of interleukins (IL-1 to IL-6).
- They suppress the action of T-cells, which if activated release IL-2.
- They have minimum effect on antibody formation.

4. **Other effects**

   a. **On CNS:** They stimulate the brain producing mood elevation, euphoria, nervousness, restlessness and even psychosis in large doses. They correct apathy, depression and irritability of patients with Addison's disease.

   b. **On CVS:** They decrease capillary permeability and maintain tone of arterioles and myocardial contractility. They have a permissive effect on pressor action of adrenaline and angiotensin. They play a vital role in adaptation to stress.

   c. **On GIT:** They increase secretions of gastric acid and pepsin in the stomach and may aggravate peptic ulcer.

   d. **On blood:** They cause an increase in the number of circulating neutrophils and a decrease in the number of lymphocytes and eosinophils in the blood. This is brought about by a redistribution of the cells between the blood and other compartments. There is no lysis of lyphocytes in normal persons but in patients with acute lymphoblastic leukaemia, the lymphocytes are rapidly destroyed by glucocorticoids.

   e. **On skeletal muscles:** They correct muscle weakness in patients with Addison's disease. In large doses they may cause myopathy (muscle weakness and pain).

   f. **On bones:** They produce osteoporosis of bones in large doses.

   g. **On growth and cell division:** They inhibit growth and cell division in neonates and children but not in adults, where replenishment rather than growth of cells is involved.

Pharmacokinetics

Glucocorticoids (natural and synthetic) are well-absorbed from GIT when given orally. To achieve high concentrations in the body, hydrocortisone and its synthetic congeners are administered IV. For prolonged effects IM injections are given. They are also absorbed from the sites of local application, e.g. synovial space, conjunctival sac and skin. After absorption, they are strongly (90%) bound with plasma proteins (globulin and albumin). They are metabolized in the liver by the hepatic oxidizing enzymes of microsomes forming metabolites, which are conjugated with glucuronic acid and sulphuric acid and excreted in urine as glucuronides and sulphate esters. The biological half-lives of glucocorticoids vary from compound to compound.

Clinical Uses

Indications of glucocorticoids are:

1. **For substitution (replacement) therapy in:**

   a. Acute adrenal insufficiency.

b. Chronic primary adrenal insufficiency (Addison's disease).

c. Adrenal insufficiency secondary to anterior pituitary insufficiency.

d. Congenital adrenal hyperplasia (adreno-genital syndrome).

e. After adrenalectomy (both adrenals are removed). In these conditions glucocorticoids are used along with a mineralocorticoid (fludrocortisone).

2. **Pharmacotherapy in nonendocrine diseases:**

a. Arthritis (rheumatoid arthritis and osteoarthritis).

b. Rheumatic fever with carditis.

c. Renal disease (nephrotic syndrome).

d. Collagen diseases (dermatomyositis, polyarteritis nodosa and systemic lupus erythematosus).

e. Anaphylactic shock/acute angioneuritic oedema.

f. Pulmonary diseases (acute bronchial asthma, status asthmaticus and sometimes in chronic bronchial asthma).

g. Allergic diseases (hay fever, serum sickness, urticaria, contact dermatitis, drug reactions, bee stings, eczema and psoriasis).

h. Intestinal diseases (ulcerative colitis, Crohn's disease and coeliac disease).

i. Hepatic diseases (subacute hepatic necrosis and acute or chronic infective hepatitis).

j. Ocular diseases (interstitial keratitis, phlyctenular conjunctivitis, spring catarrh, iritis, iridocyclitis and uveitis).

k. Blood dyscrasias (autoimmune haemolytic anaemia and idiopathic thrombocytopaenic purpura).

l. Malignancies (acute lymphoblastic leukaemia, Hodgkin's disease and other lymphomas).

m. Cerebral oedema and encephalitis.

n. Miscellaneous conditions (Bell's palsy, infective polyneuritis, myasthenia gravis, complete heart block and organ transplantation (to prevent acute homograft rejection).

Types of Pharmacotherapy of Glucocorticoids

- **Pulse therapy:** It is used in threatened acute homograft rejection of an organ (e.g. renal), eye threatening Graves' exophthalmos and similar emergency conditions. In it, methylprednisolone is administered in IV bolus doses of 500 to 1000 mg once daily for three consecutive days.

- **Intensive short-term therapy:** It is used in emergency conditions like anaphylactic shock, status asthmaticus, circulatory collapse (unresponsive to pressure amines), acute necrotizing vasculitis, water intoxication, acute hypercalcaemia (due to vitamin D intoxication) and hormone therapy of metastatic breast cancer. In it, large doses of a glucocorticoid (e.g. prednisolone 100 to 200 mg/day in divided doses) is to be used for 48 to 72 hours.

- **Prolonged high dose suppressive therapy:** It is used in acute rheumatic fever with carditis, ulcerative colitis, nephrotic syndrome, acute homograft rejection, pamphigus, malignancies, collagen diseases and allergic or infective diseases. In it the initial doses of a glucocorticoid (e.g. prednisolone) may be as high as 100 to 200 mg/day in divided doses and continued for 7 to 10 days. This is followed by maintenance dose of 10 to 20 mg/day. The patients need close supervision for adverse reactions, which are common. A rapid reduction in the dose can cause an acute exacerbation of the disease, being treated.

- **Low dose, chronic, palliative therapy:** It is used in rheumatoid arthritis and osteoarthritis along with salicylates or other NSAIDs. In it, small doses of a glucocorticoid (e.g. prednisolone 5 to 10 mg/day) is used to avoid adverse effects. As the therapy is very prolonged (sometimes lifelong), so close supervision of the patient is needed. The dose should be abruptly raised to 3 to 5 times during stress like surgery or acute infection in such patients.

- **Low dose, chronic suppressive therapy (to suppress pituitary ACTH secretion):** It is used in congenital, virilizing adrenocortical hyperplasia. In it, small dose of a glucocorticoid (e.g. betamethasone or dexamethasone 0.5 mg daily at bed time) is used to suppress secretion of pituitary ACTH. The therapy is to be continued lifelong. It rarely causes any adverse effects.

- **Topical therapy (by local application):** It is valuable in many dermatological, ocular and external ear conditions. It is used as ointment, cream or drops.

- **Intra-articular and intratendinous therapy (by local infiltration):** It is used in painful osteoarthritis, bursitis and facial nodules. Its advantage is that it produces minimum systemic absorption and toxicity.

Uses of Glucocorticoids for Diagnostic Tests

- Dexamethasone suppression test of adrenal function (to inhibit release of cortisol) for diagnosis of Cushing's syndrome and endogenous depression.
- Prednisolone test to distinguish intra- and extrahepatic obstructive jaundice.
- Cortisone test in hypercalcaemia.

Contraindications of Glucocorticoids

These are given as follows:

- **Absolute contraindication:** Cushing's syndrome (precipitate the condition).
- **Relative contraindications:**
  a. Peptic ulcer (healing is retarded and relapse is common).
  b. Hypertension (may be aggravated).
  c. Diabetes mellitus (may be difficult to control).
  d. Heart disease with CCF (may be aggravated).
  e. Herpes simplex keratitis (aggravated).
  f. Psychosis (aggravated).

g. Osteoporosis (aggravated).

h. Glaucoma (may be aggravated).

They should be used cautiously in:

- Pregnancy (chance of teratogenicity).
- Tuberculosis, viral, fungal and other infections (become activated).
- Epilepsy (may be aggravated in children).
- Renal failure (aggravated).

Some Preparations and Dosage of Glucocorticoids

- Hydrocortisone hemisuccinate/acetate (Efcorlin, Wycort) injection (25, 50 mg/mL)—50 to 100 mg IV or IM.
- Cortisone acetate (Corlin) injection (25 mg/mL) 1 tablet (25 mg)—50 to 100 mg IM or orally.
- Prednisolone acetate (Wysolone, Deltacortil) tablet (5, 10 mg)—15 to 60 mg orally daily in divided doses. Prednisolone sodium phosphate injection (10 mg/mL)—20 to 80 mg IV.
- Methylprednisolone acetate/hemisuccinate (Medrol) injection (20, 40 mg/mL)—20 to 40 mg IM or IV. Methylprednisolone tablet (4 mg)—4 to 40 mg daily in divided doses.
- Triamcinolone (Ledercort) tablet (4 mg)—4 to 24 mg daily in divided doses. Triamcinolone diacetate injection (5 mg/mL)—5 to 40 mg IM or intra-articularly.
- Betamethasone sodium phosphate (Betnesol, Betnelan) tablet (0.5 mg)— 1 to 5 mg daily in divided doses. Betamethasone sodium phosphate injection (4 mg/mL)—4 to 20 mg IM or IV (in acute condition).
- Dexamethasone sodium phosphate (Decadron, Wymesone) tablet (0.5 mg)—1 to 5 mg daily in divided doses. Dexamethasone sodium phosphate injection (4 mg/mL)—4 to 20 mg IM or IV (in acute condition). Some topical (skin) preparations—hydrocortisone acetate/butyrate cream/ointment (0.1 to 0.2%), betamethasone dipropionate/valerate cream, fluticasone cream (0.05%)

flucinolone acetonide cream (0.05%) (Flucort) and clobetasol propionate cream (0.05%) (Dermoryl).

Adverse Reactions

Short-term therapy (1 to 2 weeks) with small or moderate doses of a glucocorticoid usually does not produce any adverse effects. Prolonged therapy with larger doses (more than 30 mg/day) of a glucocorticoid produces many adverse effects. The important adverse effects of glucocorticoid therapy are:

- GIT effects like acute erosive gastritis with haemorrhage, peptic ulcer, intestinal perforation and pancreatitis.
- Musculoskeletal effects like myopathy, osteoporsis and even pathological fracture of bones.
- CNS effects like insomnia, headache (due to raised intracranial pressure), convulsions (due to aggravation of epilepsy) and behavioural disturbances (mental depression and psychosis).
- Ocular effects like glaucoma and posterior subcapsular cataract (especially in children).
- CVS and renal effects like hypertension and oedema due to salt and water retention and hypokalemic alkalosis.
- Metabolic effects like precipitation of diabetes mellitus, hyperlipidaemia and hypophosphataemia.
- Endocrine effects like Cushing's syndrome and hirsutism.
- Miscellaneous effects like retardation of linear growth in children, suppression of inflammation and immune responses, alopecia, hypercoagulability of blood, thromboembolic complications, subcutaneous atrophy, delayed wound healing, menstrual disorders and teratogenicity (cleft lip or plate).

Acute Adrenocortical Insufficiency

Sudden (abrupt) withdrawal of a glucocorticoid after prolonged use is dangerous and can precipitate acute adrenocortical insufficiency due to suppression of hypothalamopituitary-adrenal axis during prolonged high dose glucocorticoid therapy leading to atrophy of adrenal cortex. It may also arise as a result of acute infection, injury or surgery in patient of Addison's disease. It is manifested as malaise, fever, weakness, pain in muscles and joints and reactivation of the disease.

Treatment

Administration of hydrocortisone hemisuccinate (100 mg IV every 4 to 6 hours), 5% dextrose saline (in adequate amounts), vasopressor drugs (to maintain BP) and antibiotics (to control infection).

Prevention: The drug should be withdrawn slowly (in tapering doses) taking several days or weeks (depending upon the duration of therapy) in order to enable the adrenal cortex to regain its functional activity.

MINERALOCORTICOIDS

Natural mineralocorticoids are aldosterone and desoxycorticosterone and synthetic mineralocorticoids are fludrocortisone and deoxycorticosterone. Aldosterone is about 30 times more potent than deoxycorticosterone or desoxycorticosterone. Aldosterone is not used clinically because it has a short plasma half-life. Desoxycorticosterone and fludrocortisone are used clinically as they have longer plasma half-lives. They have no glucocorticoid activity.

Physiological Functions and Pharmacological Actions

Mechanism of Action

They act by binding with specific intracellular (cytosolic) receptors of the target cells. The steroid receptor complex thus formed enters the nucleus and binds with a specific site of a specific DNA to modify gene transcription and forming mRNA for the synthesis of specific enzymes like Na^+/K^+-ATPase, which promotes exchange of Na^+ and K^+ in the distal renal tubular cells. They produce following effects:

- **Effects on electrolyte and water metabolism:** They act on the distal renal tubule to promote reabsorption of Na^+ with concomitant increase in excretion of K^+ and H^+. Thus repeated or prolonged administration of a mineralocorticoid produces retention of sodium and water, increase in extracellular fluid volume, hypokalaemia and some degree of alkalosis.
- **CVS effects:** They produce hypertension due to sodium and water retention. They can produce cardiotonic action *in vitro*.

Clinical Uses

They are used for replacement therapy in Addison's disease (along with a glucocorticoid, e.g. hydrocortisone).

Preparations and Dosage

- Desoxycorticosterone acetate (Percorten) injection (5 mg/mL)—2.5 to 10 mg IM daily.
- Fludrocortisone acetate (Floinef) tablet (0.1 mg).
  Initial dose —1 to 2 mg daily.
  Maintenance dose—0.1 to 0.2 mg daily.

Adverse Reactions

They can produce oedema and hypertension due to sodium and water retention, muscle weakness due to hypokalaemia (by potassium loss) and systemic alkalosis due to loss of H^+ in urine.

CORTICOSTEROID ANTAGONISTS

These are of two groups:

1. **Synthesis inhibitors**—These are:
   a. **Metyrapone/Metopirone:** It blocks the synthesis of glucocorticoids by inhibiting the enzyme, 11β-hydroxylase.
   b. **Trilostane:** It blocks the synthesis of mineralocorticoids only.
   c. **Aminoglutethimide:** It blocks the synthesis of all corticosteroids by inhibiting the enzyme, desmolase which converts cholesterol to pregnenolone.
   d. **Ketoconazole:** It has action like aminoglutethimide.
   e. **Mitotane (O, P'-DDD):** It blocks the synthesis of all corticosteroids by causing necrosis of the adrenal cortex. These drugs have limited clinical use in Cushing's syndrome.

2. **Receptor antagonists**—these are:
   a. **Spironolactone:** It is a competitive receptor antagonist of aldosterone. It is used in primary or secondary hyperaldosteronism.
   b. **Mifepristone:** It is a competitive receptor antagonist of glucocorticoid and progesterone. It is used in Cushing's syndrome (hypercorticism) to block the effects of corticosteroids.

60

Male Sex Hormones and Anabolic Steroids

MALE SEX HORMONES (ANDROGENS)

These are steroidal hormones secreted by the Leydig's cells (interstitial cells) of the testis and in small amount by the ovary and adrenal cortex.

Classification

These are of two groups:

1. Natural androgens, e.g. testosterone, dehydroepiandrosterone (DHEA) and androstenedione.
2. Semisynthetic and synthetic androgens, e.g. methyltestosterone, fluoxymesterone, mesterelone and stanolone.

Testosterone is the major natural androgen. It is synthesized from cholesterol through following steps (shown in **Fig. 60.1**).

Secretion of testosterone is stimulated by luteinizing hormone (LH) of the anterior pituitary. Follicle-stimulating hormone (FSH) of the anterior pituitary stimulates spermatogensis in the seminiferous tubules. High plasma concentration of testosterone inhibits the secretion of LH. Suppression of LH secretion may lead to atrophy of Leydig's cells decreasing testosterone secretion. Thus gonadotropins (LH and FSH) play an important role in initiating and maintaining the normal testicular functions, which are:

- Development of male genital organs like penis and scrotum and secondary male sex characters like growth of facial, pubic and body hairs and change of voice.
- Development of seminal vesicles, prostate and epididymis.
- Maintenance of spermatogenesis.
- Development of skeletal musculature and emotional get up of male type.
- Anabolic and growth promoting effects.

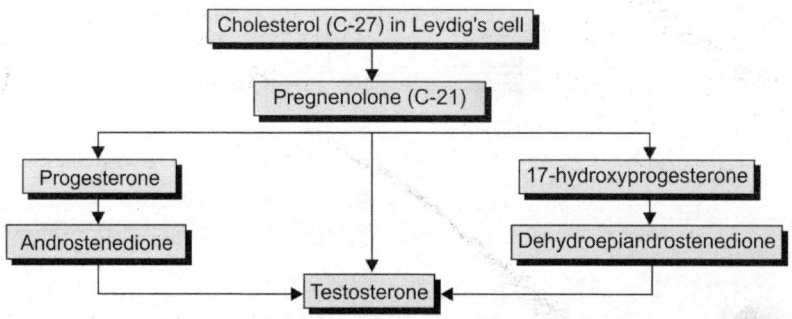

Fig. 60.1: Synthesis of testosterone

Failure of testicular function causes male hypogonadism. The daily testosterone secretion by adult males is 4 to 12 mg. This gives a plasma level of 4 to 10 ng/mL.

Physiological Functions and Pharmacological Actions

Mechanism of Action

Testosterone is converted by androgen responsive tissues to a highly active metabolite 'dihydrotestosterone', which is the active form of the hormone. Dihydrotestosterone binds with specific intracellular (cytosolic) receptors of the target cells. The steroid receptor complex thus formed enters the nucleus and binds with a specific site of a specific DNA to modify the gene transcription and forming mRNA for the synthesis of specific enzymes or other proteins to produce biological actions.

Physiological functions of testosterone: Testosterone is required for spermatogenesis, development of male sex organs and secondary sex characters, development of skeletal musculature and emotional get up of male type, anabolism and growth in males.

Pharmacological Actions

These are given as follows:

- **Androgenic effects:** Administration of testosterone in male hypogonadism reverses most of the changes. The secondary sex characters develop, muscle strength increases and sexual desire and erection of penis occur normally. Given to females, it causes increased libido and musculinization (hirsutism, growth of clitoris and male type voice). It also alters the ovarian function. It inhibits the development of proliferative phase of the endometrium. In large doses, it can inhibit ovulation and lactation. Administered during pregnancy it can cause musculinizing effect on developing female foetus.

- **Anabolic effects:** It produces positive nitrogen balance by promoting nitrogen retention. It increases skeletal muscle mass and strength and body weight. It increases appetite. Given in smaller doses it promotes growth of epiphyseal cartilage in dwarfism due to hypopituitarism and hypogonadism, probably by elevating growth hormone (HGH) levels in these children but given in large doses it causes early fusion of epiphyses leading to stunted growth in the children.

Pharmacokinetics

Androgens are well-absorbed when given orally but the natural androgen testosterone is largely inactivated in the liver by first pass metabolism and hence it is therapeutically ineffective. It is administered IM or by subcutaneous implantation. Its methyl derivatives, e.g. methyltestosterone and fluoxymesterone are administered orally as they are much less destroyed by the liver. After absorption testosterone is highly plasma protein bound (about 98%) and only 2% remains in free form. It is metabolized mainly in the liver and excreted in urine mostly as androsterone and etiocholanolone as sulphates and glucuronides. The plasma half-life of testosterone is 10 to 20 minutes.

Clinical Uses

These are given as follows:

- For substitution (replacement) therapy in hypogonadism and hypopituitarism (in children).

- For pharmacotherapy in senile osteoporosis in males, carcinoma of the breast in premenopausal females, as anabolic steroid, refractory anaemias (aplastic anaemia and anaemia of chronic renal failure) and sexual impotence.

Contraindications

- Carcinoma of prostate and breast in males.
- Pregnancy and lactation.
- Severe hepatic and renal diseases.

Preparations and Dosage

- Testosterone aqueous suspension (Aquaviron) injection (25 mg/mL)—50 to 100 mg IM once a week.

- Testosterone phenylpropionate injection (30 mg/mL)—30 to 60 mg IM every one or two weeks.
- Testosterone enanthate (Testovirondepot) injection (250 mg/mL)—250 mg IM every two to three weeks.
- Methyltestosterone tablet (5 mg)—25 to 50 mg daily.
- Fluoxymesterone (Ultandren) tablet (5 mg)—5 to 20 mg daily.

Testosterone implant and transdermal preparation are also available for long-lasting effect.

Adverse Reactions

These include precocious puberty in boys, musculinization and menstrual irregularities in females, retarded growth in children (due to early closure of the epiphyses), oedema formation (due to retention of sodium and water), prostatic enlargement, atherosclerosis (due to changes in serum lipid profile), cholestatic jaundice (by methyltestosterone and others) and liver cancer.

ANTIANDROGENS

These drugs antagonize the actions of androgens. These are of three groups:

1. Receptor inhibitors, e.g. cyproterone acetate and flutamide. They are competitive inhibitors of androgen.
2. Inhibitors of androgen synthesis, e.g. ketoconazole.
3. Inhibitors of formation of dihydrotestosterone (DHT) from testosterone, e.g. finasteride (Proscar). These drugs are used orally in precocious puberty in boys, hyper sexuality in males, acne and musculinization in females and BPH and prostatic carcinoma.

ANABOLIC STEROIDS

These are drugs with potent anabolic activity and weak androgenic activity, e.g. nandrolone, stanozolol, methandienone, ethy-lestrenol, oxymetholone and oxandralone. Chemically these are derivatives of testosterone or methyltestosterone. As testosterone has anabolic:androgenic ratio of 1:1, so it cannot be used as an anabolic agent. Hence, various steroids have been synthesized with potent anabolic action and weak androgenic action. None of the anabolic steroids is selectively anabolic without any androgenic action. At cellular level they act like testosterone.

Pharmacological Actions

They produce following effects:

- **Anabolic effects:** They promote protein anabolism, which is manifested clinically as the increase in muscle mass and the body weight. They produce positive nitrogen balance by increasing protein synthesis.
- **Anticatabolic effects:** They counteract the catabolic action of glucocorticoids on prolonged therapy. They correct protein catabolism or negative nitrogen balance produced in patients due to chronic debilitating diseases, protein deficiency, refractory anaemias, prolonged immobilization after severe burn or fracture of long bone and severe stress.
- **Other effects:** They reduce bone resorption and may prevent osteoporosis like testosterone. They improve appetite and produce a feeling of well-being. They are taken by athletes for increasing muscle strength.

Clinical Uses

They are used in chronic illness (to improve appetite and the sense of well-being), senile osteoporosis, refractory anaemias, severe hypoproteinaemia, breast cancer in females and to promote growth in hypogonadal children.

Contraindications

- Prostatic and male breast cancer
- Pregnancy
- Severe cardiac, renal and hepatic diseases.

Adverse Reactions

These are similar to those of androgens.

Some Preparations and Dosage of Anabolic Steroids

- Nandrolone phenpropionate (Durabolin) injection (25 mg/mL)—25 to 50 mg IM once weekly.

- Nandrolone decanoate (Decadurabolin) injection (25 mg/mL)—25 to 50 mg once monthly.
- Stanozolol (Stromba) tablet (2.5 mg)—2.5 to 5 mg daily.
- Ethyl estrenol (Orabolin) tablet (2 mg)— 2 to 4 mg daily.
- Methandienone (Dianabol) tablet (2.5 mg)—2.5 to 5 mg daily.

61

Female Sex Hormones and Ovulation Inducing Drugs

FEMALE SEX HORMONES

These are oestrogens and progestins.

Oestrogens

These are steroidal compounds with oestrogenic activity.

Classification

These are of two groups:
1. Natural oestrogens, e.g. oestradiol, oestrone and oestriol.
2. Semisynthetic and synthetic oestrogens, e.g. ethinyl oestradiol, dienestrol, mestranol, diethyl stilbestrol, quinestrol and chlorotrianisene.

Last three compounds are nonsteroidal.

The natural oestrogen 'oestradiol' is secreted by the theca cells of matured graafian follicle and corpus luteum (of ovary) and placenta. It is also secreted in small amount by the testis and adrenal cortex. It is converted to oestrone and oestradiol in the liver.

Secretion of oestradiol is controlled by pituitary gonadotropins (FSH and LH).

Physiological Functions of Natural Oestrogens

These are given as follows:
- Development of reproductive tract (uterus and fallopian tube) in the female.
- Development of secondary female sex characters like breasts (ductal growth), body contour, hair, skin and voice and emotional get up of female type.
- Stimulation of proliferative (preovulatory) phase of the endometrium.
- Along with progesterone, control of normal menstrual cycle and preparation of the uterus for pregnancy.
- Vasodilation of capillaries in general and particularly of those of the endometrium.
- Metabolic effects like retention of nitrogen, sodium and water in tissues.
- Cardioprotection in women of the reproductive age (probably by lowering serum LDL levels).
- Maintenance of integrity of bones (preventing osteoporosis) in women of reproductive age.
- Promotion of the union of epiphyses with the metaphyses, thus controlling the height in females.

Mechanism of Action

Like other steroids, oestrogens act by binding with specific intracellular (cytosolic) receptors of the target cells. The steroid receptor complex thus formed enters the nucleus and binds with specific site of a specific DNA to modify gene transcription and forming mRNA for the synthesis of specific enzymes or other proteins to produce biological actions.

Pharmacological Actions

These are given as follows:

- **Effects on female reproductive organs:** In adolescent females with primary hypogonadism, oestrogens used with progestins stimulate the development of sex organs and secondary sex characters and stimulate growth. In adult females, oestrogens used with progestins in a cyclical manner induce an artificial menstrual cycle and are used as oral contraceptives. In postmenopausal women, oestrogens reduce menopausal symptoms, atrophic vaginitis and osteoporosis.

- **Metabolic effects:** Oestrogens have mild anabolic actions and can promote growth in females. Given for a long period they may cause sodium and water retention leading to oedema and hypertension. They can impair glucose tolerance. They increase the serum levels of triglyceride and HDL but decrease the serum levels of cholesterol and LDL.

- **Effects on blood coagulation:** Oestrogens increase the coagulability of blood by increasing plasma levels of clotting factors like II, VII, IX and X and also fibrinogen. They increase platelet aggregation and decrease antithrombin level.

- **Effects on lactation:** Oestrogens suppress lactation without affecting prolactin levels. They are used to suppress postpartum lactation in case of neonatal death.

- **Antiandrogenic effects:** Oestrogens have been found to be beneficial in prostatic cancer, which is androgen dependent.

Pharmacokinetics

Oestrogens are rapidly absorbed from GIT after oral administration but the natural oestrogens are not therapeutically effective as they are rapidly inactivated in the liver during first pass metabolism. They are also absorbed when applied to the skin and mucous membranes and can produce systemic effects. After absorption, they are highly plasma protein bound (about 90%). They are metabolized mainly in the liver and excreted in urine as sulphates and glucuronides and slightly as free form (10%.) They undergo some degree of enterohepatic circulation.

Clinical Uses

These are given as follows:

- **As oral contraceptive pill (OCP):** Oestrogens either alone or in combination with progestins are used (discussed later on).

- **For replacement therapy in postmenopausal women:** To reduce menopausal symptoms (hot flushes, etc.), vaginal atrophy and osteoporosis, primary amenorrhoea (due to hypogonadism) in young girls (used along with progestins), Turner's syndrome (where ovaries have not developed) and Simmond's disease (where there is secondary ovarian failure due to pituitary failure), oestrogens are used.

- In menstrual disorders like dysmenorrhoea and severe dysfunctional uterine bleeding, oestrogens along with progestins are used.

- **For suppression of postpartum lactation:** Oestrogens in high doses may be used, but bromocriptine is better in this condition.

- **As postcoital contraceptives** (discussed later on).

- **In prostatic cancer (androgen dependent):** Oestrogens in high doses produce antiandrogenic action on the prostate.

- **Miscellaneous uses:** Oestrogens are used in acne vulgaris, female hirsutism, senile vaginitis, atrophic rhinitis and vulvovaginitis in children (along with a proper antibiotic).

Contraindications

- Premenopausal breast cancer (oestrogen dependent).

- History of thromboembolic diseases.

- Cautiously used in presence of hypertension, hepatic dysfunction, diabetes mellitus, migraine and uterine fibroid, which may be aggravated.

Some Preparations and Dosage

- Oestradiol benzoate injection (1 mg/mL)—1 to 5 mg IM twice weekly.
- Oestradiol dipropionate injection (1 mg/mL)—1 to 5 mg IM once weekly.
- Oestradiol valerate/cypionate injection (5 mg/mL)—5 to 20 mg IM every 2 to 4 weeks.
- Ethinyl oestrodiol (Lynoral) tablet (0.01, 0.05 mg)—0.2 to 2 mg daily.
- Mestranol (0.1 mg) and ethinydol diacetate (1 mg) tablet (Ovulen) (a progestin) used as oral contraceptive.
- Diethylstilbestrol (Stilbestrol) tablet (1, 5 mg)—1 to 5 mg daily.
- Estriol succinate (Evalon) tablet (2 mg)—2 to 10 mg daily.
- Conjugated oestrogen (Premarin) tablet (0.625, 1.25 mg)—1.25 to 10 mg daily, (conjugated means sulphates of natural oestrogens, e.g. oestrone).
- Transdermal oestradiol patch (Estraderm) containing 25, 50 or 100 mg of oestradiol. It is applied twice weekly.
- Dienestrol vaginal cream for local use in vagina.

Adverse Reactions

These include nausea, vomiting, headache, migraine, breast discomfort, increased vaginal secretion, oedema (due to fluid retention), thromboembolism, formation of gall stones, cholestatic jaundice and cancer of breast, uterus or bone (on prolonged use during menopause). Cervical or vaginal adenocarcinoma is produced in offspring of mothers receiving oestrogens during the first trimester of pregnancy.

Antioestrogens

Androgens and progestins antagonize several effects of oestrogens but drugs which have selective effect on oestrogen receptors are competitive antagonists of oestrogens.

These are clomiphene, tamoxifen and raloxifen.

Clomiphene

It is a nonsteroidal (triphenylethylene) compound with structural resemblance to diethyl stilbestrol. It is a partial agonist of oestrogen (also called impeded oestrogen), as it retains a weak oestrogenic activity. It is an ovulation inducing drug. It blocks hypothalamic and anterior pituitary oestrogen receptors and reduces the feedback inhibitory effect of oestrogens on the secretion and release of gonadotropins (FSH and LH).

Increase in gonadotropin activity by clomiphene induces ovulation in women producing ovulatory menstrual cycles.

Clinical Uses

It is used in the treatment of infertility in women with anovulatory sterility. It is also used for *in vitro* fertilization of ovum, in premenopausal breast cancer and oligospermia in males.

Preparation and Dose

Clomiphene citrate (Clomid, Fertyl) tablet (50 mg)—50 to 100 mg daily for 5 to 7 days starting from the 5th day of menstrual bleeding.

Adverse Reactions

It can cause hot flushes, enlargement of ovaries, breast engorgement, nausea, vomiting, vertigo and multiple ovulation leading to multiple pregnancies. It increases the risk of cancer of breast and uterus.

Tamoxifen and Raloxifen are selective-oestrogen receptor modulators (SERMs).

Tamoxifen

It is a nonsteroidal antioestrogen, chemically related to diethylstilbestrol. It is a partial agonist of oestrogen like clomiphene. It has affinity for oestrogen receptors and binds with the receptors but has poor activity. At the same time it blocks the binding of the oestrogen with its receptors. It has antioestrogenic action in breast cells but prooestrogenic action in uterine endometrial mucosa (causes proliferation). It is used for palliative treatment in oestrogen dependent premenopausal breast cancer. It is available as tablet (10 mg) and administered in the dosage of 10 to 20 mg twice daily for 2 to 5 years or even life-long. It can produce hot flushes, nausea, vomiting, bone pain, vaginal bleeding, thrombophlebitis and ocular toxicity. It can increase the risk of endometrial cancer.

Raloxifen binds with oestrogen receptors and acts in same places as mild oestrogen agonist and at others as antioestrogens. It is used to treat postmenopausal osteoporosis. It prevents bone resorption and reduces the concentration of serum cholesterol and LDL. It does not increase the risk of kterine cancer.

Progestins

These are steroidal compounds with progestational activity.

Classification

These are of two groups:

1. Natural progestin: Progesterone.
2. Semisynthetic and synthetic progestins:

 – Derivatives of progesterone, e.g. medroxy-progesterone, hydroxyprogesterone, megestrol, chlormadinone and dydro-esterone.
 – Derivatives of testosterone, e.g. ethisterone, dimethisterone, norethisterone (norethindrone), norethynodrel, norgestrel, ethinodiol and lynestrenol.

The natural progestin 'progesterone' is secreted by the corpus luteum (of ovary) and placenta. It is also synthesized in the adrenal cortex, where it acts as a precursor of various steroid hormones. Secretion of progesterone is controlled by pituitary LH. Epostane and trilostane are progesterone synthesis inhibitors.

Physiological Functions of Progesterone

These are given as follows:

• Induction of secretory phase of menstrual cycle on an oestrogen primed proliferative phase of the endometrium.

• Preparation of the endometrium for the implantation of the fertilized ovum and to induce decidual reactions.
• Maintenance of pregnancy.
• Promotion of development of the alveolar (acinar) system of the breast (along with oestrogen).
• Induction of changes in the vaginal epithelium and increase in secretion.
• Metabolic changes like midcycle rise (0.5°C) in basal body temperature (BBT) by thermogenic action (increasing heat production). This rise of temperature is corrected by ovulation.

Mechanism of Action

It is similar to oestrogens.

Pharmacological Action

These are given as follows:

• **Effects on the genital tract:** It produces secretory phase of menstrual cycle on an oestrogen primed proliferative phase of the endrometrium. Continuation of progesterone therapy prolongs the luteal phase and induces decidual changes in the endometrial stroma, characteristic of early pregnancy. It prevents cornification of the vaginal epithelium and brings about increased glycogen deposition. It makes vaginal secretion thick, viscid and scanty. It helps in the maintenance of pregnancy by decreasing uterine motility and inhibition of immunological rejection of foetus. It decreases T lymphocyte function and cell mediated immunity (CMI).
• **Effect on mammary gland:** It promotes the growth of alveolar (acinar) system of oestrogen primed mammary glands.
• **Metabolic effects:** It produces rise in BBT similar to that observed during midcycle of menstruation. Synthetic progestins such as testosterone derivatives and dydrogesterone are not thermogenic. Progesterone has some catabolic actions and promotes nitrogen, sodium and chloride loss. Synthetic progestins, however, have no such catabolic actions.

- **Antineoplastic effect:** It prevents development of oestrogen induced endometrial and breast carcinomas.
- **Central nervous system effects:** It has a sedative action on brain. It can suppress epileptiform fits. It has influence on the neurotransmitters of the brain. It reverses oestrogen induced alterations in the concentration of several neurotransmitters (NAd, 5-HT and GABA) in the brain.

Pharmacokinetics

It is not effective orally because it is rapidly metabolized in the liver by first pass metabolism. It has a very short biological half life (5 to 10 minutes). When administered IM in oily solution it is slowly absorbed and produces prolonged action. Synthetic progestins are effective orally as they are not easily destroyed during first pass metabolism in the liver. They are slowly metabolized in the liver and excreted in urine as metabolites.

Clinical Uses

These are given as follows:
- As oral contraceptive pill (OCP): Progestins either alone or in combination with oestrogens are used (discussed later on).
- For replacement therapy in progesterone deficiency like habitual or threatened abortion and dysfunctional uterine bleeding (DUB).
- In menstrual disorders like primary spasmodic dysmenorrhoea and premenstrual tension (combined with oestrogens).
- In endometriosis to cause regression of the endometrium, but now replaced by danazole (antigonadotropic compound).
- In fibrocystic disease of the breast, but danazole is better than progestins.
- In endometrial carcinoma and also in renal cell carcinoma (hypernephroma).

Some Preparations and Dosage
- Progesterone (Susten) capsule (200, 400 mg)—200 to 400 mg daily.

- Progesterone (Proluton) injection (25 mg/mL)—25 to 50 mg IM daily.
- Hydroxyprogesterone caproate (Proluton depot) injection (125 mg/mL)—125 to 250 mg IM weekly.
- Medroxy progesterone acetate (Farlutal) injection (50 mg/mL) and tablet (5, 10 mg)— 50 to 100 mg IM weekly, 10 to 40 mg orally daily.
- Dydrogesterone (Duphaston) tablet (5 mg)—10 to 25 mg daily.
- Allylestrenol (Gestanin) tablet (5 mg)—5 to 15 mg daily.
- Norethisterone (Primulut-N) tablet (5 mg)— 10 to 30 mg daily.
- Norethisterone acetate (Regestrone) tablet (5 mg)—5 to 15 mg daily.
- Lynestrenol (Orgametril) tablet (5 mg)—5 to 15 mg daily.

Adverse Reactions

Progestins are relatively safe drugs. In high doses testosterone derivatives can cause nausea, vomiting, headache, fatigue, breast discomfort, mental depression and even liver damage. If used during pregnancy, they may cause androgenic actions on developing female foetus and so should not be used during pregnancy.

Antiprogestin

Mifepristone (RU 486) is a derivative of the progestin 'norethisterone' with antiprogestin activity. It is a competitive antagonist of progesterone as well as glucocorticoids. When progesterone is present it acts as an antagonist but if progesterone is absent, it acts as a weak agonist. Hence, it is a partial agonist of progesterone. When administered in early stages of pregnancy it causes decidual breakdown leading to either no implantation of blastocyst or shedding of endometrium along with the implanted blastocyst. It also suppresses ovulation. It is used for induction of abortion, induction of labour after intrauterine foetal death and as postcoital contraceptive. It is also used in Cushing's syndrome to block the effects of cortico-steroids. It is available as tablet and injection and administered in a single dose of 600 mg orally or IM. It can be combined with a prostaglandin (Sulprostone). It can produce nausea, vomiting, abdominal pain and sometimes severe uterine bleeding.

Antigonadotropic Compounds

Danazol

It is a synthetic derivative of ethisterone. It has no oestrogenic or progestational properties but has antigonadotropic activity. It inhibits secretion of gonadotropins (FSH and LH) and thereby inhibits ovulation, spermatogenesis and testosterone secretion. It is used in endometriosis, menorrhagia, gynaecomastia, fibrocystic disease of breast and infertility (in both male and female). It is available as capsule (200 mg) and administered in the dosage of 200 to 800 mg daily. It can produce hot flushes, atrophic vaginitis, weight gain, acne, hirsutism, voice change, mental depression and liver dysfunction.

Gestrinone

It is an analog of danazol. It is used in endometriosis in the dosage of 2.5 mg twice in a week for six months, starting during a menstrual period.

Gonadotropic release hormore (GnRH) analogs (antagonists), e.g. leuprolide, naferelin and goserelin.

They are synthetic peptide analogs of GnRH. They indirectly inhibit oestrogen/androgen secretion by suppression of FSH and LH release from anterior pituitary and have palliative effect in advanced oestrogen/androgen dependent cancer of breast and prostate.

Ovulation Inducing Drugs

These are used in infertility due to ovulation failure in female. These are of four groups:

1. Antioestrogenic compounds, e.g. clomiphene citrate and cyclofenil.

2. Dopamine D_2 agonist, bromocriptine.

3. Human menopausal and chorionic gonadotropin combination (hMG + hCG).

4. Synthetic gonadotropin-releasing hormone (GnRH) analogs, e.g. leuprolide, hafarelin and goserelin.

These drugs are discussed in respective chapters.

62

Oral and Parenteral Contraceptives

CONTRACEPTIVES

These are antifertility drugs used to prevent conception (pregnancy) as a measure of birth control. They may act by the following mechanisms:

- Inhibition of ovulation.
- Modification of cervical mucus.
- Slowing down of the rate of ovum transport.
- Prevention of ovum maturation and sperm capacitation.
- Interfering with the implantation of fertilized ovum.
- By immunological methods.
- Inhibition of spermatogenesis in males.

ORAL CONTRACEPTIVES (OCRS)

These are used in women to prevent conception. These are of following types:

- Combination of oestrogen and progestin.
- Progestin alone.
- Oestrogen alone.

Combination of Oestrogen and Progestin (Combination Pills)

Pincus (1955) showed the usefulness of combination of oestrogen and progestin for oral use as contraceptive. Now various commercial combined preparations are available, which are less expensive, highly effective, relatively safe and easy to administer than other methods of contraception. These preparations contain an oestrogen (ethinyl-oestradiol or mestranol) and a progestin (norethisterone, norethynodrel, levonorgestrel, desogestrel, lynestrenol, ethinodiol diacetate, or megestrol acetate in small doses (shown in **Table 62.1**).

Methods of Administration

- **Fixed dose combination pills (monophasic pills):** The usual procedure is to administer one pill orally daily at bed time for 21 days, starting from the 5th day of the menstrual cycle. The next course is started 7 days after the last dose or 5 days after the onset of menstruation. If the patient forgets to take a pill at night, she should take it in the morning within 12 hours and then continue the usual schedule. If more than 24 hours have passed after the last (regular) pill taken, then the patient is considered unprotected by the pill and other measure to prevent conception must be taken. When used properly, it is the most effective (99 to 100%) type of oral contraceptive currently available.

- **Biphasic (sequential) and triphasic combination pills:** These are combined oral contraceptive pills containing varying proportions of an oestrogen and a progestin. The whole period is divided into two (biphasic) or three (triphasic) phases,

Table 62.1: Some fixed dose combination of oral contraceptives

Trade name	Estrogen	Progestin
Ovral-L/Microgynon	Ethinylestradiol (0.03 mg)	Levonorgestrel (0.15 mg)
Triquilar	Ethinylestradiol (0.03 mg)	Levonorgestrel (0.05 mg)
Novelon	Ethinylestradiol (0.03 mg)	Desogestrel (0.15 mg)
Ovral/Primovlar	Ethinylestradiol (0.05 mg)	Levonorgestrol (0.25 mg)
Lyndiol	Ethinylestradiol (0.05 mg)	Lynestrenol (1 mg)
Minovlar/Orthonovin	Ethinylestradiol (0.05 mg)	Norethisterone (1 mg)
Orgalutin/Noracy clin	Ethinylestradiol (0.05 mg)	Lynestrenol (2.5 mg)
Gynovlar	Ethinylestradiol (0.05 mg)	Norethisterone (3 mg)
Anovlar	Ethinylestradiol (0.05 mg)	Norethisterone (4 mg)
Voldys	Ethinylestradiol (0.05 mg)	Megestrol (4 mg)
Ovulen	Mestranol (0.01 mg)	Ethinodiol (1 mg)

each phase lasting for several days (7 or 14). This allows lower doses of both oestrogen and progestin in the early part of the menstrual cycle, thus reducing the total dose per cycle. Slightly higher doses of these drugs used in the later part of the cycle helps to prevent breakthrough bleeding. They are, however, more complex to use and offer little or no advantage over the morphasic pills.

Mechanism of Action of Combination of Oral Contraceptives

Oestrogen induces feedback inhibition of anterior pituitary 'FSH' secretion (through inhibition of hypothalamic GnRH secretion) leading to inhibition of development of mature graafian follicle (in the ovary). Progestin produces following actions:

- Feedback inhibition of anterior pituitary 'LH' secretion (through inhibition of hypothalamic GnRH secretion) leading to absence of the midcycle LH surge and inhibition of ovulation.
- Production of thick and viscid cervical mucus making mucosal plug, which prevents the passage of sperm to the ovum in the uterus.
- Alteration of the uterine endometrium from proliferative phase to secretory phase, so that even if an ovum is fertilized

by chance, it cannot be implanted in the endometrial decidua.

- Interference with the transport of fertilized ovum.

Progestin Only (Minipills)

In it, only a progestin pill is taken daily without interruption for 21 days. It has a high failure rate as the contraceptive effect is less reliable (because suppression of ovulation is inconsistent) and there is increased incidence of breakthrough bleeding.

Oestrogen Only (Postcoital Pills/Morning after Pills)

In it, only an oestrogen in high doses (e.g. stilbestrol 25 mg twice daily) is given for 5 days starting within 72 hours of coitus. It has high incidence of adverse effects like nausea and vomiting. It is reserved for accidental/expected coitus like rape. It probably acts by preventing the transport of fertilized ovum or making the endometrium unsuitable for implantation of the fertilized ovum (blastocyst).

Advantages of Oral Contraceptives

These are given as follows:

- Reduced incidence of dysmenorrhoea, menorrhagia, premenstrual tension and intermenstrual bleeding (metrorrhagia).

- Reduced incidence of benign breast disease, uterine fibroid, ovarian cysts, endometriosis and ectopic pregnancy.
- Reduced incidence of thyroid disease and rheumatoid arthritis.
- Avoidance of unwanted pregnancy and hence reduced maternal and neonatal mortalities.

Adverse Reactions of Oral Contraceptives

These are given as follows:

- Initial minor side effects (due to oestrogen component) like nausea, vomiting, headache, migraine, breast discomfort, increased vaginal secretion and slight oedema.
- Adverse effects after prolonged use. These are:
  - Weight gain (due to fluid retention) and hypertension.
  - Decreased glucose tolerance and unmasking of latent DM.
  - Acne and skin pigmentation.
  - Impaired hepatic functions and formation of gallstones (cholelithiasis).
  - Increased incidence of thromboembolic phenomena (deep vein thrombosis, cerebral thrombosis and pulmonary embolism).
  - Increased incidence of ocular diseases (corneal oedema, blurring of vision, eyelid oedema and contact lens discomfort).
  - Enlargement of uterine fibroid (fibromyomata), if present.
  - Mental depression and other behavioural changes.

Contraindications

These are given as follows:

- Presence of active thromboembolic disorders.
- Presence of atherosclerotic disorders.
- Presence of active liver disease and jaundice.
- Moderate to severe hypertension.
- Diabetes mellitus.
- Oestrogen dependent cancers, e.g. breast cancer and cervical cancer.
- Pregnancy.

Nonsteroidal Oral Contraceptive

Centchroman (Centron)

It is a chroman derivative developed by the Central Drug Research Institute, Lucknow, as antifertility drug. It acts as an oestrogen antagonist and interferes with the implantation of fertilized ovum. It is available as tablet (30 mg). It is administered in the dose of 30 mg twice in a week for 3 consecutive months or as long as contraception is desired starting from the first day of menstrual cycle. It can prolong menstrual cycle. It is contraindicated in jaundice, severe hepatic dysfunction, polycystic ovarian disease, tuberculosis, renal disease and allergic disorder.

Injectable Contraceptives

These are given as follows:

- **Depot progestin preparations,** e.g. Medroxy progesterone acetate (Dopot provera) injection (50, 150 mg/mL)—50 mg IM/month or 150 mg IM/3 months. Norethisterone enanthate (Noristerat) injection (100, 200 mg/mL)—100 mg IM/month or 200 mg IM/2 months).

- **Progestin implants,** e.g. levonorgestrel implant (Norplant): This implant consists of six flexible silastic capsules containing levonorgestrel (36 mg/capsule) in crystalline form. The capsules are inserted under the skin, usually on the inner side of the upper arm. The contraceptive effect lasts for 5 years. Initially 85 mg of the drug is released per day, which is decreased to 50 mg per day at 9 months and 35 mg per day at 18 months and 30 mg per day at 5th year after implantation.

These long-acting progestin preparations act by inhibiting ovulation and thickening cervical mucus secretion. Their disadvantages are menstrual irregularities including breakthrough bleeding and continued suppression of ovulation after stopping of therapy.

Male Contraceptives (Chemical)

These are drugs that inhibit (suppress) spermatogenesis by antiandrogenic action. These are cyproterone acetate, flutamide and gossypol. Gossypol is a nonsteroidal contraceptive agent. It destroys the seminiferous tubules but Leydig's cells are unharmed. After cessation of the drug, the testicular changes are reversed to normal. Its success rate is high. Flutamide is an antiandrogen and acts by preventing binding of the androgen with its receptors. These are under clinical trials as male contraceptives.

Section III

CHEMOTHERAPY

63

Introduction to Sulphonamides

INTRODUCTION

Chemotherapy is the use of specific chemical agents for the treatment of parasitic diseases caused by microbes, protozoa and helminths in order to inhibit their growth and multiplication or to kill them with minimum injury to the host tissues. The word chemotherapy was introduced by the famous German chemist Paul Ehrlich in 1891. He is known as the father of chemotherapy.

Drugs used for chemotherapy are called chemotherapeutic agents. Paul Ehrlich named them magic bullets for their specific and prompt actions. They have maximum parasitotropic effect and minimum organotropic effect. They are the most widely used drugs in clinical practice. They are divided into four groups:

1. Antimicrobial agents, e.g. antibacterial agents, antiviral agents and antifungal agents.
2. Antiprotozoal agents.
3. Anthelmintic agents.
4. Anticancer agents.

Due to analogy (similarity in structure) between cancer cells and microbes, drugs used in the treatment of cancers are called cancer chemotherapy.

Chemotherapeutic Index (CTI)

It is the ratio of maximum tolerated dose to minimum curative dose of a chemotherapeutic agent. The higher the index, the safer the chemotherapeutic agent, e.g. penicillins, cephalosporins, etc. Chemoprophylaxis is the use of chemotherapeutic agents for the prevention of infectious diseases during incubation period (carrier state), i.e. before the development of clinical manifestations of the disease, e.g. isoniazid in tuberculosis, dapsone in leprosy, ampicillin in typhoid fever, benzathine penicillin in rheumatic fever, rifampicin in meningococcal meningitis and chloroquine or pyrimethamine in malaria.

Classification of Chemotherapeutic Agents

It can be done by following ways:

1. **According to source**: These are three groups:
   a. Natural compounds, e.g. most antibiotics, quinine, emetine, vincristine, etc.
   b. Semisynthetic compounds, e.g. ampicillin, cephalexin, doxycycline, dehydroemetine, etc.
   c. Synthetic comopounds, e.g. sulphonamides, quinolones, dapsone, chloroquine, metronidazole, etc.

2. **According to chemical structure:** These are following groups:
   • Sulphonamides, e.g. sulphadiazine, sulphadoxine, etc.
   • Diaminopyrimidines, e.g. trimethoprim and pyrimethamine.

- Quinolones, e.g. nalidixic acid, norfloxacin, ciprofloxacin, etc.
- Nitrofurans, e.g. nitrofurantoin, nitroforazone, etc.
- Nitroimidazoles, e.g. metronidazole, tinidazole and secnidazole.
- Sulphones, e.g. dapsone and acedapsone.
- 4-aminoquinolines, e.g. chloroquine and amodiaquine.
- 8-aminoquinolines, e.g. primaquine and pamaquine.
- 8-hydroxyquinolines, e.g. diiodohydroxyquine and iodochlorhydroxyquin.
- Antibiotics, e.g. penicillins, cephalosporins, tetracyclines, etc.

3. **According to type of action:** These are of two groups:
   - Bacteriostatic drugs, e.g. sulphonamides, dapsone, tetracyclines, chloramphenicol, ethambutol, thiacetazone, etc.
   - Bactericidal drugs, e.g. penicillins, cephalosporins, carbapenems, streptomycin, gentamicin, rifampicin, isoniazid, cotrimoxazole, etc.

4. **According to mechanism of action:** These are of following groups:
   - Drugs inhibiting bacterial cell wall synthesis, e.g. penicillins, cephalosporins and carbapenems.
   - Drugs causing damage of bacterial cell membrane, e.g. polymyxin-B, amphoterian-B and nystatin.
   - Drugs inhibiting bacterial protein synthesis, e.g. tetracyclines, chloramphenicol, erythromycin, etc.
   - Drugs causing misreading of mRNA, e.g. streptomycin, gentamicin, neomycin, etc.
   - Drugs inhibiting bacterial DNA synthesis/function, e.g. rifampicin, quinolones and metronidazole.
   - Drugs inhibiting viral DNA synthesis, e.g. idoxuridine, acyclovir and zidovudine.
   - Drugs producing antimetabolite action, e.g. sulphonamides, sulphones, trimethoprim, etc.
   - Drugs damaging cellular microtubules, e.g. griseofulvin, colchicine, vinblastine, etc.

Combination of Antimicrobial Agents

Sometimes two or more antimicrobial agents are used in combination for the following advantages:

- To prevent the emergence of resistant strains of microorganism as in tuberculosis and leprosy.
- To enhance the antimicrobial activity, e.g. sulphamethoxazole and trimethoprim in bacillary dysentery, penicillin and gentamicin in enterococcal endocarditis, gentamicin and carbenicillin in Pseudomonas infection, ampicillin and cloxacillin in pyogenic infection, amoxycillin and clavalanic acid in serious bacterial infection. These are fixed dose combinations.

Bactericidal drug (e.g. ampicillin) should not be combined with bacteriostatic drug (e.g. tetracycline) because bactericidal drug can kill the bacteria when they are in the form of continuous multiplication. Bacteriostatic drug by arresting the process of bacterial multiplication, interferes with the action of bactericidal drug.

- To broaden the antibacterial spectum in cases of mixed infections (peritonitis, brain abscess, bronchiectasis and septicaemia)—to cover both gram-positive and gram-negative microorganisms.

Disadvantages of such combination of antimicrobials are

- Increased toxicity (local and systemic).
- Possibility of superinfection.
- Development of resistance against both the drugs.

Superinfection (Opportunistic Infection)

It is the appearance of a new infection during chemotherapy of a primary infection. It is a potentially dangerous condition. Most antimicrobial agents cause suppression of growth of normal microbial flora of the host present in the intestinal, upper respiratory and genitourinary tracts. These microflora contribute to host defence by elaborating substances called bacteriocin, which inhibits the growth of pathogenic microbes. Moreover, the pathogenic microbes have to compete with the normal microflora for nutrients for survival. In favourable condition, due to lack of competition a nonpathogenic microflora like *Candida albicans*, which is not inhibited by the drug get a chance to proliferate and invade the tissue. If the microflora is completely suppressed by the drug then there is greater chance of developing superinfection. It is commonly found after administration of broad- or extended-spectrum antibiotics, e.g. tetracyclines, chloramphenicol, ampicillin and amoxycillin. Tetracyclines are more dangerous than chloramphenicol and ampicillin to produce superinfection diarrhoea because of incomplete absorption from small intestine and higher amounts reaching the large intestine to cause greater suppression of gut microflora. Microorganisms that commonly produce superinfection are *Candida albicans, Staphylococci, Proteus, Pseudomonas* and *Clostridium difficile* (bacteroid). Important sites of superinfection are oropharynx, GIT, respiratory tract, genitourinary tract and skin. It is more common when host defence is lowered as in corticosteriod therapy, anticancer therapy, AIDS, agranulocytosis, diabetes mellitus and disseminated lupus erythematosus.

Prevention of Superinfection

Following measures are taken:

- Specific and narrow-spectrum antimicrobials should be used if possible.

- Unnecessary use of antimicrobials for minor, self-limiting or untreatable infection should be avoided.

- Unnecessary prolonged use of antimicrobials should be avoided.

Treatment of Superinfection

Following specific drugs are used:

- Nystatin or clotrimazole is used in *Candida albicans* oral thrush, vulvovaginitis and diarrhoea.

- Cloxacillin or methicillin is used in *Staphylococcal enteritis*.

- Gentamicin or cephalexin is used in *Proteus enteritis* and UTI.

- Carbenicillin, ceftazidime, amikacin or gentamicin is used in *Pseudomonas enteritis* and UTI.

- Vancomycin or metronidazole is used in *Clostridium difficile, Pseudomembranous enterocolitis* (*Pseudomembranous enterocolitis* is associated with the use of some antibiotics such as clindamycin, lincomycin, ampicillin, amoxicillin and cephalosporins).

Drug Resistance
(Microbial Resistance to Drugs)

It is the unresponsiveness of microorganisms to antimicrobial agents. It is similar to tolerance seen in men or animals. It may be natural resistance or acquired resistance:

1. **Natural resistance:** It is the inherent (intrinsic) resistance in some microorganisms, from the beginning, e.g. *M. tuberculosis* to penicillins, gram-positive bacteria (*Streptococci, staphylococci,* etc.) to streptomycin and gram-negative bacteria (*E. coli, Proteus,* etc.) to penicillin-G. In it, the drug fails to reach its target site due to lack of transport system. It is of little clinical importance.

2. **Acquired resistance:** It is the development of resistance in some microorganisms after prolonged use of antimicrobials. It can occur with any microorganism. Some microorganisms, e.g. *Staphylococci, E. coli, Proteus, Pseudomonas, M. tuberculosis,* etc. develop rapid resistance to antimicrobials, while other microorganisms develop slow resistance to antimicrobials. *Gonococci* develop rapid resistance to sulphonamides but slow resistance to penicillins. Some bacteria produce enzymes that reside at or within the cell surface and inactivate the antimicrobial drug, e.g. β-lactamase (penicillinase) produced by *Staphylococci, Gonococci,* etc. inactivating penicillin-G. Acquired resistance may be nongenetic or genetic.

   a. **Nongenetic resistance:** Once the infection has been brought under control by antimicrobial agents, a few bacteria may remain dormant (inactive) in the host and unable to multiply. These nonmultiplying bacteria are resistant to antimicrobial agents.

b. **Genetic resistance:** In it a stable genetic alteration occurs in the microorganisms and this may involve either chromosomal or extrachromosomal resistance. Chromosomal resistance develops following a spontaneous mutation in a locus that controls susceptability to a given chemotherapeutic agent. The microorganism also contains extrachromosomal genetic element called plasmids (episomers). Genetic mutation occurs by transfer of resistant gene (DNA/R-factor) from one bacterium to other bacterium. It can occur by following processes:

  i. **Transduction:** In it, the plasmid DNA is transferred from one bacterium to other bacterium by a bacteriophage (a virus that infect bacteria). It occurs in *Staphylococci* and some *Streptococci*.

  ii. **Transformation:** In it, the naked DNA (R-factor) is transferred from one resistant bacterium to sensitive bacterium. It is of little clinical importance.

  iii. **Conjugation (mating):** In it, the genetic material (chromosomal or plasmid DNA) is transferred from one bacterium to another bacterium during conjugation.

  iv. **Translocation:** In it, the exchange of short DNA sequence occurs either between two plasmids or between one plasmid and a portion of the bacterial chromosome within a bacterial cell.

Prevention of Drug Resistance

Following measures are taken:

- Indiscriminate and inadequate use of antimicrobials should be avoided.
- Use of specific and rapidly acting antimicrobials should be done.
- Use of combination of antimicrobial drugs should only be done where prolonged therapy is necessary, e.g. tuberculosis, leprosy and subacute bacterial endocarditis (SBE).
- Intensive treatment of infections by microorganisms that develop rapid resistance should be done.

Cross-resistance

It is the development of resistance of microorganisms to one antimicrobial drug having resistance to another antimicrobial drug due to similarity of chemical structures between these drugs, e.g. resistance to one sulphonamide means resistance to another sulphonamide, resistance to one tetracycline means resistance to another tetracycline, etc. Sometimes unrelated antimicrobials show partial cross-resistance, e.g. between penicillins and cephalosporins, tetracyclines and chloramphenicol, erythromycin and lincomycin, etc.

Choice of antimicrobial drug: It depends on:

- *Route of administration:* Oral route of administration is preferred over parenteral route.
- *Type of action:* Bactericidal action is preferred over bacteriostatic action.
- *Spectrum of activity:* Narrow-spectrum antimicrobial drug is preferred over broad-spectrum antimicrobial drug if the causative organism is known.
- *Toxicity of the drug:* Less toxic drug is preferred for use.
- *Cost of the drug:* Less costly drug is preferred for use.

Sulphonamides
Source and History

Sulphonamides are synthetic antimicrobial agents. Gerhard Domagk (1935) discovered that the azo dye 'Prontosil' when administered is broken down in the body to sulphanilamide, which is the active compound for antimicrobial activity against many microorganisms. He was awarded the Nobel prize in medicine in 1938 for this discovery. Since then many sulphonamides have been introduced for the treatment of bacterial infections but now their uses have diminished due to introduction of antibiotics, which are more effective and less toxic.

Chemistry

Sulphonamides are derivatives of para-amino benzene sulphonamide (sulphanilamide), which resembles para-amino benzoic acid (PABA) in chemical structure (as shown in **Fig. 63.1**).

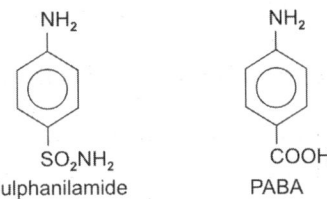

Fig. 63.1: Structures of sulphanilamide and PABA

These are white powders, mildly acidic in character and relatively insoluble in water but their sodium salts are readily soluble in water. The pH of the sodium salts with the exception of sulphacetamide sodium is very high (alkaline). Sulphonamide group (SO_2NH_2) is also present in some non-antibacterial compounds like sulphonylureas (e.g. chlorpropamide and tolbutamide), diuretics (e.g. thiazides, frusemide and acetazolamide) and anticonvulsants (e.g. sulthiame).

Classification of Sulphonamides

- Sulphonamides used for the treatment of systemic infections: These are absorbable. Depending on their duration of action, these are of three groups:
  - Short-acting sulphonamides (4 to 8 hours), e.g. sulphadiazine, sulphadimidine, sulphasomidine, sulphafurazole and sulphamethizole.
  - Intermediate-acting sulphonamides (8 to 16 hours), e.g. sulphamethoxazole and sulphamoxole.
  - Long-acting sulphonamides (1 to 7 days), e.g. sulphamethoxypyridazine, sulphadimethoxine and sulphadoxine.
  - Sulphonamides used for the treatment of bowel diseases: These are poorly absorb-

able, e.g. sulphaguanidine, phthalylsulphathiazole, succinyl sulphathiazole, sulphasalazine, mesalazine, olsalazine and balsalazine.
- Sulphonamides used topically in eye and skin infections, e.g. sulphacetamide sodium (in eye infections), silver sulphadiazine and mefenide propionate (in infected burns).

Pharmacokinetics

Sulphonamides for systemic uses are rapidly and completely absorbed from the GIT. The small intestine is the major site of absorption but small amount is absorbed from the stomach and large intestine. Peak plasma concentrations are achieved in 2 to 6 hours. In the blood, they are bound in varying degree to plasma proteins (albumin and globulin) depending on the drug. They are widely distributed in the body tissues and fluids. They can cross the BBB and the placental barrier. They are metabolized mainly in the liver by acetylation. The acetylated sulphonamide metabolites have no antibacterial activity but retain toxicity of the parent compound, e.g. they can cause crystalluria and calculus formation in the kidney. They are excreted in urine *via* glomerulus partly as metabolites and partly as unchanged (free) form. They accumulate in the body in renal failure and cause toxicity. The plasma half-life of sulphonamides vary depending upon the nature of the drug, i.e. whether short-, intermediate- or long-acting. Small amount of sulphonamides are excreted in faeces, bile, milk and other secretions. Sulphonamides for intestinal uses are poorly absorbed from the GIT and are excreted mainly in faeces.

Pharmacological Actions

Mechanism of action: Sulphonamides are bacteriostatic drugs and act by inhibiting the folic acid synthesis in the susceptible bacteria. They are structural analogs and competitive antagonists of PABA. They prevent the utilization of PABA in the synthesis of folic acid (pteroyl glutamic acid). More specifically, they are competitive inhibitors of dihydropteroate synthetase (folic acid synthetase), the enzyme responsible for the incorporation of PABA into dihydropteroic acid (the immediate precursor of folic acid). Sulphonamide-sensitive bacteria are those, that can synthesize their own folic acid. Bacteria and mammalian cells that require performed folate from outside are not affected by sulphonamides. Bacteriostasis induced by sulphonamides can be counteracted (antagonized) by PABA. Synergists of sulphonamides are trimethoprim and pyrimethamine. Antagonists of sulphonamides are PABA and PABA-containing substances like procaine, amethocaine, procainamide, pus and tissue breakdown products.

Effects on microorganisms: Sulphonamides have a wide range of antimicrobial activities. They are effective against both gram-positive and gram-negative bacteria. In the recent years many resistant strains of bacteria have developed due to widespread use of sulphonamides and so their usefulness has diminished. The cellular and humoral defence mechanisms of the host are essential for the final eradication of the infection (the bacteria are phagocytosed by the macrophages). Antimicrobial spectrum: Sensitive microorganisms are *Streptococci* (except *Strep. faecalis*), *Haemophilus influenza*, *Haemophilus ducreyi*, *Nocardia*, *Toxoplasma*, *Actinomyces*, *Bacillus anthracis*, *Donovania granulomatis* and *Chlamydia trachomatis*. *Staphylococci, Gonococci, Meningococci, Pneumococci, Vibrio coma, Pasturella pestis, Clostridia, Shigella organisms, E.coli, Proteus* and *Pseudomonas* were previously sensitive to sulphonamides but now have become resistant to sulphonamides. The minimum inhibitory concentration (MIC) of sulphonamides ranges from 0.1 µg/mL for *Chlamydia trachomatis* to 60 µg/mL for *E. coli*.

Sulphonamide resistance: Acquired bacterial resistance to sulphonamides occurs by random mutation or by transfer of resistant gene (DNA) by plasmids. The resistance is probably due to an alteration of the enzyme constitution of the bacterial cell. The alterations may be characterized by:

- An alteration of the enzyme dihydropteroate synthetase, which utilizes PABA in the bacteria.
- An increased bacterial capacity to inactivate the drug.
- Development of an alternative metabolic pathway in the bacteria to synthesize folic acid. There is no cross-resistance between sulphonamides and antibiotics.

Clinical Uses

Sulphonamides are used in following bacterial infectious diseases.

- **Urinary tract infections (UTI):** Absorbable systemic sulphonamides are used in urinary tract infections (pyelitis, pyelonephritis and cystitis) caused by *E. coli* but ineffective in presence of mixed infections. They produce effective urine and tissue levels. They are cheap and orally effective. Their long-term use has shown reasonable safety, but the development of bacterial resistance is the major problem with the use of these drugs. A short-acting sulphonamide such as sulphadiazine or sulphafurazole (sulphisoxazole) is usually administered in a dose of 2 g initially followed by 1 g 6 hourly for 7 to 10 days. Urinary pH should be kept alkaline by administration of alkali mixture during such therapy and fluid intake must be sufficient.
- **Acute bacillary dysentery:** Poorly absorbable or systemic sulphonamides are used in acute bacillary dysentery caused by *Shigella* organisms (sonnei, flexneri and boydii) but due to development of bacterial resistance, these drugs are now less preferred than cotrimoxazole, ampicillin, chloramphenicol, norfloxacin or ciprofloxacin.
- **Ulcerative colitis:** Sulphasalazine, mesalazine or olsalazine is used orally as anti-inflammatory drug in ulcerative colitis and Crohn's disease.
- **Meningococcal meningitis:** Systemic sulphonamides may be used in meningococcal Meningitis caused by *Meningococci*, but due to development of bacterial resistance to these antibiotics like ampicillin, chloram-

phenicol, gentamicin and ceftriaxone are preferred in this condition.

- **Nocardiasis:** Sulphadiazine or sulphafurazole in the dosage of 4 to 6 g daily in divided doses is used for several months in nocardiasis.
- **Toxoplasmosis:** Sulphadiazine with pyrimethamine is used in the treatment of toxoplasmosis.
- **Malaria:** Sulphadoxine with pyrimethamine is used in the treatment of malaria.
- **Trachoma and inclusion conjunctivitis:** Sulphacetamide sodium is used as eye drops (10 or 20%) but chloramphenicol or tetracyclines orally or topically is preferred.
- **Lymphogranuloma venereum and chancroid:** Systemic sulphonamides were used previously in these conditions, but tetracyclines are now the preferred drugs (used for 3 weeks).

Prophylactic Uses of Sulphonamides

These are streptococcal tonsillitis or pharyngitis and recurrence of rheumatic fever. Sulphadimidine or sulphadiazine is used in the dosage of 1 g twice daily to prevent these conditions. They have equal effectiveness as oral penicillins but there is a chance of development of streptococcal resistance to sulphonamides. In patients allergic to penicillins, they should be used without hesitation.

Some Preparations and Dosage of Sulphonamides

1. **Oral preparations:** All sulphonamides are available as tablets (0.5 g/tablet), e.g.
   - Sulphadiazine tablet (0.5 g)—initially 2 g then 1 g 6 hourly.
   - Sulphadimidine tablet (0.5 g)—initially 2 g then 1 g 6 hourly.
   - Sulphafurazole (Gantrisin) tablet (0.5 g)—initially 2 g then 1 g 6 hourly.
   - Sulphamethoxazole (Gantanol) tablet (0.5 g)—initially 1 to 2 g and then 0.5 to 1 g 12 hourly.

- Sulphadimethoxine (Madribon) tablet (0.5 g)—initially 1 g and then 0.5 g once daily.
- Sulphasalazine (Salazopyrine) tablet (0.5 g)—2 to 6 g daily in divided doses.

2. **Parenteral preparations** (given IM or IV), e.g.
   - Sulphadiazine sodium injection (250 mg/mL in 10 mL/vial)—2 g initially and then 30 to 50 mg/kg 6 hourly.
   - Sulphadimidine sodium injection (250 mg/mL in 10 mL/vial)—2 g initially and then 30 to 50 mg/kg 6 hourly.
   - Sulphafurazole diolamine injection (400 mg/mL in 10 mL/vial)—2 g initially and then 30 to 50 mg/kg 6 hourly.

3. **Some tropical preparations** (for eye and skin), e.g.
   - Sulphacetamide sodium (Albucid) eye drops (10%, 20%).
   - Silver sulphadiazine (Silverex) cream (1%).
   - Mefenide propionate (Marfanil) cream (10%).

Adverse Reactions of Sulphonamides

These are relatively common and include:
- GIT side effects like anorexia, nausea, vomiting and epigastric pain.
- **Crystalluria and haematuria (renal toxicity):** In the presence of acid urine, the acetylated sulphonamide is precipitated, mainly in the collecting tubules and calyces causing renal irritation, obstruction to the urine flow and renal colic. Crystalluria and haematuria occur leading to the development of oliguria and anuria. These renal complications can be minimized by administration of alkali mixture and plenty of fluid intake to increase urine output.
- **Hypersensitivity (allergic) reactions:** These are various types of skin rashes (mobiliform, scarlatinal, urticarial, purpuric, petechial and pemphigoid), drug fever, erythema nodosum, erythema multiforme with ulceration of the mucous membrane

(Stevens-Johnson syndrome), exfoliative dermatitis, photosensitivity, arthritis, hepatis and jaundice (hepatocellular).

- **Blood dyscrasias (haemopoietic toxicity):** Haemolytic anaemia due to deficiency of G6PD in RBCs or hypersensitivity reaction can occur. Prolonged use can produce bone marrow depression leading to anaemia, leucopenia, agranulocytosis, thrombocytopaenia and rarely aplastic anaemia.

- **Neurological toxicity:** These are peripheral neuritis, confusion, mental depression, ataxia, tinnitus, fatigue and psychotic episodes (especially in children).

- **Endocrine disorders:** Prolonged use can produce thyroid disorders like goitre and hypothyroidism by inhibiting the synthesis of thyroid hormones.

- **Miscellaneous reactions:** When administered in newborn infants especially in premature babies, they may produce kernicterus by displacing bilirubin from plasma protein (albumin) binding site, which is deposited in the basal ganglia and subthalamic nuclei of the brain causing encephalopathy. If administered in large doses in pregnant women, they may produce teratogenicity.

Contraindications of Sulphonamides

These are newborn infants, lactating mothers, pregnant women and history of hypersensitivity reactions or haemolytic anaemia.

Drug Interactions

Sulphonamides potentiate the effects of oral anticoagulants, sulphonylureas, methotrexate and phenytoin by displacing them from plasma protein binding sites with resultant toxicity. Combined preparations of only sulphonamides:

- Combined sulphadiazine (200 mg), sulphamerazine (150 mg) and sulphamethazine (150 mg) tablet (sulphatriad) for systemic use.

  Advantage: It reduces the chance of crystalluria and haematuria.

- Combined sulphacetamide (2.86%), sulphadimidine (2.86%), sulphadiazine (2.7%) cream (triple sulpha cream) for topical use in vaginitis, cervicitis and leucorrhoea.

  Advantage: It has additive effect and less irritant effect.

Combined preparations of sulphonamides with trimethoprim or pyrimethamine:

- Combined sulphamethoxazole (400 mg) and trimethoprim (80 mg) tablet (Cotrimoxazole/Septran).

- Combined sulphadiazine (410 mg) and trimethoprim (90 mg) tablet (Cotrimazine/Aubril).

- Combined sulphadoxine (500 mg) and pyrimethamine (25 mg) tablet (Croydoxin/Metakelfin). Only cotrimoxazole will be discussed here.

Cotrimoxazole (Septran, Bactrim)

It is a combined fixed dose preparation of trimethoprim and sulphamethoxazole in the ratio of 1:5. Trimethoprim is a pyrimidine derivative (diaminopyrimidine) and sulphamethoxazole is an intermediate-acting sulphonamide. When used individually they are bacteriostatic drugs but when used in combination they become bactericidal drugs. This is because they block two successive steps (sequential block) in the same metabolic pathway for the synthesis of folic acid of the bacteria, which is required for the synthesis of nucleic acids in the bacteria (as shown in **Fig. 63.2**).

Sulphamethoxazole blocks incorporation of PABA into folic acid by inhibiting folic acid synthetase and trimethoprim blocks conversion of folic acid to folinic acid by inhibiting folic acid reductase. This sequential block leads to synergistic action producing bactericidal effect.

Antibacterial spectrum: Trimethoprim has similar antibacterial spectrum as sulphamethoxazole, but it is about 20 times more potent than sulphamethoxazole. Most gram-positive and gram-negative microorganisms are sensitive to trimethoprim but *Pseudomonas*

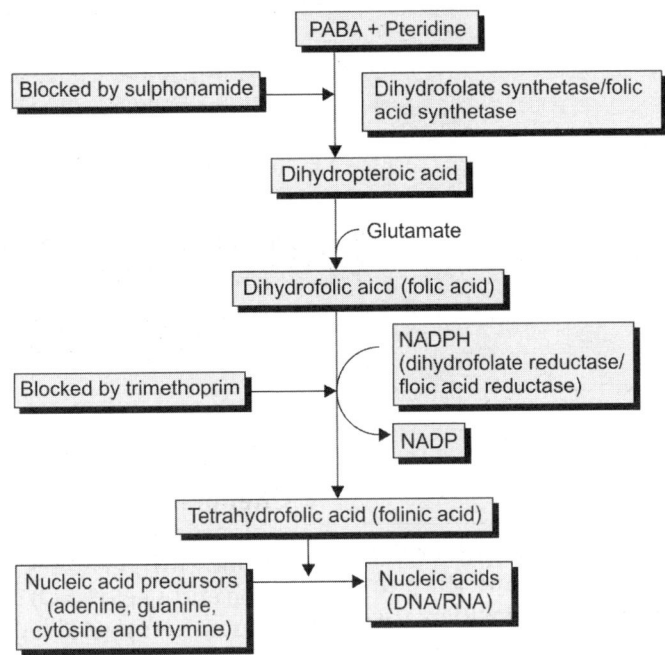

Fig. 63.2: Steps in folic acid metabolism blocked by sulphonamide and trimethoprim

aeruginosa, Bacteroides fragilis and *Steptococcus faecalis* (*Enterococcus*) are usually resistant to it. Bacterial resistance develops when the drug is used alone but when it is used in combination with sulphamethoxazole, there is a little chance of development of bacterial resistance, because the bacteria developing resistance to one of them, may still be killed by the other drug.

Pharmacokinetics

The pharmacokinetic profiles of trimethoprim and sulphamethoxazole are closely and perfectly matched to achieve a constant ratio of 1:20 in their concentrations in blood and tissues. Trimethoprim is absorbed more rapidly and completely from GIT than sulphamethoxazole. Peak blood concentrations of trimethoprim and sulphamethoxazole are reached in 2 and 4 hours respectively. Half-lives of trimethoprim and sulphamethoxazole are approximately 12 and 10 hours respectively. Thus, bacteria are always exposed to the optimum synergistic ratio of the two drugs (1:2) in the plasma producing bactericidal effect.

Clinical Uses

It is used in urinary tract infection, bronchitis, pneumonitis, shigellosis (bacillary dysentery), typhoid fever, meningitis, osteomyelitis, gonorrhoea, chancroid, prostatitis, sinusitis, otitis media and infection (pneumonia) caused by *Pneumocystis carinii* (in AIDS and neutropenic patients).

Preparations and Dosage

- Cotrimoxazole (Septran/Bactrim) tablet (trimethoprim 80 mg + sulphamethoxazole 400 mg)—2 tablets twice daily for 10 to 14 days.
- Cotrimoxazole paediatric tablet (trimethoprim 20 mg + sulphamethoxazole 100 mg) and suspension (trimethoprim 40 mg + sulphamethoxazole 200 mg/5 mL) are also available.

Adverse Reactions

These are similar to sulphonamides.

64

Quinolones and Other Drugs Used in UTI

QUINOLONES

Source: These are synthetic antimicrobial drugs like sulphonamides, but they are bactericidal drugs. They are now widely used drugs for the treatment of many infectious diseases caused by bacteria.

Classification

These are of two groups:
1. Older quinolones (1st generation, 4-quinolones), e.g. nalidixic acid, oxolinic acid, cinoxacin, enoxacin and rosoxacin.
2. Newer quinolones (2nd generation, fluoroquinolones), e.g. norfloxacin, ciprofloxacin, ofloxacin, levofloxacin, pefloxacin, lomefloxacin, sparfloxacin and gatifloxacin.

Chemistry: The basic structures of all quinolones are shown below **(Fig. 64.1).** They have one carboxylic (–COOH) group at C_3 position and a keto (=O) group at C_4 position. The parent compound nalidixic acid does not contain flourine (F) atom. Introduction of F at C_6 position increases the clinical effectiveness of the compound against many bacterial infections caused by gram-positive and gram-negative bacteria. Introduction of a piperazine ring at C_7 position changes the antibacterial and pharmacokinetic properties.

Pharmacokinetics

4-quinolones are slowly and incompletely absorbed from GIT. They do not achieve sufficient blood and tissue concentrations and

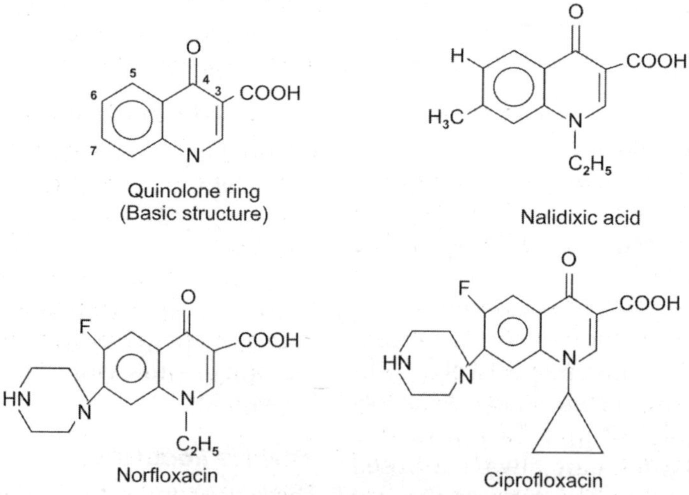

Quinolone ring
(Basic structure)

Nalidixic acid

Norfloxacin

Ciprofloxacin

Fig. 64.1: Structures of quinolones

so ineffective in systemic infections. On the other hand, fluoroquinolones are well-absorbed after oral administration and are widely distributed in the body tissues and fluids. They are concentrated in urine, bile, kidneys, lungs, bones, prostate, macrophages and neutrophils. They have greater bioavailability, tissue distribution and cellular penetration than 4-quinolones. Their peak plasma concentrations (1.5 to 6 µg/mL) are obtained within 2 hours of an oral dose. They have plasma half-lives as follows:

Norfloxacin 3 to 5 hours, ciprofloxacin 5 to 8 hours and pefloxacin 9 to 11 hours. They are metabolized in the liver and excreted in urine mainly as glucuronides.

Pharmacological Actions

Mechanism of action: They act by preventing DNA replication or transcription during cell division by inhibiting the bacterial enzyme DNA gyrase and thus causing supercoiling of separated DNA strands. This blocks DNA synthesis and bacterial cell division (by binary fission). During cell division the two strands of double helical DNA strands are separated from each other. The separated DNA strand tends to become excessively coiled (supercoiling) like a highly compressed spring. This supercoiling prevents binary fission of bacteria. DNA gyrase prevents supercoiling of DNA strands. Quinolones by inhibiting DNA gyrase help in supercoiling of DNA strands and thus prevent bacterial cell division.

Antibacterial Spectrum

4-quinolones have less antibacterial activity than fluoroquinolones because they do not achieve sufficient antibacterial concentrations in blood and tissues, but they achieve high concentrations in urine and so useful in urinary tract infections. They are also useful in GIT infections due to local antibacterial action. They have narrow-spectrum of activity and effective against only gram-negative bacteria like *E. coli, Proteus* and *Shigella* organisms. On the other hand, fluoroquin-olones have broad-spectrum antibacterial activity and effective against many gram-positive bacteria (*Streptococci, Staphylococci,* etc.) and gram-negative bacteria (*E. coli, Proteus, Shigella* organisms, *Salmonella* organisms, *Klebsiella pneumoniae, Pseudomonas aeruginosa, Campylobacter jejuni, Gonococci, Haemophilus* organisms (*influenzae, pertussis* and *ducreyi*). They are also effective against *Chlamydia, Mycoplasma, Legionella, Brucella* and *Mycobacteria.* They are ineffective against anaerobes (bacteroides) except sparfloxacin. Their minimum inhibitory concentration (MIC) is 0.2 µg/mL in blood. Ciprofloxacin is more potent than norfloxacin/pefloxacin/ofloxacin against *Ps. aeruginosa, Strepto. faecalis, Staphylococci* and *Pneumococci.*

Drug resistance: Bacteria can develop rapid resistance to 4-quinolones but slow resistance to fluoroquinolones. *Ps. aeruginosa* and *E. coli* may develop resistance to fluoroquinolones by mutation during treatment.

Clinical Uses

They are used in following bacterial infections:
- **Urinary tract infections:** They are effective in UTIs caused by sensitive microorganisms. They are also effective in prostatitis caused by sensitive bacteria.
- **Sexually transmitted diseases:** Fluoroquinolones especially ciprofloxacin is effective in gonorrhoea, softsore, urethritis and cervicitis caused by sensitive bacteria, but they are ineffective in syphilis. In pelvic infections, they may be combined with metronidazole or clindamycin to kill anaerobes.
- **GIT infections:** They are effective in bacterial gastroenteritis, traveller's diarrhoea, shigellosis and cholera. Ciprofloxacin and ofloxacin are effective in typhoid fever resistant to chloramphenicol and in carrier state of typhoid fever. Norfloxacin is used in *Campylobacter jejuni* infection in peptic ulcer.
- **Respiratory tract infections:** Fluoroquinolones are effective in Pneumonias and acute exacerbation in chronic bronchitis caused

by respiratory pathogens like *H. influenzae, Kleb. pneumoniae, Moraxella catarrhalis, Mycoplasma pneumoniae, Staphylococci* or *Legionella pneumophilia.*

- **Bone, joint and soft tissue infections:** Fluoroquinolones are effective in bone and joint infections caused by *Staph. aureus* or a gram-negative bacteria, when used in high doses for prolonged period (2 to 4 weeks). In chronic osteomyelitis and soft tissue infections they are combined with metronidazole or clindamycin to kill anaerobes.

- **Eye and ear infections:** Norfloxacin and ciprofloxacin eye/ear drops are used in conjunctivitis and otitis media caused by sensitive bacteria.

- **Other infections:** Ciprofloxacin, pefloxacin and ofloxacin are used in septicaemia, multidrug resistant tuberculosis and chloroquine resistant *Plasmodium falciparum* malaria. They are also used for prophylaxis of carrier state of meningitis (by *Meningococci* or *H. influenzae*).

Preparations and Dosage

- Nalidixic acid (Negadix, Gram-O-neg) tablet (0.5 g)—0.5 to 1 g 6 hourly. Nalidixic acid paediatric suspension (300 mg/5 mL) is also available.

- Norfloxacin (Norflox, Uriben) tablet (400 mg)—400 mg twice daily.

- Ciprofloxacin (Ciplox, Cosflox) tablet (500 mg)—500 mg twice daily. Ciprofloxacin solution (0.5 g/100 mL) is also available for IV infusion.

- Pefloxacin (Pelox) tablet (400 mg)—400 mg twice daily.

- Ofloxacin (Tarivid) tablet (200 mg)—200 to 400 mg once or twice daily.

- Lornefloxacin (Lomflox) tablet (400 mg)—400 mg twice daily.

- Sparfloxacin (Torospar) tablet (200 mg)—200 to 400 mg once or twice daily.

- Gatifloxacin (Gabact) tablet (200 mg)—same.

Adverse Reactions

These are well-tolerated drugs. They can produce:

- GIT side effects like anorexia, nausea, vomiting, abdominal discomfort and diarrhoea.

- CNS side effects like confusion, dizziness, headache, nervousness, agitation, hallucinations and rarely convulsions.

- Hypersensitivity (allergic) reactions like skin rashes, urticaria, pruritus, drug fever, eosinophilia and photosensitivity.

- Cartilage damage (arthropathy) in weight bearing joints of young children (below years) leading to stunted growth.

- Miscellaneous adverse effects like leucopenia, keratopathy (corneal opacity), renal damage and acute renal failure.

Contraindications

These are given as follows:

- Young—can cause epiphyseal cartilage damage long bones leading to stunted growth children.

- Pregnant and lactating women—can effect foetus and infant's cartilage.

- Epilepsy and other convulsive disorders—can precipitate convulsions.

- Severe renal disease—can cause acute renal failure.

- Severe hepatic disease—pefloxacin is hepatotoxic and can cause acute hepatic failure.

Drug Interactions

- Antacids and sucralfate decrease absorption of fluoroquinolones from GIT leading to decreased bioavailability and clinical efficacy.

- NSAIDs can potentiate the CNS stimulant effects of fluoroquinolones leading to nervousness, agitation, hallucinations and even convulsions.

- Ciprofloxacin inhibits the metabolism of theophylline and so increases its cardiac and CNS adverse effects.

Other Drugs Used in Urinary Tract Infections (UTIs)

Urinary antiseptics are drugs used only in urinary tract infections like pyelitis, pyelonephritis, cystitis, prostatitis and urethritis. Most urinary tract infections are caused by gram-negative bacteria like *E. coli, Proteus mirabilis, Klebsiella pneumoniae, Aerobacter aerogenes* and *Pseudomonas aeruginosa* and a few gram-positive bacteria like *Streptococcus faecalis* and *Staphylococcus aureus*. Acute urinary tract infection is usually caused by one species of microorganism (e.g. *E. coli)*, while chronic and recurrent urinary tract infections are caused by several species of microorganisms (mixed infections). For appropriate use of a drug in urinary tract infections, routine examination and culture and sensitivity test of urine must be done. Lower urinary tract infection requires short treatment (5 to 7 days), while upper urinary tract infection requires long treatment (2 to 3 weeks). Drugs used in urinary tract infections are of two groups:

- Urinary antiseptics, e.g. methenamine (Hexamine), methenamine mandelate, nitrofurantoin and nalidixic acid.
- Other antimicrobial drugs, e.g. sulphonamides, cotrimoxazole, ampicillin and other extended spectrum penicillins, gentamicin and other aminoglycosides, cephalexin and other cephalosporins, norfloxacin and other fluoroquinolones, chloramphenicol, tetracyclines and cycloserine.

Urinary antiseptics will be discussed here. Other antimicrobial drugs are discussed in respective chapters.

Urinary antiseptics inhibit the growth of many species of pathogenic microorganisms in the urinary tract. They are ineffective in systemic infections as they do not achieve effective antimicrobial concentrations in plasma in therapeutic doses. They are concentrated in the renal tubules and achieve effective antimicrobial concentrations in urine to reach the renal pelvis and urinary bladder.

- **Methenamine (Hexamine):** It is a condensation product of formaldehyde and ammonia. It is inactive as such. It is broken down to formaldehyde and ammonia in acid urine slowly. Formaldehyde is a bactericidal agent and kills many urinary pathogens at a concentration of about 20 µg/mL. It is combined with mandelic acid or hippuric acid to keep urine acidic for its better action. It is well-absorbed orally but is broken down to some extent (10 to 20%) by the gastric juice and so it is administered as enteric coated tablet. It is not metabolized in the liver. It is excreted in urine as formaldehyde and ammonia.

Clinical Uses

It is not a drug for treatment of acute urinary tract infection but it is of some value in chronic suppressive treatment (to suppress bacteriuria), when no other drug is working. It can suppress the growth of *E. coli* and many other gram-positive and gram-negative bacteria. *Proteus, Pseudomonas* and *Aerobacter aerogenes* can develop resistance to it.

Preparations and Dosage

- Methenamine (Hexamine) tablet (0.5, 1 g)—0.5 to 1 g thrice daily.
- Methenamine mandelate (Mandelamine) tablet (0.5, 1 g)—0.5 to 1 g thrice daily.
- Methenamine hippurate (Urex) tablet (0.5, 1 g)—0.5 to 1 g thrice daily.

Adverse Reactions

These are gastric discomfort, nausea, vomiting, diarrhoea, crystalluria (by mandelate), haematuria and skin rashes.

- **Nitrofurantoin (Furadantin):** It is a nitrofuran derivative. It is inactive as such. It is activated by reduction in the susceptible bacteria forming highly reactive compounds, which cause damage of the bacterial DNA strands and inhibition of bacterial enzymes leading to antibacterial action. It is bacteriostatic at low concentration (<30 µg/mL) but bactericidal at high concentration in acid urine. It is most active against *E. coli* and *Streptococcus faecalis* (*Enterococci*). Bacterial resistance to it develops slowly. It is well-absorbed orally.

It is partly metabolized in the liver and excreted in urine as metabolites and unchanged drug (about 30%). It colours urine brown, which should be informed to the patient.

Clinical Uses

It is used in both acute and chronic urinary tract infections by the sensitive bacteria. It is mainly useful in urinary tract infections, which are resistant to other drugs and in patients with mixed infections or infection with obstructive uropathy.

Preparations and Dosage

Nitrofurantoin tablet (50, 100 mg)—50 to 100 mg 3 to 4 times daily.

Adverse Reactions

It can cause nausea, vomiting, diarrhoea, skin rashes, leucopenia, agranulocytosis, haemolytic anaemia, cholestatic jaundice, neuropathy and acute pneumonitis. It should not be used along with nalidixic acid, as it antagonizes the action of nalidixic acid.

- **Nalidixic acid:** Discussed in quinolones.
- **Phenazopyridine (Pyridium):** It is an azodye with orange colour. It is not an urinary antiseptic but an urinary analgesic. It is combined with an urinary antiseptic to relieve pain, strangury and burning sensation during micturation. It is available as tablet (200 mg) and administered three times daily. It can cause nausea and vomiting.

65

Antibiotics and β-lactam Antibiotics

INTRODUCTION

Antibiotics are organic substances produced by some species of living microorganisms such as fungi, actinomycetes and bacteria, which suppress the growth and multiplication of other microorganisms or kill them in low concentrations. The term antibiotic is derived from the word 'antibiosis', which means against life. The opposite word 'symbiosis' means mutual living of two organisms.

Majority of antibiotics are obtained from natural source. Some antibiotics are now prepared synthetically, e.g. chloramphenicol, quinolones and nitroimidazoles.

Chemistry

Antibiotics have different chemical structures:

- β-lactam antibiotics (contain β-lactam ring), e.g. penicillins, cephalosporins, carbapenems and monobactams.
- Aminoglycoside antibiotics (contain aminosugars in glycosidic linkage), e.g. streptomycin, gentamicin, netilmicin, amikacin, neomycin and kanamycin.
- Macrolide antibiotics (contain a large lactone ring in which sugars are attached), e.g. erythromycin, roxithromycin, clarithromycin and azithromycin.
- Tetracyclines (contain 4 cyclic rings), e.g. tetracycline, oxytetracycline, chlortetracycline and doxycycline.

- Polypeptide antibiotics (contain many amino acids), e.g. bacitram, tyrothricin, polymyxin and colistin.
- Polyene antibiotics (contain a large ring with many double bonds), e.g. amphotericin-B, nystatin, hamycin and candicidin.
- Miscellaneous antibiotics, e.g. chloramphenicol (contains nitrobenzene ring), fusidic acid (contains steroid ring), lincomycin (a monobasic compound) and vancomycin (a glycopeptide).

Types of antimicrobial action: Antibiotics may be:

- Primarily bacteriostatics, e.g. tetracyclines, chloramphenicol, erythromycin and clindamycin.
- Primarily bactericidals, e.g. penicillins, cephalosporins, carbapenems, aminoglycosides, polypeptides and rifampicin.

Antimicrobial Spectrum

Antibiotics may be:

- Narrow-spectrum antibiotics (effective against gram-positive or gram-negative bacteria), e.g. penicillin-G, cephalexin, streptomycin and erythromycin.
- Extended-spectrum antibiotics (effective against both gram-positive and gram-negative bacteria), e.g. ampicillin, amoxicillin, carbenicillin, cefotaxime, ceftriaxone and cefeprime.

- Broad-spectrum antibiotics (effective against both gram-positive and gram-negative bacteria, *Rickettsia*, *Chlamydia*, *Mycoplasma* and *Actinomycetes*), e.g. tetracyclines and chloramphenicol.

Mechanism of Antibacterial Action

Antibiotics may act by:

- Interference with bacterial cell wall synthesis, e.g. penicillins, cephalosporins, carbapenems, bacitracin and cycloserine.
- Increasing permeability of cell membrane leading to leakage of intracellular compounds, e.g. polyene antibiotics and polypeptide antibiotics.
- Inhibiting bacterial protein synthesis by binding with 30s or 50s ribosomal subunits, e.g. tetracyclines, chloramphenicol, erythromycin and clindamycin.
- Altering bacterial protein synthesis by causing misreading of mRNA code, e.g. aminoglycoside antibiotics.
- Interfering with bacterial DNA function/synthesis, e.g. rifampicin, griseofulvin, actinomycin-D, quinolones and nitroimidazoles.

Clinical Uses

These are given as follows:

- Antibiotics used in bacterial infections, e.g. penicillins, cephalosporins, carbapenems, tetracyclines, chloramphenicol, aminoglycosides, macrolides, polypeptides and quinolones.
- Antibiotics used in tuberculosis, e.g. streptomycin, rifampicin, viomycin, capreomycin and kanamycin.
- Antibiotics used in protozoal infection (amoebiasis), e.g. tetracyclines, paromomycin, fumagillin and nitroimidazoles (metronidazole and tinidazole).
- Antibiotics used in fungal infections, e.g. griseofulvin, nystatin, amphotericin-B, hamycin and candicidin.
- Antibiotics used in maligancy (cancers), e.g. actinomycin-D, mitomycin-C, bleomycin and azaserine.

β-LACTAM ANTIBIOTICS

These are those antibiotics that contain a β-lactam ring in their chemical structure. These are penicillins, cephalosporins and carbapenems.

Penicillins

These are a family of antibiotics, that contain 6-aminopenicillanic acid in their chemical structures. Penicillin is the generic name.

History

Penicillin is the first antibiotic discovered by Sir Alexander Fleming in 1929 from a penicillium mould (fungus). Later on, two chemists Florey and Chain purified it in crystalline form and introduced it in clinical practice. Fleming, Florey and Chain were awarded Nobel Prize in medicine in 1941 for their work on penicillin.

Source

Penicillin is obtained from *Penicillium notatum* or *Penicillium chrysogenum*. As *Penicillium chrysogenum* gives greater production, so it is used as commercial source of penicillin. There are four types of natural penicillins (G, F, X and K). Of these, penicillin-G is most potent and so commonly used.

Chemistry

The basic structure (nucleus) of all penicillins is 6-aminopenicillanic acid (6-APA), which consists of a thiazolidine ring (A), fused with a β-lactam ring (B), to which a side chain is attached (as shown in **Fig. 65.1**).

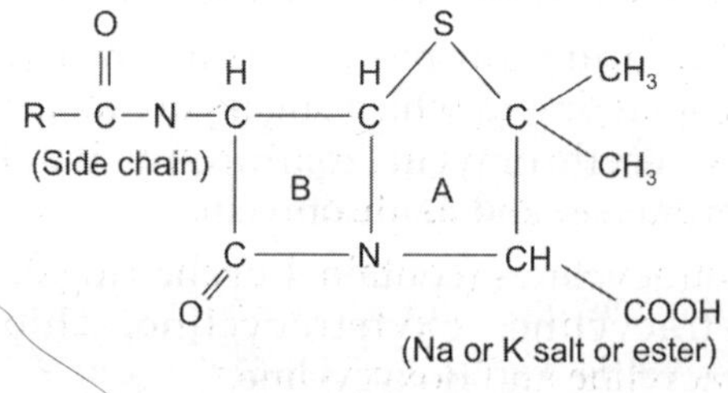

Fig. 65.1: Basic structure of penicillins

Semisynthetic penicillins are produced by altering the composition of the side chain attached to penicillin nucleus (6-APA). Both 6-APA nucleus and the side chain are essential for antibacterial activity. The side chain also determines the stability of penicillin against inactivation by gastric acid and the enzyme 'penicillinase' (β-lactamase) produced by some bacteria like *Staphylococcus aureus, E. coli, P. aeruginosa, Aerobacter aerogenes* and some strains of *H. influenzae* and *N. gonorrhoea*.

Classification

These are of two groups:

1. Natural penicillins, e.g. penicillin-G (benzyl penicillin).
2. Semisynthetic penicillins (newer penicillins). These are:
   - Acid-resistant penicillins, e.g. phenoxymethyl penicillin (penicillin V).
   - Penicillinase (β-lactamase)-resistant penicillins, e.g. methicillin, oxacillin, cloxacillin, dicloxacillin, flucloxacillin and nafcillin.
   - Extended-spectrum penicillins. These are:
     Aminopenicillins, e.g. ampicillin, amoxycillin, talampicillin, pivampicillin and bacampicillin.
   - Antipseudomonal penicillins. These are:
     - Carboxypenicillins, e.g. carbenicillin and ticarcillin.
     - Ureidopenicillins, e.g. piperacillin, mezlocillin and azlocillin.
   - Reversed-spectrum penicillins
     - Amidinopenicillins, e.g. mecillinam and pivmicillinam.
   - Penicillins with β-lactamase inhibitors, e.g. amoxicillin with clavulanic acid (Augmentin), ticarcillin with clavulanic acid (Timentin), ampicillin with sulbactum (Sulbacin) and piperacillin with tazobactum (Zosyn).

Mechanism of Antibacterial Action

Penicillins are bactericidal antibiotics. They are effective against rapidly multiplying (growing) bacteria. They act by inhibiting the bacterial cell wall synthesis. The bacterial cell wall is made up of a chemical substance called peptidoglycan, which gives rigid mechanical stability to the cell wall and protects the bacteria from the external environment. It is composed of glycan chains, which are linear strands of alternating N-acteyl muramic acid (NAMA) and N-acetyl-glucosamine (NAG). Short peptide chains (stem peptides) connect adjacent NAMAs. Each of these stem peptides is cross-linked (connected) with another stem peptide by peptide linkage. This is produced by the process called transpeptidation, which is catalyzed by the enzyme transpeptidase (as shown in **Fig. 65.2**).

Penicillin binding proteins (PBPs) are bacterial enzymes located on the cell membrane (which is inside the cell wall) and are responsible for the synthesis and cross-linkage of the peptidoglycans in the cell wall. Penicillins bind with these proteins and inactivate them, thereby preventing the synthesis and cross-linkage of peptidoglycans (by inhibiting transpeptidation reaction). This weakens the bacterial cell wall and so water from the surrounding medium (plasma) enters the cell wall deficient (CWD) bacteria as the interior is hyperosmotic. As a result lysis and death of bacteria, especially gram-positive bacteria occur. The cell walls of gram-negative bacteria (bacilli) are chemically more complex and contain β-lactamases in small amounts, which are enough to inactivate penicillin. Again, many gram-negative bacteria contain pores (porins) in their cell membrane, through which water-soluble semisynthetic penicillins like ampicillin and amoxycillin can pass and bind with PBPs leading to lysis and death of

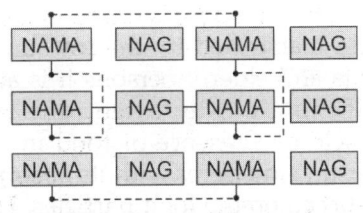

Fig. 65.2: Structure of bacterial cell wall

the bacteria. The enzyme penicillinase (β-lactamase) breaks the β-lactam ring of penicillin producing penicilloic acid, which has no antibacterial activity, but retains the antigenicity (to produce allergic reactions). The enzyme amidase breaks the side chain of penicillin and decreases the stability of penicillin against degradation by gastric acid and penicillinase.

DISCUSSION OF INDIVIDUAL GROUP OF PENICILLINS

Natural Penicillins

Penicillin-G (Benzylpenicillin): It is a narrow-spectrum penicillin. It is effective mainly against gram-positive and gram-negative cocci and some gram-positive bacilli. Gram-negative bacilli are resistant to its action. It is effective against *Streptococci* (except *Strep. faecalis*), *Staphylococci* (except those producing penicillinase), *Pneumococci, Gonococci, Meningococci, Corynebacterium diphtheriae, Clostridia organisms, Treponema pallidum, Leptospira icterohaemorrhagiae, Bacillus anthracis* and *Actinomyces bovis*. It is ineffective against *Bacteroides fragilis* and gram-negative bacteria like *E. coli, Proteus mirabilis, Aerobacter aerogenes* and *Pseudomonas aeruginosa*. It inhibits the growth of sensitive bacteria *in vitro* in a concentration as low as 1 in 50 million. It is one of the most potent antimicrobial drugs. Bacteria do not acquire resistance to it easily. Bacteria, those synthesize β-lactamase (penicillinase), e.g. *Staphylo. aureus, H. influenzae, N. gonorrhoea* and most gram-negative bacilli become resistant to penicillin.

Pharmacokinetics

It is poorly absorbed from GIT as it is lipid-insoluble and gastric acid labile. A small portion of the oral dose is found in faeces as it is mostly inactivated by the intestinal flora. In infants and elderly persons it is absorbed from GIT to a greater extent due to lower gastric acidity. Presence of food in stomach and intestine interferes with its absorption as it is adsorbed on the food particles. Hence, it should be administered one hour before or two hours after a meal. When it is administered parenterally in a aqueous solution it is rapidly and completely absorbed from the site of injection. Peak plasma concentration (8 to 10 units/mL) is reached within 30 minutes and it disappears from the plasma within 6 hours. Hence, it should be administered 6 hourly. Its minimum inhibitory concentration (MIC) in plasma (3 to 5 units/mL) persists for only 6 hours. After absorption it is widely distributed in the body tissues and fluids, mainly extracellularly. It can cross placental barrier but cannot cross BBB in normal persons as it is lipid-insoluble. In meningitis, the inflamed meninges become permeable to it. In the blood it is about 60% plasma protein bound (mainly with albumin). Its metabolic fate in the body is not definitely known. It is about 30% metabolized in the body. It is excreted mainly in urine by glomerular filtration (10 to 15%) and tubular secretion (about 80%). It is also excreted in bile, milk and saliva in small amounts. It has a plasma t½ of about 30 minutes. Probenecid (a uricosuric drug) blocks its tubular secretion leading to delay in excretion and prolonged duration of action. It is used when high plasma concentration of penicillin for long period is desirable.

Clinical Uses

It is used in following bacterial infections:

- Streptococcal infections such as pharyngitis (sore throat), scarlet fever, pneumonia, lung abscess, otitis media, mastoiditis, pyoderma and acute bacterial endocarditis. It is the drug of choice in acute nephritis and rheumatic fever.

- Staphylococcal infections such as boils, abscesses, enterocolitis, osteomyelitis, otitis media and bacterial endocarditis, but the development of penicillin-resistant staphylococci has restricted its use in these conditions.

- Pneumococcal infections such as pneumonia, empyema, pericarditis, meningitis, otitis media and osteomyelitis.

- Meningococcal infections such as meningitis and septicaemia.

- Sexually transmitted diseases (STDs)/ venereal diseases like gonorrhoea (caused by *N. gonorrhoea)* and syphilis (caused by *Treponema pallidum).*

- Diphtheria, tetanus and gas gangrene (caused by *Corynebacterium diphtheriae, Clostridium tetani* and *Clostridium welchii,* respectively) along with respective anti-serum and other measures.

- Anthrax (caused by *Bacillus anthracis)* and actinomycosis (caused by *Actinomyces bovis).*

- Miscellaneous infections such as gingivo stomatitis (caused by *Leptotrichia buccalis),* rat-bite fever (caused by *Spirillum minus),* listeria meningitis (caused by *Listeria monocytogenes)* and erysipeloid (caused by *Erysipelothrix insidiosa).*

Prophylactic uses: These are—

- Rheumatic fever (to eradicate β-haemolytic streptococci in throat).

- Bacterial endocarditis (in patients with valvular heart diseases).

- Gonorrhoea and syphilis (in sexual contacts).

- Recurrent attacks of lymphangitis (in filariasis).

- Before surgical procedures (to prevent surgical infections).

- Before tooth extraction and tonsillectomy.

- Agranulocytosis.

Preparations and Dosage

These are given as follows:

1. Short-acting preparations, e.g.

- Benzylpenicillin (sodium or potassium salt) injection (5 to 10 lakh units of the drug/vial)—5 to 10 lakh units of the drug dissolved in distilled water (3 mL) injected IM or IV every 6 to 8 hourly.

- Benzylpenicillin potassium (Pentids) tablet (200, i.e. 2 lakh units; 400, i.e. 4 lakh units and 800, i.e. 8 lakh units)—2 to 4 lakh units thrice daily, 8 lakh units twice daily.

2. Long-acting (repository) preparations: They release penicillin-G slowly from the site of injection and produce a relatively low and sustained blood level, e.g.

- Procaine benzylpenicillin (Pronapen) injection (6, 12 lakh units)—6 to 12 lakh units dissolved in distilled water (3 mL) injected IM daily.

- Fortified benzylpenicillin (crys-4) injection (3 lakh units of procaine benzylpenicillin and 1 lakh unit of benzylpenicillin/vial). The content of the vial dissolved in distilled water (3 mL) injected IM twice daily.

- Benzathine penicillin-G (Penidure) injection (combination of penicillin-G with dibenzyl-ethylene diamine) (6, 12, 24 lakh units/vial). The content of the vial dissolved in distilled water (3 mL) injected IM every 1 to 4 weeks. It is useful for prophylactic purposes as in rheumatic fever and bacterial endocarditis.

- Penicillin-G with aluminium monostearate (PAM) injection. It is now not used.

Penicillin unit: The activity of penicillin-G is expressed in unit. Crystalline sodium penicillin-G contains approximately 1600 units/mg. Thus 1 unit = 0.6 μg and 1 million (mega) unit = 0.6 g.

The activity of semisynthetic penicillins is expressed in weight (mg or g).

Adverse Reactions

Penicillin is a relatively safe (nontoxic) drug. It can occasionally produce following adverse reactions.

- **Hypersensitivity (allergic) reactions:** These occur in 1 to 2 % of patients. These include skin rashes (maculopapular, urticarial or purpuric), pruritus, serum sickness, fever, eosinophilia, lymphadeno-pathy, arthralgia, asthma, angioneurotic oedema, haematuria, albuminuria, neutro-paenia and haemolytic anaemia. Anaphylaxis is the most serious reaction (may be fatal) that occurs in 0.005% of patients. It is manifested as severe hypotension, bronchospasm with severe asthma, skin rashes, angioneurotic oedema of larynx, dyspnoea and cyanosis. This anaphylactic shock is treated by administration of adrenaline. Antihistaminics and glucocorticoids are of little value in it. Intradermal skin test with dilute solution of penicillin must be done to detect anaphylaxis (immediate hyper-sensitivity reaction). Development of flare and wheal suggests that the patient would develop anaphylactic reaction. Desen-sitization to penicillin can be done by the use of increasing amounts of pencillin given over many hours, but it is preferable to use another antibiotic (e.g. tetracycline).

Basis of hypersensitivity reactions to penicillin: The degradation products of penicillin particularly penicilloic acid combine with host protein and become antigenic. There are cross-hypersensitivity reaction between various types of penicillins.

- **Jarisch-Herxheimer reaction:** It is a nonall-ergic reaction and consists of an initial exacerbation of lesions at any stage of syphilis following the first injection of penicillin (a quick acting spirocheticidal drug). It is due to a rapid destruction of a large number of spirochetes with a release of endotoxin aggravating the local inflam-matory lesion. It occurs in majority of cases of early syphilis. It is manifested as agg-ravation of mucocutaneous lesions, malaise, fever, tachycardia, myalgia, arthralgia and lymphadenopathy (lymph nodes are en-larged and tender). It lasts for 2 to 6 hours and is harmless. The patient should be informed about this reaction. Penicillin treatment should not be stopped. A gluco-corticoid, e.g. prednisolone may be administered orally (30 mg daily) starting two days before penicillin treatment to prevent Jarisch-Herxheimer reaction. From the 7th day, the dose of prednisolone is progressively tapered and the drug is omitted with the end of penicillin treatment.
- **Superinfection (opportunistic infection by resistant intestinal microflora):** It is rare with penicillin-G, because it is a nar-row-spectrum antibiotic. It may suppress the coccal members of the bacterial flora and increase the overgrowth of resistant microorganisms such as *Klebsiella*, *Aero-bacter*, *Pseudomonas* and *Candida* leading to dermatitis, stomatitis, glossitis, vaginitis, urinary infection or pneumonia.
- **Hyperkalemia:** It may occur if excessive amount of potassium penicillin-G is admi-nistered to patients with impaired renal function.
- **Miscellaneous reactions:** It can rarely produce nephrotoxicity (interstitial nep-hritis) when high dose is used. When administered intrathecally in meningitis, it can produce CNS toxicities like headache, dizziness, myoclonic twitchings, auditory and visual disturbances, convulsions and encephalopathy. Hence, it should never be administered intrathecally. It can cause neurotoxicity when administered in large dose in uraemic patients. Oral use of penicillin-G may rarely produce nausea and vomiting. Sterile inflammatory reac-tion at the site of intramuscular injection of penicillin-G occasionally occurs. Prolonged intravenous administration of penicillin-G may cause thrombophlebitis. Accidental IV administration of procaine penicillin-G can cause anxiety, mental disturbances, para-esthesia and convulsions, probably due to procaine.

Drawbacks (disadvantages) of penicillin-G (benzyl penicillin)

- Poor oral efficacy (inactivated by gastric hydrochloric acid).
- Narrow antibacterial spectrum (effective mainly against gram-positive and gram-negative cocci and some gram-positive bacilli).
- Susceptibility to penicillinase (β-lacta-mase) produced by *Staphylococci* and other resistant bacteria.
- Short duration of action and poor pene-tration into CSR.
- Possibility of anaphylaxis.

Semisynthetic Penicillins (Newer Penicillins)

These are derivatives of 6-aminopenicillanic acid. These are produced by chemically combining specific side chains in place of benzyl side chain of penicillin-G or by incorporating specific precursors in the cultures of the mould *'Penicillium chrysogenum'*. These were developed to overcome the drawbacks (shortcomings) of penicillin-G. In addition, some β-lactamase inhibitors have been developed which have poor antibacterial activity when used alone but when combined with penicillins increase the antibacterial activity of penicillins against β-lactamase producing bacteria, e.g. *Staphylococcus aureus*, *E. coli*, etc.

Classification

Given with penicillins.

DISCUSSION OF INDIVIDUAL GROUP OF SEMISYNTHETIC PENICILLINS

Acid-Resistant Penicillins

Potassium phenoxymethyl penicillin (penicillin-V)—it differs from penicillin-G only in that it is acid stable. Given orally it is absorbed from the proximal part of small intestine and produces higher plasma concentration than the same amount of penicillin-G given orally. It is 50 to 70% plasma protein bound. It is eliminated in urine by a similar mechanism as penicillin-G. It has similar antibacterial spectrum as penicillin-G but it is only 1/5th as active against Neisseria (*Gonococci* and *Meningococci*).

Clinical Uses

It is used in less serious infections like pharyngitis, sinusitis and otitis media due to *Streptococci* and *Pneumococci* in conditions that have been brought under control by parenteral penicillin treatment and in infections which require a prolonged treatment. It is also used in prophylaxis of meningococcal infection and rheumatic fever.

Preparation and Dosage

Potassium phenoxymethyl penicillin (Crystapen-V) tablet (125, 250 mg) and suspension (125 mg/5 mL) of dry syrup—250 to 500 mg 6 hourly at least 30 minutes before taking food.

Adverse Reactions

It can cause nausea, vomiting and allergic reactions like penicillin-G. In large doses it can cause hyperkalaemia, especially when used along with a potassium sparing diuretic.

Potassium phenoxyethyl penicillin (penethicillin): It has similar pharmacological properties as potassium phenoxymethyl penicillin but it is less used.

Penicillinase (β-lactamase) Resistant Penicillins

Methicillin

It is gastric acid labile (unstable) and so administered parenterally (IM or IV) in the dose of 0.5 to 1 g every 6 hourly. It is used in the treatment of infections due to penicillinase producing *Staphylococci* but better drugs are available for this purpose. Hence it is now seldom used. It can produce nephritis, albuminuria and haematuria (nephrotoxic drug). Methicillin-resistant *Staphylococcus aureus* (MRSA) is treated by vancomycin.

Cloxacillin

It is gastric acid stable and so can be administered orally. It has weaker antibacterial activity than penicillin-G but is about 5 times more active than methicillin. It is rapidly but incompletely absorbed from GIT. Presence of food in the intestine interferes with its absorption. Hence it is administered 1 hour before or 2 hours after a meal. After absorption it is highly plasma protein bound (about 90%). It is excreted in urine and bile. It has a plasma t½ of about 1½ hours. It is used in the treatment of infections due to penicillinase producing bacteria like *Staphylococci*. It can be combined with ampicillin or amoxycillin to broaden the antimicrobial activity of the latter drugs.

Preparations and Dosage

• Cloxacillin (Klox) cap (250, 500 mg)—250 to 500 mg orally six hourly.
• Cloxacillin suspension (125 mg/5 mL of dry syrup)—50 to 100 mg/kg daily in four divided doses.

- Cloxacillin injection (250 mg/mL)—250 to 500 mg IM or slow IV injection hourly.

Adverse Reactions

It can cause nausea, vomiting and allergic reactions like penicillin-G.

Dicloxacillin

It is a derivative of cloxacillin. On oral administration it gives blood level twice that of cloxacillin due to better absorption from GIT. It is very highly plasma protein bound (about 95%). It is slowly excreted in urine. It has similar pharmacological properties as cloxacillin. It has dosage and adverse effects like cloxacillin.

Flucloxacillin

It is similar to dicloxacillin. It is less plasma protein bound than dicloxacillin and so more preferred than it for clinical use.

Nafcillin

It is more active than cloxacillin but less active than penicillin-G against penicillinase-resistant bacteria. After oral administration it is slowly, irregularly and incompletely absorbed. Hence, it is administered IM for quicker and higher plasma levels. It is mainly excreted in bile. It is administered in the dose of 0.5 to 1 g every 6 hourly. It can cause allergic reactions.

EXTENDED-SPECTRUM PENICILLINS

Aminopenicillins

These are given as follows:

Ampicillin

It has broader antibacterial spectrum than penicillin-G. It is effective against both gram-positive and gram-negative cocci and bacilli except penicillinase producing bacteria like *Staph. aureus, Ps. aeruginosa, Aerobacter aerogenes, Klebsiella pneumoniae* and indole positive *Proteus*, which are resistant to it. Anaerobes like *Bacteroides fragilis* are also resistant to it. Bacteria can develop acquired resistance to it after prolonged use and many strains of *Salmonella, Shigella, E. coli, Gonococci* and *Proteus* have developed resistance to it.

Pharmacokinetics

It is water-soluble and gastric acid stable (resistant). It is rapidly but incompletely absorbed from the intestine. Presence of food in the intestine slightly interferes with its absorption and so it is administered 1 hour before or 2 hours after a meal. Its peak plasma level is reached within 2 hours of oral administration. It persists in plasma for 6 to 8 hours and only 20% of it is bound with plasma proteins. It is excreted unchanged in urine and a high concentration is also present in bile. It undergoes enterohepatic circulation. It is partly excreted in faeces. Its tubular secretion is less pronounced than that of penicillin-G. Probenecid blocks its tubular secretion and prolongs its duration of action. It has a plasma t½ of about 90 minutes.

Clinical Uses

It is used in whooping cough, respiratory tract infections, urinary tract infections, biliary tract infections, meningitis, subacute bacterial endocarditis, gonorrhoea, Salmonella infections (typhoid and paratyphoid fevers), shigellosis (bacillary dysentery), septicaemia and mixed bacterial infections due to susceptible bacteria. It is preferred to tetracyclines in pregnant women and in infants to avoid tetracycline deposition in bones and teeth.

Preparations and Dosage

- Ampicillin (Ampilin) capsule (250, 500 mg)—250 to 500 mg 6 hourly.
- Ampicillin tablet (125, 250 mg) dry syrup (125 mg/5 mL) and injection (100 mg/mL in 10 mL vial) are also available.

Adverse Reactions

These are similar to those of penicillin-G. Skin rashes (usually maculopapular and not urticarial) are more common. Diarrhoea can occur with oral ampicillin and its derivatives and is due to irritation of the gut by the unabsorbed ampicillin and also by inhibition of the gut microflora. Interstitial nephritis rarely occurs.

Amoxicillin (Novamox)

It has similar antibacterial spectrum like ampicillin but it is less effective than ampicillin in shigellosis. It is more rapidly and completely absorbed from the intestine. Presence of food in the intestine does not interfere with its absorption. It has greater bioavailability than ampicillin. It produces higher peak and sustained plasma concentrations. It has longer plasma t½ than ampicillin. It produces less diarrhoea, because it is completely absorbed from the gut. It has clinical uses like ampicillin. It is available as capsule (250, 500 mg), tablet (125, 250 mg), dry syrup (125 mg/5 mL) and injection (100 mg/mL in 10 mL vial). It is administered in the dose of 250 to 500 mg 8 hourly. In severe or recurrent purulent respiratory infections it is administered in high dose (2 g 8 hourly). It produces less adverse effects than ampicillin.

Esters of ampicillin, e.g. talampicillin, pivampicillin and bacampicillin are prodrugs releasing ampicillin by hydrolysis into the circulation by the action of tissue esterases in the intestinal wall. They have no intrinsic antibacterial activity and so do not inhibit intestinal bacterial flora. They produce less diarrhoea than ampicillin. They are administered in the dose of 250 to 500 mg 3 to 4 times daily.

Carboxypenicillins

These are given as follows:

Carbenicillin

It has antibacterial spectrum like ampicillin but it is active against Pseudomonas aeruginosa and all strains of Proteus. It is inactivated by penicillinase. It is also acid-labile and has to be administered by parenteral route. It is about 50% plasma protein bound. It is excreted in urine within 6 hours. It is mainly used in serious urinary tract infections caused by Pseudomonas and Proteus. As Pseudomonas can develop resistance to it, so it is combined with an aminoglycoside, usually gentamicin. It is available as carbenicillin sodium (Pyopen) injection (5 g/vial) and administered in the dose of 1 to 2 g IM or slow IV 6 hourly. It can cause CCF (as it contains large amount of sodium) and bleeding (as it causes abnormal platelet aggregation).

Carbenicillin phenyl sodium (Carfecillin) and carbenicillin indanyl sodium (Geocillin) are effective orally and administerd as capsules in the dose of 1 to 2 g 6 hourly.

Ticarcillin

It is thienyl analogue of carbenicillin. It is twice as active as carbenicillin against Ps. aeruginosa, in addition to its action against gram-positive and other gram-negative bacteria. It is also active against Bacteroides fragilis, it is combined with an aminoglycoside to prevent development of resistance against the Pseudomonas species. It is acid labile and so orally ineffective. It is available as Ticarcillin sodium (Ticar) injection (5 g/vial) and administered in the dose of 1 to 2 g IM or slow IV 8 hourly. It has adverse effects like carbenicillin.

Ureidopenicillins

These are given as follows:

Piperacillin

It is penicillinase-sensitive but has a wide spectrum of antibacterial activities against gram-negative bacilli, particularly Ps. aeruginosa (against which it is three times as active as ticarcillin). It is also effective against other bacterial species including Proteus, Klebsiella, H. influenzae, Gonococci and Bacteroides fragilis. It is used mainly in serious urinary tract infections like carbenicillin. It is acid-labile and need to be administered parenterally in the dose of 1 to 2 g IM or slow IV 8 hourly. It is combined with tazobactum for synergistic action. Mezlocillin and azlocillin have similar pharmacological properties and uses as piperacillin.

Amidinopenicillins
(Reversed-Spectrum Penicillins)

These are given as follows:

Micillinam

It is not effective against gram-positive bacteria but is highly effective against gram negative bacteria like *E. coli*, *Klebsiella* species, *Shigellae* and *Salmonellae*. *Proteus* is less sensitive and *Pseudomonas* is resistant to it. It is gastric acid-labile and so administered parenterally. It can be used in urinary tract infections and typhoid fever. Pivmicillinam (Selexid) as similar antibacterial activity as micillinam. It is gastric acid stable and can be administered orally in the dose of 1.2 to 2.4 g daily in divided doses for 10 to 14 days in typhoid fever and urinary tract infections.

Penicillins with β-lactamase Inhibitors

β-lactamase (penicillinase) inhibitors (suicide inhibitors) are clavulanic acid, sulbactum and tazobactum. Clavulanic acid is a natural product obtained from *Streptomyces clavuligerus*. Sulbactum and tazobactum are semisynthetic drugs. They have similar chemical structures as clavulanic acid. When used alone they have weak antibacterial activity but when combined with penicillins like amoxycillin, ticarcillin, ampicillin and piperacillin respectively they widen the antibacterial spectrum of the latter drugs and include β-lactamase producing bacterial strains of *Staph. aureus*. *H. influenzae*, *N. gonorrhoea*, *E. coli*, *Proteus*, *Klebsiella*, *M. catarrhalis* and *Bacteroides fragilis* but *Pseudomonas aeruginosa*, *Enterobacter species* and methicillin-resistant *Staphylococci* (MRS) are resistant to them except *Tazobactam*. They are gastric acid stable and well-absorbed on oral administration. They are used in serious and mixed bacterial infections especially in urinary tract. They can be administered orally or parenterally.

Preparations and Dosage

These are available as combination products:

- Amoxicillin (250 mg) + Clavulanic acid (125 mg) capsule (Augmentin)—1 or 2 capsules administered 8 hourly.
- Ticarcillin sodium (3 g) + Potassium clavulanate (100 mg) injection (Timentin)—the content of one vial mixed with distilled water is injected IM or slow IV 8 hourly.
- Ampicillin (250 mg) + Sulbactum (125 mg) capsule (Sulbacin)—1 or 2 capsules administered 6 hourly.
- Piperacillin (3 g) + Tazobactum (375 mg) injection (Zosyn)—The content of one vial mixed with distilled water is injected IM or slow IV 6 hourly.

Adverse Reactions

These can rarely produce allergic reactions.

Cephalosporins

These are a family of antibiotics that contain 7-aminocephalosporanic acid (cephem nucleus) in their chemical structures. Cephalosporin is the generic name. There are three natural cephalosporins (C, N and P). Cephalosporin-C is the most potent. It is obtained from the mould 'Cephalosporium acremonium'. It was isolated by Brotzu in 1948 from the seawater near a sewage out fall at the Sardinian coast.

Chemistry

The basic structure of all cephalosporins is 7-aminocepehalosporanic acid (cephem nucleus) to which two side chains at R_1 and R_2 are attached to produce different cephalosporins (as shown in **Fig. 65.3**).

They are water-soluble and stable to changes in pH and temperature.

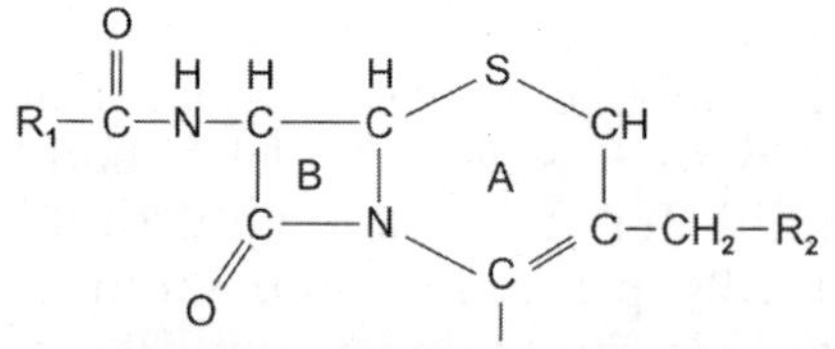

Fig. 65.3: Basic structure of cephalosporins

Classification

These are classified according to generation (i.e. chronological order of development) as follows:

- **First generation** cephalosporins, e.g. oral—cephalexin, cefadroxil and cephradine. Parenteral—cephalothin, cefazolin and cephaloridine.
- **Second generation** cephalosporins, e.g. oral—cefuroxime axetil, cefaclor and cefprozil. Parenteral—cefuroxime, cefoxitin, cefotetan, cefamandole, ceforanide and cefonicid.
- **Third generation** cephalosporins, e.g. oral—cefixime and cefpodoxime proxetil. Parenteral—cefotaxime, ceftizoxime, ceftriaxone, cefoperazone and ceftazidime.
- **Fourth generation** cephalosporins, e.g. parenteral—cefepime and cefpirome.

Pharmacological Actions

Mechanism of action: Cephalosporins are bactericidal antibiotics. They act like penicillin in inhibiting bacterial cell wall synthesis. Bacterial resistance to them can develop after prolonged use. They are resistant to β-lactamase but sensitive to cephalosporinase produced by some strains of gram-negative bacteria. Cephalosporinase destroys the β-lactam ring of cephalosporins and thus the bacteria become resistant to them.

Antimicrobial Spectrum

They possess a wide range of activity against gram-positive and gram-negative bacteria. Different generations of cephalosporins differ in their antibacterial activity.

- **First generation** cephalosporins are active against *Streptococcus pyogenes* and *Staphylococcus aureus* (except MRS) but not active against *Enterococci* and *Listeria*.
- **Second generation** cephalosporins are active against *E. coli, Klebsiella, Proteus, H. influenzae* and *Moraxella catarrhalis* but less active against gram-positive cocci than 1st generation cephalosporins. Cefoxitin and Cefotetan are also active against *B. fragilis*.

- **Third generation** cephalosporins are active against gram-positive cocci like 1st generation cephalosporins and also active against *Enterobacteriaceae, Pseudomonas aeruginosa, Neisseria gonorrhoea* and *Serratia*.
- **Fourth generation** cephalosporins have antibacterial activity like 3rd generation cephalosporins but more resistant to some β-lactamase producing bacteria.

Pharmacokinetics

Cephalosporins are administered orally or intravenously; intramuscular administration is painful. After absorption majority of cephalosporins are not metabolized in the liver except cephalothin, cefazolin and cefotaxime, which are deacetylated in the liver. Their body distribution is similar to that of penicillins. They can penetrate into CSF, synovial and pericardial fluids in sufficient concentrations. They are excreted in urine and bile. Like penicillins, probenecid slows the renal excretion of cephalosporins by blocking their renal tubular secretion. Their renal excretion is markedly reduced in renal insufficiency. Their plasma t½ varies from ½ to 4 hours depending on the compound.

Clinical Uses

Cephalosporins are widely used and therapeutically useful antibiotics. They are effective as both therapeutic and prophylactic agents. A single dose of cefazolin just before surgery is the preferred prophylaxis for surgical procedures in which skin flora are the likely pathogens. The second generation cephalosporin either alone or with aminoglycoside are considered to be drugs of choice for serious infections caused by *Klebsiella, Enterobacter, Proteus, Providencia, Serratia* and *Haemophilus species*. Ceftriaxone is now the therapy of choice for all forms of gonorrhoea. The third generation cephalosporins (cefotaxime and ceftriaxone) are the drugs of choice for the treatment of meningitis caused by *H. influenzae, Strep. pneumoniae, N. meningitis* and gram-negative enteric bacteria. Ceftazidime and an aminoglycoside (gentamicin) is the treatment of choice in *Pseudomonas meningitis*.

The generation cephalosporins are useful alternatives to penicillin for a variety of streptococcal and staphylococcal infections in patients who cannot tolerate penicillins. Cefotaxime, ceftriaxone and cefoperazone are effective in typhoid fever and cefoxitin and cefotetan have good activity against anaerobes especially *B. fragilis.* Ceftazidime and gentamicin in combination is useful in severe infections like septicaemia, osteomyelitis, septic arthritis, urinary tract infections, etc. caused by *Pseudomonas aeruginosa* and *Bacteroides fragilis.*

Some Preparations and Dosage

Oral Preparations

- Cephalexin monohydrate (Phexin, Sporidex) capsule (250, 500 mg)—250 to 500 mg six hourly. Also available as tablet (125 mg) and dry syrup (250 mg/5 mL).

- Cefadroxil (Cefadrox, Odoxil) capsule (250, 500 mg)—250 to 500 mg eight hourly. Also available as tablet (250 mg) and dry syrup (125 mg/5 mL).

- Cefuroxime axetil (Ceftum) tablet/capsule (250, 500 mg)—250 to 500 mg twelve hourly.

Parenteral Preparations

- Cefotaxime (Taxim, Cefatox) injection (0.5, 1 g/vial)—0.5 to 1 g IM or IV 8 hourly.
- Ceftriaxone (Cefaxone, Monocef) injection (0.5, 1 g/vial)—0.5 to 1 g IM or IV 12 hourly.
- Cefuroxime (Sufacef, Cefogen) injection (0.5, 0.75 g/vial)—0.5 to 1.5 g IM or IV 8 hourly.
- Ceftazidime (Fortum) injection (0.5, 1 g/vial)—0.5 to 1 g IM or IV every 8 to 12 hourly.
- Cefazolin (Reflin, Azolin) injection (0.5, 1 g/vial)—0.5 to 1 g IM or IV 8 hourly.

Adverse Reactions

Cephalosporins are generally well-tolerated antibiotics but more toxic than penicillins. Their common adverse effects are hypersensitivity (allergic) reactions like penicillin. They can cause blood dyscrasias like neutropaenia and thrombocytopaenia (by bone marrow depression). Ceftriaxone and cefoperazone can cause severe bleeding by causing hypoprothrombinaemia, thrombocytopaenia and platelet dysfunction. Intolerance to alcohol producing disulphiram like state (antabuse reaction) can occur with cefamandole, cefotetan and cefoperazone. Diarrhoea due to irritant effect on the intestine and superinfection with resistant microorganisms (*Enterococci, Pseudomonas* and *Anaerobes)* may occur with some cephalosporins (1st and 2nd generations). CNS toxicities like cerebral irritation, nystagmus and hallucinations may occur following intrathecal administration of cephaloridine. Nephrotoxicity (kidney damage, i.e. acute tubular necrosis) can occur following large doses of cephalosporins, especially cephaloridine when used with high ceiling diuretics like frusemide or aminoglycosides like gentamicin.

Carbapenems

These are imipenem and meropenem.

Imipenem

It is a β-lactam antibiotic derived by modification of a parent antibiotic thienamycin derived from *Streptomyces cattleya.* Thienamycin is unstable, but its N-formimidoyl derivative 'imipenem' is stable.

It is bactericidal antibiotic and acts like penicillins. It has a wider antibacterial spectrum than cephalosporins. It is highly active against gram-positive and gram-negative aerobes and many anaerobes. It is very resistant to hydrolysis by most β-lactamases. It is not active against *Chlamydia* and *Mycoplasma* species. It is not effective orally and hence administered parenterally. It does not penetrate intracellularly and, therefore, is inactive against intracellular microorganisms. It is rapidly hydrolyzed by a renal tubular enzyme, dipeptidase and, therefore, the concentration of the active drug in the kidney is less than that in the plasma. It is usually combined with 'cilastatin', an inhibitor of the renal tubular dipeptidase to prevent its degradation. Cilastatin has no antimicrobial activity. It is used in the treatment of mixed bacterial (aerobic and anaerobic) infections and resistant gram-negative bacterial infections (especially UTI, RTI and intra-abdominal and gynaecological infections) not responding to other β-lactam antibiotics.

Preparation and Dosage

Imipenem (0.5 g) + Cilastatin (0.5 g) injection/vial (Primaxin)—the content of one vial mixed with distilled water is injected IM 8 to 12 hourly. It can also be administered by IV infusion in the dose of 1 to 2 g daily in 3 or 4 divided doses.

Adverse Reactions

It can cause hypersensitivity (allergic) reactions and GIT disturbances (as excreted in bile). It can produce convulsions in high dosage especially in patients with CNS disorders.

Meropenem

It is dimethyl carbamolylpyrolidinyl derivative of thienamycin. It has antimicrobial activity like imipenem with activity against some imipenem resistant *Pseudomonas aeruginosa* but less active against gram-positive cocci. It does not require co-administration with cilastatin, as it is not sensitive to renal tubular dipeptidase. It is claimed to be less toxic than imipenem.

Monobactams

Aztreonam

It is a monocyclic β-lactam compound. It is obtained from *Chromobacterium violaceum*. It has activity only against aerobic gram-negative bacteria especially *E. coli, Klebsiella, H. influenzae, Proteus mirabilis* and *Ps. aeruginosa*. It is used as an alternative to aminoglycoside antibiotics in severe infections caused by gram-negative bacteria. It is administered IM in the dose of 1 to 2 g every 8 to 12 hourly. It has mild toxicity.

66

Aminoglycoside Antibiotics

INTRODUCTION

These are antibiotics that contain amino sugars linked to an aminocyclitol ring by glycosidic bonds. They are polycations and their polarity is in part responsible for their pharmacokinetic properties. They are used mainly to treat infections caused by aerobic gram-negative bacteria. They interfere with protein synthesis in susceptible micro-organisms. Although most inhibitors of bacterial protein synthesis are bacteriostatic but these antibiotics are bactericidal.

History

The first aminoglycoside antibiotic strep-tomycin was isolated from an actinomycete called 'Streptomyces griseus' by Waksman, Schatz and Bugie in 1944. Then other aminoglycoside antibiotics were isolated and some were prepared semisynthetically.

Source

This is shown in **Table 66.1**.

The difference in spelling (—*micin*) as compared with that of other aminoglycoside antibiotics (—*mycin*) is due to different origin, i.e. from micromonospora. Amikacin and netilmicin are semisynthetic derivatives of kanamycin and sisomicin respectively introduced in 1972.

Chemistry

Aminoglycosides consist of two or more amino sugars joined in glycosidic linkage to a

Table 66.1: Source of aminoglycoside antibiotics

Antibiotic	Source
Streptomycin	Streptomyces griseus
Kanamycin	Strep. kanamyceticus
Neomycin	Strep. fradiae
Tobramycin	Strep. tenebrarius
Paromomycin	Strep. rimosus
Framycetin	Strep. lavendulae
Gentamicin	Micromonospora purpurea
Sisomicin	Micromonospora inyoensis
Dihydro-streptomycin	Semisynthetic derivative of streptomycin
Amikacin	Semisynthetic derivative of kanamycin
Netilmicin	Semisynthetic derivative of sisomicin.

hexose nucleus, which is usually in the central position. This hexose (aminocyclitol) is either streptidine (found in streptomycin) or 2-deoxystreptamine (found in other aminog-lycoside antibiotics). Depending on chemical structures they are divided into several families:

- Streptomycin family, e.g. streptomycin and dihydrostreptomycin.
- Neomycin family, e.g. neomycin, framy-cetin and paromomycin.
- Kanamycin family, e.g. kanamycin, tobra-mycin and amikacin.

- Gentamicin family, e.g. gentamicin, sisomicin and netilmicin.

Antimicrobial Activity of Aminoglycosides

They are narrow-spectrum antibiotics. They are effective mainly against aerobic gram-negative bacteria especially gram-negative bacilli. They are highly active against Enterobacteriaceae (*E. coli, Proteus, Klebsiella, Shigella,* etc.). They are also active against *Pseudomonas aeruginosa, Yersinia pestis* and *Pasteurella tularensis.* They are moderately active against *Haemophilus* and *Neisseria* species. Streptomycin and kanamycin have limited antibacterial spectrum compared with other aminoglycosides but they are active against *Mycobacterium tuberculosis.* Aminoglycosides have little activity against anaerobic microorganisms or facultative bacteria under anaerobic conditions. Their activities against most gram-positive bacteria are limited. They are not active against gram-positive cocci like *Strepto. pneumoniae* and *Strepto. faecalis* (*Enterococci*). The aerobic gram-negative bacilli vary in their sensitivity to different aminoglycosides. The minimum inhibitory concentration (MIC) of different aminoglycosides are different (0.25 to 130 µg/mL).

Mechanism of Action

They are rapidly bactericidal. Bacteria killing is concentration dependent; the higher the concentration, the greater the rate at which bacteria are killed. A postantibiotic effect, i.e. residual bactericidal activity persisting after the serum concentration has fallen below the MIC is a characteristic of aminoglycosides and the duration of this effect is concentration dependent. For this property, they can be administered in one daily dosing.

They act by interfering with the bacterial protein synthesis by causing misreading and premature termination of translation of mRNA at the ribosome. The aberrant proteins produced may be inserted into the cell membrane leading to altered permeability and further stimulation of aminoglycoside transport. The progressive disruption of the cell envelope as well as other vital processes of bacteria are responsible for lethal action of aminoglycosides. The primary intracellular site of action of aminoglycosides is the 30s ribosomal subunit, which consists of 21 proteins and a single 16s molecule of RNA.

Bacterial Resistance to Aminoglycosides

Bacteria may be resistant to the antibacterial activity of aminoglycosides by following ways:
- Failure of permeation of the antibiotic through the pores in the outer cytoplasmic membrane of the bacteria.
- Low affinity of the antibiotic for the bacterial ribosome.
- Inactivation of the antibiotic by the bacterial enzymes. Plasmid mediated elaboration of aminoglycoside inactivating enzymes is involved in Enterococci (*Strepto. faecalis* and *Strepto. faecium*). As different enzymes are responsible for inactivation of gentamicin and streptomycin, so a small proportion of gentamicin resistant strains of *Enterococci* will be susceptible to streptomycin. Resistance to streptomycin indicates resistance of kanamycin, tobramycin, amikacin and netilmicin. Anaerobic bacteria are resistant to aminoglycosides due to lack of necessary transport system.

Pharmacokinetics of Aminoglycosides

Aminoglycosides are highly polar cations. They are thus very poorly absorbed from the GIT. Less than 1% of the dose is absorbed following either oral or rectal administration. They are not inactivated in the intestine and they are eliminated quantitatively in faeces. They are rapidly absorbed after intramuscular injection. Their peak plasma concentrations occur in 30 to 90 minutes. Due to polar nature, their distribution in the body is limited. They enter poorly in most cells, CNS and eye. Their concentrations in secretions and tissues are low. High concentrations are only found in renal cortex and in the endolymph and perilymph of the inner ear. Concentrations in CSF are only 10% of that of plasma. Except streptomycin, there is negligible binding of aminoglycosides to plasma protein (albumin).

They are very little metabolized in the liver. They are excreted almost entirely by glomerular filtration. A large fraction is excreted unchanged in urine. Their half-lives vary between 2 to 3 hours in patients with normal renal functions.

Clinical Uses of Aminoglycosides

These are discussed according to aminoglycosides.

Streptomycin

It is used in the treatment of tuberculosis but due to rapid development of resistance its use is now limited.

It is now used in the treatment of plague, brucellosis and tularemia. In combination with penicillin-G it is also used in the treatment of streptococcal endocarditis.

Kanamycin

It is a reserve drug for the treatment of tuberculosis, where it is used in combination with other antitubercular drugs.

Neomycin

It is used orally as an intestinal antiseptic before colonic surgery and for suppression of intestinal flora in hepatic coma to decrease toxin production and blood concentration of ammonia. It is also used topically in skin, eye and ear infections along with other antibiotics like bacitracin or polymyxin (to prevent the emergence of resistant strains and to widen the antibacterial spectrum).

Framycetin

It is only used topically in skin, eye and ear infections.

Paromomycin

It is used in chronic bacillary dysentery, chronic amoebic dysentery, for sterilization of bowel before surgery and in hepatic coma.

Gentamicin

It is used in urinary tract infections, pneumonia, meningitis, endocarditis, peritonitis, intraabdominal and pelvic infections and septic states caused by sensitive bacteria, including *Pseudomonas, Enterobacter, Klebsiella* and *Serratia*. It is also used topically in skin, eye and ear infections caused by sensitive bacteria.

Sisomicin

It has therapeutic uses like gentamicin.

Tobramycin

It is used in the treatment of bacteremia, osteomyelitis and pneumonia caused by *Pseudomonas* species. It should be used concomitantly with an antipseudomonal penicillins (e.g. piperacillin) or a third generation cephalosporins (e.g. ceftazidime).

Amikacin

It has therapeutic uses like gentamicin and tobramycin. It is preferred in the treatment of serious nosocomial gram-negative bacillary infections in hospitals, when resistance to gentamicin and tobramycin has developed.

Netilmicin

It is used in the treatment of serious infections due to susceptible Enterobacteriaceae and other aerobic gram-negative bacilli. It has been found effective against some gentamicin resistant pathogens except *Enterococci.*

Some Preparations and Dosage

- Streptomycin sulphate injection (0.5, 1 g/vial)—0.75 to 1.5 g IM daily.
- Kanamycin sulphate (Kancin, Kantrex) injection (0.5, 1 g/vial)—15 mg/kg/day IM.
- Neomycin sulphate (Uneomycin) capsule (0.5, 1 g)—4 to 8 g/day in divided doses.
- Gentamicin sulphate (Genticin) injection (80 mg/2 mL vial)—3 to 6 mg/kg/day IM or IV in 2 or 3 divided doses.
- Tobramycin (Nebcin) injection (80 mg/2 ml vial)—2 to 5 mg/kg/day IM or IV in 2 or 3 divided doses.
- Amikacin (Mikacin) injection (250 mg/2 mL vial)—10 to 15 mg/kg/day IM or IV in 2 or 3 divided doses.
- Netilmicin (Netromy cin) injection (200 mg/2 mL vial)—5 to 8 mg/kg/day IM or IV in 2 or 3 divided doses.

- Paromomycin (Humatin) capsule (0.5 g)—2 to 4 g daily in 2 or 3 divided doses.
- Framycetin (Soframycin) ointment, cream or solution (0.5%).

Adverse Reactions

All aminoglycosides can produce ototoxicity and nephrotoxicity. These side effects complicate the use of these drugs and make their administration difficult.

- *Ototoxicity*: Both vestibular and auditory dysfunctions can occur with the administration of any of the aminoglycosides. These drugs progressively accumulate in the perilymph and endolymph of the inner ear, when their concentrations in plasma are high. This causes ototoxicity (largely irreversible) due to progressive destruction of vestibular or cochlear sensory cells, which are highly sensitive to damage by aminoglycosides. They interfere with the active transport system essential for the maintenance of the ionic balance of the endolymph. Streptomycin and gentamicin mainly produce vestibular dysfunction, whereas amikacin, kanamycin and neomycin mainly produce auditory dysfunction. Tobramycin produces both vestibular and auditory dysfunctions. Netilmicin is less ototoxic than other aminoglycosides. Dihydrostreptomycin is more ototoxic than streptomycin and so no longer used (obsolete).
- *Nephrotoxicity*: About 15% of patients receiving aminoglycosides for more than 10 days develop mild renal impairment, which is reversible. This is due to marked accumulation and high retention of aminoglycosides in the proximal tubular cells. After several days there is a defect in renal concentrating ability, mild proteinuria and the appearance of hyaline and granular casts. After several additional days the GFR is reduced. Acute tubular necrosis may occur rarely.
- *Neuromuscular blockade:* All aminoglycosides have a potential curarimimetic action producing neuromuscular blockade and apnoea (respiratory arrest) on intrapleural or intraperitoneal administration. It is unusual on intramuscular administration. This is probably due to inhibition of acetylcholine release at the neuromuscular junction through competition with calcium ions. The blockade thus produced can be antagonized by calcium salts or by neostigmine. Patients with myasthenic gravis are more susceptible to neuromuscular blockade by aminoglycosides.
- *Superinfection*: Aminoglycosides administered orally especially streptomycin can produce superinfection by *Staph. aureus* and *Candida albicans*. Endocarditis due to *Candida* and *Staphylococcal enterocolitis* may occasionally be fatal.
- *Other adverse effects*: Streptomycin can produce nausea, vomiting, optic neuritis and peripheral neuritis by local irritation. All aminoglycosides can rarely produce hypersensitivity reactions like skin rashes, eosinophilia, fever, blood dyscrasias, angioneurotic oedema, exfoliative dermatitis, stomatitis and anaphylactic shock.

Common Properties (Features) of Aminoglycosides

- They are poorly absorbed from GIT when administered orally as they are highly polar cations.
- Their distribution in the body is mainly extracellular due to polar nature.
- Their penetration into CSF (except in the neonate) and eye is poor on systemic administration.
- They are found in high concentrations in the renal cortex and in the endolymph and the perilymph of the inner ear, which accounts for their nephrotoxicity and ototoxicity.
- They are excreted relatively rapidly by the kidneys by glomerular filtrations.
- Bacterial resistance to them develops rapidly and they show cross-resistance.
- They are highly active against gram-negative bacteria and are almost inactive against anaerobes. They are bactericidal antibiotics.
- They exhibit synergism when combined with penicillin or cephalosporin.

67

Macrolide Antibiotics

INTRODUCTION

These are so-named because they contain a many-membered lactone ring to which one or more deoxy sugars are attached.

History and Source

The first macrolide antibiotic 'erythromycin' was discovered by Mc Guire and co-workers in 1952 in the metabolic products of a strain of 'Streptomyces erythreus'. Roxithromycin, clarithromycin and azithromycin are semisynthetic derivatives of erythromycin.

Chemistry

Erythromycin is a macrolide antibiotic. Roxithromycin, clarithromycin and azithromycin differ from ethythromycin by addition of methyl substituents at different positions of lactone ring. These structural modifications improve gastric acid stability and tissue penetration and broaden the antibacterial activity.

Antibacterial Activity

Erythromycin is usually bacteriostatic but it becomes bactericidal in high concentrations against very susceptible microorganisms. It is most effective against aerobic gram-positive cocci and bacilli. For susceptible bacteria like Strep. pyogenes and Strep. pneumoniae, the MIC ranges from 0.015 to 1.0 µg/mL. It is usually active against Campylobacter jejuni, B. pertussis,

Mycoplasma pneumoniae, G. vaginitis, Legionella pneumophilia and Chlamydia trachomatis. It is also active against N. gonorrhoeae, N. catarrhalis and T. pallidum. It is not active against most aerobic enteric gram-negative bacilli. Roxithromycin, clarithromycin and azithromycin are also active against H. influenzae, T. gondii and M. avium complex.

Mechanism of Action

Macrolide antibiotics act by preventing bacterial protein synthesis. They bind reversibly to the 50s ribosomal subunits and prevent the translocation of the newly synthesized peptidyl tRNA from the acceptor site on the ribosome to the peptidyl (donor) site (D-site). Gram-positive bacteria accumulate about 100 times more erythromycin than do gram-negative bacteria.

Bacterial Resistance to Macrolide Antibiotics

It results from three types of plasmid mediated alteration given as follows:

- A decrease in the penetration of the drug through the cell envelope as in Strepto. epidermidis.
- Induction of production of methylase enzyme, that modifies the ribosomal target, leading to decreased drug binding.
- Hydrolysis of macrolides produced by Enterobacteriaceae like E. coli.

Pharmacokinetics

Erythromycin base is incompletely but adequately absorbed from the upper part of small intestine. It is inactivated by gastric acid and so it is administered as enteric coated tablets or as capsules containing enteric coated pellets that dissolve in the duodenum. Food delays its absorption by increasing gastric acidity. Peak plasma concentrations are only 0.3 to 0.5 µg/mL after four hours of oral administration of 250 mg of erythromycin base. Erythromycin estolate is less susceptible to gastric acid than the base and is better absorbed. High concentrations of erythromycin can be achieved (10 µg/mL) after one hour of IV administration of 500 mg erythromycin lactobionate or gluceptate. Roxithromycin, clarithromycin and azethromycin are more resistant to gastric acid hydrolysis than erythromycin and better absorbed from GIT after oral administration. They give better tissue levels. They are widely distributed in the body tissues and fluids except CSF.

Their bioavailability may be affected by food, which delays their absorption. Erythromycin diffuses readily into intracellular fluids and antibacterial activity can be achieved at all sites, except the brain and CSF. It can penetrate into prostatic fluid and a concentration of 40% of plasma is obtained. The erythromycin base is about 80% plasma protein bound and its estolate is about 90% plasma protein bound. It is metabolized in the liver and excreted in urine as metabolites and slightly (2 to 5%) as free form. Roxithromycin, clarithromycin and azithromycin are longer acting macrolides with a plasma t½ of 12 to 18 hours.

Clinical Uses

Erythromycin is an effective substitute for penicillin in the treatment of infections caused by penicillin-sensitive bacteria. It is particularly useful in patients, who are allergic to penicillins and in those bacteria have developed resistance to penicillins. It is as effective as tetracycline in the treatment of *Mycoplasma pneumoniae* and *Chlamydia pneu-*

moniae. It is the drug of choice in whooping cough and chancroid.

Erythromycin is used for the treatment of following conditions:

- Mycoplasma infections
- Legionnaires' disease
- Chlamydial infections
- Whooping cough (pertussis)
- Diphtheria
- Streptococcal infections
- Staphylococcal infections
- Campylobacter infections
- Tetanus
- Syphilis and gonorrhoea
- Chancroid
- Atypical mycobacterial infection.

Prophylactic Uses

It is used for prophylaxis of recurrence of rheumatic fever in patients who are allergic to penicillin. It is also used for prophylaxis of bacterial endocarditis following dental (tooth extraction, etc.) or respiratory (bronchoscopy, etc.) procedures.

Roxithromycin is used as an alternate to erythromycin for the treatment of pneumonia, acute bronchitis, sinusitis, pharyngitis, tonsillitis, genital infections and skin and soft tissue infections.

Clarithromycin is used mainly for the treatment of peptic ulcer and atypical pneumonia and other respiratory tract infections.

Azithromycin is used mainly for the treatment of respiratory tract infections caused by *H. influenzae* and conjuctivitis, cervicitis and urethritis caused by *C. trachomatis*.

Preparations and Dosage

- Erythromycin stearate (Erythrocin) tablet (100, 200, 500 mg)—200 to 500 mg eight hourly.
- Erythromycin estolate (Althrocin) tablet (250, 500 mg)—250 to 500 mg eight hourly.
- Roxithromycin (Roxid) tablet (150, 300 mg)—150 to 300 mg twice daily.

- Clarithromycin (Claribid) tablet (250 mg)—250 to 500 m.g twice daily.
- Azithromycin (Azithral) capsule (250 mg)—250 to 500 mg once daily. These are also available as dry syrup, granules and drops.

Adverse Reactions

Erythromycin rarely causes serious adverse effects like nausea, vomiting and diarrhoea and allergic reactions like fever, eosinophilia, skin rash, urticaria, dermatitis and lymphadenopathy. Anaphylaxis rarely occurs. Hepatic dysfunction, particularly cholestatic hepatitis and jaundice can occur with erythromycin estolate. It is probably an allergic manifestation through a direct hepatotoxic action. It usually clears up within a few days after discontinuation of treatment. It can also cause superinfection by gram-negative bacteria and *Candida*, as it causes inhibition of the gram-positive bacterial flora of the intestine. Semisynthetic derivatives of erythromycin are better tolerated than erythromycin and produce less adverse effects.

Drug Interactions

- Erythromycin can potentiate the effects of carbamazepine, valproate, theophylline, warfarin, corticosteroids, astemizole, terfenadine, digoxin, triazolam, cyclosporine and ergot alkaloids (ergotamine, ergometrine, etc.) by inhibiting the cytochrome P450 mediated metabolism of these drugs.
- It can interfere with the action of chloramphenicol and bactericidal antibiotics like penicillins.

Semisynthetic macrolides cause less drug interactions than erythromycin.

Oleandomycin, triacetyloleandomycin and spiramycin also belong to macrolide group of antibiotics. Their action is much weaker than erythromycin group of antibiotics and so they are now rarely used.

68

Broad-spectrum Antibiotics

These are tetracyclines and chloramphenicol. These are so-called, as they are active against a wide range of microorganisms including bacteria, rickettsiae, mycoplasma and chlamydiae.

TETRACYCLINES

These are tetracyclic compounds (contain 4 cyclic rings in their structures).

History and Source

The first tetracycline 'chlorotetracycline' was isolated from *Streptomyces aureofaciens* by Dugger in 1948. This was followed by oxytetracycline, isolated from *Streptomyces rimosus* by Finlay in 1950. Tetracycline was prepared by catalytic hydrogenation of chlorotetracycline by Subba Rao in 1953. Afterwards many semisynthetic tetracyclines have been introduced for clinical uses.

Chemistry

Tetracyclines are naphthacene derivatives. The naphthacene nucleus is made up by fusion of 4 partially unsaturated cyclohexane radicals as shown in **Fig. 68.1**.

Their acid salts are more stable in the dry powdered state and are preferred for therapy. They are more stable in acid pH.

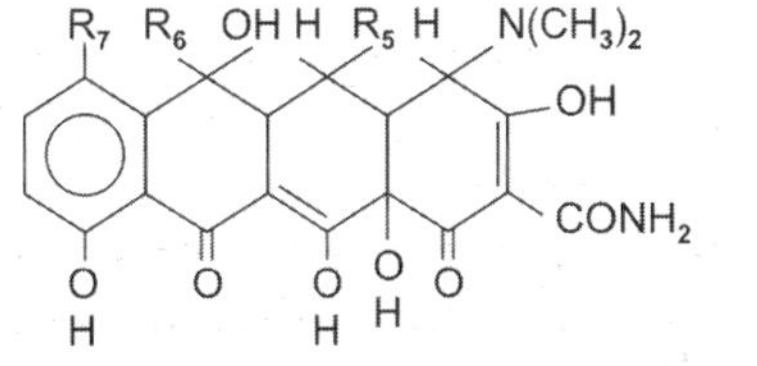

Classification of Tetracyclines

These are of two groups:

	R_7	R_6	R_5
Tetracycline	H	CH_3	H
Chlorotetracycline	Cl	CH_3	H
Oxytetracycline	H	CH_3	OH

Fig. 68.1: Basic structure of tetracyclines

- Natural tetracyclines (older tetracyclines), e.g. chlorotetracycline, oxytetracycline and tetracycline.
- Semisynthetic tetracyclines (newer tetracyclines), e.g. dimethylchlorotetracycline, methacycline, lymecycline, doxycycline and minocycline.

Antimicrobial Activity

Tetracyclines possess a wide range of antimicrobial activities against aerobic and anaerobic gram-positive and gram-negative bacteria. They are also effective against some microorganisms that are resistant to cell wall active antimicrobial drugs such as Rickettsiae, *Coxiella burnetii*, *Mycoplasma pneumoniae*, chlamydiae, legionellae, ureoplasma, some atypical mycobacteria and Plasmodium spp. They have little activity against fungi except

Actinomyces. They are also active against *Borrelia recurrentis, Leptospira icterohaemorrhagiae* and *Treponema pallidum.* Protozoa *Entamoeba histolytica* is inhibited only by high concentrations of tetracyclines. They are ineffective against viruses. They are more effective against gram-positive organisms than gram-negative organisms. They are bacteriostatic antibiotics. Bacterial strains that are inhibited by about 4 μg/mL (MIC) of tetracyclines are considered sensitive.

Mechanism of Action

They act by inhibiting bacterial protein synthesis. They bind to the 30s subunit of bacterial ribosomes and prevent the access of tRNA to the acceptor site on the mRNA ribosome complex.

Bacterial resistance to tetracyclines: It is primarily plasmid mediated. Mechanisms involved are:

- Decreased accumulation of tetracyclines as a result of either decreased antibiotic influx or aquisition of an energy dependent efflux pathway.
- Decreased access of tetracyclines to the ribosome because of the presence of ribosomal protection protein.
- Enzymatic inactivation of tetracyclines.

Many microorganisms including *Staphylococci, Streptococci, H. influenzae, Pneumococci, E. coli* and other enterobacteriaceae develop resistance to tetracyclines. There is cross-resistance between tetracyclines. Gram-positive bacteria resistant to tetracyclines are susceptible to chloramphenicol, but gram-negative bacteria resistant to tetracyclines are usually resistant to chloramphenicol.

Pharmacokinetics

Most of the tetracyclines are incompletely absorbed from the GIT. The percentage of oral dose that is absorbed (in empty stomach) is lowest for chlortetracycline (30%), intermediate for oxytetracycline, tetracycline, demethylchlortetracycline and methacycline (60 to 80%) and high for doxycycline,

minocycline and lymecycline (95 to 100%). Most absorption takes place from the stomach and upper part of small intestine in acidic medium. They are not destroyed by the gastric acid or by the intestinal flora. Their absorption is decreased by milk (contains calcium) and antacids (contain aluminium, magnesium and calcium) due to formation of insoluble chelate complexes with these metals. After absorption, tetracyclines are distributed widely in the body tissues and fluids. They accumulate in RE cells of liver, spleen and bone marrow and in bone, dentine and enamel of unerupted teeth. In the CSF, they reach only 20% of that of plasma concentrations but minocycline and doxycycline being lipophilic can attain high CSF concentrations (50% of that of plasma concentrations). Tetracyclines cross the placental barrier and enter the foetal circulation and amniotic fluid. They are also secreted in milk. They are metabolized in the liver and excreted mainly in the urine by glomerular filtration except doxycycline which is excreted mainly in faeces through liver and bile. Tetracyclines other than doxycycline can accumulate in the body in renal failure. Hence, only doxycycline can be used in renal insufficiency. For enterohepatic recycling, tetracyclines may remain in the body for long period after cessation of therapy.

Clinical Uses

Tetracyclines are indicated in:

- Rickettsial infections like murine, epidemic and scrub typhus, rickettsial pox, Q fever and Rocky Mountain spotted fever. Fever subsides within 2 to 3 days and rash disappears within 4 to 6 days.
- Chlamydia infections like lymphogranuloma venereum, pneumonia, bronchitis, sinusitis, cervicitis, epididymitis, inclusion conjunctivitis, trachoma and psittacosis.
- Mycoplasma infections like primary atypical pneumonia, bronchitis, urethritis and genital lesions.
- Sexually transmitted diseases (STDs) like gonorrhoea, syphilis and chancroid.

- Bacillary infections like *H. pylori* infection in peptic ulcer, acute bacilary dysentery (shigellosis), traveler's diarrhoea, cholera, plague and tularaemia.
- Coccal infections like skin and soft tissue infections (by gram-positive cocci), pneumococcal pneumonia and meningococcal meningitis.
- Urinary tract infections (UTIs) like cystitis, prostatis and urethritis (caused by sensitive bacteria).
- Respiratory tract infections like pharyngitis, sinusitis and chronic bronchitis.
- Acne vulgaris (benefit is produced in small dosage).
- Other infections like actinomycosis anthrax, nocardiosis, brucellosis, yaws, relapsing fever, leptospirosis, lyme disease, amoebic dysentery and drug-resistant malaria.

Some Preparations and Dosage

- Tetracycline (Achromycin)/Oxytetracycline (Terramycin)/chlorotetracyline hydrochloride (Aureomycin) capsule (250, 500 mg)—250 to 500 mg 6 hourly. They are also available as dry syrup (125 mg/5 ml), injection (100 mg/ml) and eye drops and ointment (0.5 to 1%).
- Demethylchlortetracycline (Ledermycin) capsule (150, 300 mg)—150 to 300 mg six hourly. It is also available as dry syrup (75 mg/5 ml).
- Doxycycline (Doxt) capsule (100 mg)—200 mg (single dose) on first day and then 100 mg daily.
- Minocycline (Minocin) capsule (100 mg)—100 mg twice daily.

Adverse Reactions

These are given as follows:

- **GIT side effects** like nausea, vomiting, epigastric distress, diarrhoea, stomatitis, glossitis and proctitis.
- **Hypersensitivity (allergic)** reactions like skin rashes, urticaria, fever, exfoliative dermatitis, anaphylaxis, photosensitivity and blood dyscrasias (leucopenia, thrombocytopaenia and aplastic or haemolytic anaemia).
- **Tooth and bone effects:** Tetracyclines chelate calcium forming a tetracycline calcium orthophosphate complex, which is deposited in areas of calcification in the teeth and bones. Therefore, during the period of tooth development tetracycline therapy can lead to permanent discolouration of teeth and hypoplasia of teeth enamel. Pigmentation of permanent teeth and increased risk of carries may occur in children receiving long-term therapy of tetracyclines. Hence, tetracyclines should be avoided in infants and children up to the age of 8 years. Administration of tetracyclines during pregnancy can lead to deposition in foetal bones and may reduce their linear growth producing maldevelopment of bones. Hence, tetracyclines should be avoided during pregnancy.
- **Azotaemia (rise in blood urea nitrogen (BUN)):** In patients with renal impairment, tetracyclines may cause azotaemia by inhibition of protein synthesis leading to accumulation of amino acids (due to non-utilization for peptide synthesis) and excessive formation of nitrogenous waste products. A reversible Fanconi-like syndrome manifested as nausea, vomiting, proteinuria, glycosuria, acidosis and aminoaciduria may develop after ingestion of outdated tetracycline capsules. This is caused by the degradation product 'epienhydrotetracycline', which is a toxic substance.
- **Other adverse effects**, e.g. hepatotoxicity, superinfection, increased intracranial pressure (especially in infants) and renal damage can also occur with tetracyclines.

Drug Interactions

- They interfere with the bactericidal action of β-lactam antibiotics.
- They potentiate the anticoagulant action of coumarin drugs.

- Drugs like gastric antacids, iron salts, bismuth salts and mineral products decrease bioavailability of tetracyclines.
- Drugs like carbamazepine, phenytoin and barbiturates decrease plasma half-lives of tetracyclines.

Chloramphenicol/Chloromycetin

History and Source

It was isolated from *Streptomyces venezuelae* by Burkholder in 1947. It is now prepared synthetically.

Chemistry

It is a derivative of dichloroacetic acid and contains a nitrobenzene moiety (as shown in **Fig. 68.2**).

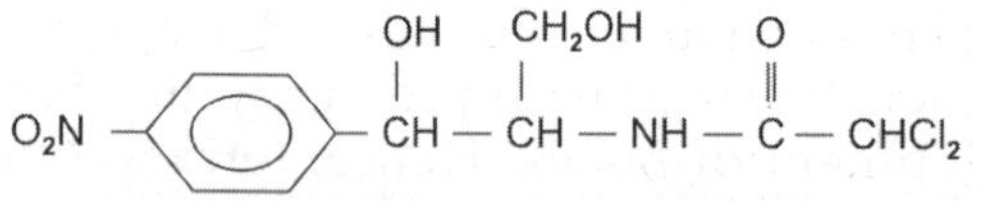

Fig. 68.2: Structure of chloramphenicol

Antimicrobial Activity

It is primarily bacteriostatic, although it may be bactericidal to certain species of bacteria such as *H. influenzae, N. meningitidis* and *Strep. pneumoniae.* It has antibacterial spectrum like tetracyclines. Thus it is effective against bacteria, rickettsiae, chlamydiae and *Mycoplasma pneumoniae.* It differs from tetracyclines in the following aspects:

- It is highly active against *Salmonella typhi,* where tetracyclines are ineffective.
- It is more active than tetracyclines against *H. influenzae, H. pertussis, K. pneumoniae* and anaerobes including *Bacteroides fragilis.*
- It is less active than tetracyclines against Cocci, Enterobacteriaceae (*E. coli, A. aerogenes, Proteus,* etc.), *Shigella* organisms, *Vibrio cholerae, Pasteurella (P. pestis* and *P. tularensis), Brucella* and Spirochetes (*T. pallidum* and *Leptospira icterohaemorrhagiae).*
- It is not active against *Mycobacteria, Actinomyces, Pseudomonas* and protozoa (*E. histolytica* and *Plasmodia)* as it fails to penetrate these bacteria, whereas tetra-

cyclines are effective. The minimum inhibitory concentration (MIC) of chloramphenicol is 8 μg/mL.

Mechanism of Action

It acts by inhibiting bacterial protein synthesis. It readily penetrates bacterial cells, probably by facilitated diffusion. It acts primarily by binding reversibly to the 50s subunit of bacterial ribosomes (near the site of action of macrolide antibiotics).

Bacterial resistance to chloramphenicol: Some bacteria like *Staph. aureus, H. influenzae, S. typhi, Shigella* and Enterobacteriaceae develop resistance to chloramphenicol by acquisition of a specific resistance (R) factor, which is a plasmid mediated enzyme 'chloramphenicol acetyl transferase' (acquired by conjugation), which causes acetylation of chloramphenicol. Acetylated derivatives of chloramphenicol cannot bind with the bacterial ribosomes and so bacteria develop resistance to chloramphenicol. *E. coli* may exhibit a cross-resistance to chloramphenicol and tetracyclines.

Pharmacokinetics

It is completely absorbed from the GIT after oral administration. It has a high bioavailability. It is widely distributed in the body including CSF and CNS. It is about 60% plasma protein bound. It is metabolized in the liver to the extent of about 90% and excreted mainly in urine as water-soluble glucuronide (by conjugation with glucuronic acid in the liver) and as free form (10%). It undergoes enterohepatic recycling. It has a plasma t½ of about 4 hours. It is administered 6 hourly to maintain a steady therapeutic level.

Clinical Uses

It is indicated in:

- **Typhoid fever:** It is the drug of choice in typhoid fever. Drugs used in typhoid fever are chloramphenicol, ampicillin/amoxicillin, pivmecillinam, cotrimoxazole, ciprofloxacin/ofloxacin and third generation cephalosporins (ceftriaxone and cefoperazone). Chloramphenicol should be used as early as possible and to be continued for a period of 14 days to prevent relapse. Ampicillin/amoxicillin is also used to treat typhoid fever but its therapeutic response is slower in onset and often inadequate. It is preferred in typhoid carriers. Cotrimoxazole is also effective in typhoid fever, but it requires administration in high dosage and to be continued for seven days after defervescence. It has low relapse rate and carrier state is uncommon. It can be combined with chloramphenicol in multidrug resistant (MDR) *S. typhi*. Ciprofloxacin, pivmecillinam, ceftriaxone and cefoperazone are other drugs effective in typhoid fever. These are used against multidrug resistant *S. typhi*.

- **Bacterial meningitis (by *H. influenzae*):** Chloramphenicol is better than ampicillin in *H. influenzae* meningitis because it easily crosses BBB. Nowadays third generation cephalosporins like ceftriaxone and cefotaxime are preferred than chloramphenicol as they are bactericidal and attain high concentrations in CSF.

- **Anaerobic infections:** Chloramphenicol is effective against most anaerobic bacteria including *Bacteroides fragilis*. It may be used alone or along with metronidazole or clindamycin in serious anaerobic infections of the bowel or pelvis (intra-abdominal or pelvic abscess). Together with ampicillin and metronidazole it is used in the treatment of brain abscess. Along with antimicrobial treatment, surgical drainage of abscess is done whenever necessary.

- **Rickettsial infections:** Chloramphenicol may be used but tetracyclines are more preferred due to less toxicity than chloramphenicol.

- **Miscellaneous conditions:** It can be used in brucellosis and plague (second choice drug after tetracyclines), whooping cough (second choice drug after erythromycin) and bacillary dysentery (second choice drug after cotrimoxazole). It is used topically in ocular infections (due to gram-

positive bacteria and *Chlamydia trachomatis*) as it penetrates satisfactorily into the intraocular fluid. It is also used topically in chronic otorrhoea (especially due to gram-negative bacteria) and in skin infections.

Preparations and Dosage

- Chloramphenicol (Chloromycetin, Parexin) capsule (250, 500 mg)—250 to 500 mg six hourly.
- Chloramphenicol palmitate dry syrup (125 mg/5 mL)—25 to 50 mg/kg/day in 4 divided doses.
- Chloramphenicol sodium succinate injection (125 mg/mL)—125 to 250 mg IM or slow IV six hourly.
- Chloramphenicol eye/ear drops (0.5% solution).
- Chloramphenicol applicap (containing 1% ointment).

Adverse Reactions

Chloramphenicol has some major adverse reactions so it should not be used where other alternatives are available. It can produce:

- **Bone marrow toxicity:** The nitrobenzene radical of chloramphenicol is responsible for bone marrow depression, which is probably an idiosyncratic reaction producing anaemia, leucopenia, agranulocytosis, thrombocytopaenia and even aplastic anaemia with pancytopaenia. It is not dose related. It occurs more commonly in those individuals who undergo prolonged therapy or repeated administration of chloramphenicol.

- **Neonatal toxicity (gray baby syndrome):** When chloramphenicol is used in neonates (especially in premature babies) in high doses (> 100 mg/kg body weight/day) then gray baby syndrome is produced. It usually begins within 3 to 7 days after treatment is started. It is manifested in first 24 hours as vomiting, refusal to suck, lethargy, abdominal distension and shallow irregular respiration. After 24 hours, the condition worsen leading to hypothermia, flaccidity, passage of loose green stools, metabolic acidosis, peripheral vascular collapse, gray cyanosis, shock and finally death. It is due to:

– Failure of conjugation of chloramphenicol in the liver due to low level of hepatic glucuronyl transferase enzyme activity in the first 2 or 3 weeks of neonatal life.

– Immaturity of the renal tubules in the neonate (infant) leading to impairment of excretion of free form of chloramphenicol.

• **Hypersensitivity (allergic) reactions:** Chloramphenicol can rarely cause skin rashes, drug fever, angioneurotic oedema, exfoliative dermatitis, atophic glossitis and haemorrhages from GIT, urinary bladder and skin.

• **Superinfection:** Chloramphenicol can rarely cause superinfection (GIT or vaginal candidiasis) as it is almost completely absorbed from GIT.

• **Miscellaneous reactions:** Chloramphenicol can cause nausea, vomiting, unpleasant taste and diarrhoea (GIT side effects). It can produce peripheral neuritis, optic neuritis, headache, mental confusion, depression and delirium (CNS side effects). Large dose of chloramphenicol can produce typhoid shock syndrome in patients of typhoid fever due to excessive release of endotoxin from the killed *S. typhi*.

Drug Interactions

• Chloramphenicol is a hepatic microsomal enzyme inhibitor. It decreases the metabolism of phenytoin, tolbutamide, warfarin and cyclophosphamide leading to their toxic effects.

• Microsomal enzyme inducers like phenobarbitone, phenytoin and rifampicin increase the metabolism of chloramphenicol leading to decreased therapeutic effects of chloramphenicol.

69

Miscellaneous Antibiotics

INTRODUCTION

These are minor antibiotics that are less used in systemic microbial infections, e.g.

- Lincosamide antibiotics, e.g. lincomycin and clindamycin
- Polypeptide antibiotics, e.g. polymyxins and bacitracin
- Vancomycin
- Spectinomycin
- Fusidic acid (sodium fusidate)
- Rifampicin
- Cycloserine.

DISCUSSION OF DRUGS

Lincomycin (Lincocin)

It is isolated from *Streptomyces lincolnensis*. It is effective orally and parenterally. It is bacteriostatic and acts by inhibiting bacterial protein synthesis by binding with 50s subunit of bacterial ribosomes. It has a spectrum of antibacterial activity like penicillin and erythromycin. It can be used in staphylococcal, streptococcal and pneumococcal infections in patients allergic to penicillin or erythromycin. It has been found more effective than penicillin or erythromycin in the treatment of osteomyelitis and prostatitis due to its better penetration into bones and prostatic tissue, but it is now rarely used due to following disadvantages:

- Rapid development of bacterial resistance especially by *Staph. aureus.*
- Development of pseudomembranous colitis and monilial superinfection during treatment.
- Depression of neuromuscular transmission and potentiation of competitive neuromuscular blocker when used concomitantly. It has been replaced by clindamycin for clinical use.

Clindamycin

It is a semisynthetic derivative of lincomycin. It is bacteriostatic at low concentrations and bactericidal at higher concentrations. It acts like lincomycin by binding with 50s subunit of bacterial ribosomes and suppressing bacterial protein synthesis. It has similar antibacteral activity to erythromycin against *Streptococci, Staphylococci* and *Pneumococci*. It is active against many strains of *Staph. aureus* except methicillin-resistant strain. It is more active than erythromycin or chloramphenicol against many anaerobic bacteria, especially *B. fragilis*. It shows good activity against *Pneumocystis carinii* pneumonia and *Toxoplasma gondii* encephalitis. Bacterial strains are considered sensitive to clindamycin when the minimum inhibitory concentration (MIC) for them is < 0.5 μg/ml. It has some activities against both chloroquine-sensitive and chloroquine-resistant strains of *Plasmodium falciparum* and *Plasmodium vivax*.

Pharmacokinetics

It is much better absorbed orally than linco-mycin and food does not interfere with its absorption. It is more protein bound than lincomycin (60%). It is distributed widely in body tissues and fluids including bones and prostatic tissues. Its penetration in CSF is poor. It is partly metabolized in the liver. About 60% of the drug is excreted unchanged in faeces and urine.

Clinical Uses

It is used in staphylococcal, pneumococcal and streptococcal infections not responding to penicillin or erythromycin and in individuals allergic to these antibiotics. It is used in the treatment of acute and chronic osteomyelitis and prostatitis due to its better penetration into bones and prostatic tissues. It is also useful in prophylaxis and treatment of anaerobic infections, especially by *B. fragilis*. It is used in combination with an amino-glycoside and penicillin or cephalothin in the treatment of peritonitis due to faecal contamination. It is used in the treament of encephalitis by *T. gondii* in AIDS patients. It is not useful for the treatment of brain abscess due to poor penetration into brain tissue.

Preparations and Dosage

- Clindamycin (Clinimycin) capsule (150 mg)—150 to 450 mg 6 hourly.
- Clindamycin dry syrup (150 mg/5 mL)—10 to 20 mg/kg/day in 3 or 4 divided doses in children.
- Clindamycin injection (300 mg/2 mL)—600 mg IM or IV infusion 8 hourly.
- Clindamycin ointment (1%, Clindac-A) for acne vulgaris.

Adverse Reactions

It can cause diarrhoea due to pseudomem-branous colitis (by superinfection with *Cl. difficile* and *Cl. sordellii*, which produce exotoxins with a necrotizing effect on the colonic mucosa). This is treated by van-comycin or metronidazole after stopping the offending drug. It can also produce hyper-sensitivity reactions like skin rashes, exudative erythema, multiforme (Stevens-Johnson syndrome), granulocytopaenia, thrombo-cytopaenia and anaphylaxis. Its other adverse effects include neuromuscular block and thrombophlebitis (at injection site).

Polymyxins

These are a group of closely related poly-peptide antibiotics elaborated by various strains of *Bacillus polymyxa*, an aerobic spore forming rod-shaped microorganism found in soil. Polymyxin-B and polymyxin-E (Colistin) being less toxic of these antibiotics are used in therapy as sulphate. Colistin is obtained from *Aerobacillus colistinus*. The antibacterial activity of polymyxin-B and colistin are similar and restricted to gram-negative bacteria including *Enterobacter*, *E. coli*, *Klebsiella, Salmonella, Pasturella, Bordetella* and *Shigella*, which are usually sensitive to concentrations of 0.05 to 2.0 µg/mL. Most strains of *Ps. aeruginosa* are inhibited by less than 8 µg/mL *in vitro*. They are bactericidal antibiotics and act by damaging the bacterial cell membrane by a detergent action. They are not absorbed orally. They are poorly absorbed from mucous membranes and the surface of large burns. Administered parenterally, highly toxic and produce nephrotoxicity, ototoxicity, hepatotoxicity and neuromuscular bockades. Polymyxin-B sulphate is used only topically. Colistin sulphate (Colymycin-S) is used orally as suspension in infants and children with diarrhoea caused by bacteria susceptible to the drug. The dose is 5 to 15 mg/kg daily in 3 divided portions. It can cause nausea, vomiting and diarrhoea (due to superinfection with *Proteus*). Infections of skin, mucous membranes, eye and ear caused by polymyxin-B sensitive bacteria respond to local application of it in solution, cream or ointment. Otitis externa and corneal ulcer caused by *Pseudomonas* may be cured by its topical use. It is used in combination with a variety of other compounds for synergistic action. It is more toxic than colistin and so not used orally. Hypersensitivity reactions due to liberation of histamine may occur with these drugs. Development of bacterial resistance to these drugs rarely occur.

Bacitracin

It is a polypeptide antibiotic obtained from *Bacillus subtilis*. It was isolated in 1943 from the damage tissue and street dirt debrided from a compound fracture in a young girl named Tracy and hence the name bacitracin. It has antibacterial spectrum like penicillin. A variety of gram-positive cocci and bacilli, *Neisseria*, *H. influenzae* and *T. pallidum* are sensitive to 0.1 unit of bacitracin/mL. Actinomyces and fusobacterium are inhibited by concentrations of 0.5 to 5 units/mL. Enterobacteriaceae, *Pseudomonas*, *Candida spp.* and *Nocardia* are resistant to the drug. It is bactericidal and acts by inhibiting bacterial cell wall synthesis. Microorganisms do not readily develop resistance to it. It is not much absorbed orally. Administered parenterally produces serious nephrotoxicity (acute tubular necrosis and anuria). It is now used only topically as an antiseptic. It is used in various superficial infections of skin, eye, ear and mucous membranes. It is available as ophthalmic and dermatologic ointments and also as powder for preparation of topical solutions. It is used in combination with neomycin or polymyxin-B or both. Hypersensitivity reactions from topical use are uncommon. When administered orally it can produce nausea, vomiting and abdominal pain.

Vancomycin

It is isolated from *Streptomyces orientalis*. It has a complex chemical structure. It is effective against gram-positive bacteria but not against gram-negative bacteria. Every strains of *Staph. aureus* including methicillin-resistant *Staph. aureus* (MRSA) strain are inhibited by it at a concentration of 1 to 5 µg/mL. Enterococci (e.g. *Strep. faecalis)* and *Cl. difficile* (causative organism of antibiotic induced pseudomembranous colitis) are also susceptible to it. It acts by inhibiting the synthesis of bacterial cell wall in sensitive bacteria by binding with high affinity to the D-alanyl-D-adenine terminus of cell wall precursor units. It is bactericidal for rapidly dividing microorganisms. Enterococci may develop resistance to vancomycin due to production of an enzyme that modifies the cell wall precursor, so that it no longer binds vancomycin. It is not absorbed orally. Its IM injection is very painful. It is used IV very slowly, otherwise Redman syndrome (RMS) can develop. It is widely distributed in different tissues of the body. It is excreted by the kidney in urine. It is used in antibiotic induced pseudomembranous colitis and diarrhoea caused by *Cl. difficile*, where it is given orally in the dose of 125 to 250 mg 6 hourly. It is also used in MRSA infections and penicillin allergic patients, where it is administered by slow IV infusion in the dose of 1 g 12 hourly.

It can produce thrombophlebitis at the injection site, ototoxicity (in high doses) and RMS (by quick IV infusion). RMS (Redman syndrome) is characterized by redness of face and trunk, hypotension and pruritus due to release of histamine from mast cells, because it is a histamine liberator. It can be prevented by pretreatment with antihistamine.

Spectinomycin

It is isolated from 'Streptomyces spectabilis'. Chemically it is an aminocyclitol, which is closely related to aminoglycosides. It is effective against a number of gram-negative bacteria including *N. gonorrhoeae*. It is inferior to other drugs to which such bacteria are susceptible. It acts by inhibiting protein synthesis in gram-negative bacteria by binding with 30s ribosomal subunit. Its action is similar to that of aminoglycosides but it is not bactericidal and does not cause misreading of polyribosome nucleotides. A high degree of bacterial resistance may develop to it as a result of mutation. It is rapidly absorbed after IM injection. It does not significantly bound to plasma protein and all of the administered dose is excreted in urine in 48 hours. It is only used in the treatment of gonorrhoea caused by strains resistant to first line drugs or if there are contraindications to the use of these drugs. It is administered IM in a single dose of 2 g. It can produce allergic reactions (urticaria, chills and drug fever), dizziness, nausea and insomnia. Its injection is painful.

Fusidic Acid/Sodium Fusidate

It is obtained from the parasitic fungus *'Fusidium coccineum'*. It has a steroidal structure but is devoid of hormonal effects. It is effective mainly against gram-positive bacteria, including penicillinase producing *Staph. aureus.* It is used in the treatment of resistant staphylococcal infection. It is bactericidal. It can be used as an alternative drug to antistaphylococcal penicillins in the treatment of acute and chronic osteomyelitis but staphylococci rapidly develop resistance to it. Hence, it is used concurrently along with an antistreptococcal penicillin. It is administered orally as capsule (0.5 g) in the dose of 0.5 to 1 g 8 hourly. It can be used by IV infusion as diethanolamine fusidate. It is very effective in staphylococcal skin infections like pyoderma and folliculitis, where it is applied as ointment or cream (2%) twice daily. It can be combined with systemic penicillin or erythromycin when used as ointment or cream. It can cause skin reactions, nausea, vomiting, epigastric pain, diarrhoea and hepatic dysfunction. It may aggravate peptic ulcer and exert a catabolic effect. Rifampicin and cycloserine are discussed as antitubercular drugs in the next chapter.

70

Drug Therapy of Tuberculosis

INTRODUCTION

Tuberculosis is a chronic granulomatous infectious disease caused by *Mycobacterium tuberculosis, M. bovis* or atypical mycobacteria (collectively called *tubercle bacilli*). Robert Koch in 1882 discovered the causative organism of tuberculosis. Tuberculosis is a systemic disease. The commonest form in man is chronic pulmonary tuberculosis. It can also involve other organs of the body including the brain. Though it is a chronic disease but it can be acute fulminating forms like tuberculous pneumonia and generalized miliary tuberculosis. Drug therapy is the most important aspect of the management of tuberculosis. Many chemotherapeutic agents are now available for the treatment of tuberculosis.

Classification of Antitubercular Drugs

These are of two groups:
- Standard drugs (first line drugs/primary drugs).
  - Tuberculocidal drugs, e.g. isoniazid, rifampicin, pyrazinamide and streptomycin.
  - Tuberculostatic drugs, e.g. ethambutol and thiacetazone.
- Reserve drugs (second line drugs/secondary drugs).
  - Tuberculocidal drugs, e.g. capreomycin, kanamycin, clarithromycin, azithromycin, rifabutin and fluroquinolone, ciprofloxacin, ofloxacin and sparfloxacin.

- Tuberculostatic drugs, e.g. ethionamide, cycloserine and para-amino salicylic acid (PAS).

Reserve drugs are used in resistant cases of tuberculosis. Antitubercular drugs are always used in combinations of 2, 3 or 4 drugs, as single drug administration leads to rapid development of drug-resistant tubercle bacilli. Chemoprophylaxis with isoniazid is the only exception to this rule. Multidrug therapy (MDT) in tuberculosis: The objectives are—

- To delay the emergence of drug-resistant tubercle bacilli.
- To enhance the antibacterial action of the drug
- To shorten the duration of drug therapy.
- To reduce the toxicity of individual drugs by using them in minimum therapeutic dosage.

The aim of chemotherapy of tuberculosis involves three goals:

- Killing of rapidly multiplying tubercle bacilli in order to make them sputum negative rapidly, so that the patient is non-contagious and safe for the community.
- Killing of persisting tubercle bacilli in order to cure the disease and to prevent relapse.
- Prevention of emergence of resistance of tubercle bacilli to the drugs, so that the bacilli remain susceptible to the drugs.

Antitubercular drug regimens (WHO recommendations). These are:

- **Long-term optimum therapeutic regimen (12–18 months):** Initially isoniazid (300 mg) + Ethambutol (800 mg) or streptomycin (0.75g) IM or thiacetazone (150 mg) daily for the first two months.

This is followed by:

Isoniazid (300 mg) + Thiacetazone (150 mg) daily for 10 to 15 months. This is a cheap regimen but the relapse rate is high (20%).

- **Short-term optimum therapeutic regimen (6 months):** This type of treatment is possible only when strict supervision by the clinician can be maintained in the first two months of the regimen (during the intensive phase of treatment). Initially, isoniazid (300 mg) + Rifampicin (450 mg) + Ethambutol (800 mg) + Pyrazinamide (1.5 g) daily for two months. This is followed by:

Isoniazid (300 mg) + Rifampicin (450 mg) daily or 4 months. This is recommended by WHO. This is an expensive regimen but the cure rate is high (98%).

Besides these drug regimens, there are many other drug regimens of tuberculosis, including direct observation treatment (DOT). Instead of supplying the drugs to the patient for self-administration at home, the patient is called at outdoor clinic, and administered the drugs under supervision to ensure that the drugs are actually consumed. The drugs are administered thrice weekly in higher doses, e.g. isoniazid, 600 mg; rifampicin, 450 mg; pyrazinamide 1500 mg; Ethambutol, 1200 mg and Streptomycin, 1 g.

Adjuvant Therapy

The patient should take nutritious diet and should avoid smoking and other respiratory irritants. Secondary respiratory infection must be treated with appropriate antibiotics. Diabetes mellitus if present must be treated with insulin or oral antidiabetic drugs. Dry, hacking and spasmodic cough is treated by cough suppressant like codeine phosphate. Haemoptysis due to pulmonary haemorrhage and pulmonary insufficiency due to emphysema, chronic bronchitis or pulmonary fibrosis should be properly treated.

DISCUSSION OF INDIVIDUAL DRUGS

Isoniazid

Chemically it is the hydrazide of isonicotinic acid (isonicotinic acid hydrazide/INH) and is structurally closely related to pyridoxine. It is a highly potent antitubercular drug but atypical mycobacteria are insensitive to it. It does not act against any other microorganism. It is the main drug in antitubercular regimens. It is given in combination with other antitubercular drugs to prevent emergence of mycobacterial resistance. In tubercular meningitis it is given in double doses.

Mechanism of Action

It is primarily tuberculocidal but may be tuberculostatic at lower concentration. It kills actively growing tubercle bacilli rapidly but inhibits dormant tubercle bacilli, which are persisters. It acts on both extracellular and intracellular (inside the macrophage) tubercle bacilli. It can easily penetrate the caseous tissue. It probably acts by inhibiting the enzyme 'mycolase synthetase', which is required for the synthesis of mycolic acid, an essential component of membrane lipids of mycobacterial cell wall. It thus interferes with the synthesis of mycobacterial cell wall.

Drug resistance: In a susceptible mycobacterial population 1 in 10^7 are resistant mutants, which do not allow isoniazid penetration. To prevent emergence of mutants, isoniazid should not be used alone but always used in combination with other antitubercular drugs.

Pharmacokinetics

It is rapidly and completely absorbed from GIT. It is widely distributed in all body tissues and fluids including brain and CSF. It crosses placental barrier and is secreted in milk. It is metabolized in the liver mainly by acetylation, which is under genetic control. In slow acetylators neurotoxicity (peripheral neuritis) is more common, while in rapid acetylators hepatotoxicity (due to the metabolite acetyl hydrazine) is more common. Plasma half-lives of isoniazid in slow and rapid acetylators are 3 hours and 1½ hours respectively. However, the rate of acetylation of isoniazid does not affect the daily dose. To prevent peripheral neuritis, pyridoxine (vitamin B_6) is combined with isoniazid in the treatment of tuberculosis. Isoniazid binds with pyridoxine or pyridoxal phosphate (the active metabolite of pyridoxine) to form hydrazones of pyridoxine and, therefore, inhibits pyridoxal kinase which converts pyridoxine to pyridoxal phosphate.

Pyridoxine $\xrightarrow[\text{ATP} \qquad \text{ADP}]{\text{Pyridoxal kinase}}$ Pyridoxal phosphate

Absence of pyridoxal phosphate leads to peripheral neuritis, which can be corrected by administration of pyridoxine (5 to 10 mg daily). Isoniazid is excreted in urine mainly as metabolites acetyl isoniazid, isonicotinic acid, isonicotinoyl hydrazone and glycine conjugate and slightly as unchanged form.

Clinical Uses

It is used in the treatment of all types of tuberculosis. It is the drug of choice in tubercular meningitis. It is the only drug for chemoprophylaxis of tuberculosis.

Preparations and Dosage

- Isoniazid (Isonex) tablet (100, 300 mg)—300 mg daily, 600 mg daily in tubercular meningitis. Children—10 mg/kg/day.
- Isoniazid syrup (100 mg/5 mL) for children.
- Isoniazid injection (100 mg/mL) for children and intrathecal administration.

Adverse Reactions

It has low incidence of toxicity (about 5%) incomparison to other antitubercular drugs. It can produce neurotoxicity and hepatotoxicity, which are related to dose and duration of therapy. Neurotoxicity is due to pyridoxine deficiency caused by competition between isoniazid and pyridoxine or pyridoxal phosphate for the enzyme pyridoxal kinase. It is manifested as peripheral neuritis (causing anaesthesia, paraesthesia and burning pain along the distribution of sensory nerves in the extremities) and convulsions (due to CNS stimulation) and psychotic episodes (in patients with history of epilepsy or psychosis). Hepatotoxicity is manifested as clinical jaundice due to multilobular hepatic necrosis. It is more in elderly persons and alcoholics.

Allergic reactions like skin rashes, drug fever, lymphadenopathy and jaundice can also occur with isoniazid. It can also cause haemolysis of RBCs in patients deficient with G6PD enzyme in RBCs.

Drug Interactions

Isoniazid is a hepatic microsomal enzyme inhibitor. It inhibits the metabolism of drugs like phenytoin, carbamazepine and ethosuximide leading to their toxicity.

Rifampicin

It is a semisynthetic derivative of the antibiotic 'Rifamycin-B' produced by *Streptomyces mediterranei*. Chemically it is a macrocyclic compound. It is a highly potent antitubercular drug effective against all types of tubercle bacilli including dormant bacilli. It is also effective against lepra bacilli and many gram-positive and gram-negative bacteria (*Staph. aureus, N. meningitidis, H. influenzae, E. coli, Klebsiella, Pseudomonas, Proteus* and *Legionella*). It is used only in tuberculosis and leprosy. In other infections it is rarely used due to danger of emergence of resistant bacteria.

Mechanism of Action

It is a tuberculocidal drug. It is as effective as isoniazid and better than other antitubercular drugs. It is effective against both extracellular and intracellular tubercle bacilli. It is also effective against atypical mycobacteria. It acts by inhibiting DNA dependent RNA polymerase and thus inhibiting RNA synthesis in the sensitive bacteria.

Drug resistance: Rifampicin resistance is either due to bacterial permeability barrier or to a mutation of DNA dependent RNA polymerase. If it is used alone, mycobacteria develop rapid resistance to it. Hence it is used in combination with other antitubercular drugs. There is no cross-resistance with other antitubercular drugs.

Pharmacokinetics

It is well-absorbed from GIT. Food interferes with its absorption resulting in lower plasma levels. When a dose of 600 mg is given orally ½ hour before breakfast, the peak plasma concentration is achieved within 2 hours and the effective therapeutic concentration persists for more than 12 hours. It is widely distributed in various body tissues and fluids including brain and CSF. It is highly plasma protein bound (about 85%). It crosses placental barrier. It is metabolized in the liver forming desacetyl rifampicin, which is as active as rifampicin against tubercle bacilli. It undergoes enterohepatic circulation. It is excreted mainly in urine and faeces. It makes urine, faeces and saliva orange red in colour during excretion.

Clinical Uses

It is mainly used in the treatment of tuberculosis and leprosy in combination with other drugs. It can be used for the treatment of brucellosis and serious staphylococcal septicaemia. It is used for chemoprophylaxis of meningococcal meningitis and *H. influenzae* meningitis.

Preparations and Dosage

- Rifampicin (Rifampin) capsule (450, 600 mg)—450 to 600 mg daily. Children—15 mg/kg/day.
- Rifampicin syrup (100 mg/5 mL) for children.

Adverse Reactions

It has low incidence of toxicity (less than 5%). It can cause skin rashes, diarrhoea, dizziness, ataxia, leucopenia and eosinophilia. It can produce flu-like syndrome during high dose (900 mg) intermittent therapy (biweekly). It has been reported to produce hepatitis by liver damage especially in elderly patients, alcoholics or persons with hepatic dysfunction. It causes teratogenic effects in animals and it is better to avoid rifampicin during pregnancy.

Drug interactions: Rifampicin is a hepatic microsomal enzyme inducer. It increases metabolism of drugs like hydrocortisone, digoxin, dapsone and oral contraceptives leading to decreased therapeutic efficacy of these drugs.

Pyrazinamide

Chemically it is pyrazinoic acid amide. It is a structural relative of nicotinamide (pyrazine analog of nicotinamide). It is active only against *M. tuberculosis* like isoniazid. It is a tuberculocidal drug but its mechanism of action is not known. It is effective against *M. tuberculosis* of human type but is ineffective against the bovine and atypical forms of tubercle bacilli. It shows antitubercular activity in an acidic pH (< 6.0) and is effective only against tubercle bacilli within macrophages (where pH is acidic). When combined with isoniazid and rifampicin, it exerts a potent sterilizing effect on the tuberculous lesions during the first two months of therapy but later on it adds little effect. Resistance to it develops rapidly if used alone and hence it is used in combination with other antitubercular drugs.

Pharmacokinetics

It is well-absorbed from GIT. It is widely distributed in the body tissues and fluids including brain and CSF. It is metabolized in the liver by deamination. It is excreted in urine as metabolites and unchanged form.

Clinical Uses

It is used only in tuberculosis in combination with other antitubercular drugs.

Preparations and Dosage

- Pyrazinamide (P-zide) tablet (750 mg)—1.5 g daily (25 mg/kg/day).
- Pyrazinamide syrup (250 mg/5 mL) for children—30 mg/kg/day. Morphazinamide (Dynazide) is more potent than pyrazinamide.

Adverse Reactions

It can produce metallic taste, anorexia, nausea, vomiting, malaise, skin rashes, fever, arthralgia, exanthema and rarely photosensitivity (producing bright red brown discolouration of the exposed parts of the body) and acute hypertension. Toxic hepatitis with jaundice may occur at any time during the course of treatment. Hence, it should not be used in hepatic dysfunction. On prolonged therapy it can cause hyperuricaemia and precipitation of gout by inhibiting uric acid excretion in urine.

Ethambutol

Chemically it is dextrorotatory isomer of ethylene diamine butanol. The levorotatory form is inactive against mycobacteria but is equally toxic. It is a tuberculostatic drug but its mechanism of action is not known. It is effective against mycobacteria resistant to isoniazid, streptomycin, ethionamide and PAS as well as against atypical mycobacteria. It acts mainly against rapidly multiplying mycobacteria in the walls of tuberculous cavities. When it is used with other antitubercular drugs resistance to it develops slowly and the development of resistance to other drugs is greatly delayed. There is no cross-resistance with other antitubercular drugs.

Pharmacokinetics

It is well-absorbed from GIT. It is distributed widely in the body tissues and fluids, the CSF level is only 50% of the plasma level. It penetrates into RBCs, which probably serve as a depot from which the drug is released into circulation. It is partly metabolized in the liver. About 50% of the orally administered drug is excreted unchanged in urine within 24 hours and about 15% of the drug is excreted in urine as metabolites. A part of the drug is excreted in faeces.

Clinical Uses

It is only used in tuberculosis in combination with other antitubercular drugs.

Preparation and Dosage

Ethambutol tablet (400, 800 mg)— 15 to 25 mg/kg/day) (800 mg daily).

Adverse Reactions

It is oculotoxic drug. It can produce visual disturbances (optic neuritis, red-green blindness, loss of vision and retinal damage) if administered for prolonged period. Most of these symptoms are reversible if the drug is withdrawn after 2 months. It should be avoided in children because of difficulty in identifying early reduction in visual acuity in them. Other adverse effects of ethambutol include nausea, anorexia, giddiness, peripheral neuritis, retrobulbar neuritis, allergic reactions, hyperuricaemia (like pyrazinamide) and mental disturbances.

Thiacetazone/Amithiazone

Chemically it is a derivative of thiosemicarbazone and related to isoniazid. It is a tuberculostatic drug with low efficacy. Its mechanism of action is not known. It is cheap and used as a companion drug to isoniazid in long course regimen of tuberculosis. It is well-absorbed from GIT and widely distributed in body tissues and fluids. It is partly metabolized in the liver and excreted largely in unchanged form in urine. It is used only in tuberculosis in combination with other antitubercular drugs to prevent development of resistant mycobacteria. It is available as tablet (50, 150 mg) and used in the dose of 150 mg daily (2 mg/kg/day). It can produce anorexia, nausea, vomiting, skin rashes, drug fever, exfoliative dermatitis, hepatitis and blood dyscrasias (granulocytopaenia and agranulocytosis). Hepatotoxicity is the most serious adverse reaction of thiacetazone, but due to genetic reason it is less common in Indians.

Ethionamide

Chemically it is closely related to isoniazid. It is a tuberculostatic drug and probably acts by inhibiting protein synthesis in the mycobacteria. It is effective against tubercle bacilli resistant to other antitubercular drugs. It is also effective against atypical mycobacteria. Resistance to it develops rapidly if used alone and hence it is used in combination with other antitubercular drugs. It is rapidly absorbed from GIT. It is widely distributed in body tissues and fluids and achieves a significant concentration in the CSF. Its metabolic fate is unknown. About 1% of the drug is excreted in the active form in urine. It is used in tuberculosis as a reserve drug (second line drug) along with other drugs. It is available as tablet (125, 250 mg) and used in the dose of 0.75 to 1 g daily in two divided doses. It can cause GIT irritation (producing anorexia, nausea, vomiting and diarrhoea), allergic reactions (skin rashes and thrombocytopaenia), hepatitis, peripheral neuritis, optic neuritis and pellagra like symptoms (stomatitis and diarrhoea). Concurrent administration of pyridoxine (vitamin B_6) along with it is necessary to prevent neurotoxicity. Prothionamide is more potent than ethionamide.

Streptomycin

It is discussed along with aminoglycoside antibiotics. It is a tuberculocidal drug. It is less effective than isoniazid and rifampicin but more effective than all other antitubercular drugs. It kills rapidly multiplying tubercle bacilli at neutral pH in the walls of the tuberculous cavities but cannot penetrate into macrophages and caseous material. It is used as one of the drugs in multidrug therapy against tuberculosis. It is administered IM in the dose of 0.75 g daily. It can produce ototoxicity, nephrotoxicity and neuromuscular blocks.

Cycloserine

It is obtained from *Streptococcus orchidaceus*. Chemically it is related to the amino acid alanine. It is a tuberculostatic drug and acts by inhibiting the synthesis of bacterial cell wall. It is active against *M. tuberculosis*, resistant to isoniazid or streptomycin and against atypical mycobacteria. It is well-absorbed orally and distributed to various body tissues and fluids including brain and CSF. It is metabolized in the liver and excreted in urine as both metabolites and unchanged drug. It is used in tuberculosis as a reserve drug (second choice drug) along with other drugs. It is available as tablet (125, 250 mg) and administered in the dose of 0.5 to 1 g daily in two divided portions. In children a dose of 10 to 15 mg/kg/day is used. It can cause neurotoxicity, hepatotoxicity, convulsions and psychosis. Toxicity is its major drawback. Other antitubercular drugs like capreomycin, kanamycin and PAS are now rarely used due to toxicity. Newer drugs clarithromycin, azithromycin, rifabutin and fluoroquinolones (ciprofloxacin, ofloxacin and sparfloxacin) may be useful in the treatment of infections with *M. tuberculosis* and *M. avium* complexes.

71

Drug Therapy of Leprosy

INTRODUCTION

Leprosy is a chronic granulomatous infectious disease caused by *M. leprae* and affecting skin and peripheral nerves. Clinically there are four main types of leprosy, *viz.* lepromatous, tuberculoid, indeterminate and dimorphic (border line). They are determined by the degree of cell mediated immunity (CMI) in the host against the lepra bacilli. In lepromatous leprosy, the CMI is low (lepromin test negative), the lepra bacilli are plenty in the lesions and the disease progresses rapidly. It affects mainly face, nose, ears, eyes and lymph glands. The typical lesion is a small hypopigmented, circular, erythematous patch without itching or hypoalgesia. Gradually, the skin becomes furrowed and nodulated, giving the appearance of 'leonine fades'. Later on ulceration occurs due to tissue destruction involving eyes, nose and larynx. Peripheral nerves are affected last in this condition. In tuberculoloid leprosy, the CMI is adequate (lepromin test strongly positive), the lepra bacilli are scanty in the lesions and the disease progresses slowly. Peripheral nerves are predominantly affected and thickened. The typical lesion is a large, flat and hypopigmented skin area with red raised margin with loss of sensation (anaesthesia).

In indeterminate form of leprosy the lesions are slight and do not indicate about the type of disease. In dimorphic (borderline) leprosy, the CMI is low and it becomes lepromatous leprosy if left untreated. Lepromatous leprosy and borderline leprosy have plenty of bacilli in the lesions and are called multibacillary leprosy, whereas tuberculoid leprosy and indeterminate leprosy have scanty bacilli in the lesions and are called paucibacillary leprosy.

Classification of Antileprotic Drugs

These are of four groups:

- Sulphones, e.g. dapsone (DDS) and acedapsone (DADDS).
- Phenazine dye, e.g. clofazimine.
- Antitubercular drugs, e.g. rifampicin, ethionamide.
- Newer drugs, e.g. minocycline, clarithromycin, pefloxacin and ofloxacin. Of all these drugs, only rifampicin, clarithromycin and ofloxacin are leprocidals and others are leprostatics.

Multidrug therapy (MDT) in leprosy: The objectives are—

- To prevent the emergence of bacterial resistance to drug especially to dapsone.
- To shorten the duration of drug therapy and to increase the patient's compliance.
- To make the patient noninfectious as early as possible.
- To prevent deformity and disability of the patient.

Antileprotic drug regimens (WHO recommendation). These are:

- **Three-drug regimen:** Multibacillary leprosy is treated by Dapsone (100 mg daily, self-administered) + Rifampicin (600 mg once monthly, supervised) + Clofazimine (50 mg daily, self-administered and 300 mg once monthly, supervised).

  Duration of treatment: Two years, follow-up five years.

- **Two-drug regimen:** Paucibacillary leprosy is treated by Dapsone (100 mg daily, self-administered) + Rifampicin (600 mg once monthly, supervised).

  Duration of treatment: Six months, follow-up two years.

DISCUSSION OF INDIVIDUAL DRUGS

Dapsone

Chemically it is diaminodiphenyl sulphone (DOS).

It is the most commonly used sulphone, because it is cheaper and most active drug. All other sulphones are converted in the body to dapsone, but none is superior to dapsone. It is the drug of choice in the treatment of leprosy.

Mechanism of Action

It is a leprostatic drug. It is chemically related to sulphonamides and has similar mechanism of bacteriostatic action. It acts by inhibiting folate synthesis in the bacteria by competing with PABA (preventing incorporation of PABA into folic acid of the bacteria). Its antibacterial action can be antagonized by PABA containing substances. It arrests the growth of many bacteria sensitive to sulphonamides. Its specificity for *M. leprae* is probably due to difference in its affinity for folate synthetase. Doses of dapsone needed for treating other bacterial infections are too toxic for use and so not used.

Drug resistance: Both primary and secondary resistance of *M. leprae* to dapsone may occur. Low dosage dapsone therapy and irregular treatment are mainly responsible for the development of such resistance. Dapsone should be used in combination with at least one drug (rifampicin) to prevent resistance.

Pharmacokinetics

It is almost completely absorbed from GIT. It is widely distributed in the body tissues and fluids. It is 70% plasma protein bound. It is more concentrated in skin (particularly leprotic skin), muscles, liver and kidneys and retained there for 2 to 3 weeks. It is metabolized in the liver by acetylation, glucuronidation and sulphate conjugation. It undergoes enterohepatic circulation, which prolongs its action. It is a cumulative drug. It has a plasma half-life of 1 to 2 days. It is excreted in urine mainly as metabolites and slightly as unchanged form. It is also excreted in milk and faeces.

Clinical Uses

These are given as follows:

- Treatment of leprosy: It is the most widely used drug in all types of leprosy. It is the primary drug and always used in combination with rifampicin.
- Chemoprophylaxis of leprosy: It is the only drug used.
- Treatment of chloroquine resistant falciparum malaria: It is used in combination with pyrimethamine.
- Treatment of *Pneumocystis carinii* pneumonia in AIDS patients.

Preparations and Dosage

- Dapsone (Novopone) tablet (50, 100 mg)—50 to 100 mg daily.
- Dapsone injection (20% w/v suspension in arachis oil)—0.2 mL IM weekly initially and gradually increased to a maximum of 0.8 mL weekly.
- Acedapsone (Diacetyl dapsone/DADDS) injection (a repository preparation)—225 mg IM monthly injections are used in unreliable patients.

Adverse Reactions

It is a potentially toxic drug. It can produce:

- GIT upsets like anorexia, nausea and vomiting.
- Allergic reactions like skin rashes, pruritus, fever, exfoliative dermatitis, photosensitivity and hepatitis with cholestatic jaundice.
- Blood dyscrasias like haemolytic anaemia (in patients with G6PD deficiency in RBCs), agranulocytosis and methaemoglobinaemia.
- Other toxicities like headache, nervousness, psychosis, paraesthesia, peripheral neuropathy, goitrogenesis and liver damage.
- Lepra reaction: It is the acute exacerbation of leprosy during dapsone treatment. It is of two types:

Type 1 reaction: It occurs usually in tuberculoid leprosy. In it, the existing lesions show increased erythema and swelling and the constitutional symptoms are not marked. It is a delayed type of hypersensitivity reaction and occurs in patients with good CMI towards *M. leprae.* It may lead to complete healing of lesions by decreasing the number of lepra bacilli.

It does not require treatment.

Type 2 reaction (erythema nodosum leprosum, ENL): It occurs usually in lepromatous leprosy and borderline cases. It is a serious reaction leading to aggravation of existing lesions with appearance of many crops of bright erythematous nodules and raised patches. The basic lesion is a vasculitis following deposition of (antigen + antibody) immune complexes in skin and other tissues. There is associated constitutional symptoms like fever, neuralgia, exfoliative dermatitis, hepatitis, orchitis and lymphadenitis. This reaction responds to clofazimine in the dose of 100 mg three times a day. Alternative drugs that can be used are chloroquine (150 mg base three times a day), thalidomide (400 mg daily) and prednisolone (20 to 30 mg daily in divided doses) to suppress the lesions by anti-inflammatory action. Dapsone treatment is continued in full doses throughout both types of lepra reaction.

Rifampicin

It has been discussed with antitubercular drugs. It is a leprocidal drug and highly effective in leprosy. It acts by inhibiting DNA dependent RNA polymerase and thus inhibiting RNA synthesis in the sensitive bacteria. It is a costly drug and administered along with dapsone. It has been found that supervised administration of rifampicin (600 mg) once a month is equally effective as daily administration of rifampicin (600 mg) in leprosy (as it kills 80% of lepra bacilli). Bacterial resistance to rifampicin can develop rapidly if used alone. It is used in all types of leprosy. It is administered orally as capsule. Its adverse reactions and drug reactions have been discussed previously.

Clofazimine

Chemically it is a phenazine dye congener. It is a leprostatic drug. It acts on *M. leprae* and *M. avium intracellulare.* It probably acts by binding with DNA of mycobacteria (preventing template function of DNA), so that RNA formation for bacterial protein synthesis does not occur. It has also antiinflammatory action. Mycobacteria develop resistance to it if used alone and hence it is used in combination with dapsone and rifampicin.

Pharmacokinetics

It is absorbed moderately (to the extent of about 50%) from GIT. It is distributed well in body tissues and fluids. It is being lipid-soluble, accumulates in adipose tissue and penetrates the cell membrane and macrophages easily. It is stored in reticuloendothelial tissues and skin and released from there very slowly. It penetrates CSF poorly. It is slowly metabolized in the liver and is excreted in urine and bile. It has plasma half-life of 70 hours.

Clinical Uses

It is used in lepromatous leprosy and atypical mycobacterial infection (caused by *M. avium* complex) especially in AIDS patients. It is also used for the treatment of type 2 lepra reaction during dapsone therapy.

Preparation and Dose

Clofazimine (Clofazine) capsule (50, 100 mg)—50 to 100 mg daily or 300 mg monthly supervised.

Adverse Reactions

It is generally well-tolerated. It can cause GIT upset (anorexia, nausea, abdominal pain and diarrhoea), reddish or brown black discolou-ration of the skin, hair and secretions, photo-sensitivity and dryness and itching of skin.

Ethionamide

It has been discussed with antitubercular drugs. It is more expensive and more toxic than dapsone but has faster bacteriostatic action against *M. leprae* than dapsone. It may be used as a substitute of dapsone or clofazimine in multi-drug regimen of leprosy. Prothionamide is more potent than ethionamide.

Newer drugs like minocycline, clarithromycin, pefloxacin and ofloxacin have been found to possess antileprotic activities. These are under clinical evaluation. These are used in patients intolerant/allergic to sulphones.

72

Drug Therapy of Malaria

INTRODUCTION

Malaria is an acute and chronic parasitic disease caused by the intracellular protozoan of the genus Plasmodium and is characterized by fever with rigors, anaemia and spleno-megaly. There are four species of *Plasmodia*, *viz. P. vivax, P. falciparum, P. ovale* and *P. malariae*. Malarial parasites are transmitted to humans by the bite of female anopheline mosquitoes, the definite host for plasmodia. In India, most malaria are caused by *P. vivax* and some by *P. falciparum*. The *P. vivax* induced malaria is usually not lethal but shows relapses. The clinician must take measures, so that relapse does not occur. The *P. falciparum* induced malaria is serious and

often becomes fatal, but once cured does not show relapse. *P. ovale* and *P. malariae* induced malaria are rarely found in India. *P. vivax* causes benign tertian malaria and *P. falciparum* causes malignant tertian malaria.

Life Cycle of Malarial Parasite (MP)

It comprises two phases, *viz.* schizogony in man (host) and sporogony in female anophe-line mosquito (vector). The salivary glands of the infected mosquito contain a large number of sporozoites and during sucking of blood, the sporozoites are inoculated into the blood-stream of man. These sporozoites disappear rapidly from the circulation and invade the parenchymatous cells of the liver and the

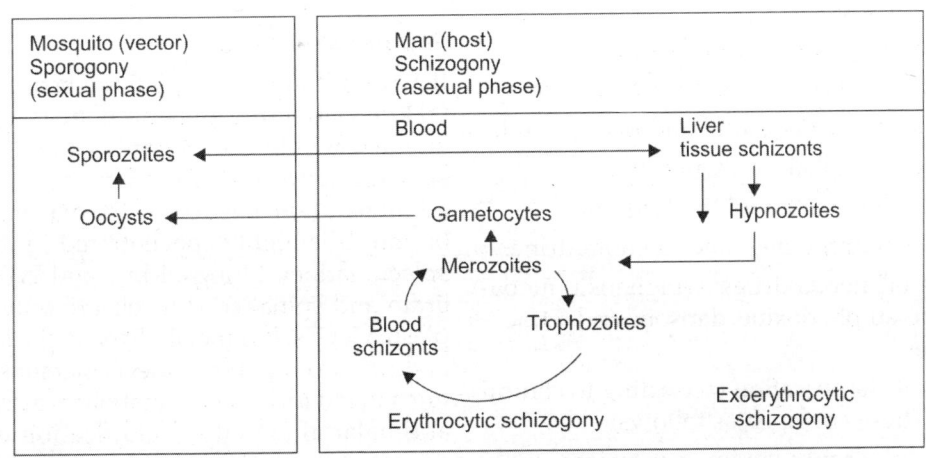

Fig. 72.1: Life cycle of malarial parasite (Plasmodium)

reticuloendothelial cells and multiply there to form tissue schizonts (primary exocytic form or pre-erythrocytic stage). The incubation period for *P. falciparum* is 5 to 7 days and for *P. vivax* is 8 days to several months. On completion of pre-erythrocytic stage, several thousands merozoites are released into the bloodstream, which invade the erythrocytes (RBCs) and there they undergo further development and multiplication giving rise to erythrocytic schizonts (asexual erythrocytic stage) known as trophozoites. The infected RBCs eventually rupture releasing parasites along with metabolic and toxic products into the bloodstream. These parasites then undergo following phases:

- Invade fresh erythrocytes again producing erythrocytic schizogony repeatedly.
- Undergo differentiation into male (microgametocyte) and female (macrogametocyte) sexual forms, which when taken by another mosquito develop into zygote.
- In *P. vivax* malaria, some of them enter new liver cells and continue exoerythrocytic stage. They are called hypnozoites, which are responsible for relapse of malaria.

Classification of Antimalarial Drugs

This can be done in two ways:

1. **Chemical classification** (according to chemical structure). These are:
   - 4-aminoquinolines: Chloroquine and amodiaquine.
   - 8-aminoquinolines: Primaquine.
   - Diaminopyrimidines: Pyrimethamine.
   - Biguanides: Proguanil and cycloguanil.
   - Cinchona alkaloids: Quinine
   - Quinoline methanol: Mefloquine.
   - Phenanthrene methanol: Halofantrine.
   - Miscellaneous drugs: Qinghaosu, mepacrine, sulphadoxine, dapsone and tetracyclines.

2. **Clinical classification** (according to clinical use). These are given as follows:
   - Causal prophylactics, e.g. primaquine, pyrimethamine and proguanil. They are tissue schizonticides acting on exoerythrocytic stage of plasmodia in liver cells and prevent erythrocytic invasion. True causal prophylactics which destroy the sporozoites before their invasion of liver cells are not available.
   - Clinical curatives/suppressives, e.g. chloroquine, amodiaquine, quinine, mefloquine, halofantrine, qinghaosu, proguanil, mepacrine, pyrimethamine, sulphadoxine, dapsone and tetracyclines. They are blood schizonticides acting on erythrocytic stage of plasmodia and terminate clinical attack.
   - Radical curatives, e.g. primaquine with chloroquine in *P. vivax* malaria. They are blood and tissue schizonticides to eradicate both erythrocytic and exoerythrocytic forms of *P. vivax* and prevent relapse of *P. vivax* malaria.
   - Gametocidal drugs, e.g. primaquine, pyrimethamine and proguanil. They are effective against gametocytes of all species of plasmodium. Chloroquine, quinine and mefloquine are effective against gametocytes of *P. vivax*.

DISCUSSION OF INDIVIDUAL DRUGS

Chloroquine

It is a 4-aminoquinoline derivative. It is the most frequently used antimalarial drug.

Pharmacokinetics

It is rapidly and completely absorbed from GIT. Its effective plasma concentration is attained within 2 to 3 hours of oral administration and within 15 minutes of IM administration. It is about 55% plasma protein bound. It is highly concentrated in the liver, spleen, kidneys, lungs, RBCs and WBCs. The brain and spinal cord levels are only 20% of plasma levels. It is metabolized in the liver and is slowly excreted in urine as metabolites and unchanged form. The metabolites also exhibit antimalarial activity. Acidification of urine decreases excretion of chloroquine (a basic drug).

Due to its high affinity for tissue proteins, it persists in the body for a considerable time. It has a plasma half-life of about five days.

Pharmacological Actions

It produces following actions:

- **Antimalarial action:** It is a suppressive and clinical curative drug in malaria. It kills the asexual erythrocytic forms of *P. vivax* and *P. falciparum*. It is also effective against the gametocytes of *P. vivax*, *P. ovale* and *P. malariae* but not of *P. falciparum*. It has no effect on the sporozoites, pre-erythrocytic and persistent tissue forms of plasmodia. As a suppressive, it is superior to quinine and mepacrine. Resistance to chloroquine by *P. falciparum* has developed in endemic areas producing serious problem.

Mechanism of Antimalarial Action

It is a blood schizonticidal drug. It has high affinity for nucleoproteins. It is selectively taken up by RBCs. Plasmodia live on haemoglobin of RBCs. Chloroquine being a basic drug accumulates in the acidic food vacuoles of plasmodia and interferes with the degradation (digestion) of haemoglobin by the parasitic lysosomes and thus prevents the plasmodia to utilize haemoglobin.

It forms a toxic complex with heme, which damages the plasmodial membranes. It prevents the formation of parasitic pigment hemozoin by inhibiting the heme polymerase. It also inhibits nucleoprotein synthesis of plasmodion presenting incorporation of phosphate into the RNA and DNA leading to death of immature plasmodia.

- **Other antiparasitic actions:** It is effective against *E. histolytica*, *G. lamblia*, *Clonorchis sinensis* (Chinese liver fluke) and *Diphyllobothrium latum* (fish tapeworm).

- **Miscellaneous actions:** It has antiinflammatory, antihistaminic and local anaesthetic activities. In high dosage it has cardiac depressant action and anticholinesterase activity.

Clinical Uses

It is used in:

- **Malaria:** It is the drug of choice for the treatment of acute attack of malaria except in chloroquine-resistant *P. falciparum* malaria. It is also used for suppressive prophylaxis of both *P. vivax* and *P. falciparum* malaria.

- **Amoebiasis:** It is effective in extraintestinal amoebiasis like amoebic hepatitis but ineffective in intestinal amoebiasis, because it is completely absorbed from small intestine and a very little amount reach the large intestine (where *E. histolytica* is present).

- **Giardiasis:** It is effective in giardiasis when administered in the dosage of 250 mg daily for five days.

- *Clonorchis sinensis* **infestation:** It is administered in the dosage of 250 mg daily for six weeks.

- **Taeniasis:** It is more effective against fish tapeworm than pork and beef tapeworms. It is administered in a single total dose of 2 g in the morning in empty stomach, followed later by a saline purgative.

- **Collagen diseases** like rheumatoid arthritis and disseminated lupus erythematosus (DLE). It is administered in the dose of 250 to 500 mg daily for prolonged period.

- **Lepra reaction:** It is effective in controlling lepra reaction during dapsone therapy (discussed previously).

Preparations and Dosage

- Chloroquine phosphate/sulphate (Lariago/Resochin) tablet (250 mg of the salt/150 mg of the base). In acute attack of malaria—1 g (4 tablets) to be taken initially followed by 0.5 g (2 tablets) after 6 hours and then 0.5 g (2 tablets) daily for 2 days. For suppressive prophylaxis—0.5 g (2 tablets) once weekly (in endemic area).

- Chloroquine phosphate/sulphate injection (40 mg of the base/mL). In acute attack of malaria—200 to 300 mg of the base IM or slow IV (diluted with 100 mL of 5%

dextrose saline). The total parenteral dose within 24 hours should not exceed 900 mg of the base. It is used especially in cases of cerebral malaria for rapid action.

Adverse Reactions

It is a relatively safe drug. It can cause mild headache, nausea, vomiting, anorexia, abdominal pain, skin rashes, pruritus, deafness, neuromyopathy, photosensitivity, pigmentation and visual disturbances (blurring of vision, diplopia and temporary loss of accommodation), which are reversible. On prolonged use in high doses as in rheumatoid arthritis and DLE, it may cause lenticular opacity, subcapsular posterior cataract and retinopathy (causing loss of vision) which are irreversible. It can also cause insomnia, acute psychotic episodes and seizures (by stimulating CNS) and cardiac depression and abrupt fall of BP (on IV administration). Unlike quinine, it can be used safely during pregnancy. It has no teratogenic effect.

Contraindications

It is contraindicated in patients with psoriasis and porphyria. It should be used cautiously in the presence of severe liver, gastrointestinal, neurological and haematological diseases.

Amodiaquine has similar properties as chloroquine but more toxic.

Primaquine

It is an 8-aminoquinoline derivative. It has only antimalarial action. It is effective against:

- Hypnozoites (dormant parasites), which cause the persistent tissue phase of P. vivax and P. ovale.
- Primary exoerythrocytic forms of P. falciparum.
- Gametocytes of all species of plasmodia. It has no effect on the erythrocytic forms of plasmodia.

Mechanism of Action

It probably acts by forming an active metabolite, which acts as a powerful oxidizing agent and causes damage to both erythrocytes and plasmodia. This may be the mechanism of both antimalarial and haemolytic actions.

Pharmacokinetics

It is rapidly absorbed from GIT. Its effective plasma level reaches in 1 to 2 hours. It is highly concentrated in the liver, lung and skeletal muscle. It is rapidly metabolized in the liver by oxidation and is excreted in urine within 24 hours. Only 1% of the drug is excreted unchanged in urine.

Clinical Uses

It is used for radical cure of relapsing malaria caused by P. vivax and P. ovale. It is given after full curative dose of chloroquine to cover the erythrocytic phase. It is ineffective as suppressive/clinical curative of malaria. It is not used for prophylaxis of malaria due to its toxicity.

Preparation and Dosage

Primaquine phosphate (Quinaprim) tablet (7.5, 15 mg of base)—for radical cure of P. vivax malaria—15 mg of the base daily for 14 days is given after chloroquine treatment in clinical curative dose.

In case of P. falciparum malaria it is now used for five days after chloroquine treatment as gametocidal.

Adverse Reactions

It can cause epigastric distress, abdominal cramps, anaemia, leucopenia, agranulocytosis, methaemoglobinaemia and cyanosis. In patients with G6PD deficiency it can cause intravascular haemolysis of RBCs producing haemoglobinuria and haemolytic anaemia. It is contraindicated during pregnancy (may cause of haemolysis of G6PD deficient foetuses) and in patients with collagen diseases (RA and DLE) (may aggravate the diseases).

Pyrimethamine

It is a diaminopyrimidine derivative. It is effective against the erythrocytic forms (blood schizonts) of all types of plasmodia but the action is slow. It is effective against the primary tissue phases of *P. falciparum* and *P. vivax*. It is ineffective against the exoerythrocytic forms and gametocytes of the plasmodia. It can be used for prophylaxis of malaria because of slow action in weekly dosage. This action is enhanced when used in combination with sulphadoxine, due to sequential blockade of folic acid synthesis in the plasmodia (sulphadoxine inhibits DHF synthetase and pyrimethamine inhibits DHF reductase).

Pharmacokinetics

It is well-absorbed from GIT. It is concentrated in the liver, kidneys, lungs and spleen. It is slowly metabolized in the liver and excreted in urine for more than 14 days. It has a plasma half-life of 4 days.

Clinical Uses

It is used for:
- Treatment of acute attack of malaria, especially in chloroquine-resistant *P. falciparum* malaria. It is used in combination with sulphadoxine.
- Prophylaxis of malaria in endemic area. It is used in combination with sulphadoxine in weekly dosage.
- Toxoplasmosis: It is used in the dosage of 25 mg twice daily for one week followed by 25 mg once daily for three weeks along with sulphadiazine (4 g daily) for 4 weeks.

Preparations and Dosage

- Pyrimethamine (Daraprim) tablet (25 mg)—used in toxoplasmosis.
- Pyrimethamine (25 mg) + Sulphadoxine (500 mg) tablet (Croydoxin-FM/Malocide) or Sulphadimethopyrazine (500 mg) tablet (Metakelfin).

  For clinical cure: 2 to 3 tablets in single dose.
  For prophylaxis: 2 tablets weekly.

Adverse Reactions

It is well-tolerated but may cause megaloblastic anaemia, thrombocytopenia and agranulocytosis in some persons on prolonged use.

Proguanil/Chloroguanide

It is a biguanide derivative. It is a prodrug. It cyclizes and gets converted into a triazine compound 'cycloguanil' which is the active product. It is an effective blood schizonticide against *P. vivax* and *P. falciparum* but its action is slower than chloroquine. It is effective against the primary pre-erthyrocytic tissue form of *P. falciparum*. It is not directly gametocidal but it prevents the development of gametes in the gut wall of mosquito. It has no action against the persistent tissue form of *P. vivax*. It acts by binding with the enzyme 'DHF reductase' in the plasmodia and thus preventing the completion of schizogony. Plasmodia especially *P. falciparum* develop rapid resistance to it. It is slowly but adequately absorbed from GIT, mostly from the intestine. Its effective plasma concentration is attained in 6 hours. It is about 75% plasma protein bound. It achieves a higher concentration within RBCs than in plasma. It is slowly metabolized in the liver and excreted in urine in several days. It has a plasma half-life of about 15 hours. It is used for prophylaxis of malaria. It is available as proguanil (Palhdrin) tablet (100 mg) and administered 100 mg daily. It can produce GIT upset, mouth ulcers, skin rashes, leucopenia and haematuria. It has no hypoglycaemic action though it is a biguanide.

Quinine

It is the chief alkaloid of cinchona bark. It is the oldest of the antimalarial drugs. Chemically it is a quinoline derivative. It is a levoisomer. Its dextroisomer quinidine has antimalarial and antiarrhythmic actions.

Pharmacological Actions

These are given as follows:
- **Antimalarial action:** It acts primarily as blood schizonticide. It has little effect on sporozoites or pre-erythrocytic forms of plasmodia. It is also gametocidal for *P. vivax* and *P. malariae* but not for *P. falci-*

parum. It is not used for prophylaxis of malaria. As a suppressive and curative drug it is more toxic and less effective than chloroquine. It is especially valuable for the treatment of severe illness due to chloroquine-resistant and multidrug-resistant strains of *P. falciparum.*

Mechanism of Action

It acts like chloroquine in destroying plasmodia in RBCs.

- **Action on skeletal muscle:** It has curare like relaxant action on the skeletal muscle. It can antagonize the actions of physostigmine and neostigmine on skeletal muscle as effectively as curare. It can cause symptomatic relief of myotonia congenita, a disease opposite to that of myasthenia gravis. It produces alarming respiratory distress and dysphagia in patients with myasthenia gravis.
- **Other actions:** It has mild analgesic and antipyretic actions. It has mild quinidine like depressant action on the heart. It stimulates uterine muscle during the third trimester of pregnancy (ecbolic action).

Pharmacokinetics

It is rapidly and completely absorbed from GIT. Its absorption is delayed by antacids. Its plasma peak level reaches in 1 to 3 hours. It is about 70% bound to plasma proteins. It is metabolized in the liver and completely excreted in urine in 24 hours. It is not a cumulative drug. It has a plasma half-life of 10 hours.

Clinical Uses

It is used in:

- **Malaria:** It is used for suppressive treatment and cure of chloroquine-resistant and multidrug-resistant *P. falciparum* malaria. In severe illness, prompt use of loading dose of IV quinine is imperative and can be life-saving. Oral medication to maintain therapeutic concentration is then given as soon as it can be tolerated. For the treatment of infections with multidrug

resistant strains of *P. falciparum* slower acting blood schizonticides like sulphonamide or tetracycline are given concurrently to enhance the action of quinine.

- **Nocturnal leg cramps:** It relieves recumbency leg muscle cramps (night cramps) in a dose of 200 to 300 mg at bed time.
- **Myotonia congenita (a hereditary myopathy characterized by tonic spasm of skeletal muscle):** It relieves muscle spasm.
- **Varicose veins:** It is used with urethane as a sclerosing agent in varicose veins.

Preparations and Dosage

- Quinine sulphate/hydrochloride (Quiningu) tablet (300 mg)—300 to 600 mg thrice daily for 5 to 7 days.
- Quinine sulphate/hydrochloride injection (300 mg of salt/mL)—300 to 600 mg IM or slow IV infusion with 5% dextrose saline. Tetracycline hydrochloride (250 mg 6 hourly) or doxycycline hyclate (100 mg twice daily) for 7 days can be used as adjuvant drug with quinine.

Adverse Reactions

It may cause gastric irritation (producing, nausea, vomiting and abdominal cramps), cinchonism (characterized by headache, ringing in the ear, blurring of vision, tinnitus, deafness, vertigo, disturbance of colour vision, photophobia and amblyopia) and idiosyncrasy (manifested as intense flushing, pruritus, angioneurotic oedema and asthmatic attacks). It can cause myocardial depression and cardiac arrest when given IV. It may cause hypoglycaemia by releasing insulin from the pancreatic beta cells. It can cause acute haemolytic anaemia in patient deficient of G6PD in RBCs. It aggravates the symptoms of myasthenia gravis. It may rarely cause abortion and acute renal damage. It is contraindicated in pregnancy, myasthenia gravis and idiosyncratic patients.

Mefloquine

It is a quinoline methanol compound. It exists as a recemic mixture of four optical isomers with about the same antimalarial potency. It is a highly effective blood schizonticide, especially against mature trophozoite and schizont forms of plasmodia. It has no activity against early hepatic stages and mature gametocytes of *P. falciparum* or latent tissue forms of *P. vivax*. It may have some sporonticidal activities. It acts like quinine and chloroquine in destroying plasmodia present in RBCs. *P. falciparum* may develop resistance to it and so it is better to use along with sulphadoxine or pyrimethamine.

Pharmacokinetics

It is well-absorbed from GIT. It is highly bound to plasma proteins. It is highly concentrated in many organs like liver, lungs and intestine. It is metabolized in the liver and undergoes enterohepatic circulation. It is excreted in urine and faeces. It has a plasma half-life of about two weeks.

Clinical Uses

It is used for the prophylaxis and treatment of malaria caused by chloroquine-resistant and multidrug-resistant *P. falciparum*. It is especially useful as a prophylactic agent for nonimmune persons, who stay only for brief period in an endemic area.

Preparation and Dosage

Mefloquine hydrochloride (Larimef) tablet (250 mg)—1 to 1.5 g given orally as a single dose. This is followed by 250 mg once weekly for prophylaxis in endemic area.

Adverse Reactions

It can cause abdominal pain, nausea, vomiting, loss of balance and neuropsychiatric disturbances. It is contraindicated in pregnancy, young children and individuals with history of seizures.

Halofantrine

It is a phenanthrene methanol compound. It is as effective as chloroquine against chloroquine-sensitive strains of *P. falciparum*. It is also effective against strains of *P. falciparum* resistant to chloroquine, pyrimethamine and quinine. More mature parasites are particularly vulnerable to halofantrine. It does not affect latent tissue forms or *P. vivax* or gametocytes of any Plasmodium species. Its mechanism of action is unknown. It may act like chloroquine or quinine in destroying plasmodia present in RBCs.

Pharmacokinetics

It is slowly and variably absorbed from GIT. Its plasma peak level is reached in 4 to 6 hours. It should not be taken with fatty foods. It is slowly metabolized in the liver and excreted in urine. It has a plasma half-life of 2 to 3 days.

Clinical Uses

It is used as an alternative drug to quinine and mefloquine to treat acute attacks of malaria due to chloroquine-resistant and multidrug-resistant strains of *P. falciparum*.

Preparations and Dosage

- Halofantrine (Halofen) tablet (500 mg)— 500 mg 6 hourly for 3 doses and repeated after one week, if necessary.
- Halofantrine injection for parenteral use is also available.

Adverse Reactions

It causes nausea, vomiting, abdominal pain and diarrhoea. In large doses it can cause ventricular arrhythmias and cardiac arrest. It is contraindicated in pregnancy and heart diseases.

Qinghaosu

It is obtained from Chinese plant 'Qingho'. Chemically it is a sesquiterpene lactone. Its active compound is artimisinin. It is an effective blood schizonticide against *P. vivax* as well as chloroquine-sensitive and chloroquine-resistant strains of *P. falciparum*. Its mechanism of action is unknown. It may act like quinine. It is rapidly absorbed from GIT and reaches a peak plasma level in 1 to 2 hours. It is metabolized in the liver and excreted in urine.

Clinical Uses

It is used for the treatment of acute attacks of malaria especially by chloroquine-resistant *P. falciparum* and in cerebral malaria.

Preparations and Dosage

- Artesunate (Falcigo) tablet (50 mg)—100 mg twice daily on the first day followed by 50 mg twice daily for 4 to 6 days.
- Artesunate (Falcigo) injection (60 mg/mL)—120 mg IM or IV on first day followed by 60 mg once daily for next four days.
- Artemether (Paluther) injection (80 mg/mL)—160 mg IM or IV on first day, followed by 80 mg daily for four days.

Adverse Reactions

It causes abdominal pain, nausea, vomiting, anorexia and neutropenia. Very high doses can cause CNS toxicity.

Mepacrine (Quinacrine) is no longer used as an antimalarial due to toxicity and availability of better drugs for the treatment and prophylaxis of malaria.

Management of cerebral malaria: It is a serious disease with high mortality. It is an emergency condition requiring prompt treatment and good nursing care.

Specific treatment: Quinine sulphate/hydrochloride injection (containing 300 mg of the salt/mL) is given IM or slow IV infusion with 5% dextrose saline solution in the dose of 300 to 600 mg and repeated 8 hourly or chloroquine sulphate/phosphate injection (containing 40 mg of base/mL) is given IM or slow IV infusion with 5% dextrose saline solution in the dose of 200 to 300 mg and repeated 8 hourly or artesunate (60 mg/mL) or artemether (80 mg/mL) injection is given IM or IV in the dose of 2 mL on the first and then 1 mL for 4 days.

Supportive Treatment

- For shock and deep coma—5% dextrose saline IV infusion sufficiently. Dexamethasone acetate injection is given IV in the dose of 8 mg followed by 4 mg 8 hourly.
- For convulsions—Diazepam injection (10 mg) is given IV slowly.
- For hyperpyrexia—ice sponging. Paracetamol injection (0.5 g) IM is given. If not controlled chlorpromazine injection (50 mg) IM or IV infusion is given.

Malarial Vaccines

These are made by recombinant DNA technology. These are sporozoite vaccine, merozoite vaccine and gamate vaccine effective against different stages of *P. falciparum*. These are on clinical evaluation and may be useful in future to control *P. falciparum* malaria.

73

Drug Therapy of Kala-Azar

INTRODUCTION

Kala-azar (visceral leishmaniasis) is a proto-zoal disease caused by *Leishmania donovani* and is characterized by irregular fever, hepatosplenomegaly, anaemia, leucopenia and hyperglobulinaemia. It is transmitted by the bite of female sandfly 'Phlebotomas argentipes' (vector).

Oriental sore (cutaneous leishmaniasis) is caused by *Leishmania tropica* and muco-cutaneous leishmaniasis is called by *Leishmania braziliensis*. In these cases also phlebotomas sandfly acts as vector.

Life Cycle of *Leishmania donovani*

It exists in two forms:

- **Leishmania form:** It is found within the reticuloendothelial cells of the liver, spleen and lymph nodes and within the macrophages of the infected persons.

- **Leptomonad form:** It is developed from the leishmania form within the digestive tract of the sandfly after feeding blood of an infected person. It has a flagella and shows motility. It takes about 10 days for the development of leptomonad form from leishmania form. Leptomonad form of the parasite is injected by the sandfly into man during biting. After entering into reticulo-endothelial cells and macrophages, the leptomonad form of the parasite is converted to leishmania form. Diagnosis of

kala-azar is made by demonstration of the leishmania form of the parasite in the peripheral blood or in the aspirate obtained by sternal, splenic, liver or lymph node puncture.

Classification of Antikala-azar Drugs

These are of three groups:

- Pentavalent antimony compounds, e.g. sodium antimony gluconate, urea stib-amine, ethyl stibamine and meglumine antimonate.

- Diamidine compounds, e.g. pentamidine and dihydroxystilbamidine.

- Miscellaneous compounds, e.g. ampho-tericin-B, ketoconazole and allopurinol.

DISCUSSION OF INDIVIDUAL DRUGS

Sodium Antimony Gluconate/Sodium Stibogluconate

It is the drug of choice in kala-azar. It is a water-soluble pentavalent antimony com-pound containing 1/3rd antimony by weight. It is parasiticidal to the leishmania. Its exact mechanism of action is unknown. It probably acts by inhibiting sulphydryl enzymes and bioenergetics of *Leishmania amastigotes*. It is less toxic than other antimony compounds.

Pharmacokinetics

It is rapidly absorbed from the site of IM injection and is excreted unchanged in urine

505

within 6 to 8 hours. A small portion enters tissues and remains stored for long period. It is a cumulative drug.

Clinical Uses

It is used in kala-azar, oriental sore and mucocutaneous leishmaniasis.

Preparation and Dosage

Sodium antimony gluconate (Solustibosan) injection (100 mg antimony/mL in 30 mL vial)—20 mg/kg body weight IM or slow IV daily for 20 to 30 days. In oriental sore, it is infiltered around the sore.

Adverse Reactions

It can cause GIT upset (nausea, vomiting), metallic taste, headache, haemolytic anaemia, skin rashes, delayed muscle pain, stiffness of joints and rarely shock and cardiorespiratory arrest. It elevates hepatic transaminases. It is contraindicated in case with pulmonary tuberculosis and in severe hepatic and renal diseases.

Urea Stibamine

It was synthesized by the interaction of stibonic acid and urea by UN Brahmachari of Kolkata. It contains 40% of metallic antimony. It is more toxic than sodium stibogluconate and so now rarely used.

Ethyl Stibamine

It is a complex mixture of para-aminobenzene stibonic acid, para-acetyl aminophenyl stibonic acid, antimonic acid and diethylamine. It contains about 44% of metallic antimony. It is less toxic than urea stibamine but less preferred than sodium stibogluconate.

Meglumine Antimonate

This antimony compound is used by IM or IV route in the dose similar to sodium antimony gluconate. It contains 85 mg antimony per ml. It is not available in India but available in some countries.

Diamidine Compounds

These drugs are more potent leishmanicidals but are more toxic than the pentavalent antimony compounds. They are reserved drugs for cases that have failed to respond to antimonials. They are also used for the treatment and prophylaxis of African trypanosomiasis caused by various species of trypanosome (*T. gambiense, T. rhodesiense* and *T. brucei*).

Pentamidine

It is the commonly used diamidine compound. It is parasiticidal to leishmania. Its exact mechanism of action is unknown. It probably acts by inhibiting aerobic glycolysis and amino acid transport in the parasite.

Pharmacokinetics

It is rapidly absorbed from the site of injection. It is distributed in all tissues except brain. It is stored in tissues especially liver, kidney and spleen for several months and slowly released from there for excretion in urine, mostly in unchanged form. It is a cumulative drug.

Clinical Uses

It is used in kala-azar, oriental sore, mucocutaneous leishmaniasis, trypanosomiasis and *Pneumocystis carinii* pneumonia (PCP) in AIDS patients.

Preparation and Dosage

Pentamidine isethionate injection (30 mg/vial to be dissolved in D.W. to make 10% solution)—4 mg of base/kg body weight IM or slow IV infusion (over 60 minutes) in a single daily dose for 12 to 15 days. A second course may be given after an interval of 1 to 2 weeks if the infection responds less to the treatment.

Adverse Reactions

It is more toxic than antimony compounds. Its IV injection can cause dangerous reactions like breathlessness, tachycardia, dizziness, fainting, headache and vomiting. These reactions are probably due to sharp fall in BP that follows too rapid IV administration of the drug and they may be partly due to histamine release. It can also produce trigeminal neuralgia, hypoglycaemia and acute pancreatitis. Its other adverse effects include skin rashes, thrombophlebitis, thrombocytopaenia, anaemia, neutropaenia, elevation of liver enzymes and nephrotoxicity (due to inhibition of kidney DHF reductase). It is not contraindicated in cases with pulmonary tuberculosis.

Dihydroxystilbamidine

It has similar actions, uses and toxicity like pentamidine. It is available as dihydroxystilbamidine isethionate and administered IV in the dose of 250 mg daily for 10 days. A second course may be given after an interval of two weeks. It can cause late peripheral neuropathy.

Amphotericin-B, ketoconazole and allopurinol are used in those cases of kala-azar, which have failed to pentavalent antimony compounds or diamidine compounds. They are discussed in respective chapters.

74

Drug Therapy of Amoebiasis

INTRODUCTION

Amoebiasis is a protozoal disease caused by *Entamoeba histolytica* (EH). It has two forms, *viz.* trophozoite and cyst. The trophozoite form is found in the lumen of the bowel, intestinal wall, liver, lung and brain, whereas the cystic form remains only in the intestinal lumen. Thus there are intestinal and extraintestinal forms of amoebiasis. Intestinal amoebiasis is manifested as dysentery (passage of mucus and blood in stool), anorexia, abdominal pain and persistent desire to pass stools (tenesmus). Extraintestinal amoebiasis in liver is manifested as fever, hepatitis (enlarged and tender liver) and even liver abscess.

Classification of Antiamoebic Drugs

This can be done in 2 ways:

1. **Chemical classification** (according to chemical structure). These are:

   - Nitroimidazoles, e.g. metronidazole, tinidazole, secnidazole, ornidazole and satranidazole.

   - Dichloroacetamides, e.g. diloxanide furoate and etofamide.

   - Halogenated 8-hydroxyquinolines, e.g. diiodohydroxyquinoline (diiodohydroxyquin), iodochlorohydroxyquinoline (clioquinol) and broxyquinoline.

   - 4-aminoquinolines, e.g. chloroquine.

   - Ipecae alkaloids, e.g. emetine and dehydroemetine.

   - Antibiotics, e.g. tetracyclines and paromomycin.

2. **Clinical classification** (according to clinical uses). These are given as follows:

   - Drugs used only in intestinal amoebiasis (luminal amoebicides), e.g. diloxanide furoate, etofamide, diiodohydroxyquinoline, iodochlorohydroxyquinoline, broxyquinoline, tetracyclines, paromomycin and emetine bismuth iodide.

   - Drugs used only in extraintestinal amoebiasis (tissue amoebicides), e.g. chloroquine, emetine and dehydroemetine.

   - Drugs used in both intestinal and extraintestinal amoebiasis (both luminal and tissue amoebicides), e.g. metronidazole, tinidazole and secnidazole.

DISCUSSION OF INDIVIDUAL DRUGS

Metronidazole

It is a nitroimidazole derivative. It is effective against a wide variety of anaerobic protozoal parasites and anaerobic bacteria. It is directly amoebicidal, trichomonicidal and giardicidal. It has antibacterial activity against all anaerobic cocci, anaerobic gram-negative bacilli including *Bacteroides fragilis* and anaerobic spore-forming gram-positive bacilli. Nonspore forming gram-positive bacilli are often resistant to it as are aerobic bacteria. It has broad spectrum of activity against protozoa like *E. histolytica, G. lamblia, T. vaginalis* and *Balantidium coli;* helminth like *Dracunculus medinensis* (guinea worm) and anaerobic bacteria like *Bacteroides fragilis, Fusobacterium, Clostridium* and *Helicobacter* species.

Mechanism of Action

It can be considered as a prodrug in the sense that it requires metabolic activation by the sensitive organism. Once it is diffused into the cell its nitrogroup is chemically reduced by ferredoxin into a compound, which combines with DNA resulting in inactivation of DNA and producing death of the organism. Other effects of metronidazole are suppression of cellular immunity, mutagenesis, carcinogenesis and sensitization of hypoxic cells to radiation.

Pharmacokinetics

It is well-absorbed from the small intestine and little unabsorbed drug reaches the colon. It is distributed throughout the body tissues and fluids. It is only 20% plasma protein bound. It is metabolized in the liver by oxidation and glucuronidation and excreted in urine as metabolites and slightly as free form. It has a plasma half-life of about 8 hours. Hepatic dysfunction can cause accumulation of the drug.

Clinical Uses

It is used in the treatment of amoebiasis, trichomoniasis, giardiasis, balantidiasis, dracunculosis, ulcerative gingivitis (Vincent's stomatitis), pseudomembranous enterocolitis and serious anaerobic infections due to anaerobic bacteria including *Bacteroides fragilis*, Clostridium, Fusobacterium and *H. pylori*. It is used in both intestinal and hepatic amoebiases.

Preparations and Dosage

- Metronidazole (Metrogyl/Flagyl) tablet (200, 400 mg).
- Metronidazole paediatric suspension (200 mg/5 ml).
- Metronidazole vaginal tablet (500 mg).

- Metronidazole suppository (1 g).
- Metronidazole IV solution (500 mg/100 mL bottle).

For amoebiasis: Metronidazole tablet— 600 to 800 mg thrice daily for 5 to 10 days. Metronidazole paediatric suspension—35 to 50 mg/kg/day in three divided doses for 5 to 10 days. Metronidazole suppository can also be used.

For giardiasis: Metronidazole tablet—200 to 400 mg thrice daily for 7 days. Metronidazole paediatric suspension—5 to 10 mg/kg/day in three divided doses for 7 days.

For trichomoniasis: Metronidazole tablet— 2 g single dose or 200 to 400 mg thrice daily for 7 days. Metronidazole vaginal tablet can also be used.

For balantidiasis/dracunculosis/ulcerative gingivitis: In same dose as in giardiasis.

For pseudomembranous enterocolitis: Metronidazole tablet 800 mg thrice daily for 5 to 7 days. It is more effective, less toxic than vancomycin.

For serious anaerobic infections: Metronidazole IV solution—15 mg/kg is infused IV slowly for one hour, followed by 7.5 mg/kg every 6 hours till oral therapy can be instituted.

Adverse Reactions

It can produce side effects like headache, nausea, dry mouth, metallic taste, vomiting, diarrhoea, abdominal pain, furred tongue, glossitis, stomatitis, dizziness, vertigo, encephalopathy, convulsions, ataxia, numbness and paraesthesia of extremities (sensory neuropathy). It can also cause urticaria, flushing, pruritus, dysuria, cystitis, neutropaenia and disulphiram like reactions with alcohol. It has been reported to produce carcinogenicity and teratogenicity. It should be used with caution in patients with active disease of CNS due to its neurological toxicity.

Tinidazole (Tizole, Tini) is an analogue of metronidazole with a longer plasma half-life (about 14 hours). It has actions and uses like metronidazole. It has better patient compliance due to better oral absorption, longer half-life, lesser dose required and lower incidence of side effects. It is available as tablet (300, 500 mg) and administered in the dose of 300 to 500 mg twice daily for 5 to 7 days.

Secnidazole (Secnil, Seczole) is another analogue of metronidazole with a longer plasma half-life (about 21 hours). It is available as tablet (500 mg) and administered in the dose of 1 g in a single dose. It is better tolerated than metronidazole and tinidazole. Ornidazole and satranidazole are newer nitroimidazoles with pharmacological properties like tinidazole.

Diloxanide Furoate

It is a dichloroacetamide. It is directly amoebicidal but its mechanism of action is unknown. It kills trophozoites responsible for production of cysts. It is rapidly absorbed from intestine. It is metabolized in the liver by glucuronidation and excreted in urine. Given alone it is effective for the treatment of asymptomatic passers of cysts of EH. It is ineffective when used alone in the treatment of extraintestinal amoebiasis. It is used along with an appropriate systemic or mixed amoebicide to produce a cure of amoebiasis. It is available as Diloxanide furoate (Furamide) tablet (500 mg) and used in the dose of 500 mg thrice daily for 10 to 20 days. Children dose is 20 mg/kg/day in divided portions for 10 days. It is well-tolerated and side effects are mild. It can occasionally cause flatulence, vomiting, pruritus and urticaria.

Halogenated 8-hydroxyquinolines

These are effective luminal amoebicides (kill both trophozoites and cysts of EH). They are not effective in extraintestinal amoebiasis. Their mechanism of action and pharmacokinetics are not known. They are used particularly to treat asymptomatic cyst passers of EH. They are also used in combination with metrogyl/tinidazole to treat intestinal amoebiasis. They are widely and often indiscriminately used for the treatment of diarrhoea.

Preparations and Dosage

- Diiodohydroxyquinoline (Lodoquinol, Diodoquin) tablet (300 mg)—300 to 600 mg thrice daily for 15 days.
- Iodochlorohydroxyquinoline (Clioquinol, Enteroquinol) tablet (250 mg)—250 to 500 mg thrice daily for 15 days.

Adverse Reactions

They are well-tolerated. They can occasionally cause nausea, vomiting, diarrhoea, headache, vertigo, fever and skin rashes. When used in high dosage (exceeding 2 g/day) for long period they can produce serious toxicity like subacute myelooptic neuropathy (SMON), which is a myelitis like illness. In children, optic atrophy and permanent loss of vision can occur. They are banned in Japan and some other countries.

Chloroquine

It is an antimalarial drug effective against trophozoites (but not cysts) of E. histolytica (direct amoebicide). It is used in extraintestinal amoebiasis, because it is highly concentrated in the liver and lungs. It is ineffective in intestinal amoebiasis because it is almost completely absorbed from small intestine and does not reach large intestine, the site of amoebiasis. It is administered in the dose of 300 mg base twice daily for 2 days, followed by 150 mg twice daily for 2 to 3 weeks. It is relatively safe than emetine.

Emetine

It is an alkaloid obtained from the root of ipecac (Cephaelis ipecacuanha). It is a directly acting systemic amoebicide. It is effective against trophozoites (but not cysts) of E. histolytica. It was previously used from the treatment of extraintestinal amoebiasis and severe invasive intestinal amoebiasis but now replaced by the mixed amoebicide metronidazole/tinidazole, which is as effective and far safer. It cannot be administered orally as it produces emesis (vomiting). It has to be administered IM, keeping the patient at bed rest, avoiding strenous works and monitoring of pulse rate and BP, to avoid cardiotoxicity produced by the drug. It is now rarely used.

Dehydroemetine

It has similar properties as emetine but less toxic. It is administered IM in the dose of 60 mg (1 mL) daily for 6 to 10 days.

Antibiotics

Tetracyclines act indirectly by destroying normal intestinal microflora (*E. histolytica* lives symbiotically by utilizing food from normal intestinal microflora). They are used as adjuvant drugs with other directly acting luminal amoebicides.

75

Antifungal Drugs

INTRODUCTION

These are drugs used in the treatment of fungal infections (mycoses), which may be superficial or deep (systemic). Fungal infections are common, not only as primary diseases, but also secondary to therapy with oral antibiotics. Individuals suffering from diabetes mellitus, cancers, AIDS and those on corticosteroids, immunosuppressants, in-dwelling catheters and implants are more prone to develop fungal infections. Anti-bacterial antibiotics have little effect on fungal infections except actinomycosis, which responds to penicillin.

Classification of Antifungal Drugs

These are of two groups:

1. Systemic antifungal drugs: These are:

- Antibiotics, e.g. amphotericin-B and griseofulvin.
- Antimetabolite, e.g. flucytosine (a pyrimidine derivative).
- Azoles, e.g. ketoconazole, itraconazole and fluconazole (imidazoles and triazoles).

2. Topical antifungal drugs: These are:

- Azoles, e.g. econazole, miconazole, clotrimazole, terconazole, butoconazole, trioconazole, oxiconazole and sulconazole (imidazoles and triazoles).
- Antibiotics, e.g. nystatin, amphotericin-B, hamycin and natamycin (polyene antibiotics).

- Miscellaneous drugs, e.g. tolnaftate, benzoic acid, salicylic acid, undecylenic acid, zinc undecylenate, ciclopirox olamine, ichthammol, selenium sulphide, haloprogin, naftifine and terbinafine.

Types of fungal infections (mycoses)

These are of following types:

- Superficial mycoses, e.g. dermatophytosis (tinea or ringworm infection of skin and appendages like hair and nailbeds caused by dermatophytes like microsporium, epidermophyton and trichophyton), candidiasis (monilial infection of mucous membrane of mouth, pharynx, oesophagus, intestine, vagina, vulva and skin caused by *Candida albicans)* and other fungal infections (caused by tinea versicolor and tinea nigra).

- Subcutaneous mycoses, e.g. maduramycosis/madura foot (caused by some species of fungi producing subcutaneous granuloma (nodules) or chronic skin ulceration).

- Systemic (deep) mycoses, e.g. Aspergillosis (by *Aspergillus fumigatus)*, Blastomycosis (by *Blastomyces dermatitidis)*, Coccidioidomycosis (by *Coccidioides immitis)*, Cryptococcosis (by *Cryptococcus neoformans)*, Histoplasmosis (by *Histoplasma capsulatum)*, Mucormycosis (by *Mucor, Absidia)*, Sporotrichosis (by *Sporotrichum schenckii)*.

Essentials of the fungal cell: A fungal cell has a rigid cell wall which contains a large amount of polysaccharides. Inner to the cell wall lies cell membrane, where ergosterol (a plant sterol) is present but not cholesterol (present in mammalian cell membrane).

DISCUSSION OF ANTIFUNGAL DRUGS

Amphotericin-B

It is a polyene antibiotic (containing many double bonds in chemical structure). It is obtained from *Streptomyces nodosus*.

Antifungal Activity

It has a wide antifungal activity. It inhibits the growth of *Aspergillus fumigatus, Blastomyces dermatitidis, Coccidioides immitis, Cryptococcus neoformans, Histoplasma capsulatum, Sporotrichum schenckii, Mucor* and *Abisidia* in low concentrations. *Candida albicans* responds to it at a slightly higher concentration. Depending upon the concentration, it can be fungistatic or fungicidal. It acts by binding with ergosterol present in the fungal cell membrane leading to the development of hydrophilic pores, through which cell contents like sugar and potassium are drained out producing death of cells. Bacteria do not possess sterol in cell membrane and so not affected by amphotericin-B. *Candida albicans* can develop resistance to amphotericin-B.

Pharmacokinetics

It is not absorbed orally and so it is administered parenterally. For intestinal candidiasis, it can be given orally for local action. It is administered usually IV, because its IM injection is painful. It is widely distributed in body tissues and fluids but penetration in CSF is poor. It binds to sterols in tissues and lipoproteins in plasma and stays in the body for long period (about 15 days). It is about 60% metabolized in the liver and is slowly excreted in bile and urine as metabolites and unchanged form.

Clinical Uses

It is used in most systemic mycoses caused by sensitive fungi or yeasts. Topically it is useful in the treatment of Candida lesions at mucous membrane and skin (candidiasis). It is administered intrathecally in fungal meningitis. It has also been used to treat resistant cases of visceral leishmaniasis (kala-azar) and mucocutaneous leishmaniasis (oriental sore).

Preparations and Dosage

- Amphotericin-B (Fungizone) injection (50 mg/5 mL vial)—0.05 to 0.5 mg/kg/day by slow IV infusion with 5% dextrose solution and gradually increasing the dose, for 6 to 10 weeks.
- Amphotericin-B lotion (3%)—it is applied topically twice or thrice daily.
  Amphotericin-B liposomal preparations are superior than ordinary preparations.

Adverse Reactions

It is a highly toxic antibiotic. A variety of reactions may develop after its IV use. These include thrombophlebitis at the site of injection, nausea, anorexia, vomiting, headache, vertigo, fever, flushing, skin rashes, anaphylactic reactions, hypotension, cardiac arrhythmias, ventricular failure, convulsions, myalgia, peripheral neuritis, anaemia, leucopenia, thrombocytopaenia (myelotoxicity) and nephrotoxicity (manifested as increased blood urea nitrogen, hypokalemia, presence of urinary casts and sometimes haematuria due to renal damage). Hepatocellular jaundice and acute hepatic failure may occur in some cases. Intrathecal administration of the drug may result in arachnoiditis. On oral administration it may cause haemorrhagic gastroenteritis. Superinfection with bacteria can also occur.

Griseofulvin

It is an antibiotic obtained from *Penicillium griseofulvum*. Chemically it is a heterocyclic benzofuran compound.

Antifungal Activity

It is the first chemical compound to cure effectively superficial mycoses caused by various types of dermatophytes (ringworm) such as microsporium, epidermophyton and trichophyton when administered orally. It is not effective against bacteria, *Candida albicans* and any of deep fungi. It is fungistatic and not fungicidal. It acts by inhibiting the biosynthesis of microtubules of fungal cells leading to stoppage of spindle formation during mitosis. This causes stoppage of fungal reproduction and ultimately death of fungal cells. It accumulates particularly in the fungally infected keratinized areas of skin (stratum corneum) and its appendages (hair and nailbed). It is deposited in keratin precursor cells. When such cells differentiate, it is tightly bound to and persists in keratin and makes them resistant to fungal invasion. As the fungus containing keratin cell is shed off, it is replaced by normal cell. Ringworm infections of hair and nailbed require prolonged treatment with griseofulvin.

Pharmacokinetics

Given orally, microfined particles of griseofulvin are absorbed much faster than those of ordinary large particles of the drug. Fat in food helps in its absorption. Its metabolic fate is unknown. It is excreted in small amount in urine, while large amount is excreted unchanged in faeces. Its plasma half-life is about 24 hours, but it persists in the infected keratin tissue of skin for several weeks.

Clinical Uses

It is used in dermatophytosis (ringworm infection of skin, hair and nailbed). It is not effective topically but effective when used systemically (orally). It is very effective in epidermophytosis (involving skin of foot) and onychomycosis (involving nailbed). The duration of treatment with griseofulvin depends on the site of infection, e.g. body skin (by *tinea corporis*) requires 3 to 4 weeks treatment; scalp (by *t. capitis*), groin (by *t. cruris*) feet (by *t. pedis*) and hands (by *t. manus*) require 4 to 6 weeks treatment and nails (by t. unguium) requires 6 to 12 months treatment.

Preparation and Dosage

Griseofulvin (Grisovin) tablet (125, 250 mg)— 250 to 500 mg daily in two divided doses after meals. Children dose—10 mg/kg/day.

Adverse Reactions

It can cause nausea, vomiting, epigastric distress, diarrhoea, headache, paraesthesia, peripheral neuritis, vertigo, mental confusion, lethargy, blurred vision, allergic reactions (skin rashes, neutropaenia and fever) and photosensitivity reactions.

Drug Interactions

- Phenobarbitone retards the absorption of griseofulvin from the GIT.
- It increases the metabolism of warfarin and so higher dose of warfarin is necessary when used concurrently with griseofulvin.
- It can cause antabuse like reaction with alcohol.

Flucytosine

It is a fluorinated pyrimidine derivative.

Antifungal Activity

It is useful in deep (systemic) fungal infections due to yeast. It is fungistatic and not fungicidal. It acts by converting to antimetabolite '5-fluorouracil' and then to 5-fluorodeoxyuridylic acid, which inhibits thymidylate synthetase during DNA and RNA syntheses resulting in stoppage of fungal reproduction (duplication). *Histoplasma capsulatum* and *Blastomyces dermatitidis* are resistant to it.

Pharmacokinetics

It is well-absorbed from GIT and reaches adequate concentrations in blood and CSF. It is almost entirely excreted in urine in unchanged form by glomerular filtration.

Clinical Uses

It is mainly used in cryptococcal meningitis, systemic candidiasis and aspergillosis. It is used in combination with amphotericin-B due to following reasons:

- When it is used alone, the fungus develops rapidly resistance to it.
- When used in combination with AMB, the dosage required for both drugs is less and so less adverse reactions are produced.
- When used in combination with AMB, synergistic action is produced.

Preparations and Dosage

- Flucytosine (Alcobon) capsule (500 mg)— 50 to 100 mg/kg/day.
- Flucytosine injection for IV infusion is also available.

Adverse Reactions

It can cause GIT upsets (nausea, vomiting and anorexia), hepatic damage (causing hepatocellular jaundice) and bone marrow depression (causing anaemia, leucopenia and thrombocytopaenia, i.e. pancytopaenia). It is less toxic than amphotericin-B.

Azoles

Ketoconazole

It is an imidazole compound. It is water-soluble and orally effective.

Antifungal Activity

It is a broad-spectrum antifungal drug effective against many superficial and deep (systemic) fungi including *Candida albicans, Tinea versicolor, Blastomyces dermatitidis, Histoplasma capsulatum, Coccidioides immitis, Cryptococcus neoformans* and *Aspergillus fumigatus*. It is a fungicidal drug. It acts by interfering with the formation of ergosterol in the cell membrane of fungi by inhibiting the enzyme lanosterol 14α-demethylase. Ergosterol is a cell membrane stabilizing agent of fungi. Its absence in cell membrane leads to death of fungi.

Pharmacokinetics

It is well absorbed from GIT. Its absorption is retarded in presence of H_2-blockers (cimetidine and ranitidine). In circulation, it is highly plasma protein bound. Its CSF penetration is unreliable. It is metabolized in the liver and excreted in urine as metabolites and unchanged form.

Clinical Uses

It is used in candidiasis, pityriasis versicolor, blastomycosis, histoplasmosis, coccidioidomycosis, cryptococcosis and aspergillosis. It is ineffective in fungal (cryptococcal) meningitis.

Preparation and Dosage

Ketoconazole (Fungicide) tablet (200 mg)— 200 mg twice daily for 5 days.

Adverse Reactions

It can cause GIT upset (nausea, vomiting and anorexia), allergic reactions (skin rashes and pruritus) and endocrine disturbances (gynaecomastia, libido and menstrual irregularities due to suppression of androgenic and cortical steroid biosyntheses).

Contraindications

Lactating mothers (it is secreted in milk), pregnant women and persons suffering from severe liver diseases. It can cause hepatic dysfunction.

Itraconazole (Sporanox)

It is a triazole compound. It has pharmacological properties like ketoconazole. It is orally effective and has longer duration of action than ketoconazole. It is administered once daily as tablet (200 mg) for 5 days. It has uses like ketoconazole, but it is effective in cryptococcal meningitis. It is claimed to be less toxic than ketoconazole.

Fluconazole

It is a triazole compound. It is effective both orally and parenterally. It has pharmacological properties like ketoconazole. It is well-absorbed from GIT. It penetrates readily into CSF. It has a long plasma half-life (about 30 hours). It is excreted in urine mostly in unchanged form. It has uses like ketoconazole but it is effective in cryptococcal meningitis. It is administered once daily as fluconazole (Zocan, Syscan) tablet (150 mg) for 7 days. It can produce GIT upset (nausea and vomiting) and allergic reactions (skin rashes and pruritus) and abnormalities of liver functions. It does not produce any endocrine disturbance.

Other Azoles

Econazole and miconazole are imidazole compounds, whereas clotrimazole, terconazole, butoconazole, trioconazole, oxiconazole and sulconazole are triazole compounds. They are ineffective orally and used topically as cream, powder, lotion or vaginal tablet in superficial fungal infections. Miconazole has been used IV in deep (systemic) fungal infections, but it is more toxic than other azoles. Used systemically it can produce anaphylactic reactions, cardiac arrhythmias and myelotoxicity like leucopenia and thrombocytopaenia. Locally, they can produce irritation of tissue.

OTHER POLYENE ANTIBIOTICS

Nystatin (for topical use)

It is obtained from *Streptomyces noursei*. It is effective only against *Candida albicans*. It can be fungistatic or fungicidal depending on the concentration. It acts by combining with the ergosterol of the fungal cell membrane leading to development of pores in the cell membrane, through which contents of the fungal cell are drained out leading to death of the cell. It is not absorbed orally and so applied topically. It is not administered parenterally due to high toxicity (myelotoxicity and nephrotoxicity). It is administered 8 hourly as tablet (5 lakh units) in gastrointestinal candidiasis for local action. It is used as nystatin (Mycostatin) vaginal tablet (1 lakh units) in vulvovaginal candidiasis for local action. It is also available as ointment (1 lakh units/g) and suspension (1 lakh units/mL) for topical application. It can cause nausea, vomiting and diarrhoea on oral administration.

Haymycin is obtained from *Streptomyces pimprina* and natamycin (Pimaricin) is obtained from *Streptomyces natalensis*. They are mainly fungicidal. They are not absorbed orally and too toxic for parenteral use. They are available as cream, ointment, powder, suspension or tablet for topical use. They are used in superficial fungal infections. They can cause local irritation of tissue and nausea and vomiting if administered orally.

OTHER TOPICAL ANTIFUNGAL AGENTS

Tolnaftate

It is effective in the treatment of ringworm infections of skin (dermatophytosis) caused by *Trichophyton* and *Epidermophyton*. It is not effective in the treatment of candidiasis. It is used as 1% solution or cream of tolnaftate (Tinaderm). It is nonirritating, nonstaining and odourless.

Benzoic Acid and Salicylic Acid

They are effective in the treatment of ringworm infections of skin (dermatophytosis) like tolnaftate. Salicylic acid has weak antifungal (fungistatic) activity but it has keratolytic property. Compound benzoic acid ointment (Whitfield's ointment) containing 6% benzoic acid and 3% salicylic acid in an emulsifying ointment base is a commonly used and effective preparation in the treatment of dermatophytosis.

Undecylenic Acid and Zinc Undecylenate

They are effective in the treatment of ringworm infection of skin (dermatophytosis), particularly in *tinea pedis*. They produce maximal antifungal (fungistatic) activity in an acidic medium. Compound undecylenic acid ointment (Desenex ointment containing 5% undecylenic acid and 20% zinc undecylenate in an emulsifying ointment base) is an effective preparation in the treatment of dermatophytosis.

Ciclopirox Olamine

It is an effective antifungal drug in the treatment of cutaneous candidiasis, dermatophytosis and tinea versicolor. It is available as 1% cream. It can cause mild local irritation of skin.

Ichthammol/Ammonium Ichthosulphonate

It is used as 10% cream or ointment in the treatment of resistant cases of dermatomycoses and other chronic skin diseases. It can cause irritation of skin.

Selenium Sulphide

It is used in the treatment of tinea versicolor and dandruff. It is available as 2.5% suspension of selenium sulphide (Selsun) and applied once daily for five days. It has unpleasant odour. It can cause mild irritation of skin.

Haloprogin, naftifine and terbinafine have antifungal activities like topically used azoles. They are used topically as ointment, cream or lotion in superficial fungal infections.

76

Antiviral Drugs

INTRODUCTION

These are drugs used in the treatment of viral diseases. Viruses, unlike bacteria, have no cell wall. A virus consists of either double-stranded DNA or single-stranded RNA called a **genome,** which is enclosed in a protein coat called capsid. Some viruses also possess a lipoprotein envelop, that like the capsid may contain antigenic proteins. A virus is active only when it is within a host cell and becomes inactive (inert) when it is outside a host cell. Hence, viruses are obligate (bound to remain) intracellular parasites. Host cells may be mammalian (in mammalian virus), bacterial (in bacteriophage), insect (in arbovirus) or plant (in plant virus). A virus cannot prepare its own food and metabolize. It has to depend on the host cell for these purposes. When a virus enters the host cell, the host cell ceases to function for its own benefit but works to provide prepared materials (metabolic products) like nucleic acid, protein, etc. for the reproduction of the virus. The subsequent release of the infectious progeny of the virus from the host cell is called replication of virus. There are various stages in viral replication, which are cell entry (attachment and penetration), uncoating (release of viral genome), transcription of viral genome, translation of viral proteins, assembly of viral components and release of new virion from host cells (by budding or cell lysis). An effective antiviral drug must inhibit virus specific replicative events or preferentially inhibits virus directed rather the host cell directed nucleic acid or protein synthesis. DNA viruses, e.g. poxviruses (causing smallpox), herpesviruses (simplex and chickenpox, shingles A, B and C and herpes), adenoviruses (conjunctivitis and sore throat), hepadnaviruses (hepatitis A, B and C), human immunodeficiency viruses (AIDS) and papillomaviruses (warts). RNA viruses, e.g. rubella viruses (causing German measles), rhabdoviruses (rabies), picornaviruses (poliomyelitis, meningitis and common cold), arena viruses (meningitis and lessa fever), orthomyxoviruses (influenza) and paramyxoviruses (measles and mumps).

Classification of Antiviral Drugs

These are of three groups:

- Antiherpesvirus drugs, e.g. aciclovir, famciclovir, ganciclovir, valaciclovir, foscarnet, idoxuridine, sorivudine, trifluridine and vidarabine.

- Antiretroviral (anti-HIV) drugs, e.g. zidovudine, stavudine, lamivudine, didanosine and zalcitabine and protease inhibitors like saquihavir, ritonavir, indinavir and lopinavir.

- Other antiviral drugs, e.g. amantadine, rimantadine, ribavirin, methisazone and interferon-α.

DISCUSSION OF INDIVIDUAL DRUGS

Aciclovir

Chemically it is acicloguanosine related to the purines. It is effective against all types of herpesvirus except cytomegalovirus (CMV). It is virustatic and acts by inhibiting DNA synthesis in herpesviruses. It enters the virus infected cells and is acted upon by herpesvirus specific thymidine kinase (an enzyme) produced by the virally infected cell forming acicloguanosine monophosphate, which is then phosphorylated to acicloguanosine triphosphate by cellular kinases. This acicloguanosine triphosphate inhibits competitively the DNA polymerase of the herpesvirus and prevents synthesis and lengthening of new viral DNA strands during viral DNA replication. The noninfected host cell lacks thymidine kinase and so no formation of acicloguanosine monophosphate occurs.

Antiviral Spectrum

Aciclovir is effective against herpes simplex virus type-1 (HSV-1), herpes simplex virus type-2 (HSV-2), varicella zoster virus (VZV) and epstein barr virus (EBV) but not the cytomegalovirus (CMV), as it lacks the enzyme thymidine kinase. Resistance to aciclovir may develop after prolonged use. It is due to mutation in viral genome leading to production of altered DNA polymerase in the virus.

Pharmacokinetics

It is partly absorbed from GIT after oral administration and has a bioavailability of about 30%. Its CSF level is 50% of that of plasma. It is excreted in urine as metabolities and unchanged form. It has a plasma half-life of about 6 hours.

Clinical Uses

It is used in the treatment of herpes simplex virus infections like oral herpes, mucocutaneous herpes, genital herpes, herpes keratitis and herpes encephalitis. It is also effective in the treatment of infections due to VZV and EBV. In viral encephalitis it is administered IV. It can be used prophylactically to reduce the chance of HSV infections in immunocompromised patients (AIDS, after organ transplantation, etc.) either orally or IV.

Preparations and Dosage

- Aciclovir (Cyclovir, Cubivir, Zovirax) capsule (200 mg)—200 mg 4 to 6 hourly for 10 days.
- Aciclovir injection (250 mg/vial)—for IV infusion (5 mg/kg/8 hourly).
- Aciclovir cream (5%)—for topical application.

Adverse Reactions

It can cause following side effects:

On oral use: Headache, nausea/malaise, tremors and insomnia.

On IV use: Skin rashes, sweating, vomiting and hypotension.

On topical use: Stinging and burning sensation after each application.

Other Aciclovir Analogs (Congeners)

- Famciclovir (Famvir) is effective orally (250 mg capsule).
- Ganciclovir (Cytovene) is effective IV (250 mg/vial).
- Valaciclovir (Valtrex) is effective orally (500 mg capsule).

Foscarnet (Foscavir)

Chemically it is a trisodium phosphonoformate. It is effective against all types of herpesvirus and also human immunodeficiency virus (HIV). It acts by inhibiting viral DNA synthesis by interacting with herpesvirus DNA polymerase or HIV reverse transcriptase. It is particularly useful in cytomegalovirus (CMV) retinitis in patients with AIDS, as an alternative to ganciclovir. It is given by IV infusion (60 mg/kg/8 hourly) for 2 to 3 weeks. It can produce hypocalcaemia, CNS side effects (headache, tremors, irritability, hallucinations and convulsions), bone marrow depression (anaemia, leucopenia and thrombocytopaenia) and nephrotoxicity (albuminuria, renal, casts and even haematuria).

Idoxuridine

Chemically it is 5'-iodo-2'-deoxyuridine (IDUR), which is related to thymidine. It is effective against DNA viruses like herpesviruses and poxviruses. It acts by inhibiting the synthesis of DNA by preventing the utilization of thymidine (by competition) in the causative viruses. It inhibits both viral and host cells DNA synthesis and hence it has high degree of toxicity when used systemically. On prolonged use viruses can develop resistance to it. It is used mainly topically in the treatment of herpes keratitis (ulcerations of the cornea). As cornea is avascular, so systemic toxicity cannot occur. It is used as 0.5% drops or ointment of idoxuridine (Ridinox) applied 1 to 2 hours. It can cause local irritation, oedema of eyelids and photophobia. It has been used by IV infusion in herpes encephalitis in man with some success but it produces leucopenia, thrombocytopaenia, alopecia and liver damage.

Sorivudine

It is an analog of pyrimidine nucleoside. It is particularly effective against Varicella zoster virus (VZV). It acts by inhibiting viral DNA synthesis acting like aciclovir. It is used in the treatment of herpes zoster in patients with AIDS. It is administered orally or IV. It can cause GIT upset (nausea, vomiting and diarrhoea), headache and elevation of hepatic enzymes.

Trifluridine

Chemically it is trifluorothymidine. It is too toxic for systemic use and so used only topically in the treatment of herpes keratitis as 0.5% ophthalmic ointment. It appears to be more effective than idoxuridine for this purpose.

Vidarabine/Vira-A

Chemically it is adenine arabinoside. It is effective against DNA viruses like herpesviruses and vaccinia viruses. It acts by inhibiting viral DNA synthesis by stopping viral replication. It is used in herpes simplex, varicella zoster and smallpox. It is usually administered topically as 3% ophthalmic ointment in herpes keratitis. It can be administered by IV infusion (10 mg/kg/12 hourly). It has more toxicity than aciclovir. It can cause GIT upset (nausea, vomiting and diarrhoea), bone marrow depression (anaemia, leucopenia and thrombocytopaenia) and neurological toxicities (headache, tremors and insomnia).

Zidovudine

Chemically it is 3'-azido-3'-deoxythymidine (azidothymidine/AZT). It is a synthetic thymidine analog with antiviral activity against HIV-1, HIV-2, Human T-lymphotropic virus-1 (HTLV-1) of leukaemia and other retroviruses. It is nucleocidal for HIV viruses. It has strong affinity for viral DNA polymerase (reverse transcriptase) but has a very low affinity for mammalian DNA polymerase. It is acted upon by a virus specific mammalian thymidine kinase (an enzyme) and is converted to active form azidothymidine triphosphate (by phosphorylation), which competitively inhibits viral reverse transcriptase (RNA dependent DNA polymerase) and prevents any further elongation of the viral DNA (single-stranded RNA → double-stranded DNA). Thus viral DNA terminates prematurely and replication is prevented.

Pharmacokinetics

It is well-absorbed when given orally. It can also be administered IV. It is distributed well in body tissues and fluids. It can easily penetrate BBB and attains a good concentration in CSF. It is mostly (80%) metabolized in the liver and is excreted in urine, mainly as glucuronide. It has a plasma half-life of about one hour.

Clinical Uses

It is used in acquired immunodeficiency syndrome (AIDS) caused by HIV infection but complete cure is not possible by any retroviral drug.

Preparation and Dosage

Zidovudine (Retrovir) capsule (200, 250 mg)—200 or 250 mg given 4 to 8 hourly for 4 weeks or more.

Adverse Reactions

It can cause GIT upset (nausea, vomiting and diarrhoea), bone marrow depression (anaemia, granulocytopaenia and thrombocytopenia), CNS toxicity (headache, insomnia, agitation and seizures) and myopathy (myalgia, etc.).

Stavudine (Zerit), zalcitabine (Hivid) and didanosine (Videx) are alternative drugs to zidovudine in AIDS caused by HIV infection. They are more toxic than zidovudine and so used in resistant cases of AIDS to zidovudine. They are used orally.

Saquinavir, ritonavir, indinavir and lopinavir are retroviral protease inhibitors effective in HIV infection. This protease acts at the late step of HIV replication, i.e. maturation of the real virus particles, when the RNA acquires the core proteins and enzymes. These drugs bind to the protease molecule and interfere with its cleaning function. They are more effective viral inhibitors than zidovudine, etc. They are administered orally as tablets. They are less toxic than zidovudine.

Amantadine and Rimantadine

These are tricyclic amines with antiviral activity against influenza virus. They stop viral replication by preventing uncoating of virus. A virus inorder to replicate has to enter the susceptible host cell, where it is uncoated. They are used as prophylactic agents against attacks of influenza caused by influenza-A virus. Amantadine is also used in the treatment of parkinsonism as dopamine facilitator. It is available as capsule (100 mg) and administered in the dose of 200 mg daily for 5 to 7 days. It is excreted mostly in unchanged form in urine. It can produce CNS toxicity (dizziness, slurring of speech, ataxia, insomnia and seizures) and allergic reactions (skin rashes and pruritus).

Methisazone

It is a thiosemicarbazone. It is mainly effective against smallpox viruses. Its mode of action is unknown. It is used as a prophylactic agent to reduce the incidence of smallpox in contacts. It is administered orally in doses of 2 to 3 g daily in divided doses. It has low toxicity.

Interferon-α and Ribavirin

These are broad-spectrum antiviral agents effective against both DNA and RNA viruses. The exact mechanism of action of interferon is not known. It probably acts indirectly by binding with specific cell surface receptors and inducing the production of cellular enzymes which subsequently block viral replication. It is administered IM or IV. Ribavirin inhibits viral replication by inhibiting nucleic acid synthesis by converting to active compound ribavirin triphosphate. It is administered orally or as aerosol. These are relatively safer drugs. Interferons (α, β and γ) are cytokines (glycoproteins) produced by cells that are infected by viruses. They cause synthesis of a protein that exerts an inhibitory effect at the ribosomal level and interferes with the synthesis of viral coaded functional enzymes and structural coat proteins necessary for viral replication. They are biological response modifiers and immunomodulators.

INTRODUCTION

These are drugs that act either locally to expel parasitic worms (helminths) from the GIT or systemically to eradicate adult helminths or developmental forms that invade organs and tissues. They may be either vermicide (kill the worm) or vermifuge (expel the worm) to the infesting helminths. The choice of the drug depends on the efficacy, ease of administration (usually single dose is preferred), lack of side effects or toxicity and cost of the drug. Before starting the treatment, the helminths must be identified, usually by finding the ova, adult worm or larva in the faeces, urine, blood or tissues of the host for proper application of the drug.

Classification of Anthelmintics

These are of three groups. First drug is the drug of choice.

1. Drugs effective against nematodes:
   - *Ascaris lumbricoides* (roundworm)—Albendazole, mebendazole, pyrantel pamoate, piperazine citrate, levamisole and tetramisole.
   - *Ancylostoma duodenale* and *Necator americanus* (hookworms)—Mebendazole, albendazole, thiabendazole, pyrantel pamoate and bephenium hydroxynaphthoate.
   - *Trichuris trichiura* (whipworm)—Mebendazole, albendazole, thiabendazole and pyrantel pamoate.

- *Enterobius vermicularis* (pinworm)—Mebendazole, albendazole, pyrantel pamoate and piperazine citrate.
- *Strongyloides stercoralis and Trichostrongylus colubriformis* (threadworm)—Ivermectin, mebendazole, albendazole and thiabendazole.
- *Trichinella spiralis* (pork roundworm)—Albendazole, mebendazole, thiabendazole and corticosteroids.
- *Wuchereria bancrofti, Brugia malayi, Onchocerca volvulus and Loa loa* (filarial worms)—diethyl carbamazine and ivermactin.
- *Dracunculus medinensis* (guinea worm)—Metronidazole, niridazole, mebendazole, and thiabendazole.

2. Drugs effective against cestodes (flatworms):
   - *Taenia saginata* (beef tapeworm) and *T. solium* (pork tapeworm)—Praziquantel, niclosamide and albendazole.
   - *Diphyllobothrium latum* (fish tapeworm)—Niclosamide, praziquantel and albendazole.
   - *Hymenolepis nana* (dwarf tapeworm)—Praziquantel and niclosamide.
   - *Echinococcus granulosus* (hydatid worm, dog tapeworm)—Albendazole and mebendazole.

3. Drugs effective against trematodes:
   - *Schistosoma haematobium, S. mansoni* and *S. japonicum* (schistosomes)—Praziqunatel, oxamniquine and metrifonate.

• *Fasciola hepatica, Fasciolopsis nana, Paragonimus westermani* and *Clonorchis sinensis* (flukes)—Praziquantel, bithional and chloroquine.

The treatment of hookworm infestation is incomplete unless anaemia is treated by an oral iron preparation (e.g. ferrous sulphate) for 3 to 4 weeks. Wearing of footwear should be encouraged in endemic areas to avoid larva penetration into foot.

DISCUSSION OF INDIVIDUAL DRUGS

Mebendazole

It is a benzimidazole compound. It exerts broad-spectrum anthelmintic activity against *Ascaris lumbricoides, Ancylostoma duodenale, Necator americanus, Strongyloides stercoralis, Trichostrongylus colubriformis, Trichuris trichiura, Enterobius vermicularis, Trichinella spiralis* and *Echinococcus granulosus*. It is a vermicide. It acts by irreversibly inhibiting the uptake of exogenous glucose by the helminths. It takes 2 to 3 days to immobilize and kill the helminths, which are slowly cleared from the gut by defecation. It does not require a purgative in the postdrug period. It is poorly absorbed (10%) from the gut. About 90% of it is excreted in faeces and 10% is excreted in urine, partly as metabolite.

Clinical Uses and Adverse Reactions

It is used in ascariasis, ancylostomiasis, necatoriasis, enterobiasis, trichuriasis, strongyloidiasis, trichostrongyliasis and hydatid cyst. It is particularly useful in mixed (multiple) worm infestations. It is available as mebendazole (Mebex) tablet (100 mg) and suspension (100 mg/5 mL). It is given orally in the doses of 100 mg twice daily for three days in roundworm, hookworm, pinworm and whipworm infestations. In threadworm infestation a single dose of 100 mg is sufficient. In hydatid cyst it is used in high doses (400 to 600 mg three times a day for 3 to 4 weeks). It can cause nausea, abdominal pain and diarrhoea. In large doses, it may cause vertigo, dizziness, headache and arthralgia. It is

contraindicated (not safe) in pregnancy (as it is embryotoxic).

Albendazole

It is a benzimidazole compound like mebendazole. It exerts broad-spectrum anthelmintic activity like mebendazole and has similar mode of action. It has the advantage of single dose administration. It is superior to mebendazole against threadworm, tapeworm and hydatid worm. It is used in neurocysticercosis of brain caused by larva or *T. solium*. It is moderately absorbed (about 30%) from the gut, metabolized in the liver by sulphoxide formation, which is excreted slowly in urine.

Clinical Uses and Adverse Reactions

It is used in mixed (multiple) worm infestations with roundworm, hookworm, pinworm, threadworm and whipworm. It is also used in tapeworms and hydatid worm infestations. It is available as albendazole (Zentel) tablet (400 mg) and suspension (200 mg/5 ml). It is given orally in the dose of 400 mg (single dose) in roundworm, hookworm, threadworm and whipworm infestations; 400 mg for three days in pinworm and tapeworms and 400 mg twice daily for four weeks in hydatid cyst. Its dose and duration of treatment is same in adult and children above two years of age (below 2 years the dose is half). It is well-tolerated even in debilitated patients. It may cause mild GIT side effects (nausea, vomiting and dizziness) in few patients. It is contraindicated in pregnancy, and persons suffering from hepatic damage.

Thiabendazole

It is a benzimidazole compound like mebendazole. It exerts broad-spectrum anthelmintic activity like mebendazole but its use is restricted because it is highly absorbed (about 50%) from the gut producing many adverse reactions.

Clinical Uses and Adverse Reactions

It is now only used in stongyloidiasis, trichostrongyliasis, trichuriasis and hydatid cyst. It probably acts by interfering with the carbohydrate metabolism of the worms. It is available as thiabendazole (Mintezole) tablet (500 mg) and emulsion (200 mg/mL). It is given orally in the dose of 25 mg/kg in two divided doses for 5 to 7 days. It can cause allergic reactions (skin rashes, pruritus and fever), anorexia, nausea, vomiting, epigastric distress, dizziness, drowsiness, hypotension, hypoglycaemia, disturbances of colour vision, hepatic damage and crystalluria.

Pyrantel Pamoate

It is a tetrahydropyrimidine derivative. It is highly effective against roundworm, whipworm and pinworm and a little less effective against hookworms. It is a vermifuge and acts by causing contracture followed by spastic paralysis of the worms (it has a depolarizing neuromuscular blocking action on the worms), which are then expelled from the gut. Piperazine antagonizes the action of pyrantel by opposite action. It is absorbed to the extent of 20% from the gut, which is metabolized in the liver and excreted in urine. About 80% of it is excreted in faeces.

Clinical Uses and Adverse Reactions

It is used in ascariasis, trichuriasis and enterobiasis. It is available as pyrantel pamoate (Nimocid) tablet (250 mg) and suspension (250 mg/5 mL). It is given orally in the dose of 500 mg (single dose) for roundworm, whipworm and pinworm and 250 mg twice daily for three days in hookworms. It can cause nausea, vomiting, abdominal discomfort and headache. It is contraindicated in pregnancy, children below two years and persons with hepatic damage.

Bephenium Hydroxynaphthoate

It is a quaternary ammonium compound. It is effective against hookworms and roundworm. It has a moderate effect against whipworm and threadworm. It is a vermifuge and acts by causing initially contraction and then relaxation (paralysis) of the worm muscles. It is more effective against *Ancylostoma duodenale* than *Necator americanus*. It is poorly absorbed

from the gut, which is excreted in urine in unchanged form. It is mostly excreted in faeces. It is used in ancylostomiasis, necatoriasis and ascariasis.

Clinical Uses and Adverse Reactions

It is available as bephenium hydroxynaphthoate (Alcopar) granules in a packet (2.5 g base in 5 g granules). It is given orally in the morning in empty stomach mixed with water and fruit juice or syrup. It has a bitter taste and can cause nausea, vomiting and diarrhoea.

Piperazine Citrate

It is a piperazine salt. It is effective against roundworm and pinworm. It is a vermifuge and acts by causing flaccid paralysis of the muscles of the worms. Such narcotized worms are easily expelled from gut by peristaltic movements. It is absorbed to the extent of 30% from the gut, which is partly metabolized in the liver and is excreted in urine.

Clinical Uses and Adverse Reactions

It is used in ascariasis and enterobiasis. It is available as piperazine citrate (Antepar) granules (4.5 g of base) and syrup (7.5 g/5 mL in 30 mL bottle). It is given orally in the dose of 4.5 g of base (single) dose for roundworm and 2.5 g of base (50 mg/kg) daily for seven days for pinworm. It is well-tolerated and safe in pregnancy. It may cause nausea, vomiting and abdominal discomfort and in large dose muscular incoordination, weakness and even convulsions. It is contraindicated in epilepsy and renal insufficiency.

Levamisole and Tetramisole

Levamisole is *l*-tetramisole and is more preferred than tetramisole (*d-l* isomer/recemic mixture) as an anthelmintic against roundworm and hookworm. It is a vermifuge and acts by causing spastic paralysis of the worm muscles (by a depolarizing type of neuromuscular block). It also inhibits production of succinate by the worms. It is poorly absorbed from the gut and mostly excreted in faeces.

Clinical Uses and Adverse Reactions

It is used in ascariasis, ancytostomiasis and necatoriasis. It is available as tablet (50, 150 mg). It is given orally in the dose of 150 mg (single dose) for roundworm and 150 mg twice daily for hookworms in adults. Children dose is 50 mg. It is well-tolerated. It may cause nausea, vomiting and giddiness.

Ivermectin

It is a semisynthetic macrocyclic lactone, which is obtained from *Streptomyces avermintili*. It is effective against *Strongyloides stercoralis, Onchocerca volvulus, Wuchereria bancrofti* and *Brugia malayi*. It is microfilaricidal/larvicidal. It kills microfilaria but not the adult filarial worms. It probably acts as a GABA agonist by binding with GABA receptors at central synapses, and thus causing paralysis and detachment of the worm, which is then removed by the reticuloendothelial cells (macrophages). It is well-absorbed from the gut. It is metabolized in the liver and excreted in urine.

Clinical Uses and Adverse Reactions

It is used in strongyloidiasis, onchocerciasis and filariasis. It is available as ivermectin (Mectizan) tablet (2.5, 5 mg). It is given in the doses of 150 µg/kg (single dose) and repeated every 6 to 12 months (to prevent the disease). It can cause itching, skin oedema, athralgia, headache and fever. It may cause blindness due to death of the microfilaria in the eye producing ocular inflammatory lesions.

Diethyl Carbamazine Citrate

It is a piperazine derivative. It is very effective against microfilaria of *W. bancrofti, B. malayi, O. volvulus* and *Loa loa*. It is also effective against their adult worms. It causes rapid disappearance of microfilariae from the human peripheral blood (within seven days) but the microfilariae present in lymph nodes and hydrocoele (transudate) are not killed. It probably acts by sensitizing the microfilariae, so that they become susceptible to phagocytosis by the tissue (fixed) reticuloendothelial

cells but not by the circulating monocytes. It also diminishes the muscular activity of the adult worms, so that they are dislodged. Prolong treatment may kill adult worms, except *O. volvulus*. It is also effective against roundworm but prolonged treatment is required. It is rapidly absorbed from the gut. It is uniformly distributed in the body except fat. It is metabolized in the liver and excreted in urine within 30 hours.

Clinical Uses and Adverse Reactions

It is used in lymphatic filariasis, onchocerciasis and tropical pulmonary eosinophilia. It is available as Banocide/Hetrazan tablet (50, 100 mg) and syrup (50 mg/5 mL). It is given orally in the doses of 50 to 100 mg (6 mg/kg) thrice daily for 3 to 4 weeks. It can be used as a preventive of filaria in filaria affected area. It is given once in a year for 5 years. The dosage is: for 2 to 5 years—100 mg, 6 to 14 years—200 mg and 15 years and above—300 mg. It is contraindicated in children below 2 years, pregnant women and severly ill patients. It can produce side effects like anorexia, nausea, vomiting, headache, weakness and dizziness. Allergic reactions (due to release of foreign proteins in the tissues by the death of microfilariae or adult worms) include skin rashes, pruritus, fever, tachycardia, lymphadenopathy, myalgia and hypotension. Administration of antihistaminics or corticosteroids can minimize systemic allergic effects. In very large doses it can cause muscle tremors and convulsions.

Niclosamide

It is a halogenated salicylanilide derivative. It is effective against the intestinal tapeworms, *viz. T. saginata, T. solium, D. latum* and *H. nana*. It is a vermicide and acts by inhibiting oxidative phosphorylation in the mitochondria and thus interfering with ATP synthesis, respiration and glucose uptake in the tapeworms leading to death of the worms. The segments of the worm containing eggs may be digested within the intestine releasing the ova. From the ova the larvae are released. The ova or larvae are not digested. The larvae of *T. solium* penetrate the gut wall and invade the body tissue causing development of visceral cysticercosis. To prevent this, a saline purgative should be used after 1 to 2 hours of drug treatment and scolex is to be searched in the stool. It is not absorbed from the gut and excreted in faeces.

Clinical Uses and Adverse Reactions

It is used in intestinal tapeworm infestations (taeniasis). It is available as Niclosan tablet (500 mg). It is given orally in the dose of 1 g (2 tablets) in the morning in empty stomach. The tablets should be chewed and not swallowed to produce thorough mixing of the drug with the intestinal contents. Another 1 g is taken after 1 hour. The children dose is 0.5 to 1 g. *H. nana* infestation requires treatment for five days. It can be safely used in pregnancy and patients with poor health. It is well-tolerated. It may cause nausea, abdominial discomfort and headache.

Praziquantel

It is a pyrazinoisoquinoline derivative. It is effective against most cestodes (tapeworms) and trematodes (schistosomes and flukes). It is not effective against *Echinococcus granulosus* (hydatid worm) where albendazole and mebendazole are effective. It is a vermifuge and acts by causing increased permeability of the Ca^{++} ions through the cell membranes (including muscle fibres) of the susceptible worm leading to increased Ca^{++} entry into the cells of the worm and producing severe muscle contraction followed by spastic paralysis and detachment of the worm. It also produces vacuoles within the segmental cells of the worm leading to death of the cells. It is rapidly absorbed from the gut and has high bioavailability. It can cross BBB. It is metabolized in the liver and is excreted in urine.

Clinical Uses and Adverse Reactions

It is used in schistosomiasis, cysticercosis of brain or other viscera, intestinal taeniasis, *D. latum* and *H. nana* infestations in man. It is available as cysticide tablet (150, 600 mg). It is given orally in the doses of 10 to 20 mg/kg (single dose) in intestinal taeniasis, 40 to 60 mg/kg (single dose) in schistosomiasis and 40 to 60 mg/kg in two divided doses for 14 days in cysticercosis of brain. It is well-tolerated. It may cause headache, drowsiness, lassitude, nausea, vomiting, diarrhoea, fever, urticaria, skin rashes, myalgia and eosinophilia. It is contraindicated in ocular cysticercosis, because the host response can produce irreversible eye damage.

Oxamniquine

It is a tetrahydroquinoline derivative. It is only effective against *Schistosoma mansoni*. It is a vermifuge.

It is well-absorbed from the gut. It is metabolized in the liver and excreted in urine. It is used in African schistosomiasis. It is available as vansil capsule (250 mg). It is given orally in the doses of 20 to 30 mg/kg/day for 2 to 3 consecutive days. It is better tolerated when given after meal. It can cause nausea, abdominal pain, dizziness, headache and diarrhoea. Rarely it causes hallucinations and convulsions. It colours urine red. It is contraindicated in pregnancy.

Metrifonate

It is an organophosphorus compound. It is effective against *S. haematobium, A. lumbricoides, A. duodenale, N. americanus* and *T. trichiura*. It is a cholinesterase inhibitor and probably acts as a vermicide because of this property. It is well-absorbed from the gut. It is a prodrug, which is converted into dichlorovas in the body, which is a cholinesterase inhibitor. It is used in schistosomiasis caused by *S. haematobium*. It is available as Bilarsil tablet (100 mg). It is given orally in the dose of 7.5 to 10 mg/kg as a single dose and repeated every two weeks for 3 doses. It is well-tolerated. It may cause nausea, vomiting, weakness, dizziness and vertigo.

Niridazole

It is a heterocyclic nitrocompound. It is effective against schistosomes (*S. japonicum, S. mansoni* and *S. haematobium), Dracunculus medinensis* (guinea worm) and *E. histolytica*. It acts by inhibiting exogenous glucose uptake by the parasite. It is well-absorbed from the gut, metabolized in the liver and excreted in urine.

Clinical Uses and Adverse Reactions

It is used in schistosomiasis (bilharziasis) and dracontiasis. It is rarely used in amoebiasis due to high toxicity. It is available as Ambilhar tablet (500 mg). It is given orally in the dose of 25 mg/kg/day in two divided doses for 5 to 10 days. It can cause nausea, vomiting, diarrhoea, insomnia, headache, dizziness, epistaxis, convulsions and even psychosis.

Bithionol

It is a synthetic drug effective against *Fasciola hepatica* (liver fluke) and *Paragonimus westermani* (lung fluke). It is well-absorbed from the gut, metabolized in the liver and excreted in urine. It is used in *Paragonimus westermani* and *Fasciola hepatica* infestations. It is available as Bitin tablet (500 mg). It is given orally in the dose of 30 to 50 mg/kg/day in two divided doses for 5 to 10 days. It can produce nausea, vomiting, diarrhoea, dizziness, headache, hepatitis and leucopenia. Metronidazole and chloroquine are discussed in respective chapters (as antiamoebic and antimalarial drugs respectively).

78

Antineoplastic (Anticancer) Drugs

INTRODUCTION

These are drugs used in the treatment of neoplastic diseases (cancers). Though many anticancer drugs have been developed during the last four decades, but the chemotherapy of cancers is still less fruitful than the chemotherapy of microbial infections. This is because, the anticancer drugs lack the specificity of the antimicrobial drugs and have a lower margin of safety. Moreover, the host defence system in the form of antibodies, phagocytosis, etc. present in microbial infections is usually lacking or ineffective in persons with cancer cells and so the anticancer drugs cannot destroy all the cancer cells without producing toxicity. Thus, even after satisfactory initial treatment with anticancer drugs, the possibility of reoccurrence of cancers is always present. Like microbial cells, cancer cells also can develop resistance to drugs. Anticancer drugs either damage the target cancer cells or inhibit their growth. They damage the rapidly dividing cells, whether they are normal or cancer cells. Thus, they produce high tissue toxicity. They produce prolonged remission of some cancers, e.g. acute leukaemias, Wilm's tumour, Ewing's sarcoma, retinoblastoma, rhabdomyosarcoma, choreocarcinoma, Hodgkin's disease (lymphoma), lymphosarcoma, Burkitt's lymphoma, testicular carcinoma and mycosis fungoides. They produce palliation (decrease of symptoms for some period) of some cancers, e.g. breast carcinoma, ovarian carcinoma, prostatic carcinoma, lung (broncho) carcinoma, head and neck cancers, chronic lymphatic leukaemia and chronic myeloid leukaemia. Cancers that are resistant to anticancer drugs are liver carcinoma, pancreatic carcinoma, cholorectal carcinoma and malignant melanoma.

Classification of Anticancer Drugs

These are of five groups:

1. **Alkylating agents:** These are given as follows:

   - Nitrogen mustards, e.g. mechlorethamine, cyclophosphamide, ifosfamide, melphalan and chlorambucil.

   - Ethylenimines, e.g. triethylene melamine (TEM), hexaethylmelamine (HEM) and triethylene thiophosphoramide (Thio-TEPA).

   - Alkyl sulphonates, e.g. busulphan.

   - Nitrosoureas, e.g. carmustine, lomustine, semustine and streptozotocin.

   - Triazines, e.g. dacarbazine.

2. **Antimetabolites:** These are given as follows:

   - Folic acid analogs (antagonists), e.g. methotrexate (amethopterin).

   - Purine analogs (antagonists), e.g. 6-mercaptopurine, 6-thioguanine and Azathioprine.

- Pyrimidine analogs (antagonists), e.g. 5-fluorouracil, fluorodeoxyuridine and cytosine arabinoside (cytarabine).

3. **Natural (plant) products:** These are given as follows:
   - Antimitotic drugs, e.g. vinblastine, vincristine (oncovin) and taxanese by paclitaxel (Taxol).
   - Epipodophylotoxins, e.g. etoposide and teniposide.
   - Enzymes, e.g. L-asparaginase.
   - Cytotoxic antibiotics, e.g. actinomycin-D (dactinomycin), mitomycin-C, bleomycin, mithramycin (plicamycin), daunorubicin and doxorubicin (adriamycin).

4. **Hormones and hormone antagonists:** These are given as follows:
   - Glucocorticoids, e.g. prednisolone and others.
   - Androgens, e.g. testosterone and fluoxymesterone.
   - Antiandrogens, e.g. flutamide and finasteride.
   - Oestrogens, e.g. diethylstilbestrol, ethinyl estradiol and fosfeterol.
   - Antioestrogens, e.g. tamoxifen and clomiphene.
   - Progestins, e.g. hydroxyprogesterone and medroxyprogesterone.
   - Gonadotropin-releasing hormone (Gn-RH) analogs, e.g. leuprolide, naferelin and gosarelin.

5. **Miscellaneous agents:** These are given as follows:
   - Platinum coordination complexes, e.g. cisplatin and carboplatin.
   - Radioactive isotopes, e.g. radioiodine (^{131}I), radiogold (^{198}Au) and radiophosphorus (^{232}P).
   - Biological response modifiers, e.g. interferon-α and interleukin-2.
   - Other drugs, e.g. hydroxyurea, procarbazine, mitotane (O, P-DDD), aminoglutethimide, etc.

Cell Cycle Kinetics (Cytokinetics)

An understanding of the cell cycle is necessary to know the mechanism of action of anticancer drugs. All somatic cells, whether normal or cancer cells divide by mitosis. There are five phases in cell cycle, which are G_0 phase (resting phase/non-proliferating phase), G_1 phase (pre-DNA synthesis phase), S phase (DNA synthesis phase) G_2 phase (post-DNA synthesis phase) and M phase (mitosis phase). It is shown in **Fig. 78.1**.

Most anticancer drugs act on those cells which are in proliferating phase. These drugs are divided into two groups:

- **Cell cycle specific (CCS) drugs:** They act on proliferating (dividing) cells and not on resting cells, e.g. antimetabolites, vinca alkaloids, taxanep, etoposide, tinoposide and hydroxyurea.
- **Cell cycle nonspecific (CCNS) drugs:** They act on both proliferating and resting cells and so more toxic than the former drugs, e.g. alkylating drugs, cisplatin, cytotoxic antibiotics, procarbazine, dacarbazine and radioactive isotopes.

Sites of action of anticancer drugs: It is shown in **Fig. 78.2**.

General Toxicity of Anticancer Drugs

Anticancer drugs produce damaging effects on rapidly multiplying cells, whether they are normal or cancer cells, because they act on nucleic acids and their precursors. Thus, bone marrow, lymphoreticular tissue, GIT, skin and gonads are mostly affected.

1. **Bone marrow:** They produce myelosuppression (depression of bone marrow). This results in leucopenia, agranulocytosis, anaemia and thrombocytopaenia and in severe case of aplastic anaemia.

2. **Lymphoreticular tissue (RE system):** They produce lymphocytopaenia and inhibition of lymphocyte function resulting in suppression of cell mediated as well as humoral immunity. They breakdown the host defence mechanisms and increase the susceptibility to infections particularly

opportunistic infections by fungi (*Candida albicans* and fungi causing deep mycosis), virus (*Herpes simplex* and *Zoster*), protozoa (*Pneumocystis carinii*), etc.

- **GIT:** They cause nausea, vomiting, stomatitis, anorexia, diarrhoea, shedding of mucosa and haemorrhage (due to decrease in the rate of renewal of mucous lining).

- **Skin:** They cause alopecia (hair loss) by damaging the cells in hair follicles. They also cause dermatitis.

- **Gonads:** They cause damage of gonadal cells and produce oligospermia and sterility in males and amenorrhoea (due to inhibition of ovulation), menstrual irregularities and premature menopause in females. Besides these toxicities, they also produce:

  - **Hyperuricaemia** (due to massive cell destruction leading to liberation of uric acid, gout and urate stones).

  - **Hepatotoxicity** (by damaging liver cells).

  - **Foetal toxicity:** Given to pregnant women, they produce severe damage of developing foetus leading to abortion, foetal death or foetal abnormalities (teratogenicity). Hence, they are contraindicated in pregnancy.

  - **Carcinogenicity:** They can produce secondary cancers such as leukaemias, lymphomas and histocytic tumours after prolonged use. This may be due to depression of cell mediated and humoral blocking factors against cancers.

Combination Chemotherapy in Cancers

The use of combination of drugs in cancer is a consequence of limited success obtained by the use of single drug. It has enhanced the life span of patients suffering from some cancers. It is based upon kinetic, biochemical and toxicological considerations of anticancer drugs.

- **Kinetic basis of combination of anticancer drugs:** In cell destruction mechanism, a given dose of a drug destroys a constant fraction of cells. Thus combination chemotherapy is essential to increase the therapeutic potential of the drug in damaging cancer cells.

- **Biochemical basis of combination of anticancer drugs:** It produces sequential inhibition of different enzymatic reactions leading to production of an essential metabolite. It also produces simultaneous (concurrent) inhibition of parallel metabolic pathways.

- **Toxicological basis of combination of anticancer drugs:** It decreases toxicity of the individual drugs due to use of minimum therapeutic doses. It damages cancer cells in different phases of cell cycle by different drugs with different mechanisms of action.

- It also decreases development of resistance of cancer cells to the drugs.

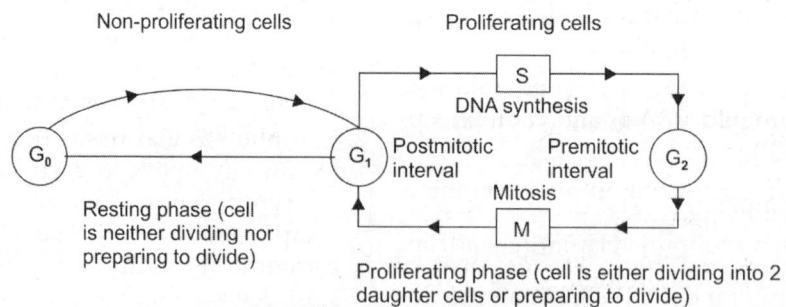

Fig. 78.1: Cell cycle

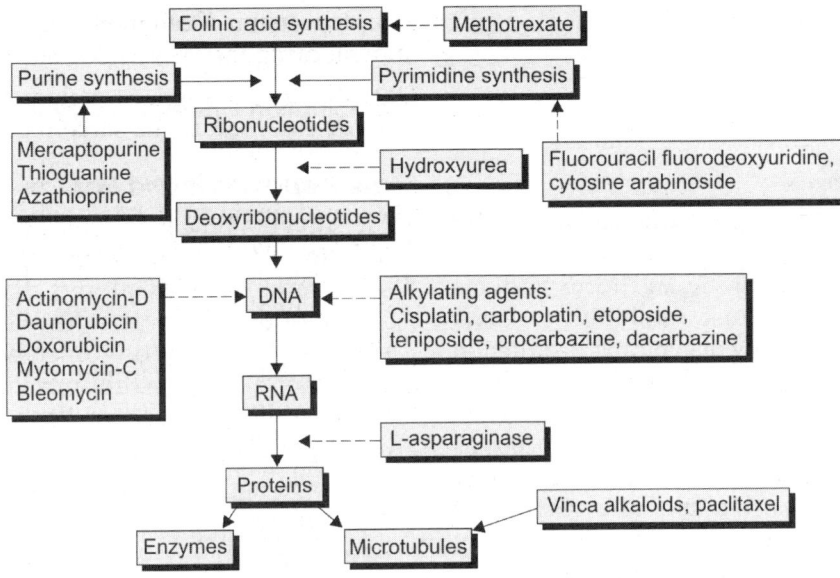

Fig. 78.2: Sites of action of anticancer drugs

SOME IMPORTANT DRUG REGIMENS FOR CANCERS

Hodgkin's Disease (Lymphoma)

1. MOPP regimen (contains mechlorethamine + oncovin + procarbazine + prednisolone).
2. COPP regimen (contains cyclophosphamide + oncovin + procarbazine + prednisolone).
3. ABVD regimen (contains adriamycin + bleomycin + vinblastine + dacarbazine).

Acute Lymphatic Leukaemia

- POMP regimen (contains prednisolone + oncovin + methotrexate + purinethol).
- VAMP regimen (contains vincristine + amethopterine + mercaptopurine + prednisolone).
- COAP regimen (contains cyclophosphamide + oncovin + arabinoside cytosine + prednisolone).

Ovarian Carcinoma

- PAC regimen (contains cisplatin + adriamycin + cyclophosphamide).

- CHAC regimen (contains cyclophosphamide + hexamethyl melamine + adriamycin + cisplatin).

In choosing a drug regimen one must always keep in mind, its cost effectiveness, because cancer chemotherapy is very expensive at present.

DISCUSSION OF INDIVIDUAL GROUP OF DRUGS

Alkylating Agents

These compounds were formerly known as radiomimetics, because they induce changes similar to irradiation. In neutral or alkaline solution, they undergo intramolecular cyclization to form highly reactive quaternary ammonium derivatives called ethylene immonium cations (as shown in **Fig. 78.3**). These cations alkylate (react with) covalently with groupings like amino, sulphydryl, hydroxy or phosphate of the cellular constituents such as DNA, RNA and amino acids and render them unavailable for the normal metabolic reactions.

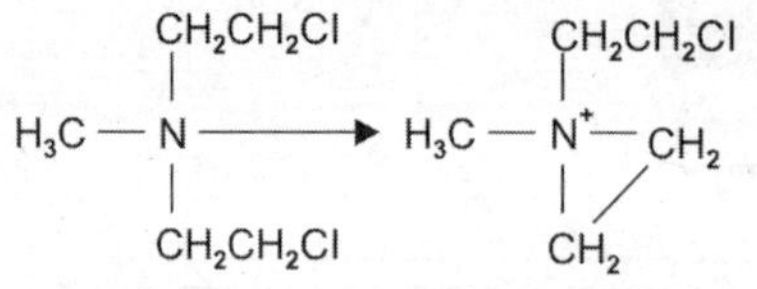

Nitrogen mustard   Ethylene immonium ion

Fig. 78.3: Mechanism of action of nitrogen mustard

They are nucleophilic and form adducts with DNA. They cause inhibition of DNA replication, miscoding of gene and production of defective proteins and breakage of DNA strands. They are cell cycle nonspecific. They cause damage of rapidly proliferating cells as well as nonproliferating cells. They show cross-resistance, i.e. if a tumour is resistant to one alkylating agent, it will be relatively resistant to other alkylating agents.

Uses of Alkylating Agents

Mechlorethamine: Hodgkin's disease, non-Hodgkin's lymphomas.

Cyclophosphamide/ifosfamide: Acute/chronic lymphatic leukaemia, Hodgkin's disease, non-Hodgkin's lymphomas, multiple myeloma, neuroblastoma, breast/ovary/lung carcinoma, Wilm's tumour, cervical carcinoma, testicular carcinoma, soft tissue sarcoma.

Melphalan: Multiple myeloma, breast carcinoma, ovarian carcinoma.

Chlorambucil: Chronic lymphatic leukaemia, Hodgkin's disease, non-Hodgkin's lymphomas.

Triethylene melamine/Hexamethylmelamine/Triethylene thiophosphoramide: Breast/ovarian/bladder carcinoma.

Busulphan: Chronic myeloid leukaemia.

Carmustine: Hodgkin's disease, non-Hodgkin's lymphomas, primary brain tumours, multiple myeloma, malignant melanoma.

Lomustine: Hodgkin's disease, non-Hodgkin's lymphomas, primary brain tumours, small cell lung carcinoma.

Semustine: Primary brain tumours, gastric/colonic carcinoma.

Streptozotocin: Malignant pancreatic insulinoma, maligant carcinoid tumour.

Dacarbazine: Malignant melanoma, Hodgkin's disease, soft tissue sarcomas.

Some Preparations and Dosage

- Mechlorethamine hydrochloride (Mustine) injection (10 mg with 90 mg of anhydrous sodium chloride/vial and dissolved in 10 mL of distilled water, just before injection)—0.1 mg/kg/day injected into the tubing of a rapidly running intravenous normal saline infusion for 3 to 4 days.
- Cyclophosphamide (Endoxan, cycloxan) tablet (50 mg) and injection (100 mg/vial and dissolved in 5 mL of distilled water)—2 to 3 mg/kg/day orally or IV for 6 to 8 days followed by daily oral maintenance dose of 100 mg for 30 to 40 days.
- Melphalan (Alkeran) tablet (2.5 mg)—4 to 6 mg daily for 2 to 3 weeks.
- Chlorambucil (Leukeran) tablet (2.5 mg)—4 to 10 mg daily for 3 to 6 weeks.
- Busulphan (Myleran) tablet (2 mg)—4 to 8 mg daily for 3 to 4 weeks and then adjust according to leucocyte count.
- Carmustine injection—100 to 200 mg/sq metre BSA/day IV.
- Lomustine capsule (40, 100 mg)—100 mg/sq metre BSA in single dose in every six weeks.
- Dacarbazine injection—3 to 5 mg/kg/day IV.

Adverse Reactions

IV alkylating agents can cause thrombophlebitis. Common adverse effects of alkylating agents are anorexia, nausea, vomiting (by stimulating CTZ) and myelosuppression. Their other adverse effects have been discussed with general toxicity of anticancer drugs. Cyclophosphamide can also produce haemorrhagic cystitis.

Antimetabolites

These are compounds which are structural analogues (similar to) of natural chemical substances (folic acid, purines or pyrimidines) that take part in normal cellular activities. They either compete with the natural substances for specific enzymes or become incorporated into nucleic acids (DNA and RNA) forming frudulent (false) macromolecules, which cannot produce reproduction of cancer cells. Thus they cause lethal synthesis of DNA and RNA by acting as false substrates. Most of these antimetabolites are cell cycle specific and act on S phase (DNA synthesis phase).

Methotrexate/Amethopterine

It is a 4-amino-substituted folic acid analogue which acts as a folic acid antagonist. It competes with folic acid for the enzyme dihydrofolate (DHF) reductase and prevents the formation of tetrahydrofolate (THF) reductase, that is required for the biosynthesis of purine, thymidylate and then DNA in the cells. Lack of DNA leads to stoppage of cellular reproduction and cellular death. It also inhibits RNA and protein synthesis in the cells.

Mercaptopurine and Other Purine Antagonists

They are structural analogues of purines (adenine, guanine, hypoxanthine, etc.). After entering the cells they are converted to active products like mercaptopurine ribose phosphate, thioguanine ribose phosphate, etc. which inhibit the biosynthesis of purines by inhibiting the enzyme phosphoribosyl transferase and thus leading to inhibition of biosynthesis of DNA and RNA in the cells.

Fluorouracil and Other Pyrimidine Antagonists

They are structural analogues of pyrimidines (uracil, thymine, cytidine, etc.). After entering the cells, they are converted to active products like fluorouridine triphosphate, fluorodeoxyuridine monophosphate, etc. which inhibit the biosynthesis of pyrimidines (by inhibiting the enzyme, thymidylate synthetase) and thus leading to inhibition of biosynthesis of DNA and RNA in the cells.

Uses of Antimetabolites

Methotrexate: Acute lymphatic leukaemia, Hodgkin's disease, choriocarcinoma, breast/lung/head and neck carcinoma, mycosis fungoides, osteogenic sarcoma.

Mercaptopurine/Thioguanine: Acute lymphatic leukaemia, chronic myeloid leukaemia, choriocarcinoma, breast/ovarian/lung carcinoma.

Fluorouracil: Breast/GIT/pancreatic/ovarian/urinary bladder carcinoma, premalignant skin lesions.

Cytosine arabinoside: Acute myeloid leukaemia, acute lymphatic leukaemia, chronic myeloid leukaemia, non-Hodgkin's lymphomas.

Some Preparations and Dosage

- Methotrexate (Biotrexate, Neotrexate) tablet (2.5 mg) and injection (50 mg/vial)— 2.5 to 10 mg daily for five days. 15 to 30 mg/sq metre BSA IM or IV twice weekly for 3 weeks.
- Mercaptopurine (Purinethol) tablet (50 mg)—2.5 mg/kg body weight daily and then adjusted according to leucocyte count.
- Fluorouracil (Fluracil) capsule (250 mg) and injection (250 mg/5 mL)—10 to 15 mg/kg body weight daily orally or IV for 3 to 5 days followed by 7.5 mg/kg orally every second or third day till toxicity is seen.
- Cytosine arabinoside (Cytarabine) injection (100 mg/5 mL)—3 to 6 mg/kg body weight IV daily in two divided doses for 5 to 10 days.

Adverse Reactions

Methotrexate can cause myelosuppression leading to megaloblastic anaemia and pancytopaenia. It can produce GIT side effects like nausea, vomiting, anorexia, diarrhoea, desquamation and bleeding. It may also cause hyperuricaemia and hyperuricosuria due to massive destruction of the cells of lymphoid tissue. Its toxicity is treated by folinic acid but not folic acid (ineffective). Mercaptopurine can cause myelosuppression and GIT side effects like methotrexate. It may also cause hyperuricaemia and hyperuricosuria like methotrexate. It may sometimes cause jaundice by hepatic damage. Other anti-metabolites cause myelosuppression and GIT side effects like methotrexate.

Natural (Plant) Products

Vinca alkaloids (Vinblastine and Vincristine) are obtained from the plant *Vinca rosea* (periwinkle). They are mitotic inhibitors. They block cell proliferation during mitosis by binding with microtubular protein 'tubulin' and cause disruption of mitotic spindle. As a result the chromosomes fail to move apart during mitosis and arrest mitosis at M phase. They are cell cycle specific drugs and act on various phases of cell cycle. Paclitaxel is an alkaloid obtained from the plant *Taxus brevifolia/ baccatta*. It is cell cycle specific drug and arrest mitosis in G_0 and M phases.

Podophyllotoxin is an alkaloid obtained from the plant *Podophyllum peltatum*. Etoposide and teneposide are semisynthetic derivatives of podophyllotoxin. They cause mitotic arrest at S-G_2 phase. L-asparaginase is an enzyme obtained from the bacteria *E. coli*. It causes degradation of amino acid 'asparagine' to aspartic acid and ammonia. Some cancer cells require asparaginine for their survival and so there occurs inhibition of protein synthesis and cell death when L-asparaginase is administered. Cytotoxic antibiotics are obtained from microorganisms (Streptomyces species). They intercalate with DNA and inhibit RNA synthesis. Bleomycin produces superoxide by reacting with iron and oxygen which damage DNA and cause cell death.

Uses of Natural Products

Vinblastine: Hodgkin's disease, non-Hodgkin's lymphomas, breast/testicular carcinoma.

Vincristine: Acute lymphatic leukaemia, Hodgkin's disease, non-Hodgkin's lymphomas, Wilms' tumour, neuroblastoma, small cell lung carcinoma, rhabdomyosarcoma.

Paclitaxel: Advanced ovarian carcinoma, breast/lung/oesophageal/head and neck carcinoma.

Etoposide/Teniposide: Small cell lung carcinoma, acute myeloid leukaemia, breast/lung/testicular carcinoma, Hodgkin's disease, non-Hodgkin's lymphomas.

L-asparaginase: Acute lymphatic leukaemia, malignant lymphoma.

Actinomycin-D: Rhabdomyosarcoma, choriocarcinoma.

Mitomycin-C: Breast/GIT/pancreatic/urinary bladder/cervical/head and neck carcinoma.

Bleomycin: Squamous cell carcinoma of skin, testicular/cervical/oesophageal/head and neck carcinoma.

Doxorubicin/Daunorubicin: Acute lymphatic leukaemia, acute myeloid leukaemia.

Some Preparations and Dosage)

- Vinblastine sulphate (Cytoblastin) injection (10 mg/vial)—0.1–0.2 mg/kg body weight IV once weekly. The dose can be raised by 0.05 mg at weekly interval.
- Vincristine sulphate (Cytocristin) injection (1 mg/mL in vial)—0.025 to 0.075 mg/kg body weight IV once weekly.
- Paclitaxel (Intaxel) injection (30 mg/vial)— 175 mg/sq metre BSA by IV infusion over three hours and repeated every three weeks.
- Etoposide (Etosid) injection (100 mg/ 5 mL)— 50 to 60 mg/sq metre BSA/day by IV infusion over one hour and repeated every three weeks.
- L-asparaginase (Eispar) injection (10,000 units/vial)—50 to 100 units/kg/day IV or IM for 3 to 4 weeks.
- Actinomycin-D (Dacmozen) injection (0.5 mg/vial)—15 mg/kg/day IV for five days.
- Mitomycin-C injection (10 mg/vial)—2 mg/sq metre BSA/day IV for five days.
- Bleomycin (Bleocin) injection (15 mg/ vial)— 30 mg IV or IM weekly for 4 to 6 weeks.

Adverse Reactions

These are as general toxicity discussed before. L-asparaginase can cause allergic reactions, hepatotoxicity pancreatitis and mental depression.

Hormones and Hormone Antagonists

These are not cytotoxic drugs. They act by altering hormonal milles and thus causing inhibition of cell growth of hormone dependent tumours by opposite actions. They are only palliative and can be used as adjuvant to cytotoxic chemotherapy and/or surgery. They are used in:

Glucocorticoids: Acute lymphatic leukaemia, chronic lymphatic (by lympholytic action) leukaemia, Hodgkin's disease, non-Hodgkin's lymphomas.

Androgens: Breast carcinoma (premenopausal).

Antiandrogen (Flutamide): Prostatic carcinoma.

Oestrogens: Breast carcinoma (postmenopausal), prostatic carcinoma.

Antioestrogen (Tamoxifen): Breast carcinoma (pre- or postmenopausal).

Progestins: Endometrial carcinoma (metastatic).

GnRH analog (Leuprolide): Prostatic carcinoma.

These are discussed in endocrine pharmacology.

Miscellaneous Agents

Platinum coordination complexes (cisplatin and carboplatin) act like alkylating agents. They bind with DNA strands by cross-linking causing damage of cells. They are used in testicular/ovarian/urinary bladder/lung/thyroid/uterus/head and neck carcinomas, neuroblastoma and osteogenic sarcoma. They are available as injection (10 mg/vial) and administered IV like mechlorethamine. They produce severe nausea and vomiting, anaemia, renal damage and anaphylactic like reactions.

Radioactive isotopes: They emit radiation and produce ionization in the cells leading to cell destruction. They are used in:

- *Radioiodine (sodium ^{131}I)*—50 to 200 millicuries orally: Thyroid carcinoma, thyrotoxicosis.
- *Radiophosphorus (sodium phosphate ^{32}P)*—3 to 5 millicuries IV: Polycythemia vera, chronic lymphatic/myeloid leukaemia.
- *Radiogold (^{98}Au)*—100 to 150 millicuries into pleural or peritoneal cavity: Malignant pleural and peritoneal effusions.

They produce myelotoxicity, damage of liver, lymph nodes, gonads, lungs and GIT. They are mutagenic and carcinogenic.

Biological Response Modifiers

Interferon-α and interleukin-2 have been found useful in some cancers like leukaemias, malignant melanoma and renal cell carcinoma (hypernephroma). They are immunomodulator and thus increase T-lymphocyte activity and stimulate proliferation of natural killer cells, which are known to be deficient in cancer patients. They are administered orally, or as aerosol. They are safer drugs in short-term treatment.

Hydroxyurea and Procarbazine

Hydroxyurea is a substituted urea. It acts by inhibiting DNA synthesis (by inhibiting ribonucleotide reductase enzyme, which converts ribonucleotide to deoxyribonucleotide). It is used in chronic myeloid leukaemia and melanoma. It is administered as capsule (100 mg) in the dose of 100 to 300 mg daily. It can cause myelosuppression, hyperuricaemia and dermatitis. Procarbazine (N-methylhydrazine) is used in Hodgkin's disease and oat cell carcinoma of lung. It is converted to an active metabolite in the liver which depolymerizes DNA and causes damage of DNA and chromosomes. It is administered as capsule (50 mg) in the dose of 100 to 300 mg daily. It can produce myelotoxicity and CNS toxicity (restlessness, disorientation, drowsiness). Mitotane and aminoglutethemide are discussed with corticosteroids.

Section IV

IMMUNOPHARMACOLOGY

79

Introduction to Immunomodulators

INTRODUCTION

Immunopharmacology is the study of drugs that are used to modulate immune responses. In human beings, the immune response is composed of cell mediated (cellular) immunity and humoral (antibody) immunity. The ability of an individual to produce an immune response forms the basis of hypersensitivity (allergic) reactions and autoimmune diseases.

The primary objectives of immunotherapy are:

- To produce desired immunity by immunization with specific antigens or by administration of specific antibodies or cytokines.
- To control undesired immune reactions produced by drugs.

Thus, immunotherapy is indicated in:

- Allergic reactions
- Autoimmune diseases
- Infectious diseases
- Cancers
- Organ/tissue transplantation.

The presence of a normal functioning immune system is extremely important for a healthy life. It protects the body against invading microorganisms, toxins and foreign cells (transplants). Any hyporeactivity, hyperreactivity, absence or abnormal reactivity of this system leads to a variety of diseases.

The immune system has two divisions, *viz.* innate immune system and adaptive immune system. The innate immune system consists of macrophages and natural killer cells, which recognize and kill the foreign antigens. The adaptive immune system consists of lymphocytes, which are activated when they recognize the specific antigenic determinants (epitopes). There are two types of lymphocytes, *viz.* T lymphocytes (T cells) and B-lymphocytes (B cells). T lymphocytes are derived from thymus and responsible for cell mediated immunity. B lymphocytes are derived from bone marrow and responsible for humoral (antibody) immunity. T lymphocytes have four subtypes, *viz.* helper T cells, suppressor T cells, cytotoxic T cells and lymphokine producing T cells. Helper T cells (CD4+ cells) and suppressor T cells (CD8+ cells) are involved in complex ways in antibody production (CD means cluster of differentiation, which is a type of receptor present on the cell surface of T cells). Cytotoxic T cells and lymphokine producing T cells are involved in cell mediated immune response.

The recognition of the antigens by the T cells leads to proliferation of these cells, infiltration of these immune cells at the site of action and cellular immunity. The infiltration T cells exert their cytotoxic action by the release of various types of lymphokines such as transfer factor (TF), migration inhibitory factor (MIF), chemotactic factor (CF), lympho-toxin (LT), interleukin-2 and interferon-α.

The recognition of the antigens by the B cells leads to proliferation of the cells, conversion to plasma cells and production of specific antibodies called immunoglobulins (IgG, IgA, IgM, IgD and IgE). The specific antibody binds with the specific antigen leading to its inactivation or even phago-cytosis. There is a heat-labile serum com-ponent called complement, which causes bacteriolysis and phagocytosis. The important properties of immunoglobulins are shown in **Table 79.1**.

Immunomodulators

Drugs may modulate immune mechanism by either suppressing or stimulating one or more of the following processes.

- Antigen recognition and phagocytosis
- Lymphocyte proliferation
- Formation of antibodies
- Antigen-antibody reaction

- Release of mediators due to immune response
- Modification of target tissue response.

Immunomodulators are immunosuppres-sants and immunostimulants.

Immunosuppressants

These are drugs that suppress undesirable immunological responses. Since immunity confers resistance to disease, the use of drugs for suppressing it appears odd at first sight, but as the immunity is the ability of the body to recognize self from non-self (foreign), so suppression of immunity leads to failure to recognize and to tolerate antigens produced by its own tissues (autoimmunity).

Immunosuppressants are of three groups:

- **General immunosuppressants:** They suppress all immune responses, e.g. cytotoxic agents like azathioprine, cyclo-phosphamide, mycophenolate mofetil, methotrexate and chlorambucil.
- **Specific immunosuppressants:** They suppress only cell mediated immunity,

Table 79.1: Biological properties of immunoglobulins (Ig)

Property	IgG	IgA	IgM	IgD	IgE
Site	Serum, amniotic fluid	Serum, secretions, GIT	Serum	Serum	Serum
Placental transfer	Yes	No	No	No	No
Complement fixing	Yes	No	Yes	No	No
Plasma t½ (days)	23	6	5	3	2
Beneficial effects	Neutralizes toxins, enhances phago-cytosis, immuno-protection of foetus	Neutralizes toxins, protects external body surfaces	Neutralizes toxins, participates in agglutinating and cytotoxic reactions	Serves as antigen receptor on B cells	Mediates changes in vascular permeability in allergic disorders
Injurious effects	Antigen-antibody reaction can cause tissue injuries like Arthus reaction and serum sickness	No	Like IgG	No	Can cause anaphylactic reactions

e.g. cyclosporine, tacrolimus, antilymph-ocytic serum (ALS) or antilymphocytic globulin (ALG) and Rho(D) immune globulin.

- **Partial immunosuppressants:** They suppress the unwanted reactions due to immunoresponses, probably by their anti-inflammatory actions, e.g. glucocortico-steroids, salicylates, phenylbutazone, sulphasalazine and methoxalen.

Uses of Immunosuppressants

- Treatment of autoimmune diseases, e.g. autoimmune haemolytic anaemia, idio-pathic thrombocytopenic purpura, acute glomerulonephritis, ulcerative colitis, rheumatoid arthritis and systemic lupus erythematosus (SLE). Drugs used are pred-nisolone, cyclosporine, azathioprine, cyclophosphamide and methotrexate.

- Prevention of Rh haemolytic disease of newborn (neonate)-Rho (D) immuno-globulin is used prophylactically in Rho (D) negative mother during pregnancy.

- Organ transplantation like kidney, liver, heart and bone marrow to prevent graft rejection. Effective drugs are cyclosporine, tacrolimus, prednisolone, azathioprine, cyclophosphamide and antilymphocytic globulin (ALG).

DISCUSSION OF SOME DRUGS

Cyclosporine

It is a polypeptide antibiotic derived from a fungus 'Cylindrocarpon lucidium'. It is now synthesized. It has immunosuppressive activity. It causes marked inhibition of T cells proliferation (specific T cells inhibitor). It blocks an early stage in the activation of cytotoxic T lymphocytes after the recipient is exposed to the antigen. It is not effective once an immune response has commenced. It is a selective (specific) immunosuppressant and acts by binding with specific receptors (cyclophilins) within lymphocytes leading to decreased production of interleukin-2 (IL-2) and fall of T lymphocyte count.

Pharmacokinetics

It is well-absorbed from GIT. Its bioavail-ability after oral administration is 30 to 50%. In the circulation it is 50% bound to ery-throcytes, 10% to leucocytes and 40% to plasma proteins. It is almost completely metabolized in the liver and excreted in urine as metabolites.

Clinical Uses

It is used as an immunosuppressive agent in organ transplantation to prevent graft rejection. It is used in combination with a glucocorticoid (prednisolone) in this situation. It is also used in rheumatoid arthritis and myasthenia gravis. It is a expensive drug.

Preparations and Dosage

- Cyclosporine (Imosporin) capsule (50, 100 mg): It is used in the doses of 10 to 15 mg / kg/day starting 6 to 12 hours prior to organ transplantation and continued in the same doses for 1 to 2 weeks, after which the dose is reduced to 5 to 8 mg/kg/day.

- Cyclosporine injection (50 mg/mL) for IV administration is also available.

Adverse Reactions

It can produce nephrotoxicity, hepatic dys-function, hypertrichosis, gingival hyper-trophy, neuropathy, myopathy, hypertension, tremor, GIT disturbances, hyperuricaemia, increased susceptibility to infection and development of malignant lymphomas (caused by Epstein-Barr virus). It does not cause myelosuppression.

Tacrolimus

Tacrolimus is a macrolide antibiotic with mechanism of action like cyclosporine. It is more potent than cyclosporine. It is under clinical evaluation in organ transplantation to prevent graft rejection.

Azathioprine

It is a cytotoxic antimetabolite chemically related to 6-mercaptopurine. It is a prodrug and is converted in the body to the active metabolite 6-mercaptopurine. It has immuno-suppressive activity. It acts by inhibiting DNA synthesis and thus preventing proliferation of lymphocytes (particularly T cells) that occur in response to the newly introduced antigens (in the case of organ transplants). It is a non-selective (general) immunosuppressant. It is well-absorbed after oral administration. It is metabolized in the liver and excreted in urine mainly as metabolites.

Clinical Uses

It is used as an immunosuppressive agent in organ transplantation to prevent graft rejection. It is also used in autoimmune diseases like haemolytic anaemia, acute glomerulonephritis, rheumatoid arthritis and myasthenia gravis.

Preparation and Dosage

Azathioprine (Imuran) tablet (50 mg): Initially 5 mg/kg/day, then 1 to 3 mg/kg/day in divided doses for three months.

Adverse Reactions

It can cause myelosuppression, malaise, dizziness, vomiting, skin rashes, fever, muscle pain, arthralgia, disturbed liver function, cholestatic jaundice, cardiac arrhythmias, hypotension, alopecia and rarely pancreatitis and pneumonitis.

Cytotoxic Agents

Cytotoxic agents like cyclophosphamide, mycophenolate mofetil, methotrexate and chlorambucil are also used as immuno-suppressants but they are less preferred due to their myelosuppressive and other adverse reactions.

Glucocorticoids

Glucocorticoids (prednisolone, etc.) are potent immunosuppressants as well as antiinflam-matory agents. They cause reduction of blood lymphocyte count by lympholytic action, reduction of endogenous proinflammatory substances (PAF, PCs, LTs, histamine and bradykinin), reduction of circulating IgG and reduction of production of IL-2 by helper T cells (CD4+ cells), which are decreased in numbers. They are used as immunosup-pressive agents in organ transplantation to prevent graft rejection. They are also used in autoimmune diseases like rheumatoid arth-ritis, SLE, haemolytic anaemia, iodiopathic thrombocytopaenic purpura and ulcerative colitis.

Antilymphocytic Serum

Antilymphocytic serum (ALS) or semipuri-fied antilymphocytic globulin (ALG) is obtained from horses immunized against human thymus, lymph nodes or spleen cells (lymphoid cells). It acts by destroying T lymphocytes (T cells) or rendering them nonfunctional. It is administered in the dose of 1000 units/kg (1 to 5 mL of serum) IM along with another immunosuppressant (gluco-corticoid or azathioprine) in patients undergoing organ transplantation to prevent graft rejection. It reduces the doses of other immunosuppressants and decreases their adverse reactions. It can produce pain and induration at the site of injection, fever, thrombocytopaenia, anaphylactic reaction and development of malignant lymphomas.

Rho (D) immune globulin is discussed in the next chapter.

Immunostimulants

These are drugs that augment or facilitate immune mechanisms. They are beneficial for individuals with immune deficiency. They act by increasing the humoral (antibody) res-ponses, enhancing phagocytic activity of macrophages or modifying the cell mediated immune responses. They are used in immuno-deficiency disorders such as AIDS, chronic infectious diseases and cancers particularly leukaemias (involving lymphatic system).

They are cytokines (interferon-α and interleukin-2), levamisole, BCG vaccine and immunoglobulin. Cytokines are natural substances (proteins) that are produced in response to a variety of stimuli including antigens. Interferon stimulates proliferation of

T cells and activates macrophages and natural killer cells. It is now prepared by recombinant DNA technology. It is used in several cancers including hairy cell leukaemia, chronic myeloid leukaemia and Kaposi's sarcoma and several viral infections (hepatitis and HIV). Interleukin-2 (IL-2) stimulates the production of T helper and T cytotoxic cells. It is used in metastatic melanoma and renal cell carcinoma. It can produce hypotension and shock.

Levamisole: It is an anthelmintic with potent immunostimulant property. It can increase delayed hypersensitivity and/or T cell mediated immunity. It has been used in Hodgkin's disease, colorectal cancer and rheumatoid arthritis with some success.

BCG vaccine: Bacille Calmette-Guérin (BCG) and its active component 'muramyl dipeptide' are useful products that have been found to produce an immunostimulant effect. BCG increases the phagocytic activity of T cells and natural killer cells. It has been used along with conventional therapy in urinary bladder cancer, lung cancer and metastatic melanoma with some success. It can cause hypersensitivity reactions, shock, chills, fever, malaise and immune complex disease.

Immunoglobulin

It is prepared commercially from pooled human plasma obtained from donors. It contains all of the immunoglobulin subclasses and has antibody titres for common bacterial, viral and fungal pathogens. It is used in various immunodeficiency states including hypogammaglobulinaemia; haemorrhagic diseases such as idiopathic thrombocytopaenic purpura and autoimmune haemolytic anaemia and in infectious diseases like measles and hepatitis. It is also used in the prevention of infection in chronic lymphatic leukaemia and multiple myeloma. It can cause hypersensitivity reactions and anaphylactic shock.

80

Immunization: Vaccines and Sera

INTRODUCTION

Immunization is the method of increasing the lymphocyte mediated specific immunity in the subject for the prevention or treatment of many infectious diseases. It is either active or passive.

Active Immunization

It is done by administration of vaccines and toxoids, which contain antigens. Administration of antigens to the host induces formation of specific antibodies and induces cell mediated immunity. This active immunity is very effective in the prevention of many infectious diseases and is longer-lasting than passive immunity.

Passive Immunization

It is done by administration of immune sera containing preformed antibodies or antitoxins obtained from the sera of animals (horse and rabbit) or humans, who have been actively immunized. It is given to individuals not exposed to the pathogen earlier or does not possess adequate immunity, but as a help to tide over an emergency situation. Its main advantage is the immediate availability of readymade antibodies against micro-organisms, but it produces short-lasting immunity. Moreover, administration of animal sera may produce hypersensitivity reactions and even fatal anaphylactic shock. Administration of human immunoglobulins

(Igs) do not produce such reactions and the immunity produced is also relatively longer-lasting.

Immunizing Agents for Producing Active Immunity

1. **Vaccines:** These are chemical substances which after administration lead to specific protection against diseases. These are prepared from live attenuated microorganisms, killed microorganisms, toxoids or combination of these. Some are prepared by recombinant DNA technology, e.g. human BCG vaccine and human hepatitis-B vaccine:

   a. **Live vaccines:** These are BCG vaccine, oral polio vaccine (OPV), mumps vaccine, etc. These are prepared from attenuated microorganisms, which have lost their ability to produce disease but their immunogenic potential is intact. A single dose is sufficient for immunization and the immunity produced by them is long-lasting.

   b. **Killed or inactivated vaccines:** These are pertussis vaccine, rabies vaccine, hepatitis-B vaccines, typhoid-paratyphoid A and B vaccine, cholera vaccine, influenza vaccines, etc. These are administered SC or IM. These are relatively nontoxic and safe but efficacy is less.

   c. **Combination vaccines:** These are diphtheria, pertussis and tetanus (DPT) vaccine; measles, mumps and rubella (MMR) vaccine, etc.

In these, 2 or 3 vaccines are combined together. Their advantages are single administration and low cost.

2. **Toxoids:** These are tetanus toxoid, diphtheria toxoid, mixed diphtheria and tetanus (DT) toxoid (double antigen) and mixed diphtheria, tetanus and pertussis (DTP) toxoid (triple antigen). These are prepared by adding formalin to toxins of microorganisms and incubating them at 37°C for 3 to 4 weeks. When administered SC or IM they produce antibody response. National/ universal immunization programme schedule is shown in **Table 80.1**.

Immunizing Agents for Producing Passive Immunity

1. **Antisera:** These are tetanus antitoxin (ATS), diphtheria antitoxin (ADS), gas gangrene antitoxin (ACS), rabies antiserum, antisnake venom serum, etc. These are derived from the animals (horse and rabbit), who have received a vaccine, toxin or toxoid. The sera of these animals contain antibodies against microorganisms or other toxins.

2. **Immune human sera:** These are prepared from immune or hyperimmunized and convalescent adults. These are now preferred than ATS or ADS of animal origin.

3. **Immunoglobulins (human):** These are prepared from pooled human blood plasma having higher levels of antibody titre. These are seperated human gamma globulins, *viz.* IgG, IgA, IgM, IgD and IgE, which carry the antibodies. Recombinant DNA technology and hybridoma technique have nowadays enabled mass production of specific human immunoglobulins.

DISCUSSION OF SOME IMMUNIZING AGENTS

Vaccines

I. Viral Vaccines

Polio Vaccine

There are two types of polio vaccine, *viz.* oral polio vaccine (OPV) and inactivated polio vaccine (IPV). Oral polio vaccine (sabin vaccine) is a live attenuated vaccine of poliomyelitis virus types 1, 2 and 3 strains. It is available either in monovalent (containing single strain) or in trivalent form (containing all the strains), which is commonly used. It provides both systemic immunity and local (intestinal) immunity to reinfection by the poliomyelitis virus. It is administered orally in the dose of 0.5 mL at 6, 10 and 14 weeks in infants and repeated at 18 months (booster dose). It does not produce any serious adverse effects. Vaccine associated paralysis is very rare. It is contraindicated in presence of acute infection, diarrhoea and immunodeficiency disorders. Inactivated polio vaccine (salk vaccine) is given by SC or IM injection in the dose of 0.5 mL in 3 doses at an interval of 4 to 6 weeks between the 1st and 2nd doses and 12 months between the 2nd and 3rd doses. It produces active immunity against paralytic poliomyelitis by producing serum antibodies specific for types 1, 2 and 3 polio virus. It produces only limited resistance to growth of the virus in the intestine and does not affect

Table 80.1: Immunization programme schedule in children and pregnant women

Age	Vaccine/Toxoid
At birth	BCG vaccine
6 weeks	DTP + OPV
10 weeks	DTP + OPV
14 weeks	DTP + OPV
9 months	Measles vaccine
18 months	DTP + OPV (booster/reinforcing dose)
5 years	DT (booster dose)
10 years	Tetanus toxoid + TAB vaccine
16 years	Tetanus toxoid + TAB vaccine

Note: Pregnant women (24 to 32 weeks), tetanus toxoid, 2 doses at 1 month apart.

the carrier state (excretion of virus in faeces). For these reasons, it is less favoured than oral polio vaccine. However, for a small selected number of cases it is superior to oral polio vaccine. As oral polio vaccine (OPV) contains live (though attenuated) virus, it can produce poliomyelitis in immunocompromised persons (e.g. persons receiving immuno-suppressants), but inactivated polio vaccine (IPV) contains killed poliovirus and so does not produce poliomyelitis. Its adverse effects are mild and consists of local pain, erythema, induration, fever and rarely allergic reactions. Pulse polio is the oral polio vaccine in mass scale below the age of 5 years in 2 doses at 2 months interval.

Measles Vaccine

It is available as a freeze dried product of live attenuated measles virus grown in chick embryo. It produces active immunity against measles in about 95% of the recipients with a single dose. It is administered SC in a dose of 0.5 mL at the age of 9 months (for primary vaccination). A second dose can be given at the age of 15 months. It produces a non-communicable mild measles infection. It can produce mild febrile response with skin rash, cough and coryza. It is contraindicated in pregnancy, children with active tuberculosis and those allergic to egg proteins.

MMR Vaccine (Tresi Vac/Trimovax)

It is a combined preparation of live attenuated virus of three viral diseases (measles, mumps and rubella, i.e. German measles). It is very popular. It is administered by deep SC or IM injection in a dose of 0.5 mL at the age of 4 to 5 years of age (before entry to the primary school) irrespective of previous measles vaccination or history of measles, mumps or rubella. It produces adverse effects like measles vaccine. It is contraindicated in children with altered immunity and those on high doses of corticosteroids or immuno-suppressants. It is also contraindicated in pregnancy, children with active tuberculosis and those allergic to egg proteins, neomycin or kanamycin.

Influenza Vaccine

It is available as highly purified absorbed, bivalent influenza vaccine. It contains antigens from inactivated influenza virus A and virus B. It produces active immunity within 2 to 3 weeks. A single dose of 0.5 mL SC or IM gives protection for 6 months in adults. Children need two doses 4 to 6 weeks apart. It can produce allergic reactions and polyneuritis.

Rabies Vaccine (Antirabies Vaccine)

It is the killed/inactivated rabies virus vaccine. It is of three different types, *viz.* nervous tissue vaccine, purified chick embryo cell (PCEC) vaccine and human diploid cell vaccine (HDCV).

1. **Nervous tissue vaccine:** In it, the virus is obtained from infected animals (sheep and rabbit) brain. It is cheap. It is the oldest variety of rabies vaccine still in use. It is administered SC in the abdominal wall in the dose of 2 to 5 mL for 14 days. The injection site should be changed with every dose and the patient is instructed to avoid fatigue provoking activities. It produces active immunity for about 3 months. It is, however, incomplete and unpredictable. It can produce local induration, erythema, lympadenopathy and neuroparalytic com-plications (polyneuritis, myelitis and ence-phalomyelitis).

2. **Purified chick embryo cell vaccine:** It is obtained by growing the virus in primary cultures of chick fibroblasts. It is available in ampoule (RABIPUR) of 1 mL containing 2.5 IU. It is administered IM in the dose of 1 mL for 6 doses on 0, 3, 7, 14, 30 and 90 days (presuming the day of dog bite is day 0). It gives a very high degree of protection against rabies. It can produce mild adverse effects like local reaction, fever and allergic reactions.

3. **Human diploid cell vaccine:** It is obtained from human fibroblast culture and gives a better antibody response than the older vaccines. It produces long-lasting imm-unity. Moreover, it is free from serious adverse effects. It is now considered as the

vaccine of choice in rabies. It is available as MERIEUX rabies vaccine (MIRV) containing 2.5 IU per mL ampoule. It is administered IM in the dose of 1 mL for 3 doses on 0, 7 and 28 days. Booster (reinforcing) doses can be given every 2 to 3 years in those who continue to be at risk. There is no contraindication of this rabies vaccine.

Hepatitis-B Vaccine (Engerix-B)

It contains inactivated B virus surface antigen (HBs Ag). It is now prepared biosynthetically from yeast cells using recombinant DNA technology. Active immunity against the infection develops after 6 months and lasts for 5 to 7 years. Hence for immediate protection, specific hepatitis-B immunoglobulin should be used. Hepatitis-B virus (HBV) has many antigens, of which hepatitis-B surface antigen (HBs Ag) formerly called Australian antigen is very important. When it is introduced into the body of the host, it stimulates the production of corresponding antibody called anti-HBs. The vaccine is indicated in high risk persons. It is administered IM in the dose of 1 mL and repeated one month and 6 months later. It is quite safe and produces minimum adverse effects.

Smallpox Vaccine (Vaccine Lymph)

It contains live attenuated virus of vaccinia. It is now not available for use in clinical practice: Routine smallpox vaccination was abandoned in 1971 due to complete eradication of smallpox in India.

II. Bacterial Vaccines

Typhoid Vaccine

There are two types of typhoid vaccine, *viz.* oral typhoid vaccine and polysaccharide typhoid vaccine. Oral typhoid vaccine (Typhoral) is a live attenuated vaccine of typhoid-*Ty 21a* strain of *Salmonella typhi*, which is nonpathogenic. It has antigenicity but no virulence. It is administered orally as enteric coated capsule. One capsule is given one hour before meal on days 1, 3 and 5 irrespective of age (every alternate day for 3 days) every three years as immunity persists for three years. The bacilli released from the capsule are taken by peyer's patches of intestine and multiply producing local (intestinal) immunity forming IgA antibodies, which prevent the pathogenic *S. typhi* to invade the intestine. The antibodies on being absorbed into the circulation give rise to active humoral immunity against *S. typhi*. It is safe and convenient but is costly. It can produce mild abdominal pain, diarrhoea, skin rash and fever. It is contraindicated in existing active disease, immunosuppressed patients, acute febrile conditions and diarrhoea. Polysaccharide typhoid vaccine (Typhim Vi) is prepared from purified Vi capsular polysaccharide of *S. typhi*. It is administered in the dose of 0.5 mL SC or IM. It produces immunity for at least three years. It can produce local pain, swelling and fever. It does not give protection against *S. paratyphi* A and B.

Typhoid-Paratyphoid A and B Vaccine (TAB Vaccine)

It is a suspension of heat killed *S. typhi* and *S. paratyphi* A and B. Children below three years do not require primary immunization with this vaccine, as typhoid and paratyphoid fevers are rare in these children. It is used in 2 doses of 0.5 mL and 1 mL respectively at 2 to 4 weeks interval. Booster doses are given once in three years in endemic areas. It can produce local pain, swelling and fever.

Cholera Vaccine

It is a suspension of heat killed strains of *Vibrio cholerae*. It is administered SC or IM in the doses of 0.5 mL followed by 1 mL at 1 to 4 weeks interval. Immunity appears within 7 to 10 days and lasts for 3 to 6 months. It can produce local pain and low grade fever for 1 to 2 days.

BCG Vaccine

Bacillus Calmette-Guérin is a strain of bovine tubercle bacillus with greatly attenuated virulence. This live vaccine was developed in France by Calmette and Guerin. It increases the patient's resistance to tuberculosis by producing artificial primary tuberculosis infection with an organism which causes only a local lesion and swelling of adjacent lymph nodes. Before vaccination, a tuberculin test is carried out by intradermal injection of five test units of purified protein derivative (PPD) obtained from the *Mycobacterium tuberculosis*. If the test is negative, then 0.1 mL of BCG vaccine is injected intradermally in the deltoid region. It produces the formation of a papule followed by an ulcer within 4 to 6 weeks. Gradually healing of the ulcer occurs but the papule may be detectable up to a period of one year. After vaccination, the tuberculin test becomes positive within 6 to 12 weeks indicating the development of immunity against tuberculosis.

Ideally BCG vaccine should be given within first six months of life. Pretesting with PPD is not necessary if BCG vaccine is given immediately after birth. It is the safest vaccine among vaccines in current use. It can be administered even in tuberculin positive children, in which the reaction may be accelerated.

III. Toxoids

Tetanus Toxoid

It is a detoxified preparation (by formaldehyde) of *Clostridium tetani* produced exotoxin. It is available in two forms, *viz.* purified toxoid aluminium hydroxide and purified toxoid aluminium phosphate. It produces greater and longer-lasting immunity than that obtained with tetanus antitoxin. It has markedly reduced the incidence of tetanus. For primary immunization, it is administered either alone or with diphtheria and whooping cough (pertussis) antigens (toxoids) within the first year but after three months of age. When used alone it is administered SC or IM in 3 doses of 0.5 mL on 0, 1 and 2 months (at one month intervals). A booster (reinforcement) dose of 0.5 mL may be given five years after the 3rd dose. It is available as 0.5 mL in ampoule, 5 mL vial and 10 mL vial. It can rarely produce allergic reactions.

Diphtheria Toxoid

It is a detoxified preparation (by formaldehyde) of *Corynebacterium diphtheriae* produced exotoxin. It produces active immunity against diphtheria. It has markedly reduced the incidence and severity of diphtheria. It is absorbed on aluminium hydroxide. It is available in combination with tetanus and pertussis antigens (triple antigen, DTP) or with tetanus antigen (double antigen, DT). Primary immunization is done by administration of 3 doses (0.5 mL each) of triple antigen (DTP) on 6, 10 and 14 weeks. A booster dose (0.5 mL) given at 18 months of age. Again at five years a booster dose (0.5 mL) of double antigen (DT) is given. It can produce local reactions, formation of nodules and cysts and fever.

Triple Antigen (Trip Vac)

It is a mixture of toxoids of diphtheria, tetanus and pertussis (DTP). It is available as 0.5 in ampoule. It is given in the dose of 0.5 mL SC or IM to actively immunize all children at 6, 10 and 14 weeks of age. A booster dose is given at 18 months of age. It can cause fever, irritability and loss of appetite in children. It is contraindicated during acute febrile illness and in children with history of convulsions or epilepsy.

Double Antigen (Dual Vac)

It is a mixture of toxoids of diphtheria and tetanus (DT). It is available as 0.5 mL in ampoule. It is given in the dose of 0.5 mL SC or IM at the age of five years (preschool) and in younger children where pertussis vaccine is contraindicated as a substitute of triple antigen. It has adverse effects and contraindications like triple antigen.

IV. Antisera

Diphtheria Antitoxin (ADS)

It is a serum preparation obtained from horses, which have been actively immunized against *C. diphtheriae* toxins. It contains the antitoxin globulins that have the power of neutralizing the toxin of these organisms. It has a potency of 1000 IU per mL. It neutralizes the diphtheria toxin locally at the site of infection and also that circulating in the blood, but it cannot neutralize the toxin fixed to the tissues and it does not reverse the pathological changes already produced by the toxin. It is also given in Schick positive persons who are in contact with diphtheria patients. It is available as 1000 IU and 20,000 IU in 5 mL and 10 mL ampoules.

Prophylactic dose: 500 to 1000 IU IM or SC.

Therapeutic dose: 20,000 to 40,000 IU IM and partly IV.

It can cause allergic reactions, vasovagal attacks, fever, serum sickness and anaphylactic shock.

Tetanus Antitoxin (ATS)

It is a serum preparation obtained from horses, which have been actively immunized against *Cl. tetani* toxins. It contains the antitoxin globulins, which neutralize tetanus toxin. It is given in contaminated wounds of more than 12 hours duration. Wound excision and dressing of wound are also essential. It is available as 750; 1500; 5000; 10,000; 20,000 and 50,000 IU per ampoule or vial.

Prophylactic dose: 1500 to 3000 IU IM or SC.

Therapeutic dose: 50,000 to 100,000 IU IM and partly IV.

It can cause allergic reactions, fever, serum sickness and anaphylactic shock.

Gas Gangrene Antitoxin (AGS)

It is a polyvalent gas gangrene antitoxin containing antitoxins against *Cl. welchii, Cl. septicum* and *Cl. oedematiens*. It is available as 4000 IU/mL in 5 mL ampoule.

Prophylactic dose: 10,000 to 20,000 IU IM or SC.

Therapeutic dose: 30,000 to 75,000 IU IM or SC.

It has adverse reactions like tetanus antitoxin. Nowadays gas gangrene is treated by high dose of IV penicillin-G, excision and dressing of wound and hyperbaric oxygen therapy. Antitoxin is now rarely used.

Rabies Antiserum (ARS)

It is a hyperimmune horse serum containing the globulins that neutralize the rabies virus. It is usually given with rabies vaccine in patients who have received severe bites. It is available as 12 IU per mL in 5 mL ampoule. It is administered in the dose of 40 IU/kg IM and at the same time 400 IU is infiltered around the wound. It can produce severe allergic reactions and so rabies immune globulin is preferred to it.

Antisnake Venom Serum

Common poisonous snake bites are due to viper venom and elapid venom. Viper venom present in Russel's viper, saw scaled viper and daboia is cardiotoxic and elapid venom present in cobra, krait and mamba is neurotoxic, which causes muscle paralysis by neuromuscular blocking action. Lyophilized polyvalent antisnake venom serum (antivenin) is obtained from immunized horses. It contains purified antitoxin globulins that neutralize toxins present in the venom of poisonous snakes. It is reconstituted by adding 10 mL of distilled water. A sensitivity test is performed by injecting 0.1 mL of 1:10 diluted antivenom SC. If no reaction occurs within 30 minutes, then 20 to 40 mL of the antivenom is injected IV slowly (1 mL/mL) and repeated at intervals of 3 to 4 hours till symptoms of poisoning disappear. A total of 200 to 300 mL may be required in a patient depending upon the severity of bite. It can cause severe allergic reactions and anaphylactic shock. Hence, adrenaline injection is given SC or IM simultaneously. Glucocorticoid and antihistaminic injections may also be given prophylactically.

V. Immune Human Sera

Tetanus Immune Globulin

It is a sterile solution containing specific gammaglobulin prepared from human plasma having a high titre of tetanus antitoxin.

It is obtained from plasma of hyperimmunized subjects with tetanus vaccine. As it is of human origin, it produces less allergic reactions than tetanus antitoxin obtained from the animal. It has plasma half-life of 3 to 4 weeks.

Prophylactic dose: 250 to 500 IU IM.

Therapeutic dose: 5,000 to 10,000 IU IV.

Active immunization with tetanus toxoid should be carried out simultaneously.

Rabies Immune Globulin

It is prepared from plasma of donors hyperimmunized with the rabies vaccine. It is preferred than rabies antitoxin due to minimum toxicity. It is used in all persons with known or suspected exposure to rabies virus and is given along with rabies vaccine. The dose is 20 IU/kg IM or IV.

Human Anti-D (Rho) Immunoglobulin (Rhesuman, Rhiggal)

It is prepared from pooled plasma of naturally immunized women with high titre of anti-D antibodies. In a Rh negative woman with a Rh positive husband, if the foetus is Rh positive, the foetal erythrocytes may escape into the maternal circulation across the placenta, commonly during delivery or rarely during pregnancy causing maternal rhesus immunization. This antigen on RBCs may cause erythroblastosis foetalis in the subsequent pregnancy. In order to neutralize this antigen before, it causes maternal rhesus immunization and to prevent erythroblastosis foetalis in subsequent pregnancies, it is necessary to give a dose of Rho (D) Ig 500 units within 72 hours of delivery. Antenatal dose at 28 weeks of pregnancy is now recommended. It is also used after abortion. It is available as lyophilized powder in 100, 250 and 350 units vials along with water for injection. Its side effects are mild and rare. It is contraindicated in Rh positive women and in Rh negative women who develop Rh antibodies because of a previous conception or transfusion of Rh positive blood.

Human Immunoglobulins (Igs)

Plasma protein can be fractionated into four important components, *viz.* albumin and α-, β- and γ-globulins. γ-globulin carries antibodies and is known as human normal immunoglobulin (HNI). It is obtained from serum of pooled human adult blood, which is known as immune serum. It consists of IgG (95%) and small amounts of other Igs (IgM and IgA). More selective type of α-globulin against a particular infection can be obtained from the blood of individuals convalescing from that disease or from the blood of individuals recently immunized against that disease. The Ig obtained in this way is called hyperimmune serum or human specific immunoglobulin.

Clinical Uses

It is used for prophylactic and therapeutic purposes. It is administered IM or IV. It is indicated in:

- Patients suffering from hypogammaglobulinaemia (when serum γ-globulin concentration is 200 mg or less). Normal serum α-globulin concentration varies between 600–1500 mg per 100 mL. In it, HNI is administered in the dose of 0.025 to 0.05 g per kg body weight at weekly intervals for prolonged period.
- Diseases like measles and rubella (for prophylaxis), infective hepatitis (for treatment), mumps and poliomyelitis (for prophylaxis) and diphtheria (for prophylaxis and treatment). In these diseases HNI is administered in the dose of 250 to 750 mg IM or IV.

Specific immunoglobulins are available for tetanus, rabies and hepatitis-B.

Preparation

Human normal immunoglobulin (Gamafine) injection (10% 1 mL).

Adverse Reactions

It can cause pain at the site of injection. Allergic reactions can also occur. It may produce fever, nausea, flushing, shivering and joint pain and rarely bronchospasm, hypotension and collapse.

Section V

MISCELLANEOUS DRUGS

81

Vitamins

INTRODUCTION

Vitamins are organic substances that must be provided in small quantities from the environment because they cannot be synthesized in the body or their rate of synthesis is inadequate for the maintenance of nutrition and health of mammals (e.g. the production of nicotinic acid from tryptophan). The environment source of most vitamins is the diet, except the endogenous synthesis of vitamin D under the influence of ultraviolet light. Some vitamins (e.g. B complex group) are synthesized by intestinal bacteria (gut flora) but they are little utilized.

Vitamin deficiency leads to characteristics symptoms and signs. The deficiency can be primary type (due to inadequate diet) or secondary type (due to malabsorption and chronic diarrhoea or due to increased metabolic need during pregnancy, lactation and childhood). Vitamins in pure forms are used during vitamin deficiencies or diseases associated with their deficiency. All vitamins are well-absorbed from GIT.

Classification of Vitamins

These are of two groups:

1. Fat-soluble vitamins, e.g. vitamins A, D, E and K.
2. Water-soluble vitamins, e.g. vitamin B complex (thiamine, riboflavin, nicotinic acid, nicotinamide, pantothenic acid, pyridoxine, biotin, choline, inositol, carnitine, folic acid and cyanocobalamin) and vitamin C (ascorbic acid).

The individual vitamins differ widely in structure and function. Fat-soluble vitamins are stored in the body for prolonged period and are liable to cause hypervitaminosis (cumulative toxicity) after regular consumption of large amounts. On the other hand, water-soluble vitamins are stored in the body to only a limited extent and so frequent consumption is necessary to maintain saturation of tissues.

As consumed, many vitamins are not biologically active and require processing in the body (*in vivo*). In the case of several water-soluble vitamins (e.g. thiamine, riboflavin, nicotinic acid and pyridoxine) activation includes phosphorylation and also may require coupling to purine or pyrimidine nucleotides (e.g. riboflavin and nicotinic acid). In their major actions, water-soluble vitamins participate as cofactors for specific enzymes, whereas two fat-soluble vitamins (A and D) behave like hormones and interact with specific intracellular receptors in their target tissues.

DISCUSSION OF INDIVIDUAL VITAMINS

I. Fat-soluble Vitamins

Vitamin A (Anti-infective Vitamin)

Chemistry and Source

It is a long chain alcohol related to β-carotene. It occurs in nature in two forms:

1. *Retinol (vitamin A₁):* Present in fish liver oil (cod, shark and halibut fishes).
2. *Dehydroretinol (vitamin A₂):* Present in freshwater fishes and green plants like carrot, turnip, spinach and cabbage. It is inactive as such (provitamin A). One molecule of it splits into two molecules of retinol.

Daily requirement of vitamin A (in adult male): 1000 µg (4000 IU), 1 µg of retinol is equivalent to 3.3 IU of vitamin A activity, i.e. 1 IU of vitamin A = 0.3 µg of retinol.

Physiological Functions/Pharmacological Actions

It is essential for the functioning of retina (normal vision), integrity of the epithelial cells/tissues and for bone growth and reproduction. It forms part of the light-sensitive protein 'rhodopsin' (visual purple) present in the rods of retina, which are sensitive to light of low intensity. It is involved in the phenomenon of dark adaptation (visual cycle).

Bleaching of rhodopsin leads to generation of visual nerve impulse. Rhodopsin is very quickly resynthesized from opsin and retinal. A similar pigment (iodopsin) is synthesized in the cones of retina, which are sensitive to light of high intensity (bright light), colour, vision and primary dark adaptation. In vitamin A deficiency rods are affected more than cones. Prolonged deficiency of vitamin A causes night blindness (nyctalopia) due to irreversible structural changes of rods and cones in retina. It promotes differentiation and maintains structural integrity of epithelial tissues all over the body. It also promotes mucus secretion, inhibits keratinization of skin and improves resistance to infection. It promotes bone growth and foetal development. It also maintains spermatogenesis.

Deficiency States

It produces following changes:
- Xerosis (dryness) of eye, Bitot' s spot, keratomalacia (softening of cornea), corneal opacity and night blindness leading to total blindness.
- Dry and rough skin with papules (toad skin), hyperkeratinization of skin and atrophy of sweat glands.
- Keratinization of bronchopulmonary epithelium and increased susceptibility to infection.
- Atrophy of gastrointestinal mucosa leading to diarrhoea.
- Shedding of epithelial lining of urinary tract leading to increased tendency of urinary stone formation.
- Growth retardation and foetal malformation.
- Sterility due to faulty spermatogenesis and abortion in female.

Clinical Uses

It has prophylactic and therapeutic uses.

Prophylactic uses: During infancy, pregnancy and lactation and in hepatobiliary diseases and steatorrhoea.

Therapeutic uses: In established vitamin A deficiency diseases and for the treatment of acne vulgaris and other skin diseases (applied topically).

Preparations and Dosage

- Vitamin A (Aquasol A) capsule (50,000 IU), injection (100,000 IU in 2 mL ampoule).
- Vitamin A (Arovit) tablet (50,000 IU)/ injection (100,000 IU in 2 mL) and drops (150,000 IU/mL).

  Prophylactic dose: 3000 to 5000 IU/day.
  Therapeutic dose: 10,000 to 50,000 IU/day.

- Topical preparations of vitamin A are tretinonin (retinoic acid) and isotretinonin (isoretinoic acid).
- Combined vitamin A and D preparations.

Sea fish liver oil (Adexolin) capsule (5000 IU of vitamin A and 400 IU of vitamin D) and liquid (9000 IU/mL of vitamin A and 720 IU/mL of vitamin D).

Adverse Reactions

Excessive intake or high dose of vitamin A especially in children can cause hypervitaminosis-A (cumulative toxicity), which is manifested as anorexia, vomiting, headache, dry hair, loss of hair, rough skin, dermatitis, exfoliation of skin, enlarged liver and spleen (hepatosplenomegaly), bony exostosis, anaemia and oedema.

Treatment

Withdrawal of vitamin A and administration of vitamin E, which causes deposition of vitamin A in tissues.

Vitamin D (Antirachitic Vitamin)

Chemistry and Source

Vitamin D has steroid ring and is considered as a prohormone, which is biotransformed into a number of physiologically active metabolites which function as hormones. It is obtained from two sources, namely vitamin D_2 (ergocalciferol) derived by ultraviolet radiation of ergosterol in plants and vitamin D_3 (cholecalciferol) derived from 7-dehydrocholesterol in skin by ultraviolet irradiation. Cholecalciferol is converted to 25-hydroxycholecalciferon (25-OHD or calcifediol) in the liver and is then converted to 1,25-dihydroxy vitamin D_3 (calcitriol) in the kidney. Calcifediol is the main vitamin D derivative found in circulation and may represent the storage form of the hormone. Calcitriol is the active hormone, whose renal synthesis from calcifediol is regulated by parathormone and plasma levels of phosphate. Synthetic vitamin D derivatives, e.g. alfacalcidol and dihydrotachysterol are also available. These are biotransformed into calcitriol in the liver.

Daily requirement (in adult male):

Ergocalciferol (vitamin D_2)—5 µg (200 IU).

Cholecalciferol (vitamin D_3)—1 µg (40 IU).

Physiological Functions/Pharmacological Actions

The main action of vitamin D is to increase plasma calcium levels by following mechanisms:

- Stimulation of calcium absorption from GIT: Calcitriol stimulates the synthesis of carrier proteins, which bind calcium and transport it across gastrointestinal mucosa.
- Stimulation of bone reabsorption: Calcitriol mobilizes calcium from bones and exerts synergistic effect with parathormone.
- Increase in renal tubular reabsorption of calcium: Calcitriol enhances proximal tubular reabsorption of both calcium and phosphate in the kidney. Increased phosphate reabsorption is decreased by the phosphate excreting effect of parathormone.

Deficiency States

It produces rickets in children and osteomalacia in adults (especially in pregnant and lactating mothers). The growing metaphyseal cartilage and osteoid tissue are not calcified leading to rickets. Epiphysis is swollen, line of calcification disappears, bones are soft and spongy and bend under body weight. In osteomalacia, decreased bone density and gross bone deformities are produced.

Therapeutic Uses

It is used in:

- Rickets and osteomalacia for prevention and treatment.
- Hypoparathyroidism (characterized by hypocalcaemia and hypophosphataemia) for treatment.
- Vitamin D deficiency secondary to malabsorption syndrome, liver disease and chronic renal disease for treatment.
- Osteoporosis including senile and postmenopausal osteoporosis for prevention and treatment.
- Fanconi's syndrome characterized by hypophosphataemia. It raises lowered plasma phosphate levels.

Preparations and Dosage

- Many preparations containing vitamin D are available: Ergocalciferol (Calciferol, Drisdol) is pure vitamin D_2 and is available for oral and intramuscular administration. Dihydrotachysterol (DHT, Hytakerol) is a pure crystalline compound obtained from vitamin D_2 and is available for oral administration. Calcifediol (Calderol) and calcitriol (Rocaltrol) are available for oral administration.

- Liquid contains 300,000 IU/mL and injection contains 600,000 IU/mL ampoule (in Drisdol/Ostelinf orte).

  Prophylactic dose: 500 to 1000 IU/day.

  Therapeutic dose: 3000 to 4000 IU/day.

Adverse Reactions

Administration of large dose of vitamin D (exceeding 10,000 IU/day) for prolonged period (10 to 14 weeks) can produce hypervitaminosis-D, which is manifested as hypercalcaemia (producing drowsiness, nausea, abdominal pain and anorexia), osteoporosis, ectopic calcification, renal damage and renal stone.

Treatment

Withdrawal of vitamin D and administration of glucocorticoids and large fluid intake.

Vitamin E (Antisterility Vitamin)

Chemistry and Source

It is alpha tochopherol. It is present in vegetable oils, wheat germ, cereals, spinach, nuts, legumes, egg yolk and milk.

Daily requirement (in adult male): 10 to 20 mg.

Physiological Functions/Pharmacological Actions

It is necessary for normal reproduction. It is an intracellular antioxidant that acts as a cytoprotective agent. As an antioxidant it prevents oxidation of essential cellular constituents or prevents the formation of toxic oxidation products such as the peroxidation products formed from unsaturated fatty acids that have been detected in its absence. There is a relationship between vitamin A and vitamin D. The intestinal absorption of vitamin A is increased by vitamin E, hepatic and other cellular concentrations of vitamin A are elevated. This effect may be related to the protection of vitamin A by antioxidant properties of vitamin E. It also protects the various effects of hypervitaminosis A.

Deficiency States

In adults, the incidence of vitamin E deficiency is rather rare because of adequate nutritional supply and considerable storage of the vitamin. The signs of vitamin E deficiency in children include enhanced hydrogen peroxide haemolysis, creatinuria and skeletal muscle disorders (flexia and gait disturbance). Its deficiency in animals produce sterility.

Therapeutic Uses

It is used in the treatment of muscular dystrophy, cardiomyopathy, nocturnal muscle cramps, sexual impotence and recurrent abortions. It is used prophylactically in atherosclerosis and certain types of cancers.

Preparations and Dosage

Vitamin E (Evion, Tocoper) capsule (100, 200, 400 mg)—200 to 400 mg daily.

Adverse Reactions

It is nontoxic even in large dose.

Vitamin K (Coagulation Vitamin)

It is discussed with coagulants in haematologic pharmacology.

II. Water-Soluble Vitamins

Vitamin B Complex

It consists of 12 vitamins.

Thiamine (Vitamin B_1)

Chemistry and source: It is a colourless crystalline compound containing a pyrimidine and a thiazole ring linked by a methylene bridge. It is present in the outer layer of cereals (rice polishings), pulses, nuts, green vegetables, yeast, egg and meat.

Daily requirement (in adult male): 1.5 to 2 mg.

Physiological functions: It is converted in the body to active form 'Thiamine pyrophosphate', which acts as a coenzyme in carbohydrate metabolism (in the decarboxylation of α-ketoacids such as pyruvate and α-ketoglutarate and in the utilization of pentose in the hexose monophosphate shunt, the latter function involves the thiamine pyrophosphate dependent enzyme transketolase). In thiamine deficiency, the oxidation of α-ketoacids is impaired and an increase in the concentration of pyruvate in the blood occurs.

Pharmacological actions: It is practically devoid of pharmacodynamic actions when given in usual therapeutic doses.

Deficiency states: Severe thiamine deficiency leads to the condition known as beriberi. The main symptoms of thiamine deficiency are related to the nervous system (dry beriberi) and to the cardiovascular system (wet beriberi). Dry beriberi is manifested as polyneuritis (peripheral neuritis) with numbness, tingling, hyperesthesia, muscular weakness and atrophy resulting in wrist drop, foot drop, paralysis of whole limb, mental changes, sluggishness, poor memory, loss of appetite and constipation. Wet beriberi is manifested as cardiovascular disorders like palpitation, breathlessness, high output cardiac failure and generalized anasarca.

Therapeutic uses

- It is used for the prevention and treatment of beriberi.
- It is also used in peripheral neuritis (occurring in pregnancy and chronic alcoholics and by drugs like isoniazid, pyrazinamide, etc.) and GIT disorders (like anorexia, chronic diarrhoea and ulcerative colitis).

Preparations and dosage

- Thiamine hydrochloride (Berin, Betabion) tablet (50, 100 mg)

Prophylactic dose: 2 to 8 mg/daily.

Therapeutic dose: 25 to 100 mg daily.

- Thiamine hydrochloride (Berin) injection (100 mg/mL in 10 mL vial).

Therapeutic dose: 100 mg/day IM or IV till symptoms regress and then continued in maintenance dose orally.

Adverse reactions: It is nontoxic, but in hypersensitive persons it may cause anaphylactic reaction when given parenterally.

Riboflavin (Vitamin B₂)

Chemistry and source: It is a yellow flavone compound. It is present in green leafy vegetables, whole grains, yeast, milk, cheese, egg and meat.

Daily requirement: 1.5 to 2 mg.

Physiological functions: It is converted in the body to 2 physiologically active forms: flavin mononucleotide (FMN) and flavin dinucleotide (FAD), which act as coenzymes for a wide variety of respiratory flavoproteins (enzymes) concerned with tissue oxidation. Enzyme catalyzed reactions are:

Riboflavin + ATP→ FMN + ADP.

FMN + ATP→ FAD + PP (pyrophosphate).

Pharmacological actions: No overt pharmacological effects follow the oral or parenteral administration of riboflavin.

Deficiency states: Deficiency of riboflavin produces a syndrome called ariboflavinosis. It is manifested as angular stomatitis, glossitis, sore throat, cheilosis (burning sensation in mouth), seborrheic dermatitis of face, trunk and extremities, anaemia and neuropathy.

Therapeutic uses: It is used in the prevention and treatment of ariboflavinosis.

Preparations and dosage

- Riboflavin (Lipobol) tablet (20 mg).

Prophylactic dose: 5 to 10 mg daily.

Therapeutic dose: 20 to 50 mg daily.

- Riboflavin injection (10 mg/mL): 10 to 20 mg IM daily.

Adverse reactions: It is nontoxic.

Nicotinic Acid (Vitamin B₃)

Chemistry and source: It is a pyridine compound and its amide is nicotinamide (vitamin B₄). It is present in outer layer of cereals (rice polishings), nuts, pulses, fish, meat, liver and egg. Amino acid 'tryptophan' is regarded as provitamin B₃ as it is partly converted into nicotinic acid in the body.

Daily requirement: 13 to 20 mg.

Physiological functions: It is converted into nicotinamide in the body. The active forms of nicotinamide are nicotinamide adenine dinucleotide (NAD) and nicotinamide adenine dinucleotide phosphate (NADP), which act as coenzymes for a wide variety of enzymes, that catalyze oxidation-reduction reactions essential for tissue respiration.

Pharmacological actions: Nicotinic acid and nicotinamide are identical in their function as vitamins, but they differ in their pharmacological actions. Nicotinic acid but not nicotinamide in large dose is a vasodilator, particularly in skin vessels and lowers plasma lipid levels.

Deficiency states: Deficiency of nicotinic acid produces a syndrome called pellagra. It is manifested as dermatitis, diarrhoea and dementia. Tongue becomes very red, swollen and ulcerative. Anaemia and hypoproteinaemia also occur. Chronic alcoholics are particularly susceptible to develop pellagra.

Therapeutic uses

- It is used for prevention and treatment of pellagra.
- It is also used as a vasodilator in peripheral vascular diseases and as a hypolipoproteinaemic drug in atherosclerosis.

Preparations and dosage

- Nicotinic acid (Niacin) tablet (25, 50 mg). **Prophylactic dose:** 15 to 30 mg daily. **Curative dose:** 50 to 200 mg daily.
- Nicotinic acid injection (20 mg/mL)—20 to 50 mg daily.

Adverse reactions: It can cause flushing, urticaria, pruritus and fainting attack. Nicotinamide is nontoxic.

Pantothenic Acid (Vitamin B₅)

Chemistry and source: It is an organic acid. It is present in yeast, wheat, peanuts, cereals, milk and liver.

Daily requirement: 2 to 5 mg.

Physiological functions: It is converted in the body to active form coenzyme A, which serves as a cofactor for enzyme catalyzed reactions involving transfer of acetyl (2 carbon) groups in oxidative metabolism of carbohydrates, gluconeogenesis, synthesis and degradation of fatty acids and synthesis of steroids and porphyrins.

Pharmacological actions: It has no pharmacological actions even in large doses.

Deficiency states: It is uncommon in human beings. If it occurs it is manifested as fatigue, malaise, headache, paraesthesia and somnolence.

Therapeutic uses: It is used in the treatment of burning foot symptoms, postoperative paralytic ileus (intestinal atony) and streptomycin toxicity.

Preparations and dosage

- Calcium pantothenate tablet (50 mg)—50 to 100 mg daily.
- Calcium pantothenate injection (50 mg/2 mL)—100 to 200 mg IM or IV.

Adverse reactions: It is nontoxic.

Pyridoxine (Vitamin B₆)

Chemistry and source: It is a pyridine compound. It is present in meat, egg, fish, milk, soyabeans, potatoes, wheat and cereals.

Daily requirement: 2 to 3 mg.

Physiological functions: It is converted in the body to the active form 'pyridoxal phosphate' (by pyridoxal kinase), which acts as a coenzyme in several metabolic transformations of amino acids, including decarboxylation, transamination and racemization, as well as in enzymatic steps in the metabolism of sulphur-containing hydroxyamino acids. It is involved in the metabolism of tryptophan (conversion of tryptophan to 5-HT) and methionine (conversion of methionine to cysteine). It is also required for the synthesis of dopamine, histamine, GABA and delta-aminolevulinic acid (a precursor of heme) and for conversion of linolenic acid to arachidonic acid.

Pharmacological actions: It does not produce outstanding pharmacodynamic actions after oral or parenteral administration.

Deficiency states: Deficiency of pyridoxine produces seborrheic dermatitis, stomatitis, glossitis, nervous irritability, convulsions, vomiting, peripheral neuritis, carpal tunnel syndrome and microcytic hypochromic anaemia.

Therapeutic uses

- It is used for the prevention and treatment of pyridoxine deficiency states.
- It is also used in morning sickness, hyper-emesis gravidarum, convulsive seizures in children and in drug induced (by isoniazid, cycloserine, hydrallazine, etc.) peripheral neuritis (as it is an antineurotic vitamin).

Preparations and dosage

- Pyridoxine tablet (10 mg)

  Prophylactic dose: 10 mg daily.

  Therapeutic dose: 30 to 100 mg daily.

- Pyridoxine hydrochloride injection (50 mg/ 2 mL): 50 mg IM.

Adverse reactions: It is nontoxic.

Biotin (Vitamin B_7)

Chemistry and source: It is a sulphur-containing organic acid. It is present in organ meats, egg yolk, milk, fish and nuts.

Daily requirement: 100 to 300 μg.

Physiological functions: It is a cofactor for the enzymatic carboxylation of pyruvate, acetyl CoA, propionyl CoA and β-methyl crotonyl CoA. It plays an important role in both carbohydrate and fat metabolism.

Deficiency states: Its deficiency can produce dermatitis, atrophic glossitis, hyperesthesia, muscle pain, lassitude, anorexia, alopecia and mild anaemia.

Therapeutic uses: It has been used in the treatment of infantile seborrhea and in the condition of genetic abnormality of biotin-dependent enzymes in the dose of 5 to 10 mg orally daily.

Adverse reactions: It is nontoxic.

Choline (Vitamin B_8)

Chemistry and source: It is trimethyl ethanolamine. It is present in egg yolk, legumes, organ meats, milk and whole grain cereals.

Daily requirement: 200 to 500 mg.

Physiological functions: It is a precursor of acetylcholine. It is a part of lecithin. It has an important role in the transport of fat. It is a source of labile methyl groups.

Deficiency states: Its deficiency has not been demonstrated in humans. Its deficiency in rats causes fatty liver and renal degeneration.

Therapeutic uses: It has been used in the treatment of fatty liver and hepatic cirrhosis in the dose of 150 to 300 mg/kg/day orally.

Adverse reactions: It is nontoxic.

Inositol (Vitamin B_9)

Chemistry and source: It is a hexahydroxy-cyclohexane, an isomer of glucose. It is present in whole grain cereals, milk, fruits and vegetables.

Daily requirement: Unknown.

Physiological functions: It is present in the form of phosphatidylinositol in phospholipids of cell membranes and plasma lipoproteins. Inositol triphosphate (IP_3) functions as an intracellular second messenger by stimulating the release of Ca^{2+} from intracellular stores.

Deficiency states: nIts deficiency in rats can cause alopecia, retarded growth and impaired lactation.

Therapeutic uses: It has been used for the treatment of diseases associated with disturbances in the transport and metabolism of fat.

Adverse reactions: It is nontoxic.

Carnitine (Vitamin B_{10})

Chemistry and sources: It is β-hydroxy-γ-trimethylammonium butyrate. It is present in meat and dairy products.

   Daily requirement: Unknown.

Physiological functions: It is important for oxidation of fatty acids. It also facilitates the aerobic metabolism of carbohydrate. It enhances the rate of oxidative phosphorylation.

Deficiency states: Its deficiency can produce functional abnormalities of cardiac and skeletal muscles.

Therapeutic uses: It is used in the treatment of systemic carnitine deficiency in the dose of 1 to 2 g/day in divided doses orally.

Adverse reactions: It is nontoxic.

Ascorbic Acid (Vitamin C)

Chemistry and source: It is a six carbon ketolactone, structurally related to glucose and other hexoses. It is a reducing agent and *l*-form is biologically active. It is present in fruits and fresh vegetables. Citrus fruits (lemon and orange) and black currants are the richest sources. Human milk contains more vitamin C than cow's milk.

   Daily requirement: 50 to 100 mg.

Physiological functions: It functions as a cofactor in a number of hydroxylation and amidation reactions by transferring electrons to enzymes that provide reducing equivalents.

Thus, it is required for or facilitates the conversion of certain proline and lysine residues in procollagen to hydroxyproline and hydroxylysine in the course of collagen synthesis, the oxidation of lysine side chains in proteins to provide hydroxytrimethyllysine for carnitine synthesis, the conversion of folic acid to folinic acid, microsomal drug metabolism and the hydroxylation of dopamine to form noradrenaline. It is involved in the synthesis of adrenal steroids and catecholamines and in the metabolism of cyclic nucleotides and prostaglandins. It directly stimulates collagen synthesis and is very important for maintenance of intracellular connective tissue. Normal wound healing and capillary integrity are dependent on vitamin C. It is an antioxidant and protects vitamins A and E and polyunsaturated fatty acids.

Pharmacological actions: It possesses low pharmacological actions.

Deficiency states: Deficiency of vitamin C causes scurvy, which is manifested as swollen and bleeding gums, increased capillary fragility, petechial and subperiosteal haemorrhage, deformed teeth, brittle bones, impaired wound healing, anaemia and growth retardation.

Therapeutic uses: It is used for prevention and treatment of scurvy, to promote wound healing, in iron deficiency anaemia, as urinary acidifier (4 to 8 g/day) and to increase body resistance in common cold and cancer.

Preparations and dosage: It is available as tablet, injection and liquid preparations (Suckcee, Limcee, Celin).

   Prophylactic dose: 50 to 100 mg daily.

   Therapeutic dose: 1 to 2 g daily.

Adverse reactions: It is nontoxic.

82

Minerals

INTRODUCTION

Minerals are chemical elements or compounds occurring naturally as a product of inorganic processes. About 5% of body weight of human beings is made up of minerals. They serve as essential nutrients in the body. They are divided into two groups:

1. Essential macronutrients (required in large amounts), e.g. calcium, magnesium, phosphorous, sodium, potassium, chloride and sulphur.
2. Essential micronutrients (required in small amounts), e.g. iron, manganese, copper, cobalt, zinc, iodide, fluoride and silver.

DISCUSSION OF SOME ESSENTIAL MINERALS

Calcium (Ca)

Source

Milk and milk products, green leafy vegetables and cereals are rich sources of calcium. Drinking water contains calcium salts and contributes to the calcium intake. Daily requirement:

- Adults and infants—500 to 600 mg/day.
- Pregnant women and growing children—600 to 700 mg/day.

Distribution in the Body

An adult human body weighing 70 kg contains about 1.2 to 1.4 kg of calcium. About 99% of the body calcium is present in bones, 1% in the soft tissues and 0.1% in the body fluids. In the bone (skeleton), calcium is present mostly as crystalline hydroxyapatite and to a small extent as noncrystalline phosphates and carbonates. Intracellular calcium constitutes about 1% of body calcium and has vital function as a second messenger regulating a variety of intracellular enzymes. The plasma calcium concentrations vary from 8.5 to 10.5 mg/dL, of which 50% remains as free ionized calcium (Ca^{2+}) and the rest is bound to plasma proteins (40%) and various anions (10%). The plasma calcium concentration is held within a narrow homeostatic range by parathormone, calcitonin and calcitriol (derived from vitamin D). Extracellular calcium is important for the maintenance of electrical excitability of nerves, skeletal muscles and cardiac muscle, formation of bone and teeth and coagulation of blood.

Pharmacokinetics

In adults, the average daily intake of calcium is about 800 mg. Of this, only 40% is absorbed by active transport process from the proximal part of small intestine with the help of a calcium binding protein in the cells of the mucosal villi, the level of which is regulated by calcitriol, the active metabolite of vitamin D. Calcium is also absorbed by passive diffusion from the distal part of small intestine. Absorption of calcium is stimulated physiologically by the parathormone, vitamin D, an acid residue in the intestine and a high protein diet. It is also stimulated by deficient calcium intake and calcium deficiency *via* hypocalcaemia. Calcium absorption is reduced by an excess of phosphates, oxalates (from vegetables), phytates (from cereals) and fatty acids (in patient with steatorrhoea) in the diet. Calcium is excreted in faeces, urine and sweat. The total amount of calcium secreted in the intestinal tract is about 200 mg daily, of which 130 mg is excreted in faeces. 99% of calcium filtered by the kidney is reabsorbed from the renal tubules in the absence of vitamin D. 1% reabsorption is under the influence of vitamin D and parathormone. Calcitonin inhibits proximal tubular reabsorption of calcium and increases its urinary excretion.

There is no tubular secretion of calcium. Daily urinary excretion of calcium varies from 80 to 160 mg. A rise in plasma ionic calcium from any cause (hyperparathyroidism, hypervitaminosis D, excessive bone reabsorption or bone destruction), produces a larger load of calcium to the renal tubules leading to increased urinary excretion of calcium (about 500 mg/day). There is significant excretion of calcium in sweat and milk.

Physiological Functions/Pharmacological Actions

- It is necessary for excitation contraction coupling and force of the muscular contractions (contractility).
- It is an important factor for proper development of action potential in the myocardium.
- It is necessary for proper neuromuscular excitability.
- It acts as a second messenger in the molecular level action of many hormones.
- It is necessary for the release of many neurotransmitters from their respective neurons.
- It is necessary for coagulation of blood (for conversion of prothrombin to thrombin).
- It is necessary for proper formation of bone and teeth. Calcium deficiency during intrauterine life and during the extrauterine

growth period leads to delayed and defective dentition and poor bone formation.

A negative calcium balance leads to osteoporosis (a bone disorder in which bones are normal in chemical composition but the total bone mass is reduced).

Clinical Conditions

1. Hypercalcaemia (high calcium level in blood)

Common causes: Hyperparathyroidism, hypervitaminosis D, milk alkali syndrome, prolonged immobilization, chronic thiazide therapy and sarcoidosis.

Clinical features: Lethargy, anorexia, weakness, muscular hypotonia, nausea, vomiting and severe constipation. Kidneys show inability to concentrate the urine and polyuria and dehydration may occur. Heart may show irregularities. Excess calcium is deposited in various tissues (arteries, cornea, muscles and kidneys). Mental changes may also occur.

Treatment

- Correction of dehydration by administration of normal saline.
- Administration of a diuretic like frusemide (80 mg IM every four hours) to increase calcium excretion in urine.
- Administration of a corticosteroid like prednisolone (20 to 40 mg/day orally) to reduce calcium absorption.
- Administration of a chelating agent like disodium edetate (30 g in 20 mL) IV to chelate calcium in blood.

2. Hypocalcaemia (low calcium level in blood)

Common causes: Vitamin D deficiency, vitamin D resistance, hypoparathyroidism and chronic renal failure.

Clinical features: Increased neuromuscular irritability with paraesthesia, tetany, convulsions and laryngeal spasm. Hypoplasia of teeth and atrophy of skin and nails may occur.

Treatment

- Administration of a calcium salt like calcium gluconate (10 to 20 mL of 10% solution IV slowly at the rate of 2 mL/minute) or calcium laevulinate (10 mL of 10% of solution IM or IV) or calcium chloride hydrate (6 to 2 g through IV drip).
- After plasma calcium level has been stabilized, oral calcium preparations, namely calcium lactate, calcium gluconate or calcium glubionate (1 to 2 g daily) can be administered.

Absorption of orally administered calcium can be increased by concurrent administration of vitamin D.

Intravenous calcium is contraindicated in digitalized patients as it exerts synergistic effect and potentiates digitalis toxicity.

Therapeutic Uses

- To prevent or correct calcium deficiency as in:
  - Growing children, pregnant women and lactating mothers.
  - Individuals with diets deficient in calcium or excessive loss of calcium in urine.
  - Patients with osteoporosis (postmenopausal or due to Cushing's syndrome).
  - Patients on long-term corticosteroid therapy.
  - Patients with vitamin D deficiency (rickets and osteomalacia). Here oral calcium salts are used.
- As an antacid, e.g. calcium carbonate.
- In the treatment of tetany and lead colic and to counteract the systemic effects of magnesium salts and hypocalcaemia. Here calcium gluconate or chloride is administered IV.
- As phosphate binders—oral calcium carbonate and calcium citrate are used as phosphate binders (in presence of aluminium hydroxide) in chronic renal failure.
- In the treatment of urticaria and nonspecific intestinal colic—an oral calcium salt may be used.

Adverse Reactions

Oral calcium salts produce constipation, hypercalcaemia (in milk alkali syndrome) and rarely intestinal obstructions due to formation of calcium concretions. Calcium chloride is irritant by all routes and so rarely used. Extravasation of calcium salts during IV administration may lead to local sloughing. IV administration of calcium in digitalized patients can cause cardiac arrhythmias and cardiac arrest.

Magnesium (Mg)

Source

It is widely distributed in nature including plants and animals. Good dietary sources are nuts, vegetables, grains, chocolate, cocoa, fish and meat.

Daily requirement: 300 to 350 mg in adults.

Distribution in the body: The adult human body contains about 20 to 30 g of magnesium. Of this, about 55% is present in bones, 25% in muscles, 15% in nonmuscle soft tissues and body fluids, 1% in the extracellular fluid and 20% in intracellular fluid. The plasma magnesium concentrations vary from 1.8 to 2.4 mg/dL, of which 33% is bound to plasma proteins. Cardiac and skeletal muscles, liver, brain and kidneys contain greater amounts of magnesium.

Pharmacokinetics

Magnesium is absorbed to the extent of 1/3rd of dietary intake from the GIT by active transport. It competes with calcium for carrier sites. Therefore, a high intake of either one of them interferes with the absorption of the other. It is mainly excreted by the kidney by glomerular filtration. It is also excreted in faeces, saliva and milk. Parthormone is essential for both gastrointestinal and renal tubular reabsorption of magnesium. Only 3 to 5% of filtered magnesium appears in urine and the rest is reabsorbed. Renal impairment may cause magnesium retention leading to magnesium toxicity.

Physiological Functions/Pharmacological Actions

- It acts as a catalyst in several metabolic reactions. It is involved in the phosphorylation of glucose in anaerobic metabolism and oxidative decarboxylation in the citric acid cycle. It is a cofactor of enzymes like membrane ATPase involved in the oxidative phosphorylation of ADP to ATP and also for the enzymes that are involved in the transfer of phosphate from ATP to a phosphate acceptor. It is involved in the uptake and storage of catecholamines within the storage granules of adrenergic nerve endings. It is also involved in the activation of ribosomes by mRNA.
- It plays an important role in neuromuscular transmission and activity. It depresses myoneuronal transmission by reducing the quantal release of acetylcholine and by antagonizing its depolarizing effect at the motor end plate.
- It has depressant effect on all types of muscles. It produces peripheral vasodilatation.
- It is a CNS depressant and produces irritability, confusion and convulsions in low concentration.

Clinical Conditions

1. Hypomagnesemia (low magnesium level in blood)

Common causes: Severe diarrhoea malabsorption syndrome, chronic alcoholism, diabetic ketoacidosis, hyperthyroidism, hyperparathyroidism, diuretic therapy, aldosteronism and renal tubular acidosis.

Clinical features: Neuromuscular hyperirritability, mental disturbances (restlessness and aggressiveness), cardiac disturbances, involuntary movements (tremors), convulsions, nystagmus, dysphagia and rarely tetany can occur.

Treatment: Administration of a magnesium salt like magnesium sulphate (5 to 10 mL of 25% solution IV slowly or IM).

2. Hypermagnesemia (high magnesium level in blood)

Common causes: Unusual increase in absorption (in excess intake) and decrease in urinary excretion (in renal impairment).

Clinical features: Muscle weakness, hypotension, atrial fibrillation, drowsiness and a curare like effect at the myoneuronal junction (skeletal muscle relaxation).

Treatment: Administration of calcium salts like calcium gluconate (10 to 20 mL of 10% solution IV slowly).

Therapeutic Uses

- *As antacids and osmotic purgatives*: Magnesium hydroxide and magnesium trisilicate are used as nonsystemic antacids and magnesium sulphate, magnesium carbonate and magnesium hydroxide are used as osmotic purgatives.
- *As anticonvulsant*: Magnesium sulphate is occasionally used to control seizures in eclampsia (toxaemia of pregnancy) where it is administered IM or IV.
- *In raised intracranial tension*: Concentrated solution of magnesium sulphate is sometimes used rectally to reduce intracranial tension.
- *In magnesium deficiency:* Magnesium hydroxide is usually used orally. Magnesium sulphate by injection (IM or IV) is rarely required.
- *In cardiac arrhythmias*: Magnesium sulphate by IV injection can be used to treat ventricular tachyarrhythmias in the immediate postmyocardial infarct period and is life-saving.
- *Local uses*: Magnesium sulphate (25 to 50%) in glycerine is used topically for relieving inflammation and acts by osmotic effect. Magnesium sulphate when given orally in poisoning by soluble barium salts, forms insoluble barium sulphate. Magnesium oxide is an ingredient of universal antidote.

Adverse Reactions

Oral magnesium salts produce diarrhoea and loss of electrolytes. Parenteral magnesium sulphate produces flushing, hypotension, cardiac depression (heart block and cardiac arrest), ganglion block, skeletal muscle paralysis, CNS depression and respiratory paralysis.

Phosphorus (P)

Source

It is abundantly present in almost all foods. Meat, milk, fish, cereals, pulses and nuts are main sources of phosphorus. A part of phosphorus in cereals is present as phytate, which is not absorbed from GIT.

Daily requirement: 800 to 1200 mg in adults.

Distribution in the body: The total phosphorus content of an adult human body is about 500 to 600 g. Of this, about 75% is present in bones and teeth and the remaining 25% is in other tissues (including skeletal muscles, skin, nervous tissues and viscera). In bones and teeth, it is present in combination with calcium in the ratio of 2:1 (Ca:P). Soft tissues contain higher amount of phosphorus than calcium. Phosphorus in the soft tissue is mostly in the form of organic esters and in the bone and tooth in the form of orthophosphate. It is a constituent of DNA and RNA and as a part of phospholipid it is an integral component of cell membranes. The red blood cells contain more phosphorus than the plasma. The plasma phosphorus is present in three forms, *viz.* inorganic phosphorus (3 to 5 mg/dL), ester phosphorus (0.1 to 0.7 mg/dL) and lipid phosphorus (7 to 15 mg/dL). The term plasma phosphate means the plasma inorganic phosphate measured as phosphorus.

Pharmacokinetics

Absorption of phosphorus is more complete than that of calcium. About 70% of dietary phosphorus is absorbed in the small intestine. A high calcium intake and presence of a large amount of aluminium hydroxide interfere with the intestinal absorption of phosphorus.

It is mainly excreted by the kidney by glomerular filtration. A large amount of filtered phosphorus is reabsorbed by renal tubules and some is secreted by distal tubular cells. The urinary excretion of phosphorus is under the control of parathormone, which diminishes its tubular reabsorption and thus increases its excretion. Phosphorus is also excreted in faeces, saliva and milk.

Physiological Functions/Pharmacological Actions

- It is necessary for the formation of healthy bones and teeth. Phosphorus needed for this purpose is available at the site by the action of alkaline phosphatase on organic phosphates. When the ion product (Ca × P) exceeds a critical level locally, then deposition of calcium phosphate as crystals occurs.

- It is essential for phosphorylation combination with phosphoric acid which is a key reaction in several metabolic processes of carbohydrates, lipids and proteins in the body. It is thus involved in enzyme regulation, storage and controlled release of chemical energy in the form of high energy phosphate bonds and regulation of delivery of oxygen by the level of diphosphoglycerate and ATP in the red blood cells.

- It forms an integral part of the nuclei and cytoplasm of cells.

- It plays an important role in the regulation of acid–base balance in the plasma and within cells.

- It is involved in H^+ excretion in urine.

Clinical Conditions

1. Hypophosphataemia (low phosphate level in blood)

Common causes: Severe dietary deprivation of phosphorus, long-term use of aluminium containing antacids, hyperparathyroidism, vitamin D deficiency (rickets and osteomalacia), phosphaturia (as in Fanconi's syndrome due to disorder of tubular reabsorption of phosphorus), chronic alcoholism and diabetic ketoacidosis.

Clinical features: Muscular weakness, anorexia, skeletal pain, haemolysis, mental changes, decreased myocardial contractility and respiratory failure.

Treatment: Administration of neutral phosphate solution orally. It is prepared as follows: disodium hydrogen phosphate (3.7 g), sodium dihydrogen phosphate (1 g) orange syrup (16 mL) ,and water (to make 60 mL). It is administered in the dose of 15 to 60 mL three times daily according to tolerance. IV neutral phosphate solution is used in severe hypophosphataemia.

2. Hyperphosphataemia (high phosphate level in blood)

Common causes: Hypoparathyroidism, acromegaly and renal failure.

Clinical featur es: Hypocalcaemia, bone resorption, and widespread metastatic calcification of soft tissues including heart and kidneys.

Treatment: Administration of aluminium hydroxide or calcium carbonate orally to reduce phosphate absorption from intestine.

Therapeutic Uses

- In hypophosphataemia due to various causes.
- In chronic hypercalcaemia, except in the presence of concurrent hyperphosphataemia.

Adverse Reactions

It can cause diarrhoea and widespread deposition of calcium phosphate with organ damage (if administered IV).

Sodium (Na)

Source

Table salt (NaCl) is added to prepare food, bread, cheese, whole grains, eggs, milk and vegetables.

Daily requirement: 5 to 15 g in adults.

Distribution in the body: It is distributed in all body tissues and fluids, mainly in extracellular fluid (ECF). It is present to the extent of about 1/3rd in the inorganic portion of the skeleton bone, which acts as a sodium reservoir. It is present in the body in association with chloride, bicarbonate, phosphate and lactate.

Pharmacokinetics

It is absorbed from small intestine, particularly from jejunum by both active transport and passive diffusion. Concurrent administration of glucose stimulates rapid sodium absorption. In the ileum, it is absorbed mainly by active transport process. It is secreted into the GIT, which is totally reabsorbed. It is excreted through urine and sweat. About 15 g of sodium is filtered out every minute at the glomeruli. Of this, 98% is reabsorbed by the renal tubules and only 2% is excreted in urine. Urinary excretion of sodium is regulated by aldosterone and renal blood flow. Aldosterone promotes sodium reabsorption and potassium excretion by acting on distal renal tubule.

Physiological Functions/Pharmacological Actions

- It is the principal cation in extracellular fluid. It maintains plasma volume, water and electrolyte balance and acid–base balance and regulates nerve and muscle functions.
- Sodium concentration of plasma is about 330 mg/dL and that of cells is about 85 mg/dL.

Clinical Conditions

1. Hyponatremia (low sodium level in blood)

Common causes: Diarrhoea, cholera, acute bacillary dysentery, hot; dry or moist climate causing cutaneous loss of sodium, burns, administration of diuretics, diabetic coma, during starvation or increased catabolism of proteins and Addison's disease.

Clinical features: Loss of appetite, vomiting, lethargy, muscle cramps, hypotension, syncope and shock.

Treatment: Administration of normal saline by IV infusion. In severe cases, 2–3 L/2–3 hours may be required. Administration of potassium and bicarbonate by IV infusion depending upon the type of fluid loss.

2. Hypernatremia (high sodium level in blood)

Common causes: Acute nephritis, nephrosis, aldosteronism, CCF, acute hypotension and drug induced (e.g. NSAIDs and reserpine).

Clinical features: Pitting oedema (due to sodium and water retention) and hypertension.

Treatment: Sodium depletion is brought about by:
- Restricting the daily dietary sodium intake.
- Increasing the sodium excretion in urine by using diuretics.
- Improving renal perfusion, e.g. digoxin in CCF and IV 5% glucose infusion in oligemic shock.

Potassium (K)

Source

Vegetables, fruits, nuts, coconut water, chicken and liver.

Daily requirement: 3 to 5 g in adults.

Distribution in the body: Potassium is the major intracellular cation and hence its distribution is related to the cell mass. About 70% of body potassium is present in muscles, 20% in the brain and large viscera and 10% in skin and subcutaneous tissues. As compared to sodium, the amount of potassium in bone is small.

Physiological Functions/ Pharmacological Actions

- It is the principal cation in the intracellular fluid (ICF).
- It maintains water and electrolyte balance, acid–base balance and regulates nerve and muscle functions.
- Potassium concentration of plasma is about 20 mg/dL and that of cells is about 400 mg/dL.

Clinical Conditions

1. Hypokalaemia (low potassium level in blood)

Common causes: Decreased intake (especially in old people), excessive sweating, vomiting, diarrhoea, sodium overload, starvation, diabetic acidosis, excessive use of diuretics, renal tubular acidosis (Fanconi syndrome) and nephrotic syndrome.

Clinical features: Lethargy, malaise, mental confusion, weakness of muscles, anorexia, thirst, neuromuscular paralysis, intestinal dilatation, paralytic ileus, hypotension, bradycardia, cardiac arrhythmias, conduction defect and renal dysfunction.

Treatment: Oral administration of adequate amount of potassium in the form of potassium chloride/bicarbonate/citrate. In severe cases, potassium is administered by slow IV drip. Potassium should never be given directly into a vein or into the tubing of an intravenous drip as this may cause sudden rise in serum potassium level and death from cardiac arrest.

2. Hyperkalaemia (high potassium level in blood)

Common causes: Acute or chronic renal insufficiency, tissue injury (due to increased catabolic processes), IV administration of potassium, Addison's disease (due to lack of aldosterone) and drug induced (e.g. NSAIDs, ACE inhibitors, spironolactone and triamterene).

Clinical features: Skeletal muscle paralysis, respiratory paralysis, cardiac arrhythmias, idioventricular rhythm and cardiac arrest (in diastole).

Treatment: Serum potassium level can be reduced by:
- Skipping potassium in diet.
- Administration of cation exchange resin orally for depleting potassium.
- Promoting the entry of potassium into cells by injecting 5 to 10 units of plain insulin and 50 mL of 50% glucose IV over 5 minutes and correcting acidosis by administration of sodium bicarbonate IV.
- Promoting potassium excretion in urine by using fludrocortisone as in Addison's disease.
- Peritoneal dialysis or haemodialysis to correct severe hyperkalaemia. It is sometimes life-saving.

Chloride (Cl)
Source
Mainly available as sodium chloride (table salt).

Daily requirement: 10 to 20 g in adults.

Distribution in the body: It is distributed in all body tissues and fluids. It is present mainly in ECF. Blood cells contain small amounts of chloride.

Pharmacokinetics
It is completely absorbed from GIT. It is mainly excreted in urine and to some extent in sweat.

Physiological Functions/Pharmacological Actions
It is involved in fluid and electrolyte balance, acid–base balance, formation of gastric HCl and chloride shift in bicarbonate transport in erythrocytes.

Deficiency States
Hypochloraemia may occur due to excessive loss of NaCl in diarrhoea, loss of gastric juice by vomiting or pyloric obstruction. Hypochloraemic alkalosis may occur in Cushing's disease or after administration of ACTH or cortisone.

Treatment
Administration of NaCl orally or parenterally. Other important minerals required as nutrients are shown in **Table 82.1**.

Table 82.1: Other important minerals (trace elements)

Mineral	Source	Functions	Pharmacokinetics	Deficiency states
Zinc (Zn)	Meat, eggs, liver, milk, oyster, cereals, pulses, nuts, fruits and vegetables	Cofactor of many enzymes such as lactate dehydrogenase, alkaline phosphatase, carbonic anhydrase and superoxide dismutase	Absorbed from small intestine. Transported by binding with plasma proteins. Excreted in faeces, urine and sweat.	Dwarfism, hypo-gonadism, impaired wound healing, decreased taste and smell acuity, dermatitis and alopecia.
Mangan-ese (Mn)	Whole grains, cereals, nuts, legumes, fruits and vegetables	Cofactor of hydrolase, decarboxylase and transferase enzymes. Glycoprotein and proteoglycan synthesis.	Transported as transmanganin (lactoglobulin), stored in liver and kidneys.	Ataxia, sterility and bone deformities in animals. Unknown in humans.
Copper (Cu)	Liver	Constituent of oxidase enzymes like cytochrome-C oxidase.	Transported by albumin, bound to ceruloplasmin.	Hypochromic micro-cytic anaemia, secon-dary to malnutrition.
Cobalt (Co)	Foods of animal origin	Required only as a constituent of vitamin B_{12}.	Like vitamin B_{12}	Vitamin B_{12} deficie-ncies.
Iodine (I)	Iodized salt, sea food	Constituent of thyroxine and triiodothyronine.	Stored in thyroid gland as thyroglobulin.	Children: Cretinism. Adults: Goitre, hypothyroidism and myxoedema.
Fluoride (F)	Drinking water, many tooth-pastes	Increases hardness of bone and teeth.	Absorbed from intestine, lungs and skin. Excreted in urine, sweat and faeces.	Dental carries, osteo-porosis.

83

Therapeutic Gases and Enzymes

THERAPEUTIC GASES

These are oxygen, carbon dioxide and helium.

Oxygen (O$_2$)

It is a colourless and odourless gas supplied in compressed form in steel cylinders painted black with a white shoulder.

Physiological Functions of Oxygen

Oxygen is vital for human survival. Inspired air contains 21% of oxygen, 0.04% of carbon dioxide and 78% of nitrogen; and expired air contains 14% of oxygen, 5.6% of carbon dioxide and 78% of nitrogen. Due to gaseous exchange in lungs, inspired oxygen enters the blood and is carried largely in combination with haemoglobin as oxyhaemoglobin and to a small extent (0.3%) as a physical solution in plasma. Oxyhaemoglobin is largely responsible for the transfer of oxygen to the tissues, where haemoglobin is reduced. When oxygen is inhaled at a higher pressure (more than one atmospheric pressure), then sufficient oxygen is carried in physical solution and transfer of oxygen to the tissues is carried out from the physically dissolved oxygen without desaturating oxyhaemoglobin. As a result carbon dioxide transport from the tissues is less. As the hydrogen ion acceptor reduced haemoglobin is not available and so carbon dioxide tension of tissues rises.

Effects of Inhalation of Pure Oxygen (100% O$_2$)

These are given as follows:

- *Respiratory effects*: Initially there is respiratory depression due to inhibition of chemoreceptor activity and decrease sensitivity of respiratory centre (RC) to carbon dioxide. Later on, there is mild stimulation of respiration.

- *Cardiovascular effects*: There is slight decrease in the heart rate and moderate decrease in cardiac output. The coronary and cerebral blood flows are probably reduced, while the pulmonary vessels are dilated increasing pulmonary circulation. There is little change in BP.

- *Other effects*: There is a decrease in the partial pressure of nitrogen within the pulmonary alveoli with subsequent diffusion of nitrogen from the body cavities and blood into the alveoli, from where it is eliminated in expiration.

Therapeutic Uses

- In hypoxia (lack of oxygen) due to any cause, e.g. acute bronchial asthma, pulmonary emphysema, pneumonia, pneumothorax, massive pleural effusion, methaemoglobinaemia, CCF, circulatory shock and barbiturate/salicylate/cyanide poisoning.

- As a diluent for gaseous and volatile general anaesthetics.
- To prevent decompression sickness (Caisson disease): It is used by workers in pressurized spaces to reduce the inhaled nitrogen concentration and thus to prevent decompression sickness.
- For hyperbaric oxygen therapy: It is the administration of pure (100%) oxygen at higher pressure (more than one atmospheric pressure) in a special chamber filled with compressed oxygen and the patient breathes oxygen through a face mask or a mouthpiece. It produces better oxygenation of tissues by overcoming the barrier to increased oxygen transport and causing an increase amount of oxygen physically dissolved in blood. It is used in respiratory disease of the newborn, acute left ventricular failure, carbon monoxide poisoning, cyanide poisoning, decompression sickness, congenital cyanotic heart disease, acute myocardial infarction, cerebrovascular accident, aerobic infections like chronic osteomyelitis with draining lesions unresponsive to medical and surgical treatments, anaerobic infections like gas gangrene (by *Cl. welchii),* open heart surgery, organ transplantation and malignant tumour resistant to radiotherapy (due to hypoxia).

Adverse Reactions

Inhalation of hyperbaric oxygen decreases heart rate and cardiac output and produces peripheral vasoconstriction including retinal blood vessels. It is more toxic to respiratory and central nervous systems. It can produce cough, nasal congestion, chest pain, nausea, vertigo, tinnitus, paraesthesia, muscular twitchings, involuntary movements, convulsions and coma. In premature infants it can cause retrolental fibroplasia (a vascular proliferative disease of retina), which may lead to blindness in some cases. It can produce carbon dioxide narcosis in patients with COPD, narcotic poisoning respiratory muscle weakness (from poliomyelitis, polyneuritis and myasthenia gravis) and raised intracranial tension causing carbon dioxide retention, papilloedema and coma. It is manifested as drowsiness and convulsions.

Carbon Dioxide (CO$_2$)

It is a colourless and odourless gas supplied in liquid form at high pressure (58 to 72 atmospheric pressure) in steel cylinders which are painted grey. Combination of oxygen and 5 to 10% carbon dioxide (carbogen) are also supplied in steel cylinders, which are painted black but have grey and white quaterings on neck and shoulder.

Physiological Functions of Carbon Dioxide

Carbon dioxide is produced in the body during tissue and food metabolism. Inspired air contains 0.04% of carbon dioxide whereas expired air contains 5.6% of carbon dioxide. It diffuses from the cells of origin into the blood, where it is carried as bicarbonate (65%), carboxyhaemoglobin (27%) and carbonic acid (8%). Many tissues have special enzymes, e.g. carbonic anhydrase for handling of carbon dioxide. It is a natural respiratory stimulant.

Effects of Inhalation of Carbon Dioxide

These are given as follows:

- *Respiratory effects*: Inhalation of 2% carbon dioxide increases the rate and tidal volume of respiration by directly stimulating the respiratory centre (RC) in the brain stem (chemical drive) as well as reflexly through stimulation of the peripheral arterial (carotid and aortic) chemoreceptors.
- *Cardiovascular effects*: Carbon dioxide by a direct action decreases the heart rate and the force of cardiac contraction. It also relaxes the vascular smooth muscle, tending to cause vasodilation. These direct circulatory effects of carbon dioxide are antagonized by the sympathetic activation induced by it, causing an increase in the peripheral release of the catecholamines. Thus, carbon dioxide increases the heart rate, cardiac output, systolic and diastolic BPs and pulse pressure. As cerebral and

coronary blood vessels are devoid of significant sympathetic control, so they are dilated after carbon dioxide inhalation. Similarly, the splanchnic and skeletal muscle blood vessels are dilated. Carbon dioxide is the most potent cerebral vasodilator.

- *CNS effects*: Inhalation of 2% carbon dioxide stimulates the cerebral cortex and reduces the electrical and chemical seizure thresholds. Inhalation of 10% carbon dioxide depresses the cerebral cortex but activates the subcortical areas that have cortical projections.

Therapeutic Uses

- *As respiratory stimulant*: Inhalation of carbogen is used in respiratory depression due to drug, disease or injury.

- In chronic obstructive pulmonary diseases (COPD) like chronic bronchitis, emphysema and bronchial asthma. Intermittent inhalation of carbogen is used to liquefy bronchial secretion and to help expectoration.

- *In hiccups*: Inhalation of 10% carbon dioxide is used to relieve intractable hiccups by a CNS depressant action.

- *Local uses*: Carbon dioxide snow, which has a temperature of −80°C is used to destroy warts and naevi by local application for 5 to 6 seconds. It is a painless procedure and the scarring is minimum. The surrounding tissue should be covered with soft paraffin for protection.

- *Miscellaneous uses*: Supersaturated solution of carbon dioxide or aerated waters are used to increase gastric juice secretion. Evolution of carbon dioxide by chemical reaction with acid in stomach often used to mask unpleasant taste of saline purgatives.

Adverse Reactions

Inhalation of 7% carbon dioxide causes headache, dizziness, mental confusion, palpitation, dyspnoea and hypertension and 15% CO_2 causes loss of consciousness (coma).

Helium (He)

It is an inert gas of low density (lighter gas). It is administered in closed circuit apparatus. It is used as helium-oxygen mixture (1:4).

Therapeutic Uses

- It is used by intermittent inhalation for treating prolonged asthmatic attacks resistant to other forms of therapy. Due to its low density, it minimizes the breathing effort.

- It is used prophylactically for prevention of Caisson's disease and in the treatment of oedema and spasm of larynx, paralysis of vocal cord, emphysema, bronchiectasis and pulmonary fibrosis.

- It is a useful noninflammable diluent for oxygen during anaesthesia and open heart surgery.

Adverse Reactions

Inhalation of helium in high concentration may produce asphyxia.

THERAPEUTIC ENZYMES

These are given as follows:
- Digestive enzymes, e.g. diastase, pepsin, papain, trypsin, lipase and pancreatin. These are discussed in GIT pharmacology.
- Fibrinolytic enzymes, e.g. plasmin (fibrinolysin), streptokinase, urokinase and tissue plasminogen activator (alteplase). These are discussed in haematologic pharmacology.
- Antineoplastic enzymes, e.g. L-asparaginase. It is discussed in cancer chemotherapy.
- Local proteolytic enzymes, e.g. hyaluronidase, chymotrypsin, α-chymotrypsin and serratiopeptidase. These will be discussed here.

Hyaluronidase (Hyalase/Hynidase)

It is a proteolytic enzyme obtained from the extract of pig or ox testes. It is present in certain snake and bee venoms and some virulent microorganisms. It acts by depolymerizing hyaluronic acid, an essential component of the intracellular ground substances, which determines the permeability of the tissues. Administered subcutaneously, it increases the tissue permeability due to spreading activity. It contains not less than 300 units of activity per mg. It is used to promote the rapid absorption of drugs and fluids given SC or IM. It is also used to promote absorption of blood or fluid in traumatic or postoperative oedema or haematoma and along with local anaesthetics. It is administered SC locally in the dose of 1500 units dissolved in 1 L of fluid. Sodium hyaluronate in highly purified form is used in ophthalmic surgical procedures. It should not be applied directly to the cornea. It is antigenic and may produce allergic reactions. There may be spreading of infection, if it is injected into or around the infected area. It is contraindicated in cancers as it can cause spreading of cancer cells.

Chymotrypsin

It is a proteolytic enzyme obtained from the extract of ox pancreas. It is used for debridement of surface wounds. It is also used in traumatic soft tissue inflammation and oedema along with conventional treatment (NSAIDs, corticosteroids). It is available as tablets containing 50,000 units of the enzymes per tablet. It is also available as combination product of chymotrypsin and trypsin tablets (soluzyme) and ointment. It produces allergic reactions rarely.

α-chymotrypsin (Alfapsin)

It is a subtype of chymotrypsin. It is mainly used in ophthalmology for dissolving the suspensory ligament of the lens to facilitate the dissection of the lens during intracapsular extraction of cataract (opaque lens). It is available as injection and sublingual tablet (5.8 mg). It is used as 0.2 to 0.5 mL of a freshly prepared 1:5000 solution injected slowly behind the lens into the posterior chamber. It is also used for the treatment of inflammation oedema due to injury, surgery, infection or dental procedures where it is administered orally in the dose of 4 to 6 tablets daily. It produces allergic reactions rarely.

Serratiopeptidase (Flanzen/Bidanzen)

It is a proteolytic enzyme obtained from the *Serratia* bacteria. It is used for the treatment of inflammation after operation and traumatic injury. It relieves pain and inflammation following tonsillectomy, episiotomy, perineal laceration and alveolar abscess. It is available as tablet (5, 10 mg) and used in the doses of 5 to 10 mg thrice daily. It can produce allergic reactions rarely.

84

Antiseptics and Disinfectants

STERILIZATION

Sterilization is a process that completely eliminates all microbres (microorganisms) from living tissues or nonliving objects by using a germicide—antiseptic or disinfectant.

Antiseptics are chemical agents which are used to inhibit growth or kill microorganisms in contact with living tissues (e.g. skin and mucous membrane) when applied to their surfaces. Disinfectants are chemical or physical agents used to kill microorganisms in contact with non-living (inanimate) objects (e.g. instruments and other appliances) when applied to their surfaces. Physical agents include heat in various forms, filtration and non-ionizing and ionizing radiations.

Chemical Agents Used as Antiseptics/ Disinfectants

They are of following groups:

- Acids, e.g. boric acid, benzoic acid, salicylic acid and acetic acid.
- Alkalies, e.g. sodium hydroxide and potassium hydroxide.
- Alcohols, e.g. ethylalcohol and isopropylalcohol.
- Aldehydes, e.g. formaldehyde and gluteraldehyde.
- Halogens and halogen-containing compounds, e.g. chlorine, iodine, chlorophores and iodophores.

- Phenols and related compounds, e.g. phenol, cresol, chlorocresol, hexachlorophene and chlorhexidine.
- Oxidizing agents, e.g. hydrogen peroxide, potassium permanganate, sodium permanganate and zinc permanganate.
- Heavy metals, e.g. mercury salts, silver salts and zinc salts.
- Dyes, e.g. acriflavine, proflavine, gentian violet and brilliant green.
- Surfactants:
  - Anionic agents, e.g. soaps, sodium lauryl sulphate and sodium cetostearyl sulphate.
  - Cationic agents, e.g. benzalkonium chloride, cetylpyridinium chloride, cetrimide and dequalinium.
  - Cetrimide + Chlorhexidine (Savlon, Cetavion).
- Nitrofurans, e.g. nitrofurazone (Furacin).
- Topical antibiotics, e.g. neomycin, bacitracin, framycetin and chloromycetin.

Mechanisms of Action of Antiseptics/ Disinfectants

They may act by:

- Oxidation of bacterial protoplasm.
- Coagulation of bacterial proteins including enzymes.
- Bacterial enzyme inhibition by binding with free sulphydryl (–SH) groups (essential for bacterial enzyme actions) or

competition with essential substrates for the important enzymes in the bacterial cell.

- Increasing the permeability of the bacterial cell membrane (by a detergent-like action).

An ideal antiseptic/disinfectant should possess the following properties:

- It should be highly germicidal with broad-spectrum activity (i.e. active against bacteria, fungi, viruses and protozoa).
- It should be noninjurious to the host cells.
- It should be active in presence of foreign substances (blood, pus, exudates and excreta).
- It should be non-irritating and non-sensitizing (no allergy).
- It should be non-staining with agreeable colour and odour.
- It should be rapidly active with sustained duration of action.
- It should be stable and compatible with soaps and other detergents.

Disadvantages of antiseptic/disinfectant are:

- It can be absorbed from the local wound producing systemic toxicity.
- It can retard the healing of wound.
- It can spread infection if not properly applied.

Evaluation of Germicidal Activity of an Antiseptic/Disinfectant

Potency of antiseptic/disinfectant is generally expressed by its phenol coefficient (Rideal-Walker coefficient). It is the ratio of the minimum concentration (maximum dilution) of the testing (unknown) agent required to kill a 24-hour culture of *Bacillus typhosus* in 7.5 minutes at 37.5°C to that of phenol under similar conditions. The higher the ratio, the greater is the germicidal activity of the testing agent. *In vitro* sensitivity tests are also available for determining the potency of unknown antiseptic.

Therapeutic index of an antiseptic is determined by comparing the concentration at which it acts on microorganisms with that which produces local irritation or tissue damage.

Discussion of Antiseptics/Disinfectants

- *Acids*: Boric acid is a nonirritant but weak antiseptic. As powder, ointment or water solution it is applied to a variety of skin lesions. It is also used as eye/ear drops and as glycerin of boric acid for painting throat and tongue lesions. Sodium borate (Borax) is used for same purposes as boric acid. Benzoic acid has antibacterial and anti-fungal actions. It is nontoxic and used as food preservative in 0.1% concentration. Salicylic acid has antibacterial, antifungal and keratolytic actions. It is used as ointment or dusting powder for the treatment of seborrhoeic dermatitis, psoriasis, acne and fungal skin diseases. It is also used for destruction of warts and corns. Whitfield's ointment containing 6% benzoic acid and 3% salicylic acid is used for the treatment of ringworm infection. Acetic acid is used as bactericidal agent in 0.25% concentration. It is particularly useful in *Pseudomonas aeruginosa* infection of external ear.
- *Alkalies*: Sodium hydroxide and potassium hydroxide are used for disinfecting excreta from poliomyelitis patients. They are caustics and can be used for removal of warts.
- *Alcohols*: Ethylalcohol and isopropyl alcohol in 70% concentrations are used as skin antiseptics. However, they exhibit poor activity against bacterial spores, fungi and viruses. Hence they are not useful for sterilizing surgical instruments.
- *Aldehydes*: Formaldehyde (5 to 10% solution) is used as disinfectant to kill bacteria as well as their spores from surgical gloves and instruments. It is not used as antiseptic because it is irritant to the mucous membranes and precipitates tissue proteins. Formalin contains formaldehyde (40%) in methanol. When applied to the unbroken skin, it hardens the epidermis and may render it tough. It is used for disinfection of excreta, sputum and brush bristles and for preservation of pathological specimens.

Gaseous formaldehyde is used as fumigator for disinfection of those articles in rooms which cannot be wetted with formaldehyde solution. It is obtained by heating formaldehyde or formalin solution. Glutaraldehyde (Cidex) is less irritant than formaldehyde and used for disinfection of rubber, plastic and metal appliances in 2% concentration.

- *Halogens and halogen-containing compounds*: Chlorine is used for purification of drinking water and to disinfect excreta or to irrigate wounds. In acid or neutral pH it becomes HOCl (hypochlorous acid), which is lethal to the microbes including viruses and protozoa. Its bactericidal action is significantly reduced in the presence of organic matter. It is used mainly as chlorinated lime (bleaching powder), sodium hypochlorite, chloramine and halozane (tablet), which are chlorophores, releasing chlorine slowly from the chlorine complex. Eusol is a solution of chlorinated lime and boric acid. It contains not less than 0.3% of chlorine. It is irritating and should, therefore, be diluted with saline before using on denuded surfaces.

Iodine is a widely used antiseptic. It is a powerful bactericidal agent. It also possesses sporicidal, fungicidal, amoebicidal and viricidal activities. A 2% solution (in alcohol) of iodine with sodium iodide (tincture of iodine) is used on intact skin for small wounds and abrasions. Its main disadvantage is that it is irritant. It is also used as compound iodine paint (Mandl's pigment) in throat infection. Iodophores are water-soluble organic compounds of iodine which release free iodine in solution, e.g. povidone iodine is a complex of polyvinylpyrrolidone and iodine. It is now preferred than iodine. It is water-soluble and nonirritant antiseptic. It is available as 10% solution and ointment. It is used as gargle (for oral infections), ointment (in cuts, wounds, bites and fungal infections) and solution (as preoperative antiseptic and in cuts, abrasion and vaginal moniliasis).

- *Phenols and related compounds*: Phenol (carbolic acid) is a bactericidal and fungicidal agent in 1 to 2% concentration in water. In concentration over 3% it is injurious to tissues. In 5 to 10% concentration it is used for disinfecting nonliving objects (floor of room and excreta). It is a deodorant (removes offensive smell). Phenyl is chlorophenol. Phenol is also used to cauterize dog bite or snake bite. For its antipruritic action it is used in calamine lotion. Phenol was introduced as an antiseptic by Lord Lister in 1867. Substituted phenols are more effective than phenol as disinfectants. These are cresol, chloroxylenol, hexachlorophene and chlorhexidine. Cresol is available as lysol (cresol with soap solution) and chloroxylenol as dettol. Both the preparations are used for disinfection of surgical instruments and other objects. Hexachlorophene (3%) is used as antiseptic in soaps and detergents. Chlorhexidine solution is used for wound cleansing and handwashing by surgeons. Savlon is a mixture of chlorhexidine and hexachlorophene. It is a very popular antiseptic/disinfectant. Chlorhexidine soaps are also available.

- *Oxidizing agents*: Hydrogen peroxide (H_2O_2) in 3% solution with water is used as mouthwash and for cleansing of wounds. It has wide antimicrobial spectrum. Its effervesence removes debris from inaccessible regions. It has short duration of action and is unstable on storage. Permanganates are antiseptic and antifungal agents. Potassium permanganate is 1 in 10,000 solution kills microorganisms. Higher concentrations, however, are irritating to tissues. Sodium permanganate solution (Condy's lotion) or zinc permanganate solution is used as gargle and mouthwash and also for vaginal irrigation and in fungal infections of skin.

- *Heavy metals*: Inorganic mercury salts like yellow mercuric oxide and ammoniated mercury are used as eye ointment and skin ointment respectively as antiseptics. Organic mercury salts like mercurochrome (1 to 3% solution) and thiomersol (0.1 to 0.3% solution) are used as antiseptics on skin and mucous membrane. They are now less used because they are quite toxic. Silver salts like silver nitrate, silver proteinate and silver sulphadiazine are antiseptics. 1% silver nitrate and 10% silver proteinate (Argyrol) are used as eye drops and silver sulphadiazine as antiseptic. Zinc is used in burns as ointment. Zinc salts like zinc sulphate, zinc chloride, zinc oxide and zinc carbonate have astringent and antiseptic properties. Zinc sulphate is used as eye drops and skin lotion. Zinc chloride is used as astringent and antiseptic lotion. Zinc oxide is used as ointment or lotion in eczema, impetigo and pruritus. Zinc carbonate tinted with ferric oxide (calamine) is the major ingredient of calamine lotion.

- *Dyes*: Acriflavine and proflavine are effective germicidals. They are used for the treatment of infected wounds and burns in 0.1 to 0.2% solution. Gentian violet is a potent antiseptic used mainly against gram-positive microorganisms. It is used to treat burns, boils, chronic ulcers and fungal infections in 0.5 to 1% solution. Brilliant green is a potent antiseptic and used in 1% solution for the treatment of wounds, burns and minor injuries.

- *Surfactants*: They are surface active agents. They are widely used as detergents, emulsifiers and wetting agents. Anionic detergents are weak antiseptics but cationic detergents are effective antiseptics at 0.1% concentration. They are also used for disinfection of surgical instruments, rubber goods and other materials in 1 to 2% concentrations. They are non-irritating and nontoxic, stable on storage and active against a wide variety of microorganisms. Alcohol increases their germicidal activity. Their action is slow and antagonized by soaps, pus and tissue constituents.

- *Nitrofurans*: Nitrofurazone (Furacin) is a furan derivative. It is effective against many microorganisms. Topically it is a safe antiseptic. It is used as 0.2% cream, ointment, solution or powder. It is very effective in burns.

- *Topical antibiotics*: Neomycin, bacitracin, polymyxin-B, framycetin and chloromycetin are used in superficial infections of skin and mucous membrane and have potent antiseptic property against a wide range of microorganisms.

85

Dermatomucosal Agents and Ectoparasiticides

Drugs acting locally on skin and mucous membranes are:

- **Demulcents:** These are inert substances which sooth inflammed or denuded skin or mucosa by preventing contact with air and irritants in the surroundings, e.g. gum-acacia, gum tragacanth, glycyrrhiza, methyl cellulose, propylene glycol, glycerine, etc. These are applied as thick colloidal or viscid solutions in water.

- **Emollients:** These are bland (nonirritant) oily substances which sooth and soften skin, e.g. olive oil, linseed oil, arachis oil, wool fat, wool alcohol, beeswax, paraffins (soft, hard or liquid), oil of theobroma (cocoa butter), etc. They form an occlusive film over the skin, preventing evaporation and thus restoring elasticity of cracked and dry skin. Some of them are used as ointment bases.

- **Adsorbants and protectives:** These are finely powdered, inert and insoluble solid substances that adsorb (bind to their surface) noxious and irritant substances and give physical protection to the skin or mucosa. These are of three groups:
  - Dermal protectives, e.g. magnesium or zinc stearate, talc, calamine, zinc oxide, bentonite, starch, boric acid, etc.
  - Gastrointestinal protectives, e.g. kaolin, pectin, activated charcoal, chalk, aluminium hydroxide, magnesium trisilicate, etc.
  - Occlusive protectives, e.g. collodion, dimethicone, etc.

- **Astringents:** These are substances that precipitate superficial proteins but do not penetrate cells. They toughen the surface making it mechanically stronger and decrease exudation, e.g. tannic acid, tannins, alcohols, bismuth carbonate, alum, aluminium hydroxychloride, zinc oxide, phenol sulphonate, etc.

- **Irritants and counterirritants:** Irritants are substances that stimulate sensory nerve endings and induce inflammation at the site of application. They produce cooling sensation or warmth, pricking or tingling, hyperaesthesia or numbness and local vasodilatation (hyperaemia), e.g. carbolic acid, hydrochloric acid, caustic soda, etc. Counterirritants are irritants that produce a remote effect through axon reflex and relieve pain and inflammation in deeper organs, e.g. camphor, thymol, menthol, turpentine oil, clove oil, eucalyptus oil, methyl salicylate, alcohol, capsicum, mustard powder, etc. They are massaged to relieve headache, muscular pain, joint pain, pleural or peritoneal pain, abdominal colics, etc.

- **Keratolytics:** These are substances which destroy and remove skin lesions like corns and warts, e.g. salicylic acid (corn cap/ointment), urea, trichloroacetic acid, silver nitrate, propylene glycol, etc.

- **Antipruritics:** These are substances that relieve pruritus or itching of skin in urticaria, eczema, psoriasis, etc., e.g. antihistaminics (orally as tablet), corticosteroids (topically as ointment or cream), caladryl lotion, etc.
- **Melanizing agents:** These are substances that increase sensitivity to solar radiation and promote repigmentation of vitiliginous areas of skin, e.g. psoralens are fluorocoumarins, which on photoactivation stimulate melanocytes and induce their proliferation. Psoralen is obtained from fruit of *Ammi majus*. It is available as psoralen tablet (5 mg), solution (0.25%) and ointment (1%), manaderm tablet (10 mg) and ointment (1%). Trioxsalen and methoxsalen are synthetic drugs and available as trisoralen/neosoralen tablet (5, 25 mg) and oxsoralen/macsoralen tablet (10 mg) and solution (1%). They sensitize the skin to sunlight, which then induces erythema, inflammation and pigmentation. They are given orally and applied topically. After two hours of administration of psoralen (10 to 20 mg) the skin is exposed to sunlight initially for 15 minutes and gradually increased to 30 minutes after some days. For topical use, solution or ointment is applied on the affected area, which is then exposed to sunlight for one minute and then occluded by bandage or sunscreen ointment.
- **Demelanizing agents:** These are substances that lighten the hyperpigmented patches on skin and used in melasma, chloasma of pregnancy and malignant melanoma, e.g. hydroquinone and monobenzene. Hydroquinone (Eldoquin) is a weak hypopigmenting agent. It inhibits tyrosinase and decreases formation and increases degradation of melanosomes. It is available as lotion and cream (2 to 6%). It is applied daily locally for a few months. It can cause skin irritation, rashes and allergy. Pigmentation may recur when it is discontinued. Monobenzene (Benoquin) is a derivative of hydroquinone. It is a potent demelanizing agent. It destroys melanocytes and may cause permanent depigmentation. It is available as ointment (20%) and lotion (5%). It is applied 2 to 3 times daily for 4 to 6 months. It can cause depigmented patches, erythema and eczema.
- **Sunscreens:** These are substances that protect the skin from harmful effects of exposure to sunlight, e.g. PABA and its esters, oxybenzone, cinnamates (cinoxate, methyl anthranilate) as solution or cream (1 to 6%). Calamine, zinc oxide, titanium dioxide, heavy petroleum jelly, etc. are physical sunscreens.
- **Depilatory agents:** These are substances used to remove hairs. They act by causing temporary softening of keratin of hair in the waving process, e.g. thioglycolic alkali salt of sodium or potassium (Depilar/Avis).

Ectoparasiticides

These are drugs used to kill animal parasites that live on body surface (skin). They are used in scabies and pediculosis. Scabies is caused by a kind of mite (sarcoptes/*Acarus scabiei*). It burrows through the epidermis and lays eggs, which form papules that itch intensely. Secondary infection may occur in the lesions, which require systemic antimicrobial therapy. The preferred site of entry of the mite is finger webs and then spread to forearms, trunk, genitals and legs. It is a highly contagious disease. Hence other members of the patient's family should be treated concurrently. Garments and bedlinens should be washed in hot water and dried in sun to prevent cross-infection and reinfection. Pediculosis is caused by a kind of lice (*Pediculus*, wingless). The lice living on head is called *Pediculus capitis*, on body is called *P. corporis* and on pubic region is called *P. pubis*. They cause itching, suck blood and transmit diseases like typhus fever and relapsing fever. Their eggs are called nits, which get attached to the hair and clothing by a chitin-like cement.

Drugs Used in Scabies and Pediculosis

• *Benzyl benzoate (Ascabiol) emulsion (25%):* It is an oily liquid with a faint aromatic odour. It is the drug of choice for scabies. After a cleansing bath, it is applied all over the body except face and neck for two consecutive days, followed by a soap water bath on the third day. It is convenient to apply and does not interfere with routine works. For pediculosis, it is applied at the site of infestation taking care so that it does not enter into eyes. It is washed with soap and water after 24 hours. It may produce irritation of skin, especially in children.

• *Crotamiton (Crotorax) cream and lotion (10%):* It can be used as an alternative scabicide or pediculocide. It is less irritant than benzyl benzoate and so preferred in children. It is applied similarly as benzyl benzoate. It has antipruritic activity. It rarely causes allergic reactions.

• *Monosulphiram (Tetmosol) lotion (25%) and soap:* It is a scabicide and pediculocide but less effective than benzyl benzoate. It can cause mild irritation. It is applied similar as benzyl benzoate. Incorporated in soap, it is used for the prophylactic treatment of scabies. It is related chemically to disulphiram and hence during its use alcohol should be avoided.

• *γ-benzene hexachloride (Gammexane/ Lindane) lotion and cream (1%):* It is available as lorexane (with cetrimide and rectified spirit). It is an effective pediculocide and scabicide. It is non-irritant and nontoxic to man when applied externally. It kills the parasite by penetrating through the chitinous cover and affecting the nervous system (neurotoxic). It is the drug of choice in pediculosis. It is applied to the scalp and hair, taking care so that it does not enter the eyes and is left for 24 hours, after which it is washed with soap and water. The treatment may be repeated after a week if required. For treatment of scabies, it is rubbed all over the body except face and neck, followed by a soap water bath after 12 hours. It can be repeated after one week if required. It may cause neurotoxicity and haematotoxicity in children after absorption.

• *Dicophane (DDT) ointment and lotion (1%):* It has action and uses like gammexane. It is applied similar to gammexane.

• *Sulphur ointment (10 %):* In the past, it was a popular scabicidal agent. It has weaker pediculocidal action and so not preferred in pediculosis. When applied to the skin it is converted to hydrogen sulphide and parathionic acid, which dissolve the cuticle of the mite and kill it. It is rubbed all over the body except face and neck for three consecutive days, followed by a soap water bath on the fourth day. It is cheap but has following disadvantages:

– It has unacceptable bad odour.

– It requires repeated applications.

– It is irritant to the skin.

• *Other drugs* like thiabendazole supension (10 %), mesulphen lotion (65 % oil) and permethrin cream (1%) are also used in scabies and pediculosis by local application.

Section VI

TOXICOLOGY

86

Heavy Metals and their Antagonists

HEAVY METALS

People always have been exposed to heavy metals in the environment. The heavy metals of greatest concern are lead, mercury, arsenic, bismuth, antimony, iron, copper and cadmium. In areas of high concentrations, metallic contamination of food and water probably lead to poisonings. Metals leached from eating utensils and cookwares can produce such poisonings. Metallic constituents of pesticides and therapeutic agents (e.g. antimicrobial agents) can also produce poisonings. The burning of fossil fuels containing heavy metals, the addition of tetraethyl lead to gasoline and the increase in industrial applications of metals have increased the incidence of heavy metal poisonings.

Pharmacological Actions

The organic and inorganic salts of heavy metals possess astringent, corrosive and caustic properties on local applications. They also act as general protoplasmic poisons and impair cell functions. They combine with one or more reactive functional groups (ligands), e.g. hydroxyl (–OH), carboxyl (–COO), sulphydryl (–SH), disulphide (S—S), amino (–NH$_2$), keto (C = O) and phosphate (PO$_4$) in cells and impair functions of enzymes and other cellular constituents. In very small quantities they are lethal to several gram-positive and gram-negative microorganisms.

This antimicrobial action in low dose is called oligodynamic action.

Adverse Reactions

All heavy metals are cumulative and potentially toxic. They cause severe gastrointestinal irritation when ingested. They cause damage to organs like liver, kidneys and gut. They also affect bone marrow and neurons. Their toxicity is mainly due to inhibition of sulphhydryl (–SH) group of enzymes.

DISCUSSION OF SOME HEAVY METALS

Arsenic (As)

Inorganic arsenicals are used mainly as rodenticides, herbicides and insecticides. Organic arsenicals were used in the treatment of syphilis, trypanosomiasis, amoebiasis and trichomoniasis in the past but now obsolete.

Pharmacokinetics

Soluble arsenical salts are rapidly absorbed from GIT.

They are also absorbed through skin. Arsenic is stored in liver, spleen, kidneys, lungs, intestine, bones, hair, brain and skeletal muscle. It is excreted slowly in urine and faeces. It can produce cumulative toxicity on repeated administration in small amounts. Arsenic deposited in hair and bones is retained for several years.

Arsenic poisoning: It is usually homicidal but may be accidental, especially in children after ingestion of arsenical insecticides or herbicides. It may be acute or chronic poisoning.

- **Acute arsenic poisoning:** It is manifested as nausea, vomiting, diarrhoea, dehydration, hypotension, circulatory collapse and renal failure. It resembles the symptoms of cholera and a careful distinction is essential before starting treatment. In severe poisoning, death may occur within 24 hours. Treatment consists of correction of fluid and electrolyte imbalance by administration of IV fluids and the specific antidote dimercaprol. Haemodialysis may be necessary in severe renal failure.
- **Chronic arsenic poisoning:** It occurs from drinking water contaminated with arsenic in the soil. It is manifested as weight loss, anorexia, fatigue, diarrhoea or constipation, oedema (particularly of eyelids and ankles), hyperpigmentation of skin, dermatitis (including exfoliative), inflammatory lesions of mucous membranes, loss of hair, brittle fingernails, jaundice, aplastic anaemia and peripheral neuropathy leading to numbness, paraesthesia, wrist and foot drop. Hyperkeratosis of the palm and sole, skin and lung cancers and encephalopathy have also been reported. Treatment consists of removal of the patient from the toxic influence and administration of the specific antidote dimercaprol.

Lead (Pb)

Lead compounds have no therapeutic use, except lead subacetate which is sometimes used as a constituent of Goulard's lotion for soothing and astringent action when applied in sprains. They are, however, used in household paints and various industries and can cause chronic lead poisoning. Poisoning with lead may also occur from lead projectiles (lead shots) when embedded in the skin or the muscle. Lead salts, internally and externally exert an astringent action by formation of lead proteinate.

Pharmacokinetics

Lead is absorbed to the extent of about 10% from GIT. It is also absorbed from the respiratory mucosa as observed in workers who inhale lead fumes or dust. It is stored in liver, kidneys, bones and muscles. It is slowly excreted in urine and sweat. It can produce cumulative toxicity on prolonged use.

- **Lead poisoning:** It may be acute or chronic poisoning in young children from licking lead paint or lead toys. It is manifested as metallic taste in mouth, vomiting, dehydration, coated tongue, paroxysmal intestinal colics and CNS symptoms like vertigo, paraesthesia, muscle cramps, weakness and paralysis of muscles (wrist or foot drop). Stools become dark colour due to presence of lead sulphide. Severe anaemia and haemoglobinuria may occur leading to death. Treatment consists of prompt gastric lavage and administration laxatives like magnesium sulphate for evacuation of lead from the gut and administration of the specific antidote sodium calcium edetate (EDTA). Antispasmodics may be used to control lead colic.
- **Chronic lead poisoning:** It occurs in workers engaged in printing and lead industries. It is manifested as persistent metallic taste in mouth, anorexia, paroxysmal intestinal colics (lead colics), constipation, greyish lead line along the gingival margin (due to periodontal deposition of lead sulphide), muscle weakness, fatigue and paralysis of muscles (lead palsy) causing wrist drop or foot drop, punctuate basophilic stippling of erythrocytes, microcytic hypochromic anaemia, jaundice, loss of memory, ataxia and encephalopathy (manifested as irrita.bility, restlessness, headache, tremors, delirium, convulsions and coma). Treatment consists of removal of the patient from the toxic influence and administration of the specific antidote, sodium calcium edetate. A less useful agent is penicillamine. Dimercaprol is of little value.

Mercury (Hg)

Inorganic mercurials are now not used in therapeutics. Organic mercurials are used as antiseptics and diuretics. They can cause acute or chronic poisoning.

- **Acute mercury poisoning:** It is usually due to accidental ingestion of mercuric chloride (corrosive sublimate) and other readily ionizable mercury salts. It is manifested as metallic taste in mouth, excessive salivation, inflammation of gums (gingivitis), vomiting, diarrhoea, hypotension, circulatory collapse, cardiac arrhythmias and renal failure. Treatment consists of administration of proteins in the form of raw eggs or milk, which form nontoxic mercury proteinates. This is followed by gastric lavage to eliminate the mercury from GIT and administration of the specific antidote dimercaprol. Penicillamine and dimercaptosuccinic acid (DMSA) may also be used. Supportive treatment for correction of water and electrolyte disturbances is also done.

- **Chronic mercury poisoning:** It is more common than acute mercury poisoning. It is due to repeated administration of small doses of mercury preparation taken internally or by external application of lotion or ointment of mercury. It is manifested as irritability, tremors, headache, fatigue, stomatitis, loss of appetite, profuse salivation, nausea, intestinal colics, diarrhoea and occasional vomiting. Gums are tender, swollen, inflamed and ulcerated (spongy gums). A blue line is seen at the junction of gum with the teeth. Tongue and cheeks are swollen and ulcerated. Skin eruptions (erythematous or eczematous) may appear. There may be progressive anaemia, ematiation, mental derangement, liver damage and kidney damage.

Treatment consists of stopping of mercury treatment and administration of the antidote dimercaprol. Penicillamine is an alternative drug. Supportive treatment for correction of water and electrolyte disturbances may be required.

Copper (Cu)

Copper sulphate is commonly used to preserve fruits and to improve colour of the green vegetables. Formerly, it was used to remove excess of granulation tissue and for the treatment of trachoma. It is a valuable antidote in phosphorus poisoning.

Copper poisoning: It may occur accidentally in children who suck it by confusing with candy. Suicidal poisoning with it may also occur.

- **Acute copper poisoning:** It is manifested as styptic metallic taste in the mouth, increased salivation, thirst, burning pain in stomach, vomiting, diarrhoea and headache. Colour of the vomit is bluish or greenish. Excessive vomiting causes signs of dehydration. Urine is suppressed or diminished in quantity. There may be jaundice due to fatty degeneration of liver. In some cases there may be convulsions, paralysis of limbs and coma. Treatment consists of administration of demulcents like egg albumin (to produce insoluble copper albuminate) followed by gastric lavage by plain water. Antidote used is penicillamine or trientine. Supportive treatment for correction of water and electrolyte disturbances is also done.

- **Chronic copper poisoning:** It may occur among workers in copper factory due to constant inhalation of copper dust. It is manifested as green or purple line in the gums, styptic metallic taste in the mouth, lassitude, giddiness, headache, dyspepsia, loss of appetite, vomiting, diarrhoea, intestinal colics, anaemia and paralysis of muscles.

Treatment consists of removal of the patient from the toxic influence and administration of the antidote, penicillamine or trientine.

Iron (Fe)

Iron preparations are used in microcytic hypochromic anaemia.

- **Acute iron poisoning:** It is seen in young children due to ingestion of a large amount of oral iron (tablets or capsules) confusing with candy. It is manifested as necrotizing gastroenteritis producing severe diarrhoea, vomiting, dehydration, intestinal colics, haematemesis, metabolic acidosis, hypotension, cardiovascular collapse, cyanosis, coma and even death. Treatment consists of gastric lavage with 1% sodium bicarbonate solution (to remove undissolved iron tablets or capsules) and administration of the specific antidote, desferrioxamine. Supportive treatment for correction of water and electrolyte disturbances is also done.

- **Chronic iron poisoning:** It occurs in persons getting repeated blood transfusion (patients of thalassaemia, etc.). It is manifested as iron overload, haemosiderosis and haemochromatosis (Bronze diabetes).

Treatment consists of intermittent blood letting by phlebotomy. The specific antidote, desferrioxamine is used in severe cases.

HEAVY METAL ANTAGONISTS

These are organic compounds which combine with the metallic ions to produce relatively nontoxic and water-soluble complexes, which are subsequently excreted in urine. The process by which these compounds combine with the metals to form relatively stable nonionized ring complexes is called chelation (Chele means claw). Hence, these compounds are called chelating agents (chelators), e.g. dimercaprol, succimer, penicillamine, sodium calcium edetate, disodium edetate, triethylene tetramine and desferrioxamine.

Properties of an Ideal Chelating Agent

- It should be highly water-soluble.
- It should form non-toxic complex with the metal.
- It should retain activity at body pH.
- It should not be metabolized in the body.
- It should be excreted rapidly from the body by glomerular filtration in the kidney.

DISCUSSION OF CHELATING AGENTS

Dimercaprol (British Antilewisite)

It was synthesized during the second world war (by Stocken and Thompson) to give protection against the arsenical vesicant war gases such as lewisite.

Chemically it is a dithiol compound having two –SH groups (shown in **Fig. 86.1**). It is a colourless oily liquid with pungent smell.

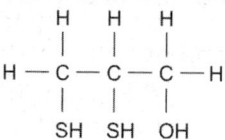

Fig. 86.1: Chemical structure of BAL

Pharmacological Actions

It forms stable and water-soluble chelate complexes with arsenic, mercury, gold, antimony, bismuth and cadmium ions, and thus protects the sulphydryl (SH) enzymes. With mercury and cadmium, the dimercaprol metal complex further reacts with another molecule of dimercaprol forming a still more stable inactive complex. Dimercaprol metal complex (2:1) is more stable than dimercaprol metal complex (1:1). These chelate complexes are excreted in urine. Dimercaprol not only protects the SH enzymes from inactivation by heavy metal but also reactivates the inhibited enzymes if administered in the early period of poisoning. It can inhibit enzymes like peroxidase, catalase and carbonic anhydrase, which have one of these metals as the prosthetic group.

Pharmacokinetics

Though it is soluble in water, but because of instability of the aqueous solution, it is administered IM in oily solution. After IM administration, peak plasma concentrations are attained in 30 to 60 minutes. Its half-life is short. Its metabolic degradation and excretion are complete within four hours.

Therapeutic Uses

It is used in acute poisoning due to arsenic, mercury, gold, antimony, bismuth and cadmium. It can be used in patients with Wilson's disease allergic to penicillamine.

Preparation and Dosage

Dimercaprol (BAL) injection (100 mg/2 mL in arachis oil) is administered IM in the dose of 2 to 3 mg/kg every 6 hourly for 2 days, twice on 3rd day and then once daily for 5 days.

Adverse Reactions

It can cause nausea, vomiting, headache, burning sensation in the mouth, salivation, lacrimation, paraesthesia of the extremities, muscle pain, muscle spasm, anginal pain, tachycardia and hypertension.

Contraindications

Iron poisoning (as it forms a toxic complex with iron) and hepatic damage. It should be used with caution in hypertensive patients.

Succimer

It is dimercaptosuccinic acid. It is chemically similar to dimercaprol but contains two carboxylic acids. It forms chelate complexes with arsenic, lead, mercury and cadmium. It can be administered orally. It is less toxic than dimercaprol because it is less permeable to cells due to lower lipid solubility. It can cause nausea, vomiting, diarrhoea, loss of appetite and skin rashes.

Penicillamine

It is a monothiol compound containing one –SH group. It is a degraded product of benzyl penicillin. Chemically it is β-dimethylcysteine. Its d-isomer is less toxic than l-isomer and so used clinically.

Pharmacological Actions

It forms stable and water-soluble chelate complexes with copper, lead, mercury and arsenic ions, and thus facilitates their excretion in urine. It also inhibits enzymes like trans-aminase and desulphhydrase, which have one of these metals as the prosthetic group.

Pharmacokinetics

It is well-absorbed from GIT after oral administration. It is rapidly excreted in urine.

Therapeutic Uses

It is mainly used in rheumatoid arthritis and acute copper poisoning. It is also used in acute lead, mercury and arsenic poisoning and to prevent copper accumulation in liver and basal ganglia in hepatolenticular degeneration (Wilson's disease), a rare hereditary disease of copper metabolism.

Preparation and Dosage

d-penicillamine (Cuprimin) capsule (125, 250 mg): 0.5 to 1 g daily in divided doses 1 hour before or 2 hours after meals (to avoid chelation of dietary metals).

Adverse Reactions

It can cause allergic reactions, bone marrow depression, nephrotoxicity and autoimmune syndrome (polymyositis and SLE).

Acetyl d-penicillamine is less toxic but weaker chelating agent than d-penicillamine. It is used in acute mercury poisoning.

Sodium Calcium Edetate (Ledclair) and Disodium Edetate

Their parent compound is ethylene diamine tetraacetic acid (EDTA).

Pharmacological Actions

They form stable and water-soluble complexes with metallic ions like calcium, magnesium, lead and iron. Sodium calcium edetate has a high affinity for lead, while disodium edetate has a high affinity for calcium. The affinity for other metals like sodium, potassium and magnesium is much less than that of lead and calcium.

Pharmacokinetics

They are poorly absorbed from GIT and so administered parenterally, usually IV. They are excreted almost completely within 24 hours by glomerular filtration and tubular secretion.

Therapeutic Uses

They are used in the treatment of acute and chronic lead poisoning and in hypercalcaemia, porphyria and iron poisoning.

Preparations and Dosage

- Sodium calcium edetate injection (20% solution in 5 mL ampoule)—20 to 40 mg/kg by IV infusion with normal saline or 5 % dextrose solution.
- Disodium edetate injection (3 g in 20 mL ampoule)—50 mg/kg by IV infusion with normal saline or 5% dextrose solution.

Adverse Reactions

They can cause thrombophlebitis, nephrotoxicity, nausea, vomiting, diarrhoea, lacrimation, fever, myalgia, dermatitis and allergic reactions (by releasing histamine).

Triethylene Tetramine (Trientine/Cuprid)

It is a copper chelating agent used in Wilson's disease to reverse the neurological changes. It is administered orally in the dose of 400 to 800 mg three times daily before meals. It is less toxic than penicillamine. It may cause iron deficiency which can be overcome by a short course of iron therapy.

Desferrioxamine

It is obtained from *Streptomyces pilosus* and is treated chemically to obtain the metal-free ligand. It is a iron chelating agent. It has high affinity for ferric iron and very low affinity for calcium. It removes iron from haemosiderin, ferritin and transferrin but not from haemoglobin or cytochromes.

Pharmacokinetics

It is poorly absorbed after oral administration and so parenteral administration is required in most cases. In severe iron poisoning, it is administered by IV infusion and in moderate cases of iron poisoning, it is administered IM of IV. In chronic iron poisoning (e.g. haemochromatosis) it is administered IM. It is metabolized mainly by plasma enzymes. It is readily excreted in urine.

Therapeutic Uses

It is the drug of choice in iron poisoning.

Preparation and Dosage

Desferrioxamine (Desferol) injection (500 mg pervial)—10 to 15 mg/kg/hour by IV infusion, 50 mg/kg IV or IM with a maximum dose of 1 g/day.

Adverse Reactions

It can cause dysuria, abdominal discomfort, diarrhoea, fever, leg cramps, tachycardia and allergic reactions including urticaria, pruritus, skin rashes and anaphylaxis.

Deferiprone

It is an orally active iron chelator which is used to clear the iron overload in transfusion siderosis and thalassaemia. It forms stable iron chelate complex, which is excreted in urine.

Preparation and Dosage

Deferiprone (Kelfer) capsule (250, 500 mg)—50 to 100 mg/kg/day in 2 to 4 divided doses.

Adverse Reactions

It is less toxic than desferrioxamine. It can cause anorexia, vomiting, altered taste, joint pain and neutropaenia.

87

Nonmetallic Environmental Toxicants

INTRODUCTION

Human beings live in a chemical environment and inhale, ingest or absorb from the skin many of these chemicals. It is important for the physician to know the potential effects of these chemicals and consider this information in making a clinical diagnosis or therapeutic plan. Contamination of air, water and food occurs due to industrialization, agricultural activity, production and use of energy, occupational exposure to chemicals and urbanization. The toxic effects of chemicals are dependent on the dose. The concentrations of chemicals in the air, water and food are usually at below levels, that produce toxic effects. Individuals most likely to experience adverse effects from chemicals are those who are exposed to chemicals at their workplace, because they often receive higher doses of chemicals than does the general population. For the safety of workers government has laid down threshold limit value (TLV) for most of the commonly used industrial chemicals.

It is expressed as parts per million (PPM). Common environmental and occupational toxic chemicals are air pollutants, solvents and vapours and pesticides.

Air Pollutants

Five major substances account for about 98% of air pollution. These are carbon monoxide (about 52%), sulphur dioxide (about 14%), nitrogen dioxide (about 14%), hydrocarbons (about 14%) and particulate matter (about 4%). These are primary air pollutants. The secondary air pollutants produced from primary pollutants by interaction with normal atmospheric components include ozone, sulphur trioxide, sulphuric acid, nitrous oxide, nitric acid, formaldehyde, acrolein, ketones and organic acids. They produce health hazards in humans and animals.

DISCUSSION OF SOME POISONOUS GASES

Carbon Monoxide (CO)

It is a colourless, tasteless, odourless and non-irritating gas, produced as a by-product of incomplete combustion of coal. The average concentration of carbon monoxide in the atmosphere is about 0.1 ppm. In heavy traffic the concentration may increase to 100 ppm.

Mechanism of Action

Carbon monoxide combines reversibly with the oxygen binding sites of haemoglobin and has affinity for haemoglobin that is about 220 times that of oxygen. The product formed 'carboxyhaemoglobin' cannot transport oxygen. Moreover, the presence of carboxyhaemoglobin interferes with the dissociation of oxygen from the remaining oxyhaemoglobin, thus reducing the transfer of oxygen to tissues. The brain and the heart are the most affected organs.

Clinical Effects

The important signs of carbon monoxide poisoning are those of hypoxia and progress in following sequence:

- Psychomotor impairment.
- Headache and tightness in the temporal area.
- Confusion and loss of visual acuity.
- Tachycardia, tachypnoea, syncope and coma.
- Deep coma, convulsions, shock and respiratory failure.

Prolonged hypoxia and posthypoxic unconciousness can result in residual irreversible damage to the brain and the myocardium.

Clinical effects of carbon monoxide may be aggravated by heavy labour, high altitudes and high ambient temperatures. The presence of cardiovascular diseases increases the risks associated with carbon monoxide exposure. Chronic exposure to low concentrations of carbon monoxide can produce development of atherosclerotic coronary disease in cigarette smokers.

Treatment

The individual is removed from the exposure site and respiration is maintained by administration of oxygen or artificial respiration. Oxygen is the specific antagonist of carbon monoxide. Hyperbaric oxygen therapy is very useful in carbon monoxide poisoning.

Sulphur Dioxide (SO$_2$)

It is a colourless irritant gas, generated primarily by the combustion of sulphur containing fossil fuels.

Mechanism of Action

Sulphur dioxide on contact with moist membranes, forms sulphurus acid, which is responsible for its severe irritant effects on eyes, mucous membranes and skin. About 90% of inhaled sulphur dioxide is absorbed in the upper respiratory tract causing bronchoconstriction and altered smooth muscle tone. Exposure to 5 ppm of sulphur dioxide for 10 minutes leads to increased resistance to airflow in human beings. Asthmatic patients are highly sensitive to sulphur dioxide.

Clinical Effects

It produces irritation of eyes, nose and throat and reflex bronchoconstriction. In severe exposure, pulmonary oedema may develop. Chronic exposure to low concentrations of sulphur dioxide can aggravate chronic cardiopulmonary disease.

Treatment

There is no specific antagonist of sulphur dioxide. Measures for relieving respiratory irritation are taken after removal of the individual from the exposure site.

Nitrogen Dioxide (NO$_2$)

It is a brownish irritant gas, sometimes associated with fires.

Mechanism of Action

It is a deep lung irritant capable of producing pulmonary oedema on acute exposure. The type I cells of the alveoli are mainly affected producing pulmonary lesions. It also irritates eyes, nose and throat in high concentration (50 ppm). Exposure of 100 ppm of nitrogen dioxide leads to pulmonary oedema and even death.

Clinical Effects

It produces irritation of eyes, nose and throat, cough, mucoid or frothy sputum production, dyspnoea and chest pain. In high concentration it produces pulmonary oedema within 1 to 2 hours. On chronic exposure to low concentrations of nitrogen dioxide emphysema of lungs is produced.

Treatment

There is no specific antagonist of nitrogen dioxide. After removal of the individual from the exposure site, certain measures are taken to relieve deep lung irritation and pulmonary oedema. These include maintenance of gas exchange with adequate oxygenation and alveolar ventilation. Drugs like broncho-dilators, antibiotics and sedatives are also used.

Ozone (O₃)

It is a bluish irritant gas that occurs normally in the earth's atmosphere, where it is an important adsorbent of ultraviolet light. It is formed by conversion of O_2 to O_3 in the atmosphere. Its concentration varies from 0.02 ppm in rural atmosphere to 0.2 ppm in urban atmosphere.

Mechanism of Action

It is an irritant of mucous membranes, especially of upper respiratory tract.

Clinical Effects

It produces respiratory tract irritation, cough and bronchoconstriction on mild exposure and shallow rapid breathing and pulmonary oedema on heavy exposure.

Treatment

There is no specific antagonist of ozone. After removal of the individual from the exposure site measures are taken to relieve deep lung irritation and pulmonary oedema like nitrogen dioxide.

Organic Solvents and Vapours

Organic solvents and their vapours are a common part of environment. Short exposures to low concentrations of solvent vapours such as gasoline, lighter fluids, aerosal sprays and spot removers may be relatively harmless, but exposure to paint removers, floor and tile cleaners and other solvents in home or industry may be dangerous. Halogenated hydrocarbons (aliphatic and aromatic) and polyhydric alcohols are widely used as industrial solvents, degreasing agents and cleaning agents. Halogenated aliphatic hydrocarbons are carbon tetrachloride, chloroform, trichloroethylene, tetrachloroethylene, trichloroethane, methyl isocyanate (MIC), etc. On acute exposure these agents cause CNS depression, neurotoxicity, hepatotoxicity, nephrotoxicity and some degrees of cardiotoxicity. On chronic exposure they cause impairment of memory, peripheral neuropathy and even carcinogenicity.

Treatment

There is no specific treatment. Treatment is symptomatic (depends upon the organ system involved).

Halogenated aromatic hydrocarbons are benzene and toluene. Benzene is used as solvent and as an intermediate in the synthesis of other chemical agents. It causes depression of CNS. Acute exposure of benzene causes euphoria, nausea, locomotor problems, headache, vertigo, drowsiness, coma and even death. Chronic exposure produces bone marrow depression leading to leucopenia, pancytopaenia, thrombocytopaenia and aplastic anaemia.

Toluene (methylbenzene) does not possess myelotoxic properties of benzene but possesses CNS depressant action. Acute exposure to toluene can cause fatigue, ataxia and loss of consciousness.

Pesticides

These include insecticides, rodenticides, herbicides and fungicides. They are used to control insects, rodents, noxious weeds and noxious fungi respectively which are harmful to plants and humans.

Insecticides kill insects in agricultural lands. These are of four groups:

- Chlorinated hydrocarbon insecticides, e.g. DDT (Chlorophenothane), γ-benzene hexachloride, cyclodienes and toxaphenes.

- Organophosphorus insecticides, e.g. malathion (Folidol), parathion, trichlorfon, ceptophos and diazinon (Tik-20).

- Carbamate insecticides, e.g. carbaryl (Sevin), dimetan, dimetilan, pyramand, propoxur (Baygon).

- Botanical insecticides, e.g. nicotine, rotenone and pyrethrum.

Rhodenticides kill rodents (rats and mice) and protect stored foodstuffs. These are hydrogen cyanide, acrylonitrile, carbon tetrachloride, strychnine, phosphorus, zinc phosphide and thalium. Herbicides destroy noxious weeds. These are of two groups:

- Chlorphenoxy compounds, e.g. dichlorophenoxy acetic acid and trichlorophenoxy acetic acid.
- Bipyridyl compounds, e.g. Paraquat.

Fungicides destroy noxious fungi and control fungal diseases in plants and seeds. These are dithiocarbamates, hexachlorobenzene and pentachlorophenol.

Treatment of Poisoning by Pesticides

- Decontamination of the individual from the poison.
- Administration of specific antidote if available, e.g. atropine and pralidoxime in case of organophosphorus compound or carbamate poisoning.
- Symptomatic and supportive treatment.

General management of drug poisoning is discussed in adverse drug reactions in general pharmacology.

Part 3

Section I

PRACTICAL PHARMACOLOGY

88

Pharmacy

INTRODUCTION

Pharmacy deals with the collection, preservation, compounding and dispensing of drugs. It may be official pharmacy or extemporaneous pharmacy.

Pharmacist is a person with a knowledge of pharmacy. He compounds and dispenses prescriptions of drugs. Weights and measures used in pharmacy are given in **Table 88.1**.

Preparations

I. Mixtures (from Latin word Mistura)

A mixture is a liquid medicinal preparation containing several doses of one or more drugs in solution or suspension and inten-

Table 88.1: Weights and measures used in pharmacy					
Metric System					
Weights (kilogram)			*Measures (litre)*		
1 kg	=	1000 g (gram)	1 L (liter)	=	1000 mL (millilitre)
1 g	=	1000 mg	1 mL	=	1 cc (cubic centimetre)
1 mg	=	1000 µg			
Imperial System					
Weights			*Measures*		
1 lb (pound)	=	16 oz. (ounce)	1 o (pint)	=	20 ft. oz. (fluid ounce)
1 oz.	=	437.5 gr. (grain)	1 fl. oz.	=	8 fl. dr. (fluid dram)
			1 fl. dr.	=	60 min (minim)
Relationship between Metric and Imperial Systems					
Weights			*Measures*		
1 g	=	15.4 gr.	1 mL	=	15 min
1 gr.	=	65 mg	1 fl. oz.	=	28.4 mL
1 oz.	=	28.4 g	1L	=	35.2 fl. oz.
Domestic Measures (Approximate Equivalents)					
1 drop	=	0.05 mL = 1 min.			
1 teaspoonful	=	4 mL = 1 fl. dr.			

Table 88.2: Latin phrases and abbreviations previously used in prescriptions

Phrase	Abbreviation	English meaning
Adde	ad	Add up to
Ana ana	a.a	Of each
Ante cibum	a.c.	Before food
Aqua	aq	Water
Bis in die	b.d./b.i.d.	Twice daily
Cum	C	With
Cras mane	c.m.	Tomorrow morning
Cras nocte	c.n.	Tomorrow night
Compositum	co	Compound
Fiat	ft	Let it be made
Gutta	Gtt	Drop
Hora somni	h.s.	At bed time
Misce	M	Mix
Mitte tales	mit. tal	Send such
Post cibum	p.c.	After food
Per os	p.o.	By month
Pro re nata	p.r.n.	As required
Omni die	o.d.	Everyday
Omni nocte	o.n.	Every night
Quantum sufficient	q.s.	Sufficient quantity
Quarter in die	q.d./q.i.d.	Four times daily
Quaque hora	q.h.	Every hour
Recipe	Rx	Take thou
Statim	Stat	Immediately
Si opus sit	S.O.S.	When necessary
Ter in die	t.d./t.i.d.	Thrice daily
Vesper	Vesp.	Evening

ded for oral administration to produce local or systemic effect.

Types of mixture: It may be:

- *Simple mixture:* It contains soluble solid ingredients, e.g. carminative mixture and alkali mixture.

- *Compound mixture:* It may be:

  - Mixture containing insoluble but diffusible solid ingredients, e.g. purgative mixture (containing magnesium sulphate and magnesium carbonate) and antacid mixture (containing aluminium hydroxide gel and magnesium trisilicate).

  - Mixture containing insoluble and indiffusible solid ingredients, which require a suspending agent (gum acacia or gum tragacanth), e.g. bismuth carbonate suspension and kaolin/creta (chalk) suspension.

Haustus (Draught) is a single dose mixture administered at bed time, e.g. Haustus sedative (containing potassium bromide).

Preparation of Mixtures

1. *Compound and dispense*
   For X,
   Rx,
   Sodium bicarbonate   – 1g
   Compound cardamom tincture   – 2 mL
   Aromatic spirit of ammonia   – 1 mL
   Water add up to   – 30 mL
   Mix and make a dose of a mixture. Send 4 such.

Direction: One dose to be taken twice daily after meal.

Date: ABC
                                   (Name of Prescriber)

Requirements
Measuring balance and weights.
Mortar and pestle.
Measuring cylinders (10 mL and 100 mL).
Mixture phial.
Paper, scissors and gum.

Ingredients: Sodium bicarbonate, compound cardamom tincture, aromatic spirit of ammonia.

Procedure: It involves 3 steps:

- *Dose marking*: 120 mL of tap water is taken in the mixture phial by means of the measuring glass. A narrow strip of white paper (2 cm breadth), whose upper margin coincides with the upper level of water and lower margin coincides with the midpoint between upper convex and lower flat surface of the dispensing phial is cut. It is folded into 4 equal parts and its corners are trimed off. It is then pasted by gum on one of the flat surfaces of the mixture phial.

- *Labelling*: A piece of white paper in rectangular shape is cut according to the flat surface of the mixture phial (covering the middle portion and leaving 1/3rd portion from the top and 1/6th portion from the bottom). The label is written and pasted on the mixture phial at the opposite side of dose marking.

THE MIXTURE
No. 1   Date:
For: X
Direction: One dose to be taken twice daily after meal.
Pharmacy: Medical
Shake the phial before use

- *Preparation of mixture*: 4 g of sodium bicarbonate is weighed by the balance and taken in the mortar. It is then made fine powder with the help of the pestle. 90 mL (3/4th of total amount) of water is added to sodium bicarbonate in the mortar. Then 8 mL of compound cardamom tincture is added to it and mixed well with the help of the pestle. 4 mL of aromatic spirit of ammonia is taken in the mixture phial and the content of the mortar is added to it. Water (tap) is slowly added to it till it reaches the upper margin of the dose slip. Then the phial is corked and shaked well. Finally it is handed over to the pharmacist.

Actions and uses

Carminatives are drugs which cause expulsion of gases from stomach and intestine and used as antiflatulent agents in flatulence, dyspepsin and intestinal colic. Sodium bicarbonate is a gastric antacid and acts by neutralizing gastric HCl as follows:

$$NaHCO_3 + HCl \rightarrow NaCl + H_2O + CO_2$$

CO$_2$ evolved is responsible for carminative action. Compound cardamom tincture contains cardamom oil (1.4%), cinnamon oil (2.8%), caraway (1.4%), cochineal (0.5%), glycerine (5%), alcohol (60%) and water (added up to 100 mL). Cochineal is the powdered dried female insects called Spanish fly (*Dactylopius coccus*). It gives red colour to the tincture/mixture. Amaranth and carmin are plant products which can be used in place of cochineal in the carminative mixture.

Aromatic spirit of ammonia contains ammonium bicarbonate (2.5%), strong solution of ammonia (7%), lemon oil (0.5%), nutmeg oil (0.3%), alcohol (75%) and water (added up to 100 mL).

Volatile oils and substances present in compound cardamom tincture and aromatic spirit of ammonia cause mild irritation of the gastrointestinal mucosa leading to increased tone and motility (peristalsis) of intestine and relaxation of sphincters leading to expulsion of gases.

2. *Compound and dispense*

For X,

Rx,

S.S. magnesium sulphate   – 60 mL

Put 2 marks

Direction: One dose to be taken next morning on an empty stomach.

Date: ABC

Requirements

Measuring balance and weights.

Mortar and pestle.

Measuring cylinders (100 mL).

Mixture phial.

Funnel and filter paper/cotton wool.

Paper, scissors and gum.

Ingredients: Magnesium sulphate.

Procedure: Dose marking and labelling are done as carminative mixture.

THE MIXTURE
No. 2   Date: For: X
Direction: One dose to be taken next morning on an empty stomach. Pharmacy: Medical College Pharmacy.
Shake the phial before use

Calculation: Solublity of magnesium sulphate is 1 in 1.5 parts of water.

2 mL of saturated solution (S.S.) of magnesium sulphate contains 1 g of magnesium sulphate and 1.5 mL of water (tap).

Therefore, 60 mL of saturated solution of magnesium sulphate contains 30 g of magnesium sulphate and 45 mL of water. [The increase in volume of the solution is due to presence of water of crystallization in magnesium sulphate ($MgSO_4.7H_2O$)].

30 g of magnesium sulphate is weighed by the balance and taken in a mortar. It is reduced to fine powder with the help of the pestle. Then 45 mL of water is added to it and mixed. It is then filtered through a filter paper or cotton wool placed in a funnel and collected in the measuring cylinder. It will be found to be 60 mL after filtration. Then it is transferred to the mixture phial and corked. Finally it is handed over to the pharmacist.

Actions and uses

Saturated solution of magnesium sulphate is a saline purgative used in acute constipation, food or drug poisoning (to remove poison from gut), after administration of an anthelmintic (to remove paralysed or dead worms from gut) and before X-ray examination of abdomen or abdominal surgery (to remove gases and hard faecal masses from gut). It acts by osmotic action and so it is an osmotic purgative. Both the ions of magnesium sulphate are poorly absorbed from the intestine. As a result they draw fluid from the intestinal wall and prevent absorption of water from the lumen of the intestine increasing the bulk of the intestinal content. This increases distention of intestinal wall and stimulates peristalsis leading to purgation (watery or liquid stools occurring in 2 to 3 hours).

Difference between Saturated and Supersaturated Solution

Saturated solution contains maximum amount of a solute dissolved in a solvent (water) at a particular temperature and pressure. Supersaturated solution contains additional amount of the solute in dissolved state in an already made saturated solution by raising temperature, pressure or both. On lowering temperature or pressure, the solute precipitates.

II. Powders (from Latin word Pulvaris)

A powder is a solid medicinal preparation containing one or more dry substances reduced to fine particles and uniformly mixed and intended for internal or external use.

Types of powder: It may be:

- *Simple powder*: It contains one active solid ingredient, e.g. atropine, aspirin, etc. and sometimes an excipient (inert substance), e.g. lactose, calcium lactate, etc. (to increase the bulk of the powder).

- *Compound powder*: It contains 2 or more active solid ingredients, e.g. aspirin, paracetamol and caffeine (APC), magnesium hydroxide and dried aluminium hydroxide gel (antacid powder).

- *Prepared powder (Pulverata)*: It contains a definite percentage of the active ingredient (alkaloid or glycoside), e.g. prepared digitalis leaf powder (contains 0.4% of digitalis glycosides, mainly digoxin), prepared belladonna herb powder (contains 0.3% of belladonna alkaloids, mainly atropine), etc.

Preparation of Powders

1. *Compound and dispense*

For X,

Rx,

Magnesium hydroxide	– 0.5 g
Dried aluminium hydroxide gel	– 0.5 g

Mix and make a powder.

Send 6 such.

Direction: One powder is to be taken thrice daily one hour after each meal.

Date: ABC

Requirements

Measuring balance and weights.

Pill tile and spatula (2, horn or iron).

Powder box.

Paper, scissors and gum.

Ingredients: Magnesium hydroxide and dried aluminium hydroxide gel.

Procedure: 3 g of magnesium hydroxide and 3 g of dried aluminium hydroxide gel are weighed separately by the balance and taken on pill tile, where they are crushed and uniformly mixed with the help of the spatula. The mixed powder is then arranged in a rectangular fashion (block) by the spatula below the scale of the pill tile and then divided into 6 equal parts by the spatula. Each part of powder is taken on separate piece of paper and then wrapped in classical manner (discussed later on). Then powders are put in a powder box, on which a label is pasted. Finally it is handed over to the pharmacist.

Label

THE POWDER
No. 1   Date: For: X
Direction: One powder is to be taken thrice daily one hour after each meal.
Pharmacy: Medical College Pharmacy.

Wrapping of powder: The powder is placed on the centre of the paper. The lower border of the paper is turned up to upper 1/7th of its width. The upper border of the paper is folded over the lower border of the paper. The upper fold is folded in such a way that it comes to the centre of the folded paper. The folded paper is turned to the opposite side and the ends are folded in such a way that their margins lie at a distance leaving 1/3rd portion in the centre.

Action and uses

Magnesium hydroxide and dried aluminium hydroxide gel are nonsystemic insoluble antacids used in hyperacidity, gastritis, reflex oesophagitis and peptic ulcer. Magnesium hydroxide is rapidly acting antacid. It quickly neutralizes gastric acid (HCl) to the end point of pH 3.5 as follows:

$$Mg(OH)_2 + 2HCl \rightarrow MgCl_2 + 2H_2O$$

In the intestine, $MgCl_2$ reacts with $NaHCO_3$ forming magnesium carbonate, sodium chloride, CO_2 and water.

$$MgCl_2 + 2NaHCO_3 \longrightarrow MgCO_3 + 2NaCl + CO_2 + H_2O$$

$MgCO_3$ is excreted in faeces and NaCl is absorbed.

Aluminium hydroxide is a slowly acting antacid, which neutralizes gastric acid (HCl) to the end point of 4.5 as follows:

$$Al(OH)_3 + 3HCl \longrightarrow 3AlCl_3 + 3H_2O$$

In the intestine, $AlCl_3$ reacts with $NaHCO_3$ forming aluminium hydroxide, hydrochloric acid and CO_2.

$$AlCl_3 + 3NaHCO_3 \longrightarrow Al(OH)_3 + 3NaCl + CO_2$$

$Al(OH)_3$ is excreted in faeces and NaCl is absorbed.

Advantages of Combination of Two Antacids

- Produces a relatively even and sustained antacid effect. $Mg(OH)_2$ is a rapid acting antacid, which neutralizes acid within a few minutes. $Al(OH)_3$ is a slow acting antacid, which produces sustained antacid effect by neutralizing acid.

- Produces synergistic (additive) effect and so less dose of each antacid is required.
- Antagonizes the side effects of each other antacid. Given alone $Mg(OH)_2$ produces loose stool due to laxative action and $Al(OH)_3$ produces constipation due to astringent action. Combination of both antacids produces normal stool.

2. *Compound and dispense*

For X,

Rx,

Sodium chloride	– 3.5 g
Trisodium citrate dehydrated	– 2.9 g
Potassium chloride	– 1.5 g
Mix and make a powder.	
Glucose	– 20 g
Send one such.	

Direction: The powder is to be dissolved in previously boiled and cooled one litre of water and to drink as directed.

Date: ABC

Requirements:

Measuring balance and weights.

Pill tile and spatula (2).

Powder box/envelop.

Paper, scissors and gum.

Ingredients: Sodium chloride, trisodium citrate, dehydrated potassium chloride and glucose.

Procedure: 3.5 g of sodium chloride, 2.9 g trisodium citrate dehydrated, 1.5 g of potassium chloride and 20 g of glucose are weighed separately by the balance and taken on pill tile, where they are crushed and uniformly mixed with the help of the spatula. The mixed powder is then taken on a piece of paper of suitable size and wrapped in classical manner. It is then put in a powder box or envelop and a label is pasted on it by gum. Finally it is handed over to the pharmacist.

Label

THE POWDER
No. 2   Date:
For: X
Direction: The powder is to be taken dissolved in previously boiled and cooled one litre of water and to drink as directed.
Pharmacy: Medical College Pharmacy.

Actions and uses

Oral rehydration solution (ORS) as powder is a substitute of normal saline and ringer lactate solution, for use in mild to moderate dehydration due to diarrhoea and vomiting causing loss of electrolytes like sodium, potassium. It prevents dehydration in diarrhoea, vomiting, burns and sunstroke. There are two types of ORS powder, *viz.*

ORS-1: It contains sodium bicarbonate (2.5 g).

ORS-2: It contains trisodium citrate dehydrated (2.9 g).

Other ingredients remain the same.

ORS-2 is more preferred than ORS-1, because trisodium citrate dehydrated is neutral and stable, whereas sodium bicarbonate is alkaline and unstable (degrades rapidly in solution). Sodium citrate is converted to sodium bicarbonate in the liver by metabolism.

Glucose helps in facilitated diffusion of sodium and potassium in the intestinal cells leading to their rapid absorption. It also supplies nutrition.

Super ORS contains an additional ingredient amino acid (glycine or alamine), which helps in intestinal absorption of sodium and potassium by cotransport like glucose.

III. Lotions (from Latin word Lotio)

A lotion is a liquid preparation containing one or more ingredients in the form of solution or suspension and meant for local application, usually externally.

Type of lotion: It may be:

1. *Simple lotion:* It contains soluble solid ingredients, e.g. potassium permanganate lotion (0.025%), mercurochrome lotion (2%) and normal saline lotion (0.9%).

2. *Compound lotion:* It contains two or more insoluble ingredients and a suspending agent, e.g. calamine lotion (B.P.).

Preparation of Lotions

1. Compound and dispense

For X,

Rx,

Potassium permanganate lotion—400 mL (1:4000)

Direction: To gargle twice daily.

Date: ABC

Requirements:

Measuring balance and weights.

Lotion bottle.

Measuring cylinder (100 mL) and glass rod.

Paper, scissors and gum.

Ingredients: Potassium permanganate.

Calculation: 4000 mL of potassium permanganate lotion contains 1 g of potassium permanganate.

∴ 400 mL of potassium permanganate lotion contains

$\dfrac{400}{4000}$ = 0.1 g = 100 mg of potassium permanganate.

Procedure: 100 mg of potassium permanganate is weighed by the balance and taken in a 100 mL measuring cylinder. Boiled and cooled water is added to it up to 100 mL marking and stirred by glass rod. Then it is transferred to a lotion bottle is discarded. Final volume (400 mL) of lotion is made by adding 300 mL of boiled and cooled water in the lotion bottle. It is then mixed by shaking the bottle after putting a cork. A label is pasted on the bottle. Finally it is handed over to the pharmacist.

Label

THE LOTION
(Poison)
No. 1   Date:
For: X
Direction: To wash the wound twice daily.
Pharmacy: Medical College Pharmacy.
For external use only.

Actions and uses

Potassium permanganate lotion is an antiseptic lotion used as gargle or mouthwash in stomatitis, gingivitis, pharyngitis and tonsillitis for vaginal wash in vaginitis and for washing of superficial infected wounds and snake bite. Potassium permanganate is an oxidizing agent. It liberates nascent oxygen when comes in contact with bacteria, and thus oxidizes bacterial protein leading to inhibition of bacterial growth or may even kill them. It has a short-lasting action. In high concentration, potassium permanganate (1:500) solution is a disinfectant (kills bacteria) and deodorant (removes bad smell) of organic matters by its strong smell. It is also used for stomach wash in alkaloidal poisoning except atropine.

2. *Compound and dispense*

For X,

Rx,

Calamine	–	15 g
Zinc oxide	–	5 g
Bentonite	–	3 g
Sodium citrate	–	0.5 g
Liquefied phenol	–	0.5 mL
Glycerine	–	5 mL
Purified water added up to	–	100 mL

Mix and make a lotion.

Direction: To be applied locally thrice daily.

Date: ABC

It is calamine lotion (B.P.).

Requirements

Measuring balance and weights.

Mortar and pestle.

Lotion bottle, glass rod.

Measuring cylinders (10 and 100 mL).

Paper, scissors and gum.

Ingredients: Calamine, zinc oxide, bentonite, sodium citrate, liquefied phenol and glycerine.

Procedure: 15 g of calamine, 5 g of zinc oxide, 3 g of bentonite and 0.5 g of sodium citrate are weighed separately by the balance and taken in a mortar. These are finally ground and mixed with the help of a pestle. Then 0.5 mL of liquefied phenol, 5 mL of glycerine and 75 mL of boiled and cooled water are added to it with the help of measuring cylinders and mixed thoroughly with the help of the pestle. The liquid is taken in a 100 mL measuring cylinder and water is added up to 100 mL marking. It is then stirred by a glass rod and poured into a lotion bottle. A cork is put and a label is pasted on the lotion bottle. Finally it is handed over to the pharmacist.

Label

THE LOTION (Poison)	
No. 1	Date:
For: X	
Direction:	To be applied locally twice daily.
Pharmacy:	Medical College Pharmacy.
Shake the bottle before use. For external use only.	

Actions and uses

Calamine lotion is an antiseptic, astringent protective and soothing lotion used in the treatment of various types of skin diseases such as dermatitis, eczema (oozing), urticaria, sunburn, impetigo, psoriasis, bed sores, napkin rashes and skin eruptions due to herpes, pox, measles, etc.

Calamine is the basic zinc carbonate (98%) coloured pink with ferric oxide (2%). It is a mild astringent, antiseptic and protective agent. Zinc oxide is a mild astringent, soothing and protective agent. Bentonite is a native colloidal hydrated aluminium silicate free from grittiness. It is insoluble in water but swells up to about 12 times of its volume in water to form a homogeneous mass (gel). It is used as a suspending agent in the lotion. Sodium citrate is highly soluble in water. It acts as a suspending agent by decreasing the viscosity produced by bentonite and converts gel into soluble form. Liquefied phenol (80% w/v of phenol) is an antiseptic and anti-pruritic agent (by local anaesthetic action). Glycerine prevents drying of lotion by virtue of its viscid character and keeps the skin moist and soft.

IV. Ointments (from Latin word Ungnentum)

An ointment is a semisolid or pasty preparation containing one or more solid ingredients incorported in a hydrocarbon or fatty base and intended for external application with or without rubbing. An ointment for use in the eye is called ophthalmic ointment (oculentum). Composition of commonly used ointment bases given as follows:

- *Simple ointment:* It contains wool fat (5%), cetostearyl alcohol (5%), hard paraffin (5%) and white or yellow soft paraffin (85%).

- *Paraffin ointment:* It contains hard paraffin (3%), white beeswax (2%), cetostearyl alcohol (5%) and white or yellow soft paraffin (90%).

- *Eye ointment:* It contains liquid paraffin (10%), wool fat (10%) and yellow soft paraffin (80%).

- *Emulsifying ointment:* It contains liquid paraffin (20%), emulsifying wax (30%) and white soft paraffin (50%).

Preparation of Ointments

1. *Compound and dispense*

For X,

Rx,

Atropine sulphate	–	100 mg
Yellow soft paraffin	–	9.9 g

Mix and make an eye ointment.

Direction: To be applied on eyelid margins twice daily.

Date: ABC

Requirements:

Dispensing balance and weights.

Ointment pot/gallipot

Pill tile and spatula.

Paper, scissors and gum.

Thread/rubber band.

Ingredients: Atropine sulphate and yellow soft paraffin.

Procedure: 100 mg of atropine sulphate and 9.9 g of yellow soft paraffin are weighed separately by the balance and kept on the pill tile at two places. These are mixed intimately with the help of two spatulas (horn) to produce a homogeneous paste. The paste is shifted to the ointment pot/gallipot at the side by a spatula. The mouth of the ointment pot/gallipot is covered by a circular paper and tied by a thread or a rubber band is applied. Then a circular label is pasted on the paper of the pot. Finally it is handed over to the pharmacist.

Label

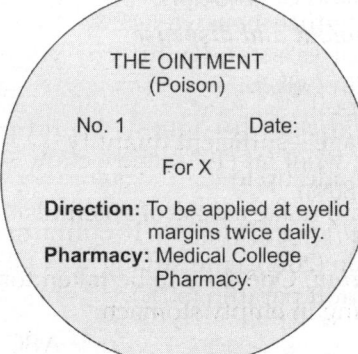

THE OINTMENT
(Poison)

No. 1   Date:

For X

Direction: To be applied at eyelid margins twice daily.
Pharmacy: Medical College Pharmacy.

Actions and uses

Atropine sulphate eye ointment is as mydriatic (to produce dilatation of pupil) and cycloplegic (to produce paralysis of accommodation) ointment, used for ophthalmologic examination of eye (dark room test), to measure the refractive error of the eye for fitting of glasses, especially in children below 5 years, who have high parasympathetic tone. It is also used in inflammatory conditions of eye like acute iritis, iridocyclitis and keratitis to give rest to the eye (in all persons).

It is contraindicated in glaucoma, as it increases intraocular tension.

2. *Compound and dispense*

For X,

Rx,

Sulphur ointment (B.P.)	– 10 g

Send.

Direction: To be used externally on the whole body surface from the neck to feet for 3 consecutive nights, followed by soap water bath and washing of garments, bed clothes, lineh, etc. on the 4th day.

Date: ABC

Requirements

Dispensing balance and weights.

Ointment pot/gallipot

Pill tile and spatula (2).

Paper, scissors and gum.

Ingredients: Sulphur powder and yellow soft paraffin (precipitated sulphur is better than sublimed sulphur because it is nongritty).

Calculation: For 10 g sulphur ointment requirements are: sulphur powder—1 g and yellow soft paraffin—9 g.

Procedure: 1 g of sulphur powder and 9 g of yellow soft paraffin are measured separately by the balance and kept on pill tile at 2 places. These are mixed intimately with the help of two spatulas (iron or horn) to produce a homogeneous paste. The paste is shifted to the ointment pot/gallipot at the side by a spatula. The mouth of the ointment pot/gallipot is covered by a circular paper and tied by a thread or a rubber band is applied. Then a circular label is pasted on the paper of the pot. Finally it is handed over to the pharmacist.

Label

THE OINTMENT
(Poison)

No. 2   Date:

For X

Direction: To be applied at external as directed.
Pharmacy: Medical College Pharmacy.

Actions and uses

Sulphur ointment is a scabicidal ointment used in the treatment of scabies. Scabies is a parasitic infestation caused by a mite, i.e. female sarcoptes (*Acarus scabiei*) which lay eggs in the burrows and crypts of webs of fingers, wrists, buttocks and genitalia and produce severe itching of skin, particularly at night (nocturnal). Applied to the skin, sulphur is slowly reduced to H_2S and oxidized to SO_2 and parathionic acid in contact with alkaline fluid. Parathionic acid is scabicidal. It is better to apply the ointment at bed time, as female parasites lay eggs at night and gives better patient compliance. The disadvantages of this ointment are bad odour, stains in clothings and requires repeated application. All the clothings and bedsheets should be boiled to prevent reinfection.

Some better scabicidal drugs than sulphur ointment are given as follows:

1. Benzyl benzoate emulsion (25%) (Ascabiol).
2. Gammabenzene hexachloride lotion (1%) (Lorexane).
3. Crotamiton cream/lotion (10%) (Crotorax).
4. Monosulphiram lotion (25%) or soap (Tetmosol).

5. Thiabendazole suspension (10%) (Mintizol).
6. Ivermectin tablet (5 mg) (Mectizen) 200 µg/kg body weight a single dose orally.

V. Emulsions (from Latin word Emulsio)

An emulsion is a mixture of two immiscible liquids, *viz*. oil and water, one of which is dispersed in fine droplets throughout the other with the help of an emulsifying agent (emulgent). Oil dispersed as fine droplets is the internal phase and water enclosing the oil droplets is called dispersion medium or external phase. An emulgent is a colloid substance which helps in the formation of stable emulsion. It forms thin films around oil droplets and prevents the coalescence of oil droplets by lowering surface tension. Commonly used emulgents are gum acacia powder and gum tragacanth powder.

Advantages of Emulsions

- Palatable due to masking of unpleasant taste of the oil.
- Greater surface area for action or absorption.

Causes of Crack of an Emulsion

- Irregular mixing of oil and water.
- Bad manipulation.
- Decomposition or precipitation of the emulgent.
  Preparation of gum, water and oil to make primary emulsion
  Fixed oil—1 : 2 : 4
  Volatile oil—1 : 2 : 2

Preparation of Emulsions

1. *Compound and dispense:*
For X,
Castor oil   – 8 mL
Mucilage—sufficient quantity
Water add up to   – 30 mL
Mix and make a dose of an emulsion. Send 2 such.
Direction: One dose to be taken tomorrow morning in empty stomach.
Date: ABC.

Requirements

Dispensing balance and weights.

Mortar and pestle.

Measuring cylinders (10 and 100 mL).

Mixture phial.

Paper, scissors and gum.

Ingredients: Castor oil and gum acacia powder.

Procedure: 4 g of gum acacia powder and 8 mL of water are taken in the mortar and triturated with the help of the pestle in clockwise direction till the mucilage is made. Then 16 mL of castor oil is added to the mucilage drop by drop with constant trituration till a clicking sound is produced or the emulsion becomes milky white. 30 mL of water is then added to the primary emulsion and mixed well. It is transferred to the mixture phial, which is labeled and dose marking given. Then water is added to make the final volume 60 mL. The phial is corked and shaked well. Finally it is handed over to the pharmacist.

Label

THE EMULSION	
No. 1	Date:
For: X	
Direction: One dose to be taken tomorrow morning in empty stomach.	
Pharmacy: Medical College	
Shake well before use	

Action and use: It is an irritant purgative used in acute constipation.

89

Pharmaceutical Preparations and Appliances

- *Tablet*: It is a hard biconvex on flat disc prepared by compressing the powder of the drug and excipient and meant for oral administration. It is of following types:
  - Plain tablet (presence of no line or coating on the surface)
  - Scored tablet (presence of a line in the middle of the surface, where it can be broken)
  - Enteric coated tablet (presence of coating of cellulose, acetate or phthalate on the surface of the tablet to protect the drug from destruction by gastric acid and to prevent gastric irritation by the drug)
  - Vaginal tablet with an applicator (for local use in vaginitis)
- *Capsule*: It is a hollow, cylindrical or oval receptacle made of gelatin and glycerine containing the drug in powder form or liquid state and meant for oral administration. It is of following types:
  - Hard capsule (hard in consistency)
  - Soft gelatin capsule (soft in consistency)
  - Controlled release capsule (spamule/ timesule).
  - Sustained release capsule (S.R. Cap).
- *Suppository*: It is a conical or torpedo-shaped body made by mixing the active drug (in powder form) with oil of theobroma (basis) and beeswax (which melts at body temperature) and meant for rectal administration. It produces local action in the rectum and avoids gastric irritation by the drug.
- *Suspension*: It is a liquid preparation contaning an insoluble drug (as powder) and a suspending agent (gum acacia/gum-tragacanth) and meant for oral administration. It is supplied in a glass or plastic bottle. It may be supplied as dry powder in a bottle, which is reconstituted by adding water to make liquid suspension.
- *Emulsion*: It is a liquid preparation containing an oil, an emulsifying agent (gum acacia/gum tragacanth) and water in the form of fine droplets and meant for oral administration. It is supplied in a glass or plastic bottle.
- *Enema*: It is a liquid preparation containing the active drug for rectal use. It is supplied in enema tube with the applicator. It may be evacuant enema (proctoclysis/exit) or retention enema of prednisolone/metronidazole/paraldehyde).
- Rectal ointment in tube (containing an active drug) with an applicator is used in piles and anal fissures.
- *Eye/Ear drops*: It is a liquid preparation containing the active drug for eye or ear use. It is supplied in a vial with a dropper.
- *Transdermal patch*: It is a thick adhesive patch of several layers containing the active drug, which is slowly released from it producing prolonged systemic effect. It is applied over the skin at different sites.

- *Ampoule*: It is a thin-walled sealed glass container holding the drug solution (in small or large volume) for injection (SC, IM or IV) in a single dose. It is out at the constricted part by a glass cutter to take out the drug in a syringe for injection.

- *Vial*: It is a thick-walled glass container with a rubber cap sealed by a tin foil and containing a drug as solution or powder, which is reconstituted (made solution or suspension) by adding purified water with the help of a needle attached to a syringe, after removing the tin foil and pushing through the rubber cap. The solution in the vial is taken in the syringe and used for injection (SC, IM or IV). A vial may be single dose or multidose vial.

- *Syringe*: It is made of glass or plastic material. It has a barrel and a piston. A needle is fitted to its nozzle. It is used for injection (SC, IM or IV) of drugs. It may be glass syringe, disposable (plastic) syringe, tuberculin syringe and insulin syringe or pen injector. The capacity of the syringe may be 1 to 100 mL.

- *Injection needle*: It is made of stainless steel with a stilet inside. The size of the needle varies with the size of the syringe. It should be disposed after use.

- *IV cannula*: It is a plastic device for administration of drug solutions into the vein through its inlets (2 or 3) from time to time and then closing the inlets by the steel stilets. The outlet is placed inside the vein and kept secured by leucoplast on the skin.

- *Inhaler*: It is a plastic or glass device for inhalation of a drug as a solution or powder placing it on the mouth or nose. It may be metered dose inhaler (delivering a measured amount of a drug as aerosol), spinhaler (delivering dry powder of a drug by puncturing of a capsule) or nebulizer (delivering compressed air-driven nebulized solution of a drug). It is used in patients of bronchial asthma and chronic obstructive pulmonary disease (COPD) for local action in the respiratory tract and to avoid systemic effects.

- *Sets*: These are devices for fluid infusion or blood transfusion. Fluid infusion set contains a glass bottle or plastic bag, rubber or plastic tube regulator of flow and stainless steel needle. It has no filtering net (strainer) inside the broad plastic tube, where fluid dropping occurs. Blood transfusion set is similar to fluid infusion set but it has a filter net (strainer) inside the broad plastic tube, where blood filtration occurs to remove foreign bodies, if present.

- Donor set contains 2 needles for collection of blood from a donor into a glass bottle containing anticoagulant solution. It is similar to fluid infusion set.

  Scalp vein (butterfly) set contains fine plastic tube and needle. It is used for administration of fluid or drug solution as well as for collection of blood for investigation in infants and young children.

- *Packages*: These are devices to contain drugs as tablets or capsules. These may be ordinary pack (looks plain), blister pack (looks like blisters), sequential pack (of oral contraceptive pills) or combipack (of anti-tubercular drugs, anti-*Helicobacter pylori* drugs, etc).

- *Sachet*: It is a small bag made of thick paper or aluminium foil containing drugs as powders or granules, e.g. ORS powder, befenium granules, etc.

- *Bottles*: These are glass or plastic containers for keeping drugs. These may be colourless or coloured bottles. Coloured bottles are used for presentation of drugs (ether, halothane, chloralhydrate, paraldehyde, etc.) which are decomposed by sunlight.

CHARTS AND TRACINGS FOR INTERPRETATION

Appropriate kymographic tracings/log dose response curves are shown in Figures 4.1, 4.2a to c, 6.1a to c, 6.2, 6.3, 6.4a and b, 6.5a, 11.1, 11.2, 11.3, 15.2, 15.3.

Section II

CLINICAL PHARMACOLOGY

90

Prescription Writing

INTRODUCTION

A prescription is a written order of a registered medical practitioner for one or more medicines together with direction to the pharmacist for their preparation and to the patient for their use at a particular time.

A complete prescription consists of six parts:

- Patient's name, sex and age.
- **Superscription:** It is written as Rx or Re, which is the symbol for the Latin word *Recipe*, meaning take thou. It is written at upper left hand corner of the prescription.
- **Inscription:** It is the body of the prescription. It enumerates the ingredients with their amounts. It consists of four groups of ingredients, *viz.* basis (chief ingredient), adjuvant (helps the basis), corrigent (corrects undesirable effects of the basis or adjuvant) and vehicle (water) or excipient (lactose, etc.).
- **Subscription:** It is the direction to the pharmacist for compounding and dispensing of drugs.
- **Signature:** It is the direction to the patient about the administration of doses of drugs, and duration of treatment. It should be written in English or Mother language.
- Initial of the medical practitioner with date. Registration number of the prescriber should be written in prescribing drugs belonging to Dangerous Drug Act (DDA), e.g. opioids, barbiturates, benzodiazepines, alcohol, cocaine, hallucinogens, etc.

EXAMPLES OF PRESCRIPTION

1. A school teacher, BD, aged 30 years presented in the chest OPD with complaints of chronic cough, chest pain, evening rise of temperature for the last 4 weeks. After clinical examination and laboratory investigation and chest X-ray, he was diagnosed as a case of uncomplicated pulmonary tuberculosis. Prescribe an antitubercular regiment for this patient.

   For Mr BD

   i. Isoniazaid tablet (each tablet containing 300 mg)

      Direction: One tablet to be taken daily before breakfast.

   ii. Rifampicin capsule (each capsule containing 450 mg)

      Direction: One tablet to be capsule daily before breakfast.

   iii. Ethambutol tablet (each tablet containing 800 mg)

      Direction: One tablet to be taken daily after breakfast.

   iv. Pyrazinamide tablet (each tablet containing 750 mg)

Direction: One tablet to be taken daily after breakfast.

The above regimen is to be continued for two months, followed by isoniazid and rifampicin in above doses for another four months.

v. Pyridoxine hydrochloride tablet (each tablet containing 10 mg)

Direction: One tablet to be taken daily in the morning along with isoniazid for six months.

Date: ABC

2. A young man of 28 years presented with high fever for 10 days. A thorough clinical examination led to a provisional diagnosis of typhoid fever that was confirmed by a positive Widal's test. Prescribe a drug for the typhoid fever of this patient.

For Mr X

Rx,

Ciprofloxacin tablet—28 tablets (each tablet containing 500 mg)

Direction: One tablet to be taken twice daily after food for two weeks.

Date: ABC

3. An adult person is suffering from frequent loose motion containing mucous and blood since last night. He is clinically diagnosed to be suffering from bacillary dysentery. Write a prescription for specific treatment of bacillary dysentery.

For Mr X

Rx,

Norfloxacin tablet—10 tablets (each tablet containing 400 mg)

Direction: One tablet to be taken twice daily for five days.

Date: ABC

4. Mr RB, complaining of epigastric burning pain particularly while the stomach remains empty for last 3 weeks. Upper GI endoscopy revealed the presence of a duodenal ulcer. Prescribe a drug for the treatment of his duodenal ulcer.

For Mr RB

Rx,

Famotidine tablet—42 tablets (each tablet containing 40 mg)

Direction: One tablet to be taken at bed time for a period of six weeks.

Date: ABC

5. Mr PD suffering from dysentery for last one day. Stool examination reveals the presence of trophozoite of *Entamoeba histolytica*. Write a prescription for the treatment of this patient.

For Mr PD

Rx,

i. Metronidazole tablet—21 tablets (each tablet containing 400 mg)

Direction: One tablet to be taken thrice daily after food for seven days.

ii. Diloxanide Furoate tablet—21 tablets (each tablet containing 500 mg)

Direction: One tablet to be taken thrice daily after food for next seven days.

Date: ABC

6. An adult patient needs bowel clearance for the radiological examination of his abdomen in the next morning. Prescribe a purgative for that patient.

For Mr X

Rx,

Bisacodyl tablet—2 tablets (each tablet containing 5 mg)

Direction: Two tablets to be taken at bed time.

Date: ABC

7. A 6-year-old child suffering from pain abdomen, weakness, anorexia and irregular bowel habits. After proper clinical and microscopical examination of stool, the child was found to be suffering from mixed worm infestation. Prescribe a drug to cure his infestation.

For Master X

Rx,

Albendazole tablet—1 tablet (each tablet containing 400 mg)

Direction: One tablet to be taken at bed time.

8. A young adult suffering from several attacks of convulsions with unconsciousness in last couple of months. After clinical and EEG study the case was diagnosed as generalized tonic-clonic seizure. Prescribe a drug for the treatment of his epilepsy.

For Mr X

Rx,

Phenytoin sodium tablet—24 tablets

Direction: One tablet to be taken thrice daily and the patient is asked to report after seven days.

Date: ABC

9. A 24-year-old female presenting with acute onset of right-sided headache accompanied by nausea, vomiting and vertigo. She is diagnosed as a case of migraine. Prescribe a drug for her treatment.

For Miss X

Rx,

Ergotamine tablet—6 tablets (each tablet containing 1 mg)

Caffeines tablet—6 tablets (each tablet containing 100 mg)

Direction: One tablet to be taken immediately followed by one tablet half hourly (if necessary) till relief of pain is achieved.

Date: ABC

10. An adult patient presented with multiple anaesthetic nodules on different parts of the body. Cutaneous smear from the anaesthetic patch revealed smear +ve for *M. lepra* Bacilli. Prescribe drugs for this patient.

For Mr X

Rx,

  i. Rifampicin capsule (each capsule containing 600 mg)

   Direction: One capsule to be taken one hour before breakfast once a month (supervised) for two years.

 ii. Dapsone tablet (each tablet containing 100 mg)

   Direction: One tablet to be taken daily after breakfast for two years.

iii. Clofazimine capsule (each capsule containing 50 mg)

   Direction: One capsule to be taken daily and six capsules (300 mg) to be taken once a month (supervised) for two years.

Date: ABC

11. A middle-aged female presented with multiple itching ring-like lesions over the abdomen, thigh and inguinal region and clinically was diagnosed to be a case of tinea corporis and tinea cruris. Prescribe treatment for this infection.

For Mrs X

Rx,

Miconazole ointment (2%)—1 tube (each tube containing 15 g)

Direction: To be applied over the affected part twice daily for one month.

12. A middle-aged female presents with history of frequency and burning sensation during micturition for last 10 days. Clinically she was diagnosed as a case of urinary tract infection. Prescribe a drug for the treatment of this patient.

For Mrs X

Rx,

Norfloxacin tablet—28 tablets (each tablet containing 400 mg)

Direction: One tablet to be taken twice daily for two weeks.

Date: ABC

13. A 30-year-old male patient presented with painless hard ulcer on his external genitalia. Clinically this was diagnosed to be a case of syphilis. Prescribe specific drug for this patient.

For Mr X

Rx,

i. Benzathine penicillin injection—1 vial (each vial containing 2.4 million units)

ii. Water for injection—1 ampoule (each ampoule containing 5 mL)

Direction: The content of the vial is to be dissolved in 5 mL of water for injection and half the quantity is to be injected deep intramuscularly with wide bore needle in each buttock.

Date: ABC

14. A 28-year-old male patient complains of purulent discharge from the urethra for last 2 days. Examination of the urethral discharge showed the presence of gram-negative intracellular diplococci, i.e. Gonococci. Prescribe proper drugs for this patients.

For Mr X

Rx,

i. Amoxicillin capsule—6 capsules (each capsule containing 500 mg)

Direction: Six capsules to be taken as a single dose at bed time.

ii. Probenecid tablet—2 tablets (each tablet containing 500 mg)

Direction: Two tablets to be taken half an hour before administration of capsules.

Date: ABC

15. An adult person presented in the eye OPD with redness mucopurulent discharge of his eyes. Clinically it was diagnosed as acute bacterial conjunctivitis. Prescribe specific treatment for the patient.

For Mr X

Rx,

i. Ciprofloxacin eye drop (0.3%)—1 vial (each vial containing 5 mL)

ii. Ciprofloxacin eye ointment (0.3%)—1 tube (each tube containing 5 g)

Direction: Two drops to be instilled in each eye thrice daily during the day time and the ointment to be applied to the lower palpebral conjunctiva of each eye at bed time till the condition improves.

Date: ABC

16. An adult male patient complaining of occasional attacks of nausea and vomiting, associated with heartburn. Patient was found to be suffering from oesophageal reflux. Prescribe a drug to control the nausea and vomiting for this patient.

For Mr X

Rx,

Metoclopramide tablet—6 tablets (each tablet containing 10 mg)

Direction: One tablet to be taken twice daily half an hour before meals.

17. An adult female presented with chronic cough with fever, bilateral non-pitting oedema for the last 6 weeks. The patient was diagnosed to be suffering from filariasis. Prescribe a drug for the treatment of this condition.

Diethyl carbamazine citrate tablet—63 tablets (each tablet containing 100 mg)

Direction: One tablet to be taken thrice daily for 21 days.

Date: ABC

18. A middle-aged male patient presented with pain and swelling of his right great toe with difficulty in walking for last two days. Clinical examination revealed that to be a case of acute gout. Prescribe a drug for the treatment of this patient.

For Mr X

Rx,

Colchicine tablet—20 tablets (each tablet containing 0.5 mg)

Direction: Two tablets to be taken immediately followed by one tablet every two hourly until relief of pain is obtained or vomiting or diarrhoea results.

Date: ABC

91

Drug Interactions with Prescriptions

EXAMPLES

1. **Rifampicin + Oral contraceptive pill (OCP):** It is a pharmacokinetic drug interaction at the level of metabolism.

   Rifampicin is a semisynthetic bactericidal agent. It is effective against mycobacterial and many other injections.

   OCP is an example of fixed dose combination of mainly ethinyloestradiol (a semisynthetic oestrogen) and norethindrone acetate (a synthetic progesterone).

   Result of interaction: Failure of contraception, menstrual irregularities like breakthrough bleeding, spotting and amenorrhoea.

   Mechanism of interaction: Rifampicin is a hepatic microsomal enzyme inducer. So the metabolism of both oestrogen and progestational components are increased and contraceptive effect of OCP is reduced.

   Remarks: This type of interaction may happen when the OCP contains less amount of oestrogen and progesterone. The patient should be advised to take OCP of high hormone content or to adopt other type of contraceptive methods.

2. **Ciprofloxacin + Theophyllines:** It is a pharmacokinetic drug interaction at the level of metabolism.

   Ciprofloxacin is one of the most commonly used fluoroquinolone bactericidal agents.

   Theophylline is a methylxanthine used in bronchial asthma.

   Result of interaction: Increased side effects of theophylline such as palpitation, hypotension, cardiac arrhythmias and convulsion.

   Machanism of interaction: The major pathway of theophylline metabolism involves 8-hydroxylation resulting in formation and excretion of 1,3-dimethyluric acid. Ciprofloxacin inhibits the metabolism of theophylline by inhibition or 8-hydroxylation pathway. So plasma conc. of theophylline is increased.

   Therapeutic plasma conc. of theophylline is 10–15 mcg/mL. Tachycardia, restlessness, agitation and emesis occur at 20 mcg/mL. Seizures or convulsion occur at 30–40 mcg/mL.

   Remarks: Concurrent adiministration of these two drugs should be avoided.

3. **Metronidazole + Alcohol:** It is a pharmacokinetic drug interaction at the level of metabolism. Metronidazole is a potent chemotherapeutic agent used for multiple infections.

   Alcohol is a common beverage.

   Result of interaction: Precipitation of antabuse/disulphiram like reactions characterized by nausea, vomiting, abdominal cramps, hypotension and uneasiness.

Mechanism interaction: Alcohol is metabolized in two steps. In the first step, alcohol is converted to acetaldehyde by alcohol dehydrogenase. In the second step, acetaldehyde is converted to acetic acid by the enzyme aldehyde dehydrogenase. Acetic acid is eliminated from the body in the form of CO_2 and water. Metronidazole inhibits the enzyme aldehyde dehydrogenase resulting in accumulation of acetaldehyde, responsible for antabuse-like manifestation.

Remarks: The patient should be advised to avoid alcohol during metronidazole therapy.

NB: Other drugs causing antabuse-like reaction with alcohol are cephalosporins, oral hypoglycaemic agents, chloramphenicol, nitrofurantoin, etc.

4. *Chloroquine + Alkali mixture*: It is a pharmacokinetic drug interaction at the level of renal excretion. Chloroquine is an antimalarial drug.

Alkali mixture is a commonly used mixture in fever to counteract pyrexia induced metabolic changes.

Result of interaction: Increased side effects of chloroquine such as hypotension, vasodilation, decreased myocardial activity, ECG changes, cardiac arrest, visual disturbances, headache, lichenoid skin eruptions, bleaching of hair, etc.

Mechanism of interaction: Chloroquine is a basic drug. It is excreted in unchanged form (50%) and as its metabolite monodesethylchloroquine (20%) through kidney. Alkali mixture makes the urine alkaline. So there occurs less ionization of chloroquine in the alkaline urine leading to extensive reabsorption of chloroquine in renal tubules and increased side effects of chloroquine.

Remarks: Alkali mixture should be avoided during chloroquine therapy.

5. *Chlorpropamide + Dicoumarol*: It is a pharmacokinetic drug interaction at the level of metabolism.

Chlorpropamide is an oral hypoglycaemic agent.

Dicoumarol is an oral anticoagulant acting only *in vivo*.

Result of interaction: Hypoglycaemic effect of chlorpropamide is increased.

Mechanism of interaction: Dicoumarol prolongs the duration of action (half-life) of chlorpropamide by inhibiting its hepatic metabolism by microsomal enzymes and also reducing its renal excretion.

Remarks: During cotherapy, the dose of chlorpropamide is to be adjusted (decreased).

6. *Lithium + Thiazide*: This is a pharmacokinetic drug interaction at the level of renal excretion.

Lithium (a monovalent cation) is a mood stabilizer with narrow margin of safety.

Thiazides are moderately potent diuretics.

Result of interaction: Increased toxicity of lithium.

Mechanism of interaction: Thiazide causes hyponatremia by excreting sodium in urine and so renal elimination of lithium is reduced due to increased tubular reabsorption of lithium in proximal tubules.

Remarks: Lithium and thiazide should not be coadministered.

7. *Propranolol+ Insulins*: This is a pharmacodynamic drug interaction. Propranolol is a non-selective β-blocker.

Insulin is the hypoglycaemic hormone released from the pancreatic β-cells.

Result of interaction: (a) Symptoms of insulin-induced hypoglycaemia might be masked, (b) potentiation of insulin-induced hypoglycaemia, (c) delayed recovery from hypoglycaemia and (d) possibility of rise in BP and precipitation of angina pectoris.

Mechanism of interaction: (a) Insulin can cause hypoglycaemia in diabetic patient particularly when there is unaccustomed exercise after insulin administration, hypoglycaemia causes adrenergic hyperactivity. So there will be tachycardia, palpitation, tremor and sweating. Propranolol blocks these effects by blocking the adrenergic receptors. Diagnosis of hypoglycaemia may be difficult and initiation of treatment is delayed. (b) Propranolol itself causes hypoglycaemia. (c) Insulin-induced hypoglycaemia is compensated by hepatic glycogenolysis. Propranolol prevents this. So recovery from hypoglycaemia is delayed. (d) Unopposed activity of adrenaline on α-adrenergic receptors can increase the peripheral resistance and rise of BP.

Remarks: Administration of propranolol in diabetic patients with insulin therapy is a relative contraindication. This type of drug interaction is less with cardioselective beta blockers like atenolol.

8. *Levodopa + Pyridoxine:* This is a pharmacodynamic drug interaction at the level of decarboxylation of levodopa.

Levodopa is used for the treatment of idiopathic parkinsonism.

Pyridoxine is vitamin B_6 and acts as a cofactor of DOPA decarboxylase enzyme.

Result of interaction: The availability of dopamine in the CNS is reduced and the anti-parkinsonian effect of levodopa is decreased.

Mechanism of interaction: Peripheral conversion of levodopa to dopamine by DOPA decarboxylase is enhanced by pyridoxine. Dopamine (a catecholamine) cannot cross blood–brain barrier. Less amount of levodopa is available to enter the CNS, and so the amount of dopamine in the basal ganglia to produce beneficial effect in parkinsonism is reduced.

Remarks: Levodopa and pyridoxine should not be coadministered.

9. *Antacid + Sucralfate:* This is a pharmacodynamic drug interaction.

Antacid neutralizes the gastric HCl and raises pH of the gastric contents. They are used in the treatment of peptic ulcer.

Sucralfate is an ulcer protective agent which strongly adheres to ulcer base and protects it from peptic digestion.

Result of interaction: The cytoprotective effect of sucralfate is reduced.

Mechanism of interaction: The sucralfate complex is formed by sucrose octasulphate and polyaluminium hydroxide. In acidic pH (below 4), there occurs extensive polymerization and crosslinking of sucralfate to form a sticky, viscid, yellow-white gel, which adheres strongly to the base of ulcer crater and protects it from peptic digestion. It adheres to the ulcer base for more than 6 hours and helps in healing of ulcer.

Antacid by neutralizing gastric HCl, raises the pH of gastric contents and prevents polymerization of sucralfate and gel formation. So the ulcer healing effect of sucralfate is reduced.

Remarks: Antacid and sucralfate should not be administered simultaneously. Sucralfate should be administered at least half an hour after antacid administration or it is better to avoid this combination.

10. *Digoxin + Hydrochlorothiazide:* This is a pharmacodynamic drug interaction.

Digoxin is a cardiac glycoside mainly used in congestive cardiac failure with atrial fibrillation and in congestive heart failure. Hydrochlorothiazide is moderately potent, moderately efficacius and diuretic.

Result of interaction: Incidence of digoxin-induced cardiac arrhythmias is increased.

Mechanism of interaction: Digoxin inhibits myocardial Na^+/K^+-ATPase. So exit of Na^+ from the cell and entry of K^+ to the cell is inhibited. This leads to increased intracellular conc. of Na^+ and there is secondary rise of intracellular Ca^{++} conc. The effect of digoxin is enhanced in presence of hypokalaemia because there is increased availability of digoxin to the cardiac cell and increased binding of digoxin with Na^+/K^+-ATPase. Moreover, hypokalaemia itself inhibits Na^+/K^+ pump.

Hydrochlorothiazide causes moderate natriuresis, kalliuresis, hypercalcaemia, and hypomagnesaemia. By inducing hypokalaemia, hydrochlorothiazide can precipitate cardiac arrhythmias. Hypercalcaemia and hypomagnesaemia also can increase the incidence of digoxin-induced cardiac arrhythmias.

Remarks: During cotherapy, potassium supplementation should be done either in the form of diet (fruit juice, coconut water and vegetables) or KCl syrup or tablet.

11. *Verapamil + Propranolol:* This is a pharmacodynamic drug interaction.

Verapamil is a calcium channel blocker. Propranolol is a non-selective β-blocker.

Result of interaction: (a) May precipitate heart failure, AV block and severe bradycardia, and (b) bronchoconstrictory effect of propranolol is compensated by verapamil.

Mechanism of interaction: (a) Both propranolol and verapamil reduce myocardial contractility, heart rate and impulse conduction. In addition, verapamil inhibits the hepatic metabolism of propranolol to some extent. (b) Propranolol bloks $β_2$-adrenergic receptors of the smooth muscle of tracheobronchial tree and increases airway resistance. Verapamil by blocking calcium entry can cause bronchodilatation.

Remarks: Cotherapy should be done cautiously particularly in paroxysmal supraventricular tachycardia.

12. *Enalapril + Spironolactone:* This is a pharmacodynamic drug interaction.

Enalapril is an ACE inhibitor.

Spironolactone is a potassium-sparing diuretic. It acts as an aldosterone antagonist.

Result of interaction: Increased incidence of hyperkalaemia and arrhythmias.

Mechanism of interaction: Enalapril, being an ACE inhibitor, inhibits the formation of angiotensin II. Subsequently, aldosterone releases from adrenal cortex is reduced leading to decreased secretion of potassium in distal tubules and collecting ducts. Spironolactone, being an aldosterone antagonist, reduces the secretion of potassium in late distal tubules and collecting ducts. So when enalapril is combined with spironolactone, there may be dangerous hyperkalaemia and cardiac arrhythmias.

Remarks: Enalapril should not be combined with spironolactone during treatment of hypertension or heart failure.

13. *Amoxicillin + Clavulanic acid:* This is a pharmacodynamic drug interaction.

Amoxicillin is an extended-spectrum aminopenicillin.

Clavulanic acid is a β-lactamase inhibitor obtained from *Streptomyces clavuligerus*.

Result of interaction: Amoxicillin becomes effective against penicillinase/β-lactamase producing strains of *Staphylococci, H. influenzae, Gonococci* and *E. coli.*

Mechanism of interaction: The antibacterial action of amoxicillin is due to the presence of β-lactam ring in their structure. Penicillinase breaks the β-lactam ring, and thus the antibacterial action of amoxicillin is reduced. Clavulanic acid has a β-lactam ring that binds to β-lactamase and inactivates them (suicide inhibitor). Thus, clavulanic acid prevents the destruction of β-lactam antibiotics and potentiates the action of amoxicillin.

Remarks: Cotherapy or fixed dose combination of amoxicillin and clavulanic acid is beneficial to the patient.

14. *Gentamicin + Gallamine:* This is a pharmacodynamic drug interaction.

Gentamicin is an aminoglycoside antibiotic.

Gallamine is a non-depolarizing neuromuscular blocking drug.

Result of interaction: Muscle relaxant effect of gallamine is increased.

Mechanism of interaction: Gallamine competes with Ach, for N_m receptors or motor end plate and causes relaxation of skeletal muscle. Excess Ach, at these sites reduces the relaxant effect of gallamine. Gentamicin inhibits the release of Ach from motor end plate, and thus increases the relaxant effect of gallamine.

Remarks

 i. Use of aminoglycoside antibiotic with gallamine should be avoided.

 ii. Dose of non-depolarizing neuromuscular blocking agents should be reduced.

15. *Aspirin + Warfarin sodium:* This is both pharmacokinetic and pharmacodynamic drug interaction.

Aspirin is a prototype non-steroidal antiinflammatory drug.

Warfarin sodium is an oral anticoagulant acting only *in vivo*.

Result of interaction: Increased bleeding tendencies from various sites.

Mechanism of interaction

 a. *Pharmacokinetic:* Aspirin may displace warfarin from plasma protein binding sites resulting in increased level of free warfarin in plasma.

 b. *Pharmacodynamic:* Warfarin sodium increases prothrombin time (PT) by inhibiting the synthesis of vitamin K-dependent clotting factors. Aspirin increases bleeding time and interferes in the normal haemostasis by inhibiting the platelet aggregation. So there is increased bleeding tendencies. Moreover, aspirin is ulcerogenic in stomach and duodenum.

Remarks: Clinical significance is conflicting. This type of interaction may occur in patient of postmyocardial infarction when warfarin and aspirin are given together after initial heparin therapy.

It is better to avoid warfarin along with aspirin. If at all an antiplatelet drug is to be given along with warfarin then dipyridamole ticlopidine may be preferred.

92

Therapeutic Problems

INTRODUCTION

During prescribing of drugs for patients, some problems are faced by doctors. These can be managed by correct diagnosis of the disease by symptoms and signs and rational treatment of the disease by appropriate drugs. Some examples of therapeutic problems are given here for proper understanding about the matter. It should be remembered that a doctor must give relief to the patient by appropriate treatment within a short period as possible.

Examples of Therapeutic Problems

1. A ten-year-old school girl suffering from mild exercise induced bronchial asthma has been treated with a metered dose inhaler containing 500 μg of terbutaline per inhalation as and when required, which effectively controls the individual attack. However, she has attacks of wheezing every 3 to 4 weeks occurring during exercise even after above treatment schedule. What treatment should now be given to reduce the frequency of attacks?

Presenting features: Attacks of wheezing every 3 to 4 weeks occurring during exercise even after treatment with terbutaline.

Relevant information: A ten-year-old school girl suffering from mild exercise induced bronchial asthma was effectively controlled by 500 μg terbutaline inhalation as and when required.

Inference: As the girl even after treatment with terbutaline inhalation has been experiencing attacks of wheezing during the exercise, the said treatment schedule is not sufficient and she needs additional treatment.

Treatment

• Terbutaline (500 μg) by inhalation to continue as and when required.
• Cromolyn sodium (5 or 10 mg) four times daily by inhalation for 6 to 8 weeks. The patient is advised to report after that period. If the frequency of attacks remains unaltered, then beclomethasone dipropionate (100 μg) by inhalation four times daily to be given and continued for a period.

2. A 16-year-old school girl is admitted to the emergency department with severe short of breath. She is diagnosed as bronchial asthma. She has been using metered dose inhalation of salbutamol, ipratropium and beclomethasone. Inspite of the above treatment, the present attack is not controlled. What will be her immediate treatment?

Presenting features: The patient is having severe short of breath.

Relevant information: A ten-year-old girl has been using metered dose inhalation of salbutamol, ipratropium and beclomethasone.

Inference: Inspite of the treatment with above drugs, she has developed acute episode of bronchial asthma.

Treatment

- Moist oxygen inhalation (with normal saline) is given at the rate of 2 to 3 L/min before, during and after administration of bronchodilators to avoid worsening of ventilation/perfusion mismatch.
- Inhalation of salbutamol (5 mg) or terbutaline (10 mg) by nebulizer. Alternatively, salbutamol (250 µg) by slow IV injection or terbutaline (200–500 µg) by SC injection can be given. Aminophylline (5 mg/kg) by slow IV injection over 20 minutes may be administered to speed up the response.
- Hydrocortisone sodium succinate—200 to 500 mg IV 4–6 hourly.
- Administration of IV fluid like normal saline or 5% dextrose saline slowly.
- Administration of antibiotic like amoxicillin capsule 500 mg 8 hourly.
- Correction of acidosis by IV sodium bicarbonate solution (to produce systemic alkalinization). It also increases the sensitivity of bronchodilators.
- Transferred to intensive care unit (ICU) of a hospital, if the condition does not improve.

3. A 69-year-old woman suffering from CCF has been treated with 0.25 mg digoxin tablet daily for last 3 months, but the heart failure is not controlled adequately.

Presenting features: Inadequate control of CCF.

Relevant information: A 69-year-old woman suffering from CCF has been treated with 0.25 mg digoxin tablet daily for 3 months.

Inference: As the CCF is not adequately controlled by digoxin alone, so she needs additional treatment.

Treatment

- Physical rest is essential.
- Moderate salt restriction (2–3 g/day).
- Digoxin tablet (0.25 mg)—0.25 mg daily to be continued.
- Frusemide tablet (40 mg)—20 to 40 mg/day to be added.

- Enalapril tablet (2.5, 5 mg)—to start with a low dose of enalapril (2.5 mg daily) is to be given after stopping diuretic for 1–2 days. If there is no hypotension, the dose is gradually increased up to 5 to 20 mg daily depending on the response.
- Cause of the heart failure has to be investigated and treated properly.
- Serum potassium level is to be investigated at regular intervals and potassium supplementation is to be done if necessary.

4. A 45-year-old male patient with history of smoking presented with exertional retrosternal compressing pain radiating to the left arm and lasts for 2–5 minutes. The pain is relieved after taking rest. After proper investigation, he has been diagnosed as a case of stable angina pectoris. What will be the treatment to control the attack?

Presenting features: Exertional retrosternal compressing pain radiating to the left arm lasting for 2–5 minutes and relieved by rest.

Relevant information: A 45-year-old male patient with history of smoking.

Inference: The patient is diagnosed to be a case of stable angina pectoris and he needs treatment for control of acute attack and also for prevention of attacks.

Treatment

- The patient is advised to stop smoking.
- Diet: Fat-restricted diet is advised.
- For termination of acute attack:

  Glyceryl trinitrate tablet (0.5 mg)—one tablet sublingually or isosorbide dinitrate tablet (5 mg)—same.

  Maximum three tablets can be taken at 5 minutes interval.

- For prophylaxis (prevention):
  - Isosorbide 5-mononitrate tablet (20 mg)—one tablet twice daily.
  - Atenolol tablet (50, 100 mg)—50 to 100 mg daily.
  - Nifedipine tablet (5, 10 mg)—5 to 10 mg thrice daily, initially and then gradually increasing up to 10 to 20 mg thrice daily.

– Low dose aspirin tablet (75, 150 mg)— 75 to 150 mg once daily.

5. A 45-year-old patient suffering from angina pectoris is on treatment with isosorbide dinitrate. He is admitted to the hospital with severe chest pain and sweating and diagnosed as a case of AMI. What will be the management of this patient?

Presenting features: The patient is admitted with severe chest pain and sweating.

Relevant information: A 45-year-old patient suffering from angina pectoris was on treatment with isosorbide dinitrate.

Inference: The patient is diagnosed as a case of AMI.

Management

- The patient should be admitted in intensive coronary care unit of a hospital and continuous ECG monitoring is to be done.
- Moist oxygen inhalation is given at the rate of 2 to 4 L/min for 6 to 12 hours.
- Low dose aspirin tablet (100 mg)—one tablet daily.
- Access for IV administration of drugs is done.
  – For relief of pain—Morphine sulphate injection 2 to 4 mg IV every 5 to 10 minutes till the pain is relieved (not exceeding a total dose of 20 mg).
  To control morphine induced vomiting, metoclopramide injection 10 mg IV.
  – To reduce myocardial oxygen demand and infarct size—Metroprolol injection— 5 mg IV every 15 minutes for 3 doses, provided the pulse rate is more than 60 minutes.
  Glyceryl trinitrate by IV infusion pump at the rate of 5 µg/min initially and then the dose is gradually increased depending on the condition of patient.
  – For reperfusion of affected vessels— Streptokinase injection 1.5 million units in 100 mL of saline by IV infusion over one hour.

– To prevent thromboembolism—Delta-parin sodium (LMW heparin) injection— 5000 units 12 hourly SC. It is followed by long-term warfarin therapy.
– To control pump failure and shock— Dopamine injection—2.5 µg/kg/min by continuous IV infusion and then the dose is gradually increased to achieve appropriate haemodynamic response.
– To control cardiac arrhythmias—proper antiarrhythmic drugs are used.

6. An overweight middle-aged man is found to be hypertensive while attending a clinic for medical check-up. His BP is 170/100 mm of Hg on two successive observations. What will be the treatment for this patient?

Presenting features: BP 170/100 mm of Hg on two successive observations.

Relevant information: The patient is middle-aged and overweight.

Inference: The patient is suffering from moderate hypertension, which has to be controlled by proper treatment.

Treatment

i. General measures
  a. Moderate salt restriction (up to 5 g/day).
  b. Dietary restriction of calories and fat for weight reduction. Restriction of alcohol intake, stoppage of smoking and regular physical exercise.

ii. Drug treatment
  a. Hydrochlorothiazide tablet (25, 50 mg)— 25 to 50 mg daily.
  b. Atenolol tablet (50, 100 mg)—50 to 100 mg once daily.
  c. Amlodipine tablet (2.5, 5 mg)—2.5 to 10 mg once daily.
  d. Enalapril tablet (2.5, 5 mg)—2.5 to 30 mg once daily may be added depending on the response.

7. A 58-year-old man with history of severe hypertension for 20 years and it was controlled with medication. He stopped taking drugs for a prolonged period. His

BP was found to be 240/135 mm of Hg with papilloedema. What will be the management of this case?

Presenting features: Severe rise of BP to 240/135 mm of Hg with papilloedema.

Relevant information: A severe hypertensive patient is well-controlled with medication for 20 years and he stopped taking his drugs for a prolonged period.

Inference: This is a case of hypertensive emergency and needs prompt reduction of BP.

Management

The patient should be admitted in intensive coronary care unit of hospital for administration of following drugs:

i. Sodium nitroprusside injection—it is diluted properly in 5% dextrose solution and then administered by controlled continuous IV infusion at a rate of 0.5 to 1.5 µg/kg/min until the BP is reduced to desired level (30% reduction of pretreatment diastolic BP but not below 90 mm of Hg in first 48 hours).

ii. Frusemide injection—20 to 40 mg IV may be added to speed up antihypertensive response.

8. A 25-year-old lady is brought to emergency unit by her family members. She is unconscious with constricted pupils and froth coming out of her mouth. She is reported to consume an organophosphorus insecticide. How to manage this case?

Presenting features: The patient is unconscious with constricted pupils and froth coming out of her mouth.

Relevant information: A-25-year-old lady is reported to consume organophosphorus insecticide.

Inference: It is a case of acute organophosphorus compound poisoning.

Management

ii. *General supportive measures*

a. Removal of contaminated clothings.
b. Maintenance of airway by aspiration of secretions and artificial respiration, if required.

c. Administration of IV fluid (5% dextrose saline).
d. Diazepam injection—10 mg IV if there is convulsion.

ii. *Drug treatment*

a. Atropine sulphate injection—2 to 4 mg IV and repeated every 10 minutes until muscarinic symptoms and signs disappear (reduction of salivary and tracheobronchial secretions, increase of pulse rate, dilatation of pupils, etc.). In first 24 hours as much as 20 mg of atropine sulphate may be required.

b. Pralidoxime chloride injection—1 to 2 g IV slowly over 5 to 10 minutes. Dose may be repeated after one hour, if muscle weakness persists (maximum dose is 12 g in first 24 hours).

c. The patient is observed for 72 hours. Atropine sulphate and pralidoxime chloride may be repeated depending on the condition of the patient.

9. A middle-aged person was watching TV in dark. Suddenly he develops severe pain in right eye, vomiting and blurring of vision. On examination, right pupil is dilated, sluggishly reacting to light with raised intraocular pressure. The condition is diagnosed as a case of acute congestive glaucoma. What will be the medical management of this condition?

Presenting features: Dilated right pupil, sluggishly reacting to light with raised intraocular pressure.

Relevant information: A middle-aged person while watching TV in dark, suddenly develops severe pain in right eye, vomiting and blurring of vision.

Inference: The patient has developed acute congestive glaucoma and needs immediate management.

Management

The treatment of choice is laser iridectomy/trabeculectomy. Before surgical treatment, the intraocular pressure should be reduced by drug therapy:

- Acetazolamide injection—500 mg IV and followed by acetazolamide tablet—250 mg 4 times daily.

- Mannitol (20% solution) by IV infusion 1.5 to 2 g/kg over a period of 30 to 60 minutes.

- Pilocarpine nitrate (2% solution)—2 drops to be instilled in right eye every 10 minutes for 1 hour and then at 30 minutes interval till the desired intraocular pressure is achieved.

- Timolol maleate (0.25 to 0.5% solution)—2 drops to be instilled in right eye 6 hourly.

NB: Initially when the intraocular pressure is very high, a miotic is usually in effective, because of pressure induced ischaemic paralysis of sphincter muscle of iris.

10. A 20-year-old diabetic man on insulin therapy suddenly developed fever and missed his usual doses of insulin and become unconscious. What measures are to be taken to manage the condition?

Presenting features: The patient is unconscious.

Relevant information: A 20-year-old diabetic man receiving insulin suddenly developed fever and missed his usual doses of insulin.

Inference: The patient has developed diabetic ketoacidosis and needs immediate management.

Management

a. *Investigations:* Urine is tested for sugar and ketone bodies. Blood is sent for glucose, ketone bodies, sodium, potassium and bicarbonate estimations.

b. *Drug treatment*

- *Insulin injection:* A loading dose of 10 to 20 g units of soluble insulin is administered IV as a bolus and followed by continuous IV infusion of soluble insulin at the rate of 10 to 15 units/hour. When the blood glucose level falls to 180 mg/100 mL, the dose of insulin is reduced to 2 to 4 units/hour.

- *Intravenous fluids:* 1 to 2 litres of normal saline is administered rapidly in first hour. Then half normal (0.45% solution) saline is infused depending on the clinical assessment of fluid state of the patient. When the blood glucose level approaches to normal, 5% dextrose solution is infused slowly (to replace intracellular deficit of water and to prevent late cerebral oedema syndrome, which may occur rarely).

- *Potassium phosphate injection:* 3 to 4 hours after instillation of therapy, 5 to 10 mEq of potassium per hour is infused with normal saline (potassium phosphate is preferred than potassium chloride, because there is also depletion of phosphate in diabetic ketoacidosis).

- *Sodium bicarbonate injection:* 500 mL of isotonic sodium bicarbonate solution is administered IV, if there is severe acidosis (blood pH below 6.0).

- *Administration of proper antibiotic:* To control bacterial infection.

11. A middle-aged diabetic patient is treated with oral antidiabetic agent (tolbutamide) underwent prolonged exercise and missed his usual breakfast. He developed unconsciousness, respiratory distress and profuse sweating with temperature. How to manage the case?

Presenting features: The patient is unconscious with respiratory distress, profuse sweating and tachycardia.

Relevant information: A middle-aged diabetic patient treated with tolbutamide underwent prolonged exercise and missed his usual breakfast.

Inference: The patient has developed hypoglycaemic coma and needs immediate management.

Management

- **Intravenous glucose injection:** 40 to 50 mL of 50% dextrose solution is administered as a bolus and followed by continuous infusion of 5 to 10% dextrose solution at a rate of 1 to 2 mL/minute until the patient is able to eat a meal.

- **Glucagon injection:** 1 mg intramuscularly may be given in severe hypoglycaemia and may be repeated after 10 minutes, if necessary.
- Oral glucose should be continued.
- Dose of tolbutamide and physical activities should be adjusted.

12. A person is willing to travel an endemic area of malaria. What chemoprophylaxis is to be given to him? Even after chemoprophylaxis, he subsequently developed chloroquine-resistant malaria. How to manage the case?

Relevant information: The person is willing to travel an endemic area of malaria. Even after chemoprophylaxis, he subsequently developed chloroquine-resistant malaria.

Inference: When the person is travelling the endemic area of malaria, he needs chemoprophylaxis against malaria. When he developed chloroquine-resistant malaria, he needs treatment with other antimalarial drugs.

Management

a. *Chemoprophylaxis*

- Chloroquine phosphate tablets—300 mg base weekly starting one week before entering the endemic area and continued for 4 weeks after leaving the endemic area.
- In chloroquine-resistant endemic area: Mefloquine hydrochloride tablet—250 mg salt (228 mg base) weekly starting one week before entering the endemic area and continued for 4 weeks after leaving the endemic area or doxycycline hyclate tablet—100 mg daily starting 2 days before entering the endemic area and continued for 4 weeks after leaving the endemic area (total duration should not exceed 4 months).

b. *Treatment for chloroquine-resistant malaria*

- Quinine sulphate tablet—650 mg salt (600 mg base) three times daily for 3 to 7 days along with doxycycline hyclate tablet—100 mg twice daily for 7 days or mefloquine hydrochloride tablet—15 mg/kg as a single dose (maximum dose 1250 mg).

NB: Instead of doxycycline along with quinine, tetracycline capsule (250 mg) 6 hourly for 7 days or pyrimethamine (25 mg) plus sulphadoxine (500 mg) tablet—3 tablets as a single dose can be used along with quinine.

- If the patient is unconscious, then quinine hydrochloride injection—20 mg salt/kg diluted in 300 mL of 5% dextrose solution is infused over first 4 hours and then 10 mg salt/kg is infused over 2 to 3 hours every 8 hours.

13. A male patient develops fever with chill and rigors. *P. vivax* is found in blood smear. What will be the treatment of the case?

Presenting features: The patient develops fever with chill and rigor.

Relevant information: *P. vivax* is found in his blood smear.

Inference: The patient has developed acute attack of *P. vivax* malaria.

Treatment

- Chloroquine phosphate tablet (250 mg salt containing 150 mg base)—4 tablets initially, 2 tablets after 6 hours and 2 tablets daily for 2 days. It is followed by primaquine phosphate tablet (15 mg base)—1 tablet daily for 14 days.

14. A patient with chronic psychiatric illness was treated with largactil (chlorpromazine) for a prolonged period. He developed tremor, bradykinesia and rigidity. What treatment should be given to the patient without stopping the drug?

Presenting features: The patient developed tremor, bradykinesia and rigidity.

Relevant information: The patient with chronic psychiatric illness was treated with largactil (chlorpromazine) for a prolonged period.

Inference: The patient has developed drug induced parkinsonism.

Treatment

- Trihexyphenidyl hydrochloride tablet (1 mg)—initially 1 mg twice daily, then the dose is gradually increased up to 15 mg daily in 2 to 3 divided doses.

  Or benztropine mesylate tablet (1 mg)—1 to 4 mg twice daily

  Or diphenhydramine tablet (50 mg)—50 mg daily.

15. A woman in second trimester of pregnancy is found to be moderately anaemic on routine antenatal check-up. What will be the treatment of the case?

   Presenting features: Moderately anaemic on routine antenatal check-up.

   Relevant information: A woman in second trimester of pregnancy.

   Inference: The woman is suffering from anaemia of pregnancy.

Treatment

Ferrous sulphate (200 mg) with folic acid (0.5 mg) tablet—1 tablet three times daily after food to be continued till the haemoglobin level rises above 10 g% and then 1 tablet daily is to be continued for 3 months after delivery.

16. A 6-year-old boy while playing in a village ground was bitten by a snake. The snake was identified as poisonous one. How to manage the case?

   Relevant information: A 6-year-old boy while playing in a village ground was bitten by a poisonous snake.

   Inference: It is a case of snake bite poisoning.

Management

i. General measures

- Two tourniquets are to be applied, one immediately above the bite and another still higher over a single bone. The tourniquets should be relaxed for 10 to 15 seconds at regular intervals of 10 to 15 minutes to prevent gangrene.
- The wound is washed with potassium permanganate solution.
- 3 mL of polyvalent antisnake venom serum is infiltered in the local tissue around the site of bite.
- The affected limb is immobilized.
- Tetanus toxoid injection—0.5 mL intramuscularly.

ii. Specific treatment

- Polyvalent antisnake venom serum (lyophilized) injection—the content of each ampoule (10 mL) is dissolved in 10 mL of distilled water. Then after proper skin sensitivity test, 20 mL (2 ampoules) of reconstituted antivenom is diluted in 500 mL of 5% dextrose saline and infused over 2 hours. It may be repeated every 2 hours depending on the severity of poisoning.
- If the patient develops analphylactic reaction or serum sickness, adrenaline injection—0.2 to 0.5 mL subcutaneously, hydrocortisone sodium succinate injection—100 mg intravenously and pheniramine maleate injection—2.5 mg intramuscularly are to be administered.
- If the patient develops drowsiness, respiratory distress, oliguria, haematuria and skeletal muscle paralysis, the patient is to be sent to referral hospital and treated by blood transfusion, artificial respiration and dialysis.

  - Skin sensitivity test is done by injecting 0.02 to 0.1 mL of 1:10 diluted antivenom subcutaneously. If the patient is sensitive, antivenom is given continuously along with adrenaline, hydrocortisone and pheniramine maleate.
  - AVS is not effective against the toxin fixed to the tissues and cannot reverse the damage caused by the toxin.

National Essential Drugs List (1996)

Essential drugs list consists of drugs which are the most needed for the healthcare of the majority of the population and, therefore, should be available at all times in adequate amounts and in proper dosage forms.

Essential drugs list is a national policy decision of each country. Such guiding lists should be understood as a tentative identification of a common care of basic needs, which has universal relevance and applicability. In certain situations, there is a need to make available additional drugs essential for rare diseases. A list of essential drugs does not mean that no other drugs are useful. The list of essential drugs prepared by experts committee of clinicians and pharmacologists of India is given herewith. It will be useful for various healthcare institutions and agencies in deciding their own most needed drug list.

- **Anaesthetics and muscle relaxants**
  - a. *General anaesthetics and oxygen*: Ether, halothane, isoflurane, ketamine, nitrous oxide, oxygen, thiopentone sodium.
  - b. *Local anaesthetics*: Bupivacaine, ethylchloride, lignocaine.
  - c. *Preoperative medication and sedation*: Atropine sulphate, chloralhydrate, diazepam, morphine, promethazine.
  - d. *Muscle relaxants (peripherally acting)*: Atracurium, neostigmine, pancuronium, succinylcholine, vecuronium.
- **Analgesics, antipyretics, NSAIDs and drugs used to treat gout**
  - a. *Nonopioid analgesics*: Acetylsalicylic acid, allopurinol, diclofenac, ibuprofen, indomethacin, paracetamol.
  - b. *Opioid analgesics*: Codeine, buprenorphine, morphine, pethidine, pentazocine.
- **Antiallergics and drugs used in anaphylaxis**

Adrenaline, chlorpheniramine, dexamethasone, hydrocortisone, prednisolone, promethazine.

- **Antidotes and other substances used in poisonings**

Activated charcoal, atropine, antisnake venom, desferrioxamine, dimercaprol, naloxone, penicillamine, pralidoxime, sodium calcium edetate, sodium nitrite.

- **Anticonvulsants/antiepileptics**

Carbamazepine, diazepam, ethosuximide, phenobarbitone, penytoin sodium, sodium valproate.

- **Anti-infective drugs**
  - a. *Antihelminthics*: Albendazole, diethylcarbamazine, mebendazole, niclosamide, praziquantel, pyrantel pamoate.
  - b. *Antibacterials*:
    - i. *Penicillins:* Amoxicillin, ampicillin, benzylpenicillin, benzathinepenicillin, cloxacillin, piperacillin, procaine benzylpenicillin.
    - ii. *Other antibacterials*: Amikacin, cephalexin, chloramphenicol, ciprofloxacin, cotrimoxazole, doxycycline, erythromycin, gentamicin, metronidazole, nalidixic acid, neomycin, nitrofurantoin, norfloxacin, sulphadimidine, tetracycline.
    - iii. *Antileprotic drugs*: Clofazimine, dapsone, rifampicin.
    - iv. *Antitubercular drugs*: Ethambutol, isoniazid, pyrazinamide, rifampicin, streptomycin, thiacetazone.
    - v. *Antifungal drugs*: Amphotericin B, griseofulvin, ketoconazole, nystatin.
    - vi. *Antiamoebic and antigiardial drugs*: Chloroquine, diloxanidefuroate, metronidazole, tinidazole.

vii. *Antikala-azar drugs*: Meglumine antimoniate, pentamidine, sodium stibogluconate.

viii. *Antimalarial drugs*: Chloroquine, primaquine, quinine, sulphadoxine with pyrimethamine.

ix. *Antiviral drugs*: Aciclovir, idoxuridine.

• **Antimigraine drugs**

Acetylsalicylic acid, ergotamine, paracetamol, propranolol.

• **Antineoplastic and immunosuppressant drugs and drugs used in palliative cure**

a. *Immunosuppressants*: Azathioprine, cyclosporin.

b. *Cytotoxic drugs*: Actinomycin-D, l-asparaginase, bleomycin, busulphan, cisplatin, cyclophosphamide, cytosine arabinoside, danazol, doxorubicin, etoposide, folinic acid, fluorouracil, melphalan, mercaptopurine, methotrexate, mitomycin-C, procarbazine, vinblastine, vincristine.

c. *Hormones and antihormones*: Ethinylestradiol, prednisolone, tamoxifen.

• **Antiparkinsonism drugs**

Biperiden, levodopa with carbidopa, trihexyphenidyl.

• **Drugs affecting the blood**

a. *Antianaemic drugs*: Ferrous sulphate, folic acid, hydroxycobalamin, iron dextran.

b. *Drugs affecting coagulation:* Heparin sodium, protamine sulphate, phytomenadione, warfarin sodium.

• **Blood products and plasma substitutes**

a. *Plasma substitutes*: Dextran 70, polygeline.

b. *Plasma fractions*: Albumin (human), factor VIII concentrate, factor IX complex (containing factors II, VII, IX and X) concentrate.

• **Cardiovascular drugs**

a. *Antianginal drugs*: Diltiazem, Glyceryl trinitrate, isosorbide mononitrate, isosorbide dinitrate, propranolol.

b. *Antiarrhythmic drugs*: Amiodarone, atenolol, diltiazem, lignocaine, isoprenaline, mexiletine, nifedipine, procainamide, propranolol, quinidine, verapamil.

c. *Antihypertensive drugs*: Amlodipine, atenolol, captopril, enalapril, chlorthalidone, hydrochlorothiazide, methyldopa, nifedipine, propranolol, reserpine, sodium nitroprusside.

d. *Cardiac glycosides*: Digoxin.

e. *Drugs used in cardiovascular shock*: Dopamine, dobutamine.

• **Dermatological (topical) drugs**

a. *Antifungal drugs*: Benzoic acid with salicylic acid, miconazole, nystatin, sodium thiosulphate.

b. *Local antiinfective drugs*: Bacitracin with neomycin, framycetin sulphate, gentian violet, povidone iodine, silver nitrate, silver sulphadiazine.

c. *Antiinflammatory and antipruritic drugs*: Betamethasone, calamine, hydrocortisone.

d. *Keratoplastic and keratolytic drugs*: Coaltar, dithranol, glycerine, salicylic acid.

e. *Scabicidal and pediculocidal drugs*: Benzylbenzoate, gammabenzene hexachloride.

• **Diagnostic agents**

a. *Ophthlamic drugs*: Fluorescein, tropicamide.

b. *Radiocontrast media*: Barium sulphate, iopanoic acid, calcium ipodate, meglumine iotroxate.

• **Disinfectants and antiseptics**

a. *Antiseptics*: Acriflavin, chlorhexidine, ethylalcohol (70%), gentian violet, hydrogen peroxide, povidone iodine.

b. *Disinfectants*: Calcium hypochlorite, chlorinated lime (bleaching powder).

• **Diuretics**

Acetazolamide, furosemide, hydrochlorothiazide, mannitol, spironolactone.

- **Gastrointestinal drugs**

  a. *Antacids and antiulcer drugs*: Aluminium hydroxide, cimetidine, ranitidine, magnesium hydroxide.

  b. *Antiemetics*: Domperidone, metoclopramide, prochlorperazine, promethazine.

  c. *Antiinflammatory drugs*: Sulphasalazine.

  d. *Antispasmodic drugs:* Dicyclomine, hyoscine-N-butylbromide.

  e. *Antidiarrhoeals*: Furazolidone, loperamide, norfloxacin, oral dehydration salts powder.

  f. *Purgatives*: Bisacodyl, isphagula, senna.

- **Hormones, other endocrine drugs and contraceptives**

  a. *Adrenal hormones and synthetic analogs*: Dexamethasone, hydrocortisone, methylprednisolone, prednisolone.

  b. *Androgens*: Testosterone propionate.

  c. *Oestrogens*: Ethinyl Oestradiol.

  d. *Progestins*: Norethisterone.

  e. *Contraceptives*: Centocroman, condoms with spermicide, ethinylestradiol with norethisterone, ethinylestradiol with levonorgestrel, medroxyprogesterone acetate, norethisterone.

  f. *Antidiabetic drugs*: Glybenclamide, glipizide, insulin (short-, intermediate- and long-acting) preparations, metformin.

  g. *Thyroid hormones and antithyroid drugs*: Carbimazole, levothyroxine, potassium iodide, propylthiouracil.

- **Immunological agents**

  a. *Diagnostic agents*: Tuberculin, purified protein derivative (PPD).

  b. *Sera and immunoglobulins*: Antisnake venom sera, anti-D immunoglobulin, antitetanus immunoglobulin, diphtheria antitoxin, immunoglobulin (human), rabies immunoglobulin.

  c. *Vaccines*: BCG vaccine, diphtheria pertussis tetanus (DPT) vaccine, diphtheria

tetanus (DT) vaccine, hepatitis B vaccine, measles vaccine, measles mumpsrubella vaccine, poliomyelitis vaccine (oral), rabies vaccine, tetanus vaccine (toxoid).

- **Ophthalmological preparations**

  Atropine, chloramphenicol, ciprofloxacin, fluorescein, gentamycin, homatropine, phenylephrine, pilocarpine, prednisolone, sulphacetamide, tetracaine, timolol maleate.

- **Oxytocics and antioxytocics**

  a. *Oxytocics*: Ergometrine, methylergometrine, oxytocin.

  b. *Antioxytocics*: Terbutaline, isoxsuprine.

- **Psychotherapeutic drugs**

  a. *Antipsychotic drugs*: Chlorpromazine, fluphenazine, haloperidol.

  b. *Antidepressant drugs*: Amitriptyline, clomipramine, fluoxetine, trazodone, imipramine.

  c. *Mood stabilizers*: Lithium carbonate.

- **Drugs acting on respiratory tract**

  a. *Antitussives*: Codeine phosphate, dextromethorphan, noscapine.

  b. *Antiasthmatics*: Aminophylline, adrenaline, beclomethasone, cromolyn sodium, ephedrine, salbutamol.

- **Solutions correcting water, electrolyte and acid–base disturbances**

  a. *Oral solutions*: Oral rehydration salts solution, potassium chloride solution.

  b. *Parenteral solutions*: Glucose (5%, 50%) solution, glucose (5%) with normal saline solution, normal saline solution, ringer lactate solution.

- **Vitamins and minerals**

  a. *Vitamins*: Ascorbic acid (vitamin C), vitamin B complex, vitamin A, vitamin D, retinol, thiamine, nicotinamide, pyridoxine, riboflavin.

  b. *Minerals*: Calcium salts, iron salts (ferrous), zinc sulphate, manganese sulphate.

Bibliography

1. *Adverse Reaction to Drugs* (1/e) by OL Wade.
2. *Antibiotics and Chemotherapy* (7/e) by FO'grady, HP Lambert, RG Finch and D Greenwood.
3. *Basic and Clinical Pharmacology* (7/e) by BC Katzung.
4. *BN Ghosh's The Text Book of Pharmacology and Therapeutics* (3/e) by SS Bhattacharya and RC Majumdar.
5. *Clinical Pharmacokinetics* (3/e) by M Rowland and TN Tozer.
6. *Clinical Pharmacology* (8/e) by DR Laurence, PN Bennet and NJ Brown.
7. *Conn's Current Therapy* (1999) by RE Rakel.
8. *Drug Treatment* (3/e) by GS Avery.
9. *Fundamentals of Experimental Pharmacology* (2/e) by MN Ghosh.
10. *Goodman and Gilmaris The Pharmacological Basis of Therapeutics* (10/e) by JG Hardman, LE Limbird and Alfred Goodman Gilman.
11. *Goth's Medical Pharmacology* (14/e) by WG Clark, DC Brater and AR Johnson.
12. *Lewis's Pharmacology* (5/e) by James Crossland.
13. *Martindale: The Complete Drug Reference* (34/e) by sean C Sweet main.
14. *Modern Pharmacology* (4/e) by CR Craig and RE Stitzel.
15. *Pharmacology* (4/e) by HP Rang, MM Dale and JM Fitter.
16. *Pharmacology* (4/e) by Leonard S Jacob.
17. *Pharmacology and Pharmacotherapeutics* (15/e) by RS Satoskar, SD Bhandarkar and Nirmala N Rage.
18. *Pharmacology in Medicine—Principles and Practices* (1/e) by SN Pradhan, RP Maickle and SN Dutta.
19. *Practical Pharmacology* (1/e) by K Ahmad.
20. *Principles of Drug Action* (3/e) by WB Pratt and P Taylor.
21. *Therapeutic Drugs* (2/e) by Collin Dollery.

Index